Perspectives
on Nursing Theory

Perspectives
on Nursing Theory

Second Edition

Edited by

Leslie H. Nicoll, PhD, MBA, RN

Brighton Medical Center • University of Southern Maine
Portland, Maine

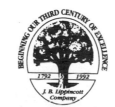

J. B. Lippincott Company
Philadelphia
New York   London   Hagerstown

Sponsoring Editor: *David P. Carroll*
Production: *TAPSCO, Inc.*
Compositor: *TAPSCO, Inc.*
Printer/Binder: *R. R. Donnelley & Sons, Inc.*

Second Edition

6 5 4 3 2 1

Library of Congress Cataloging-in-Publication Data

Perspectives on nursing theory/edited by Leslie H. Nicoll.—2nd ed.
    p. cm.
    ISBN 0-397-54911-3 (hardcover).—ISBN 0-397-54910-5 (soft cover)
    1. Nursing—Philosophy. I. Nicoll, Leslie H.
    [DNLM: 1. Nursing Theory—collected works. WY 86 P467]
RT84.5.P47 1992
610.73′01—dc20
DNLM/DLC
for Library of Congress   91-32512
                                                               CIP

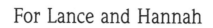

For Lance and Hannah

Contributors

MARJORIE V. BATEY, PH.D., F.A.A.N.
Professor
Community Health Care Systems Department
School of Nursing
University of Washington
Seattle, Washington

JANET L. BEATON, R.N., B.N., M.A., PH.D.
Director, Graduate Program
School of Nursing
University of Manitoba
Winnipeg, Manitoba, Canada

JAN BECKSTRAND, PH.D., R.N.
Assistant Dean of Clinical Research
Indiana University School of Nursing
Director of Clinical Research for Nursing Services
Indiana University Hospital
Indianapolis, Indiana

JEANNE QUINT BENOLIEL, R.N., D.N.SC., F.A.A.N.
Professor
College of Nursing
Rutgers: The State University of New Jersey
Newark, New Jersey

MYRTLE IRENE BROWN, PH.D., R.N., F.A.A.N.
Columbia, South Carolina

HELEN A. BUSH, PH.D., R.N.
Professor of Nursing
Texas Woman's University
Denton, Texas

BARBARA A. CARPER, ED.D., R.N., F.A.A.N.
Undergraduate Program Coordinator
College of Nursing
University of North Carolina
Charlotte, North Carolina

PEGGY L. CHINN, PH.D., R.N., F.A.A.N.
Professor
Health Sciences Center
Center for Human Caring
University of Colorado
Denver, Colorado

ROSEMARIE MARROCCO COLLINS, PH.D., R.N.C.S.
Director
Pastoral Counseling Service
Marianist Center
Folsom, Pennsylvania

LUCY H. CONANT, PH.D., R.N.
Farmer
Chester, Massachusetts

MARY E. CONWAY, R.N., PH.D., F.A.A.N.
Dean and Professor
School of Nursing
Medical College of Georgia
Augusta, Georgia

GRETCHEN CRAWFORD, PH.D., R.N.
Director
Nursing Education Program
New York State Nurses Association
Guilderland, New York

*DOROTHY M. CROWLEY, PH.D., R.N.
Formerly, School of Nursing
University of Washington
Seattle, Washington

HOLLY A. DEGROOT, PH.D., R.N., C.N.A.A.
Principal and Managing Partner
Catalyst Systems
Mill Valley, California
Assistant Research Nurse
School of Nursing
University of California
San Francisco, California

JAMES DICKOFF, PH.D.
Professor and Chair
Department of Philosophy
Kent State University
Kent, Ohio

SUE K. DONALDSON, PH.D., R.N.
Professor and Cora Meidl Siehl Chair in
    Nursing Research
School of Nursing
Professor
Department of Physiology
School of Medicine
University of Minnesota
Minneapolis, Minnesota

KARIN DUFAULT, S.P., PH.D., R.N.
Chairperson
Board of Directors
Sisters of Providence Health Care Corporations
Seattle, Washington

*ROSEMARY ELLIS, PH.D., R.N.
Formerly Professor
Frances Payne Bolton School of Nursing
Case Western Reserve University
Cleveland, Ohio

JACQUELINE FAWCETT, PH.D., F.A.A.N.
Professor
School of Nursing
University of Pennsylvania
Philadelphia, Pennsylvania

HARRIET R. FELDMAN, PH.D., R.N.
Professor and Chairperson
Department of Nursing
Fairleigh Dickinson University
Teaneck, New Jersey

JOHN H. FIELDER, PH.D.
Associate Professor of Philosophy
Villanova University
Villanova, Pennsylvania

JACQUELYN HAAK FLASKERUD, B.S.N., M.S.N., PH.D.
Professor
School of Nursing
University of California, Los Angeles
Los Angeles, California

JEANNETTE R. FOLTA, PH.D., R.N., F.A.A.N.
Professor and Chairperson
Department of Sociology
University of Vermont
Burlington, Vermont

*SARAH S. FULLER, PH.D., R.N.
Formerly Associate Professor
School of Nursing
Northern Illinois University
DeKalb, Illinois

---

*Deceased

SUSAN R. GORTNER, M.N., PH.D., F.A.A.N.
Professor and Director, Cardiac Recovery Laboratories
School of Nursing
University of California, San Francisco
San Francisco, California

LAURIE M. GUNTER, PH.D., R.N., F.A.A.N.
Professor Emeritus
Nursing and Human Development
Department of Nursing
The Pennsylvania State University
University Park, Pennsylvania

EDWARD J. HALLORAN, R.N., M.P.H., PH.D., F.A.A.N.
Associate Professor
Nursing Systems
University of North Carolina
Chapel Hill, North Carolina

MARGARET E. HARDY, PH.D., R.N.
Professor of Nursing
University of Rhode Island College of Nursing
Kingston, Rhode Island

ADA SUE HINSHAW, PH.D., R.N., F.A.A.N.
Director
National Center for Nursing Research
National Institutes of Health
Bethesda, Maryland

SUE E. HUETHER, PH.D., R.N.
Associate Professor
College of Nursing
University of Utah
Salt Lake City, Utah

ADA K. JACOX, PH.D., R.N., F.A.A.N.
Professor
School of Nursing
Johns Hopkins University
Baltimore, Maryland

PATRICIA JAMES, PH.D.
Professor
Department of Philosophy
Kent State University
Kent, Ohio

DOROTHY E. JOHNSON, M.P.H., R.N.
Professor Emeritus
University of California, Los Angeles
Los Angeles, California

HESOOK SUZIE KIM, PH.D., R.N.
Professor of Nursing
University of Rhode Island College of Nursing
Kingston, Rhode Island

MAEONA K. KRAMER, R.N., PH.D.
Professor
College of Nursing
University of Utah
Salt Lake City, Utah

JEANETTE LANCASTER, PH.D., R.N.
Professor and Dean
School of Nursing
University of Virginia
Charlottesville, Virginia

WADE LANCASTER, PH.D.
Director of Marketing
Health Sciences Center
University of Virginia
Charlottesville, Virginia

ROBERT C. LEONARD
Professor of Sociology
University of Arizona
Tucson, Arizona

*ROSE MCKAY, ED.D., R.N.
Formerly, School of Nursing
University of Colorado Health Sciences Center
Denver, Colorado

AFAF IBRAHIM MELEIS, PH.D., DR PS (HON), F.A.A.N.
Professor
Department of Mental Health, Community and
      Administrative Nursing
University of California
San Francisco, California

---

*Deceased

PATRICIA L. MUNHALL, R.N., ED.D., F.A.A.N.
Professor
Hunter-Bellevue School of Nursing
Hunter College of the City University of New York
New York, New York

MARGARET A. NEWMAN, PH.D., R.N., F.A.A.N.
Professor
School of Nursing
University of Minnesota
Minneapolis, Minnesota

NOLA J. PENDER, PH.D., R.N., F.A.A.N.
Director
Center for Nursing Research
University of Michigan School of Nursing
Ann Arbor, Michigan

HILDEGARD E. PEPLAU, R.N., ED.D., F.A.A.N.
Professor Emerita
Rutgers: The State University of New Jersey
New Brunswick, New Jersey

JOHN R. PHILLIPS
Associate Professor
Division of Nursing
School of Education, Health, Nursing and
    Arts Professions
New York University
New York, New York

MARY CAROL RAMOS, PH.D., R.N.
Clinician, Medical Intensive Care Unit
University of Virginia Health Sciences Center
Charlottesville, Virginia

PAMELA G. REED, PH.D., R.N.
Associate Professor
University of Arizona College of Nursing
Tucson, Arizona

DANIEL ROTHBART, PH.D.
Associate Professor of Philosophy
George Mason University
Fairfax, Virginia

ELLEN B. RUDY, PH.D., R.N., F.A.A.N.
Professor
Associate Dean for Research
Frances Payne Bolton School of Nursing
Case Western Reserve University
Cleveland, Ohio

BARBARA SARTER, PH.D., R.N., F.N.P.
Associate Professor and Director of MSN Program
University of Southern California
Los Angeles, California
Clinical Nurse Specialist
Kenneth Norris Jr. Cancer Hospital
Los Angeles, California

ROZELLA M. SCHLOTFELDT, PH.D., F.A.A.N.
Professor and Dean Emeritus
Frances Payne Bolton School of Nursing
Case Western Reserve University
Cleveland, Ohio

MARY E. SEGALL, PH.D., R.N.
Health Consultant
Presbyterian Church
Addis Ababa, Ethiopia

MARY CIPRIANO SILVA, PH.D., R.N., F.A.A.N.
Professor
Coordinator of the Ph.D. Program in
    Nursing Administration
School of Nursing
George Mason University
Fairfax, Virginia

MINDY B. TINKLE, R.N., PH.D.
Associate Professor
College of Nursing and Allied Health
University of Texas at El Paso
El Paso, Texas

FLORENCE S. WALD, M.N., M.S., F.A.A.N.
Associate Clinical Professor
School of Nursing
Yale University
New Haven, Connecticut

LORRAINE OLSZEWSKI WALKER
Luci B. Johnson Centennial Professor in Nursing
University of Texas at Austin
Austin, Texas

JEAN WATSON, PH.D., R.N., F.A.A.N.
Director
Center for Human Caring
University of Colorado Health Sciences Center
Denver, Colorado

GLENN WEBSTER, PH.D.
Associate Professor
Department of Philosophy
University of Colorado
Denver, Colorado

ERNESTINE WIEDENBACH, M.A., R.N., C.N.M.
Associate Professor Emeritus
Maternal and Newborn Health Nursing
Yale University
New Haven, Connecticut

NANCY FUGATE WOODS, PH.D., R.N., F.A.A.N.
Professor, Parent and Child Nursing
Director, Center for Women's Health Research
University of Washington
Seattle, Washington

POWHATAN J. WOOLDRIDGE
Associate Professor
State University of New York at Buffalo
Buffalo, New York

ELIZABETH WORTHY
Seattle, Washington

Foreword to the First Edition

Thinking nurses always must have used concepts, working hypotheses, assumptions, and presuppositions in their understandings of the world of nursing and nursing care. It is hard to imagine how one could practice nursing without theoretical thinking or theories, but it is only in the last thirty years that theoretical thinking in nursing has been the object of scrutiny. Since the late 1950s and early 1960s, nurse scholars and scientists have been involved in a theory-development movement in nursing. *Perspectives on Nursing Theory* contains the often-cited seminal papers that represent the critical thinking in this nursing theory-development movement.

The movement has evolved, in part, from the development of research in nursing and a concomittant evolutionary shift in nursing to conceptual language. As nursing research grew in the second half of the twentieth century a number of compelling questions arose: What is nursing research? What is nursing? What should be researched? How should nursing research be done?

Nurses who had research training in social or behavioral sciences learned the theories in those fields but also came to appreciate the importance of theories as both genesis and products of research processes. They came to appreciate the reciprocal relationship between theory development and research. As nurses became involved in research for nursing, of necessity, they became involved in theory development in nursing.

Theory is the term for the theoretical formulations that organize or interpret facts. Scientific theories are those that can be communicated and can be used and evaluated by others. They are produced by processes that are public, explicated, and open to evaluation against agreed-upon criteria. Scientifically tested theories are one important form of knowledge essential to effective professional practice of nursing.

Perspectives on Nursing Theory is an organized collection of papers that recaptures the first thirty years of theory development. From the papers one can follow something of the history of ideas and issues in nursing theory development, their evolution, and some progress in theoretical nursing. To understand the current activities and emphases, one needs to know and read the seminal papers in the field. The collection and organization of these papers in one volume is a singular contribution that facilitates the vicarious experiencing of thinking about theory and nursing. The papers also are essential to knowledge of some history of theory development in nursing.

The book is important for more than the glimpse of history it can provide. It is important because it provides knowledge about the authors of articles that are becoming "classics" in professional nursing. The authors' comments on the context and purposes that stimulated the original creation of the papers provide important information that enrich their meanings. The authors' comments not only enhance the value or understanding of the individual paper but also give insight to the continuities and changes in thinking during the evolution of theory and research development in nursing.

Many of the conceptual or methodological issues in nursing today are but clearer statements of issues recognizable in the collection of papers in *Perspectives on Nursing Theory*. The collection not only provides a wealth of issues, ideas, and positions, it compels one to recognize the fallibility of dogma or doctrine and to appreciate alternative points of view or changing views. Those who have read the papers as they were first published will find new meaning and insights as they reread them in the context of nursing developments in the 1980s. The emergence of nursing as a distinctive discipline is understandable only with the insights obtained from study of the ideas and issues discussed in the important papers in this collection.

The papers, with one exception, have been published elsewhere. Separately they are useful, but they do not provide the opportunity for a general comprehension of frames of references, of similarities, and of diversities in theoretical discussions of nursing as a practice and nursing as a field of inquiry. For this reason, the collection and comments about individual papers not only are valuable for the novice who needs to learn about nursing theory but are also a handy resource for the established scholar or teacher who wishes to study the history of ideas or of issues in nursing research or theory development. They are also a valuable resource for those scholars concerned with the importance of theoretical bases for nursing practice or with the advancement of conceptualizations of nursing as both a practice and as a scientific field of knowledge.

The organization of the collection makes evident the multiple areas of concern in knowledge development in nursing such as: the nature of nursing; the nature of nursing science; the nature, uses, and evolution of theory; theory-practice relationships; and theory-research relationships. Each of these areas deserves continued attention and study but not without regard for issues reflected in the writings of those who started and influenced discussions and developments.

As nurses move to debates on philosophy of science or on philosophies of nursing science, it is essential to be introduced to the beginnings of such thinking. Knowledge of the evolution of theoretical thinking in nursing is a necessity for the professional practitioner in nursing, the scientist nurse, or the effective, questioning teacher of nursing. The papers collected and organized here are essential readings for all who strive for excellence in any endeavor in nursing.

ROSEMARY ELLIS
Cleveland, Ohio
July, 1985

Foreword

Since publication of the first edition of *Perspectives on Nursing Theory,* the development of theories significant for the advancement of nursing's corpus of knowledge has been given increasing attention by scholars in the field. Two trends are clearly discernable. Nurses have enhanced interest in the philosophy of science and more particularly in developing an appropriate philosophy of nursing science. Nicoll has given recognition to these trends by reclassifying some of the earlier-published, classical articles under a unit heading entitled "Nursing Theory: Philosophical Considerations." It should be noted as well that nine more recently published articles selected for inclusion in this edition of *Perspectives on Nursing Theory* are so classified. Clearly nursing scholars have given increased attention to philosophical considerations necessary for developing the discipline that underlies nursing practices.

Whereas it is generally recognized that the practice domain of any group of professionals is given sanction by the societies that practitioners serve, it is the responsibility of scholars in each profession to discover, develop, and continuously refine the knowledge that is fundamental to their practices. Theory development is essential to those processes. Questions such as the nature of human beings and their natural quest for health, function, wholeness, comfort, and personal achievement are appropriate, fundamental philosophical questions to be addressed by nursing scholars. Quite obviously, they must also come to agreement about the nature of nursing, the dimensions of nursing knowledge, and the phenomena about which theoretical notions should be set forth and tested.

The history of nursing's early and continuous development as a scholarly discipline can readily be traced in this and the earlier edition of *Perspectives on Nursing Theory.* So also is it possible to discern the changes in research methods selected as nursing investigators have given recognition to the historical and social/cultural contexts of the profession's knowledge.

The two editions of *Perspectives on Nursing Theory* demonstrate Nicoll's careful selection of articles and their authors' additional comments, with a view toward documenting significant trends. They demonstrate nursing scholars' changing perspectives on theory development. Both books are veritable gold mines of information for mature and developing professionals whose career choices include their becoming scholarly practitioners, educators, administrators, investigators, authors, scientists, historians, philosophers or theorists. They all must be concerned with the inexorable relationships between theories and practices. They all must be concerned with the phenomena about which theories must be set forth and tested in order to insure the continuous development of the profession's corpus of knowledge.

ROZELLA M. SCHLOTFELDT
Cleveland, Ohio
August, 1991

Preface

This book represents thirty-five years of thinking and discussion by nurse scholars on the subject of nursing theory. As an anthology, this book is unique; it could not have existed in this form before this time. It is designed to provide an overview, a snapshot of some of the major discussions in recent years on the subject of nursing theory. For the person interested in understanding the current status of theory in nursing, this volume will be a useful and timely addition to the literature.

Perspectives on Nursing Theory is designed to meet the needs of diverse readers. It is a compilation of some of the most widely read and frequently cited articles on the subject of theory for nursing. As such, this book should prove useful to students, teachers, practicing nurses, and others who are interested in the theoretical development of nursing. This volume is comprehensive, but it is not exhaustive. It includes sixty-six articles that discuss, clarify, and amplify some of the current debates about the concept of theory; readings on *specific* theories are beyond the scope of this text.

The goal of this book is to help the reader develop a perspective on nursing theory, hence the title. An understanding of what has gone before is necessary for future development of the conceptual structures needed for the growth of the nursing discipline. To provide this perspective, several specific strategies have been employed in compiling this group of readings.

First, to truly understand the points an author is making, it is often necessary to have a contextual frame of reference for the reading of an article. Frequently, we read articles out of context and from a perspective of the time in which we read them; we forget to consider the perspective of the time in which the article was first written and published. To understand an article is to do more than just read the words on the page; it is necessary to have an appreciation for the author's thoughts, experiences, and purposes for writing the article. To assist you, the reader, in putting the essays in their proper contexts, supplemental information has been included in this volume: biographical information about the authors and statements written by the authors or their colleagues discussing the articles. These statements were written specifically to accompany the articles in this book; they represent the current thinking of the author about the article or the subject discussed, and should provide insight.

The inclusion of supplemental information with each article stemmed from a personal need. In my experience as a student reading these articles for the first time, I was often curious about the essays and the authors. The supplemental statements were designed to provide this type of information, and they succeeded beyond any of my original expectations. I had anticipated that contributors would send brief capsules that sketched out why an article was written. Instead, I received thoughtful, scholarly discussions of their work, writing, and perspectives on nursing. The willingness of authors to contribute in this way made me realize how essential this information is in understanding the nature of nursing theory.

Second, the articles are ordered within units and the units structured to provide a perspective on nursing theory. Within units articles are presented in chronological order as they first appeared in the literature. The units divide the subject of theory into major categories of debate that have become apparent over the years.

Unit One, "A Beginning Exploration of Theory in Nursing," includes articles that discuss theory in the broadest sense. These essays present the need for theory and discuss the concept of theory. Gunter's "Notes on a Theoretical Framework for Nursing Research" was the first article published in Nursing Research to discuss the subject of nursing theory. The seven chapters that comprise Unit I provide an overview of the past and present status of nursing theory.

Unit Two, "Nursing Theory: Philosophical Considerations" contains eight papers that discuss the philosophical foundations of nursing theory. Two of the older papers, Dickoff and James' "A Theory of Theories: A Position Paper" and Johnson's "Theory in Nursing: Borrowed and Unique" were presented at the "Theory Development in Nursing" symposium held at Case Western Reserve University in October 1967. This conference is widely acknowledged as one of the first forums where scholars in nursing came together to discuss the need and type of theory for nursing. The remaining chapters are more recent discussions of the relationship between theory and philosophy.

Unit Three, "Nursing, Science, and Nursing Science" presents writings that discuss the nature of science in nursing and other disciplines. A progression of thought is evident in this unit, which moves from a general discussion of science to a historic overview of the development of nursing science, its current meanings, and its future implications.

Unit Four, "Theory Building: Development, Analysis, Evaluation" presents fifteen chapters that focus on different components of theory and discuss the process of theory building. Individual chapters focus on strategies for theory development, models, model building, and conceptual issues. A framework for analysis and evaluation of conceptualizations in nursing is also included. Unit four gives a detailed picture of the different aspects of theory and provides the reader with information needed for a conceptual understanding of the subject of theory.

Units Five and Six, "Nursing Theory and Nursing Practice" and "Nursing Theory and Nursing Research" include twenty two papers that discuss the interrelationships among nursing theory, nursing practice, and nursing research. The shift from global to specific issues in these areas is evident in the progression of the chapters. The development of the scholarly debate about theory, research, and practice that is presented in these two units provides a firm foundation for understanding the issues that face nursing today.

How this book is utilized will vary according to each reader's particular situation and personal needs. A student may have assigned readings that partially determine the order in which the articles are read. However, even within that framework, I would hope that out of curiosity the student might choose to read chapters that are not required.

For the teacher and for the scholar, I hope that as you reread these essays they will continue to stimulate your thinking as they have done in the past.

If you are not a student or a teacher, but a nurse with an interest in learning more about theory, you may choose to read articles in order or by special interest. Some readers find it helpful to read all of the articles by one author at one time; others like to read all of the articles from one year in a group. I would like to emphasize that the ordering in this volume represents only one way to categorize and structure the content included. It is my perspective on theory, but it may not be yours. By reading these articles, I hope you develop your own perspective, can articulate that perspective, and will contribute to the development of nursing knowledge from an awareness of your perspective of nursing theory.

LESLIE H. NICOLL

Acknowledgments

First and foremost, I wish to express my gratitude and deep appreciation to all the contributors whose works are included here. I had an idealized vision of this book in my mind when I started this project. As a result of the cooperation and support of the contributors in providing me with information relating to the articles, biographical data, and other pertinent materials, the final version is very close to my ideal vision. I could not have done this alone; the nature of the project required support from each and every person involved, and the assistance I have received has been overwhelming. Although "thank you" hardly seems sufficient, it comes from the heart.

A special "thank you" is also reserved for David P. Carroll, Senior Nursing Editor at J.B. Lippincott. Dave has provided expert advice and expertise during the preparation of the second edition of this book and I wish to acknowledge his outstanding assistance.

I would also like to acknowledge the outstanding contribution of Margery Prazar, RN, BSN, MBA, who served as my editorial assistant. Without Margery's time, effort, and attention to detail, the second edition of this book would not exist.

In everyone's life there are influential people. In the first edition, I remembered three special teachers and their importance to me: Rosalind Wang, Anna Tichy, and Rosemary Ellis. My thinking and learning of theory has not ended, though, and two more teachers have entered my life and helped me to sharpen my thoughts: Karen W. Budd and Rozella Schlotfeldt, both of Case Western Reserve University. I am very fortunate to have studied with such clear and careful thinkers who help me to find meaning in everything I do. My husband Tony

Jendrek must be acknowledged for his neverending love, support, and encouragement. Like a powerful elixir, he provides the stimulus for me to be creative and to develop new ideas, and then provides me with the energy I need to pursue my dreams. Finally, two very important people in my life— my children, Lance and Hannah—must be acknowledged. I look into their clear blue eyes and realize the power and mystery of life. Theory is but one way to understand the world. Children are another.

LESLIE H. NICOLL

Contents

Unit One

A Beginning Exploration
of Theory in Nursing

It is common, when planning a trip, to use a map to assist in determining the route that will be taken during the journey. A map provides an overall view of the entire trip: major landmarks can be identified, the number of miles to be traveled can be calculated, and routes for the journey can be determined in advance.

For Unit One, a map analogy may be helpful. Unit One, A Beginning Exploration of Theory in Nursing, is designed to provide an overview of many of the issues that are discussed in future chapters in more depth. Each of the chapters in Unit One can be considered to be a landmark and as such provides the reader with a helpful reference point in determining the route the journey will take.

The journey, in this case, is a beginning exploration of theory in nursing. The landmarks are twelve articles from the period of 1962 to 1978. This was a time of intense growth, and these articles represent some of the debates that occurred during that 16-year period. Many consider 1978 to be a turning point in the development of nursing theory: publication of Advances in Nursing Science began in October of that year. The need for a journal that had as a Primary purpose "the stimulation of the development of nursing science" signaled to many that a profound change had occurred in the development of conceptualizations in nursing. No longer could the debate be contained within a few articles published annually in the currently available nursing journals; there was a need for a journal that was devoted solely to advances in nursing science. It is worth noting that Chapter 7, "Perspectives on Nursing Theory" by Margaret E. Hardy, was published in that first issue of ANS. Chapter 1, "Notes on A Theoretical Framework for Nursing Research" by Laurie M. Gunter, was the first article that appeared in Nursing Research that discussed theory specifically. Gunter notes in her comments that the same article had previously been rejected by Nursing Research several years before; Lucille Notter became Editor in 1961, and this article was published soon after she assumed the editorship. As you read through this volume, you will note there are repeated references to Lucille Notter. Her influence as Editor of Nursing Research from 1961 to 1973 was profound and far reaching.

Chapter 2, "Research in the Development of Nursing Theory: The Importance of a Theoretical Framework in Nursing Research" by Myrtle Irene Brown, was written as a guide to beginning nurse researchers and to impress upon them the need for a structure to relate research findings to a shared body of knowledge. Brown, who had pursued doctoral education in sociology, knew from that discipline the need for a theoretical structure to guide research efforts. Hers is one of the first articles that discussed the need for a similar structure in nursing to appear in the literature.

Chapter 3, " Towards Development of Nursing Practice Theory" by Florence S. Wald and Robert C. Leonard, was published in 1964. This article introduced the term "practice theory," and even now debate continues as to whether practice theory exists, and if so, whether it is different from nursing theory. Their contention was that the empirical approach should be used to build knowledge from systematic study of nursing experience. Although their advice is simple and direct, it seems as though it has not always been heeded in terms of knowledge development in nursing.

Chapter 4 includes several articles that must be taken as a whole for an accurate understanding of the debate that is presented. In the September-October 1971 issue of Nursing Research, Lorraine O. Walker's "Toward a Clearer Understanding of the Concept of Nursing Theory" was published. The next issue included commentary from four authors that she had criticized in her original essay, and the issue after that included Walker's response to the critiques. To this day, an exchange of this nature has not occurred again in the published nursing literature. Walker comments on the excitement and energy present in the debate during that 6-month period. While many people have very strong opinions about the views expressed, one must credit Walker, as Dickoff and James do, "with [the] courageous press to articulate a position distinctively enough to allow for that position to be appreciated . . . for what it is, and hence to be a subject for criticism."

Chapter 5, "Theory, Practice, and Research in Perspective" also by Lorraine O. Walker, was presented at the American Nurses' Association Ninth Nursing Research Conference in 1973. In many respects, the points in this essay are a further elaboration and continuation of the thoughts included in the articles in Chapter 4. Due to its pertinence in articulating Walkers' view of nursing theory, as well as the general unavailability of this article, it is included here. Walker comments that the ideas embodied in this article are those she still deals with today.

Chapter 6, "Nursing's Theoretical Evolution" by Margaret A. Newman, presents an overview of the state nursing theory in 1972. It is interesting to note that in the ten-year period from 1962, when Gunter's article first appeared, enough discussion had occurred to allow Newman to take an evolutionary look at the process. Newman continues to refine and develop this viewpoint, as she notes in her comments and as is evident in her more recent publications.

Chapter 7, "Perspectives on Nursing Theory" by Margaret E. Hardy, is an appropriate close for Unit One. As noted earlier, it was published in the first issue of ANS. Hardy provides information that permits the reader to stop and think about what has gone before and to consider what may lie ahead. In the context of the articles that are collected in this volume, this chapter is also good point to think about the discussions that have been presented and the debates that will follow.

Unit One, A Beginning Exploration of Theory in Nursing, should stimulate your interest and provide a foundation for the forthcoming readings. Like a map, it should arouse your curiosity about articles you will read and provide an overview of the topics that will be discussed.

Chapter 1

Notes on a Theoretical Framework for Nursing Research

Laurie M. Gunter

Although the number of studies done by nurses and non-nurses in nursing is increasing rapidly, the value of some of these studies as contributing to a science of nursing is difficult to assess in view of the fact that many of them are not done within an explicit theoretical system designed to discover either facts or the relationships between facts which are applicable to nursing. Nursing is functional or practical rather than theoretical in nature. This does not relieve it of the necessity for basing its practices upon scientific concepts. Theory, according to Parsons (1949), not only formulates what we know but also tells us what we want to know, that is, the questions to which an answer is needed. The structure of a theoretical system tells us what alternatives are open in the possible answers to a given question. If observed facts of undoubted accuracy will not fit any of the alternatives it leaves open, the system itself is in need of reconstruction. Therefore, research in nursing as that applied in any of the other functional sciences, will serve as testing bases for the various theoretical systems, i.e., observed "facts" which do not fit the existing theoretical systems will make it necessary to reconsider the system and the "facts."

The Aims of Nursing

Nursing care is the provision of personal care in a relationship of being "with" the patient as he experiences illness. It also includes assistance to the patient and to the physician with delegated aspects of the therapeutic regimen.

From an examination of this description of nursing, it is evident that nursing is primarily concerned with the individual (the human organism). The contributions which the nurse is prepared to make to this human organism are in the area of health and disease and stem from a theory of medical practice. The nurse

About the Author

LAURIE M. GUNTER writes "I was born in rural Navarro County, Texas, and spent my teenage years in San Antonio. With relatives and friends still in this area, I maintain close ties to both places. In the 1940s racial segregation limited my choices of colleges and nursing schools in the United States. I received my basic nursing education at Meharry Medical College, earning a diploma in 1943. At that time, this school had both a degree program and a diploma program; in terms of nursing preparation, the two programs were the same. Being very excited and desiring to become a nurse as soon as possible, and knowing that there was no difference in the nursing preparation provided, I didn't stop at that point to take a degree.

I later earned a degree in Home Economics from Tennessee A&I State University, then a master's degree in Education at Fisk University. Because schools of nursing offering the master's degree were not open to me, I then went to the University of Toronto for a year's study, for which I received a certificate in nursing education but no degree. This accounts for the fact that I have no degree in nursing. In terms of my knowledge, academic preparation, and performance, I have not found this to be a disadvantage, but I have encountered some discrimination based on my lack of a nursing degree. Later, I made a definite choice to study for a doctoral degree in Human Development at the University of Chicago because I thought the programs offered and the milieu best suited to my needs and abilities.

My professional experience included staff nursing, supervision, and education. I worked at four large universities: University of California at Los Angeles, Indiana University, University of Washington, and The Pennsylvania State University. I was at the latter institution from 1971 to 1987, as a Professor and also as Head of the Department of Nursing for various periods. At Meharry Medical College, I was Dean of the School of Nursing for 3 years.

I have had no military experience, although I volunteered on two different occasions but was rejected, primarily due to my minority status.

My major satisfaction in nursing has come from assisting in the development of the specialization known as gerontic nursing. I was Chairman of the first Interim Certification Board for Geriatric Nursing, and one of the most thrilling events in my life was witnessing certification of that first group, which helped us gain respect among our colleagues and eventually will help us improve health care for older people.

I retired from the Pennsylvania State University as professor emeritus in 1987 and now live in Seattle, where I offer gerontic consultation services as well as bed and breakfast accommodations. I also volunteer in an elementary school, am involved in the Fellowship for Reconciliation and the Lakewood Community Church, and serve on the Advisory Committee for the University of Washington School of Nursing—all this while spending as much time as possible with my lovely 7-year-old granddaughter, Alexandra. Retirement is wonderful and I enjoy it fully. Sometimes I think that old age is really the best time of all. But then I know that all ages are wonderful and to be treasured."

makes her contributions to the patient in an interpersonal relationship. It would seem then that a theoretical framework must include a theory of the organism (the nature of man and the social context in which he functions), a theory of medicine (disease), and a theory of interpersonal relations (the manner in which the nurse interacts with the patient) combined in such a way that all three are interdependent, interrelated, and integrated so as to be unique to nursing. The theories alone, will not be unique, but the combination and the special aspects stressed for each will be unique to nursing in such a manner as to distinguish it (nursing) from other functions.

Some examples of theoretical systems within which nursing care research may be conducted are presented for illustration. We need to keep in mind that these have been selected from many possibilities, each of which could lead to productive results. We also need to keep in mind that the area of organizing, administering, and supervising nursing service is not covered in this discussion.

The Social Context

One of the basic assumptions is that the societal process, the somatic process, and the self process (personal or psychological orientation of the person) are present and affect all of the reactions of an individual. The social context provides a rich field for theories which may apply to the area of illness and nursing, but only one will be considered here.

Attention is called to the sociological perspective of illness and the role of the physician by Talcott Parsons (1951). His fundamental thesis is that illness is a type of "deviant" behavior by which is meant behavior which fails in some way to fulfill the institutionally defined expectations of one or more of the rules in which the individual is implicated in the society. He sees illness as a social role, and not only a "condition." This factor may have some relationship to the genesis, progress, and recovery in illness. He distinguishes four main features of the "sick role" in our society: (a) the exemption of the sick person from certain responsibilities which he would be expected to carry under normal circumstances; (b) the sick person is, in a very specific sense, also exempted from a certain type of responsibility for his own state; (c) the partial character of this exemption, hence no one is given the privilege of being sick any longer than he can help it; and (d) being sick is also defined as being "in need of help," a specific kind of help from persons specially qualified to care for illness. Although he emphasizes the role of the physician, it would seem to apply also to other members of the health team.

He describes the attributes of the social role of the therapist as providing four main conditions: (a) "support" of an unconditional nature and essentially the acceptance of the patient as a member of a social group; (b) special permissiveness with expressions in the form of disapproval suspended on the part of the therapist; (c) the "patient's welfare" is placed above all else; and (d) the physician is protected against pressures which patients may exert upon him. In addition, he states that there are certain positive functions of illness from the social point of view. The sick person is isolated from influence upon others and he is placed in a situation in which he can re-adapt in order to return to his functions in society.

The Patient
(The Human Organism)

In observing patients undergoing treatment, the differences in response to illness quickly become apparent. One patient amazes the medical team by his continual decline to death, when chances for his recovery were thought to be good. Sudden changes from poor to good conditions and vice versa which are not directly explainable by physiological causes are still unanswered questions in the minds of the medical team, and present an indeterminate situation. Sullivan (1947) speaks of a similar situations as:

> . . . one of the greatest mysteries of human life, how some unfortunate people carry on in the face of apparently overwhelming difficulties, whereas other people are crushed by comparatively insignificant events, contemplate suicide, perhaps actually attempt it. This is to be understood on the basis not of the particular 'objective' events which bring about the circumstance of success under great hardship or self-destruction; it is to be understood on the basis of the self system, the organization of experience reflected to one from the significant people around one—which determines the personal characteristics of those events. In no other fashion can we explain the enormous discrepancy between people's reaction to comparable life situations (Sullivan, 1947, p. 11).

In this paper an attempt has been made to select some of the basic concepts and propositions from Goldstein's theory of the organism, and self psychology which will in part explain a patient's reaction to illness.

Goldstein (1939) proposes the psychological and physical should be treated as phenomena which have to be evaluated as to their significance in terms of the holistic reality for the individual, in the situation in which it is observed. The "functional" significance for the whole is alone relevant. The "psychological" is not the cause of the "somatic" nor the "somatic" the cause of the "psychological"; these factors are not independent of each other. It is convenient for experimental purposes to treat these phenomena as separate, but in interpretation they must again be viewed in terms of the whole organism. Halliday (1948) also discusses the necessity of a shift from a mechanistic to a biologic etiology—a change-over from the outlook upon illness as a localized disease to that of illness as vital reaction if proper preventive measures are to be instituted.

Goldstein (1939) further proposes that there is only one basic normal drive in the individual and that this is the drive for self-actualization. The tendency of normal life is toward activity and progress. The tendency of this mechanism (herein described as the self), he states, takes place during the organism's procedure of coming to terms with the outer world, due to the tendency, the drive for self-actualization.

The position of Goldstein above is similar to that in self psychology theory. Most of these theorists have considered the self as a more or less central core or unifying factor in personality. Lecky (1945) and Rogers (1951), in addition to Goldstein, also consider self-consistency, self-actualization, or self realization as the central and unifying drive within the individual. The biosocial approach is not unlike that of the self psychologists. Murphy (1947) states that the self has grown out of the matrix of indefiniteness which exists at the perceptual level and gradually comes into being as the process of differentiation goes on within the perceptual field. The term "self" can be organized largely in terms of socially defined habits. Questions as to what one means by the self do not result in references to organic and kinesthetic components, but to types of competence and of adjustment in which one constantly classifies and compares himself with others from his own or other social groups.

Some of the factors which seem to be important in the formation and evaluation of the self lie within the following areas: (a) family—attitudes toward one's parents, one's children, and self as parent, and as husband or wife; (b) peer group and friends—degrees of comfort and success in monosexual and heterosexual relationships, and in large and small groups of social relationships; (c) work or occupational status—degree of success and prestige among employers and fellow workers; (d) inner resources for meeting and solving one's own problems including religious attitudes and philosophy; and (e) goals, aspirations, and outlook for the future. For some individuals one or more of these areas may have more importance than another, and one's feelings toward himself may vary from highly positive ones to highly negative ones.

Disease

There are three major unifying concepts as regards the pathogenesis of disease, namely: (a) the principle of contagion by external agents (e.g., microbes), (b) the principle of deficiency in vital elements (e.g., the avitaminosis), and (c) the principle of stress caused by sudden changes requiring readaptation (Selye, 1952). Much research is now being done to show that because man lives his life in a social system he is concerned about his social role and the expectations of significant people about him and perhaps the greatest threat is his doubt about his ability to live the life of a man. These threats and conflicts are omnipresent, and constitute a large section of the stress to which man is exposed (Wolff et al., 1950).

Richter has demonstrated the effects of environmental pressures and stresses on form and function in the "domestication" of rats (Wolff et al., 1950). Outstanding are the reduction in size of the adrenals and thyroid, and the increase in size of the pituitary glands; the augmented capacity to adjust to changes in food, to meet laboratory circumstances, including man, and to withstand stress without attacking neighboring animals; and the reduction in capacity to tolerate poisons. Wild rats in captivity are loath to breed, and even eat their young. Possibly only those capable of domestication reproduce in such circumstances.

Selye (1950) proposes that all living organisms can respond to stress as such and that in this respect, the basic reaction pattern is always the same, irrespective of the agent used to produce stress. He calls this response the *General Adaptation Syndrome*, and its derailments, *the Diseases of Adaptation*. Goldstein's (1940) position is similar, in that he says that the essential element of disease is the shock to the existence of the individual.

Some agents of disease can be considered to be "unconditional pathogens" in that their influence upon the tissues is so great that they cause disease almost irrespective of any conditioning or sensitizing circumstances of sensitization. Their pathogenecity may depend upon genetic factors, the portal of entry through which they are introduced into the body, the previous weakening of resistance through malnutrition or cold, and possibly others, some of which remain unexplored.

It is thought that individuals possessing the capacity to meet effectively their daily problems of living in a manner which is socially acceptable are better equipped to deal with the stress of illness than those who have difficulty in making the grade with the usual stresses of life. Although illness itself may produce undesirable behavior patterns, most of the behavior patterns of the patient existed prior to the illness and may only be exaggerated by the present illness.

In the evaluation of a patient's reaction to illness, at least three aspects of the disease may require consideration: the disorder of the function responsible for the patient's symptoms, the pathological processes of the anatomical structures and organs, and the psychological reactions of the patient to these disorders and pathologies. Each of these aspects may require treatment and up to a certain point, may be considered separately. However, there may be situations in which all three processes are so closely integrated that evaluation of the separate aspects becomes difficult, or evaluation in one area coincides with the evaluation in all three areas. In other cases the patient may show different rates of progress in each area.

Interpersonal Relationships

As an example of one theoretical system for interpersonal relationships, direct hypotheses and postulates have been taken from Rogers's *Client-Centered Therapy* (Boston: Houghton Mifflin. 1951). While he speaks about client-centered therapy, nurses talk about patient-centered nursing, so that there may be a natural relationship between the two. Some of his postulates which seem to have relevance for nursing with some rewording are:

1. The patient has within himself:
   a. the capacity, latent if not evident, to experience and understand those aspects of his life and of himself which are causing him malfunction and pain;
   b. the capacity and tendency to reorganize himself and his relationship to life in the direction of optimal functioning and health.
2. The release of these latent capacities will be most adequately facilitated by experience in a personal relationship in a nonstressful psychological climate.
3. In order to establish a suitable psychological climate the nurse should:
   a. establish a relationship with the patient;
   b. be genuine in the relationship;
   c. experience unconditional positive regard for the patient (value him as a human being and avoid evaluating his actions as "wrong" or "bad");
   d. experience an empathic understanding of the patient's point of view (be able to see things as he sees them);
   e. respect the patient as a person who is capable of understanding his situation, and of participating in the planning for his recovery or for his health.

These conditions should provide a situation in which the patient is free from threat and stress and thereby able to utilize his inner resources for recovery from disease. Or he may utilize this period of illness for reorganization of his self-concept which will enable him to better meet his future life experiences. The nurse's ability to establish this kind of relationship will depend upon her own positive self regard and the positive regard which she receives from the nursing service administration. This will also be true of the instructor-student relationship in nursing.

Nursing Research

An attempt has been made to present some of the theories and propositions from social, psychological, medical and interpersonal relations theory which could possibly be used in nursing research for study. In summary, we have considered nursing as an interpersonal process involving the personal care of individuals as they experience illness within a therapeutic context. In order to do research in nursing we may need to understand theories of: (a) the nature of the human organism including the biological, psychological and sociological aspects of his being; (b) illness in terms of the society in which the organism functions; (c) the roles of the various therapists in the prevention of disease and the care of the ill; and (d) personal and social interaction.

Within such a framework we might study such problems as:

1. The effects of various experimental environments (physical, social and psychological) upon patient progress. Does a patient in an air-conditioned room recover faster or follow a milder course than one in an unconditioned environment? Does a patient who participates in group sessions with other patients have stronger inner resources for dealing with his illness than patients who do not have this opportunity?
2. The effects of various experimental methods of promoting health; e.g., group versus individual, audio-visual-centered versus interpersonal-centered methods?
3. Analysis of contributing factors to certain disease process; e.g., comparison of environmental factors or maternal factors affecting children with a number of referrals to the school nurse compared with a group of children who have not been referred to the school nurse.
4. Analysis of stressors in the hospital environment and effectiveness of certain experimental methods of relieving stress with nursing care measures.
5. Observation of patient-family interaction during illness with experimentation in making this relationship therapeutic.
6. Study of the nurse's role in the care of patients whose illnesses have been growth promoting (resulting in the establishment of a more healthy regimen) as compared with patients whose illnesses have had regressive effects.
7. Nursing activity as it is influenced by the patient's degree of physical and psychological dependence and his therapeutic regimen.

The above are just a few of the types of studies which could be done within the proposed framework and are used to illustrate how theory—biological, sociological or psychological—can help us to raise and to study the kinds of questions which will lead toward the improvement of nursing care.

References

Goldstein, K. (1939). *The organism*. New York: American Books.

Goldstein, K. (1940). *Human nature in the light of psychopathology*. Cambridge, MA: Harvard University Press.

Halliday, J.L. (1948). *Psychosocial medicine*. New York: W.W. Norton.

Lecky, P. (1945). *Self-consistency*. New York: Island Press.

Murphy, G. (1947). *Personality*. New York: Harper

Parsons, T. (1949). *Structure of social action*. Glencoe, IL: The Free Press.

Parsons, T. (1951). Illness and the role of the physician: A sociological perspective. *American Journal of Orthopsychiatry*, 21, 452–60.

Rogers, C. (1951). *Client-centered therapy*. Boston: Houghton Mifflin.

Rogers, C. (1954). *Some basic hypotheses of client-centered therapy*. Mimeographed manuscript, University of Chicago.

Selye, H. (1950). *Physiology and pathology of exposure to stress*. Montreal: ACTA.

Selye, H. (1952). *Second annual report on stress*. Montreal: ACTA.

Sullivan, H.S. (1947). *Conceptions of modern psychiatry* (2nd ed.). Washington, DC: William Alanson White Psychiatric Foundation.

Wolff, H., et al. (Eds.). (1950). *Life stress and bodily disease*. Baltimore: Williams and Wilkins.

The Author Comments

I based this article on part of my doctoral dissertation, which I did for the University of Chicago's Committee on Human Development. When I wrote my dissertation, I was not interested in trying to raise nursing to a professional level (believing that it already was a profession), or in trying to increase my status. Rather, I was interested in learning more about nursing research and nursing phenomena, as well as in learning how to deal with problems in my own relationships with patients. For I was acutely aware of my deficiencies, such as my poor understanding of human behavior (not unexpected, as knowledge of human behavior, sociology, and psychology were very limited in the 1940s) and my tendency toward ethnocentricity. For example, if a patient did not react rationally (from my point of view) and did not follow the medical regimen, or if I could not teach that person how to perform self-care, I tended to think that there was something wrong with the patient.

During my doctoral study, I was exposed to scholars in various disciplines, including psychology, biology, anthropology, education, psychiatry, and psychoanalysis, and studied with such nationally known authorities as Benjamin Bloom, Carl Rogers, Bruno Bettleheim, Bernice Newgarten, Robert Havighurst, Allison Davis, and Lloyd Warner. From each discipline and teacher, I tried to identify useful information that applied to nursing. You see, I view nursing as an applied science rather than as a theoretical science. This is not to imply that I'm "anti-theory," but rather that we may need to consider numerous theories to solve a problem and that our preparation should allow us to examine and select those theories that prove most pertinent to the solution.

At the University of Chicago, preparation for research was the major focus of doctoral study; all our courses and experiences ultimately contributed to this preparation. While developing my dissertation proposal, I had done a number of in-depth reviews of the literature in each of those particular areas and discovered the various authors and investigators that I mentioned in the article on a theoretical framework. I then was able to defend my proposal and proceed with the dissertation work.

Briefly, I selected this part of my dissertation for publication because I had not been exposed to the development of a theoretical framework in any nursing context. I thought this illustration might be useful to other nurses.

However, when I first submitted this article to *Nursing Research* in the 1950s, it was rejected. I got the impression that I was not communicating well with the nurse reviewers and that they simply did not understand what I was trying to say in the article. In 1961, after accepting a position at the University of California at Los Angeles, I set certain personal goals for publication. As I thought this article was soundly written, I decided to resubmit it to *Nursing Research* without any changes. This time, the journal accepted the article in 1961; they published it in 1962. Now, I would like to acknowledge that some editorial changes were made—probably by Dr. Lucille Notter—which I appreciate and believe made the article more readable.

Rereading the article today, I think back to the time we were just beginning to develop nursing research using theoretical frameworks, which would permit the testing of hypotheses and allow us to go beyond the survey method of research, the predominant method at the time. After consideration, I've concluded that I would not change much in the article if I rewrote it today. This could mean that I have not developed my thinking much since that time, or that the article is still basically sound. One of the article's deficiencies involves my definition of nursing, which has been expanded since that time to place more emphasis on health promotion. It also seems a little strange that I did not put more emphasis on human development. I cannot explain these shortcomings except to say that this was where I was at that point in time.

As I reread the article, I also think that I should have gone further in my career with the research problems suggested in the article, and that I should have used this theoretical framework more extensively. It did serve me well in terms of my doctoral dissertation, which was directed toward stress and self-concept in mothers of premature infants. In this comparative study, I showed that mothers of premature infants had more stressful life experiences than mothers of full-term infants. Sometimes I have regrets that I did not stay in this area of research. But the only reason I got into this in the first place was in an effort to delineate a test of the hypothesis that could be conducted within a reasonable period. I originally had wanted to study patients' responses to chronic diseases, but realized that I would have to involve physicians in evaluating the progress of the chronic disease. Knowing how busy physicians are and how unlikely they would be to fully support research under my leadership, I redirected the problem to include a measurement or indicator that would simply be part of the record; that is, infants' birthweights.

In this study, I saw, but did not test, the effects of smoking. This was just an informal observation that I reported to my Committee when I defended my dissertation, but I did not follow it up. In other words, I saw the effects of smoking on birthweight in the early 1950s when it had not been reported as such and so missed valuable opportunities for discovery. Sometimes when we follow a proposal or protocol so carefully that we do not allow ourselves to change the protocol or incorporate other hypotheses not spelled out before we started the study, we miss important opportunities to make new discoveries.

I might also add that I received some negative responses to the article, especially from graduate students, who thought I was trying to develop the theoretical framework for nursing research. They correctly thought that it was not possible for me to do this. I explained very carefully that this was a theoretical framework for nursing research—only one of many—and that I could have selected a whole different body of knowledge and theories; it just happened that I was exposed to a particular set of concepts and body of knowledge and was impressed by those concepts that I selected for this theoretical framework.

My current concern with the present emphasis on theory development in nursing is that we may have lost sight of the function of theory development and put too much emphasis on theory development as a way of increasing our professional status. In my view, there should be a purpose for nursing theory; I see this purpose as developing our understanding of nursing phenomena, not as a way to gain recognition or to attain status. My perspective considers the usefulness of such a theory, which I see as helping in testing hypotheses and ideas so that we may verify and apply this knowledge to improve nursing care.

In summary, the section of this article that I would modify today involves the aims of nursing. I see nursing today as a health service that incorporates generic nursing methods and specialized knowledge to establish conditions that will increase health-conducive behavior, to minimize and compensate for health-related losses, to provide comfort and sustenance when recovery is not possible, and to facilitate the medical care regimen. The article seems to imply two aspects of nursing, one having to do with the disease or assistance with the medical regimen and the other with the personal aspects of care provided within an interpersonal relationship. At the time I wrote it, there was little emphasis on increasing health-conducive behaviors and only limited emphasis on disease prevention.

—LAURIE M. GUNTER

Chapter 2

Research in the Development of Nursing Theory: The Importance of a Theoretical Framework in Nursing Research

Myrtle Irene Brown

As the amount of research conducted by nurses increases, we seek ways to assess the outcomes. Indirect measures, such as amounts of money spent, the proportion of nurses employed in research, and the number of projects completed, tell us much about the progress of nursing research, but the most useful measures are of the product of research, namely, growth in scientifically sound knowledge on which to base nursing care and education.

With our focus on evaluation of nursing research in terms of its outcomes, partial answers will be sought in this paper to two questions:

How far have we progressed through research toward the development of an integrated body of nursing theory?

How can we determine if a research project has a theoretical framework that will make possible a contribution to scientific knowledge?

Nurses have often participated in research which has contributed much to the basic sciences that are fundamental to the practice of all health professions. In the past, they have functioned primarily as collectors of data; in the future, nurses who are academically prepared will increasingly initiate and conduct research within the theoretical framework of such primary sciences as physiology, psychology, sociology, and bacteriology. Though some nurse researchers will make their major contributions to these basic sciences, we can expect that many will focus on the development of a body of nursing theory.

The Need for Nursing Theory

A clear mandate has been made to nurse researchers to build a body of scientifically tested nursing theory from which may be drawn the facts, concepts, and principles on which to base the education of nurses and the nursing care and service of patients, families, and communities. The need for such a unified and valid abstract

About the Author

MYRTLE IRENE BROWN currently resides in Columbia, South Carolina, her home for the last 20 years. She has been retired since June 1980, but retirement has not limited her professional interests. She comments "Since 1980 I have been greatly concerned with the continued development and health of older persons, including myself, working through the church and other community agencies open to me since retirement. I continue to be concerned that the direct care of chronically ill, fragile, and dependent older persons is given by uninformed aides, practical nurses, and registered nurses with little preparation in gerontology and geriatrics."

Dr. Brown is a graduate of Methodist Hospital School of Nursing in Peoria, Illinois. After graduation she continued her education at Eureka College, majoring in Sociology and receiving a B.A. in 1939. She earned a second baccalaureate degree, in Nursing Education, from the University of Minnesota in 1942, then continued her studies at the University of Minnesota, receiving an M.S. in Public Health and Child Health and Welfare in 1947. In 1961, Dr. Brown received a Ph.D. in Educational Sociology from New York University.

During her long career in nursing, Dr. Brown held various professional positions. She has worked as a nurse in the World Health Organization and as a research consultant with the American Nurses' Foundation, and has held numerous faculty positions at Schools of Nursing, Public Health, and Medicine around the country. At the time of her retirement, Dr. Brown was a Professor of Nursing and Associate Dean of Graduate Programs in Nursing at the University of South Carolina.

Dr. Brown considers her work in the areas of research and theory to have been particularly challenging. She comments "If I had continued to pursue the conduct of research after 1967, I would have wished to further identify the health and developmental needs of individuals that nursing could have promoted. In other words, I believe more research regarding the needs of clients rather than the processes of nursing and administration will provide a broader base for the unique functions of nursing. For myself, my work in promoting healthful development of patients, clients, students, and co-workers through nursing, teaching, counseling, and administering has been an area of professional pride and satisfaction."

system of thought with which to describe, plan, and evaluate nursing has been stated by nursing service administrators, nurse educators, and members of related health disciplines.

Loretta Heidgerken, who has written extensively on nursing research, clearly points out the dependence of the nursing profession on the development of such a systematic body of theory by describing the relationship between nursing practice and knowledge:

A well-developed practice has at its disposal a highly refined diagnostic typology that embraces the entire gamut of problems confronted by that discipline. That is, there are a series of generalizations (principles), both descriptive and prescriptive, which the professional practitioner can employ in his practice. These generalizations are classified into a systematic body of knowledge which is being continuously tested and validated (Heidgerken, 1962, pp. 140–143).

Philosophical considerations led the nurse educator, Martha Rogers, to a similar statement of the urgency for nursing theory which appears in her book *Educational Revolution in Nursing* (New York: Macmillan, 1961). She first noted the service obligation of the nursing profession, stating:

Society has a right to expect that the responsibility for nursing services will rest with persons possessing a substantial theoretical foundation for making judgments and assuming responsibility (Rogers, 1961, p. 5).

Then, turning to nursing education, she made the challenge even more explicit by pointing out that the central factor in further progress in baccalaureate curricula for the preparation of nurses is the growth of nursing theory. She identified research as the source of such theory: "Theoretical knowledge in nursing is dependent on research" (Rogers, 1961, p. 43).

Nursing service administrators have also voiced

the necessity for nursing concepts that are fitting to the realities of modern medical, hospital, health, and nursing care. In a report of a conference held jointly by the Hospital Association of New York State and the New York State Nurses Association (NYSNA), Sister Charles Marie noted that "the need for an adequate concept of nursing" (NYSNA, 1961, p. 31) was frequently reiterated in the various sessions by the participants.

Among the scientists from other health disciplines who have made the charge to nurses to develop the body of knowledge fundamental to nursing is Alan Treloar, Chief of the Statistics and Analysis Branch, Division of Research Grants, National Institutes of Health (1961). His presentation at the fourth annual conference on nursing education held under the auspices of the Western Council on Higher Education for Nursing carried this commission to nurses regarding the conduct of research:

> Distinctiveness becomes yours when care of the patient comes to the front in your activities, when you are working directly with and on behalf of the sick or maintaining good health in those not sick, when you are functioning in this sense as a part of the medical team. . . . This sector of the frontier of knowledge now requires, and I imagine forever will require, much intellectual work, scientific study, and careful testing of theory. This is where, through research, I believe you should be probing in force on the frontiers of knowledge (Treloar, 1961, pp. 8–9).

Though the call to nurse researchers to focus their studies on concept validation and theory testing has been repeatedly made, a review of many research reports by nurse investigators reveals few instances in which the relationship of a project to nursing theory has been made explicit.

Concept Validation Through Research

In spite of the fact that few nursing research reports state their relationships to the principles that are implicit in them, they have nevertheless gradually given meaning to some useful nursing terms. Concept formulation and validation is an early phase in the development of a body of knowledge. The examination of what a number of research projects have contributed to one abstraction, namely "patient-centered nursing," will answer in part our first question: How far have we progressed through research toward an integrated body of nursing theory?

Those early studies that assumed that the opinion of patients was an important source of data gave credence to the term "patient-centered." Prominent among these was the extensive project of Abdellah and Levine (1957, 1958), in which they devised a tool for assessing the extent of care that was satisfying to patients. The problem of that project dealt with the relationship of the amounts of patient-satisfying care and the nurse staffing patterns in various kinds of hospitals. In turn, Boyle (1960), focusing on the concept of empathy, and Whiting et al. (1958), using the Q-sort, revealed that there existed differences of perceptions of nurses and patients concerning what is important in nursing care. On the basis of such studies, it was concluded that patient-centered care was interfered with by nurses' lack of insight into patients' desires and wishes.

To overcome the problem of differences of nurses' and patients' perceptions, further studies of patients' opinions have been conducted. McGhee (1961), through interviews of patients after discharge from the hospital, sought information about the nursing care they had received and how this related to their needs.

Other nurse researchers, who were not content to use patients' subjective opinions and perceptions, have designed tools to measure more objectively the needs of patients. For example, the Patient Profile, a rating device, was developed for use in the research project "Comparative Evaluation of Hospital Beds" conducted by the University of Pittsburgh (Williams, 1960). Using essential physical needs of patients for the categories, a scale was developed which nurses could use to rate the extent of the patient's independence in meeting these needs and the extent to which the patient was dependent on nursing care to fulfill these physical needs.

Another effort to add reliability to the measurement of patient need was a checklist and other objective devices developed by Verhonick (1961) to make more precise both nurses' observations of decubitus ulcers and the evaluation of the degree of progress in healing. Verhonick went further than simply measuring change in decubitus ulcers; she employed this change in a patient-condition as the criterion for evaluating specific nursing care given.

Other studies have used changes in patients' conditions and behaviors as the criteria of outcomes when selected nursing interventions were introduced experimentally. Bowen, Rich, and Schlotfeldt (1961) studied the effects of instruction of patients with diabetes mellitus using measures of physical status as well as verbal knowledge of patients as criteria of the effectiveness of teaching.

The current program of research at the Yale University School of Nursing is centered on the study of the relationship of nurse-patient interaction and various criteria of patient behavior. Several projects now being conducted there will serve to test and modify the theories of dynamic nurse-patient interaction enunciated by Orlando (1961). The relationship of this program of research to theory, which was not made explicit in the research report of Dumas and Leonard (1963), has been identified in a series of articles in the *American Journal of Nursing* as validation of a theory of nursing practice (Dumas, Pelletier, & Dye, 1963).

These are but a limited selection of the research projects that have been focused on patients' conditions and the study of nursing aimed at changing these conditions. All but a few of these projects have been concerned with practical problems in nursing without expressed interest in nursing theory. Though these studies add meaning to the term "patient-centered nursing," this concept would be much more useful today if the investigators had shown clearly the relationship of their work to it.

If nurse researchers are to meet the challenge of building a body of nursing theory, we who conduct, promote, support, and use nursing research must add new criteria in the analysis and criticism of our own and others' investigatory efforts. Of each research project, we should ask:

In what ways and to what extent is this investigation linked to theory?

What contribution does this investigation make to a scientific body of knowledge?

Is the theoretical framework from one of the basic sciences, an applied science or, more specifically, nursing theory?

Assessing the Theoretical Framework of a Research Project

Research that is solidly conceived in a theoretical framework will have certain identifiable characteristics. The investigator who is conscious that he is helping to build a science will make explicit the relationship of his work to theory. This will be apparent in the research plan as well as in the final report. The purpose, the definition of terms, the related literature, as well as the findings and their implications, can all serve to relate a project to the body of scientific knowledge toward which its contribution is aimed.

If truth is to be served, the prospectus of a research project should include among its purposes the pursuit of knowledge for the sake of knowledge; its aims should not be limited to the search for facts needed to solve a specific practical problem. A utilitarian concern, however, does not of necessity prevent a particular project from also serving the broader purpose of building theoretical knowledge.

As Goode and Hatt (1952) have pointed out, applied research can contribute to theory. Applied research can put theory to the test in a specific situation; it may help clarify concepts; it may contribute new facts that lead to the formulation or redefinition of a theory.

Greenwood, in an analysis of the relationship of social science and social work, has also described how applied research may strengthen theory:

Should the application of theory yield practical principles it would be a corroboration of the theory with a consequent strengthening of the theoretical system of the social science. Therefore, while the immediate purpose of applied research is utilitarian, its ultimate result is to refine and build social science theory (Greenwood, 1955, pp. 20–33).

Even when planning the study of a practical problem, the investigator who is conscious of the possible role of applied research in theory-building will focus his purposes on seeking knowledge that supports generalizations which can be applied to many problems as well as the one at hand. This focus is possible only if the investigator is well-grounded in the literature and has related his project to the work of others.

The precise statement of the problem to be investigated is often less revealing of theory than the general purpose, as an investigator must sharply limit his problem and sub-problem according to his resources. If, however, he has studied related theory and formulated his problem as an hypothesis aimed at testing some aspect of theory, he will usually indicate this.

For example, Turk, in a report of an investigation of medical role relations, indicated as his frame of reference the theory "complex social systems include both common and disparate values" (Turk, 1963, p. 30). He also identified the social scientists and their works which have supported this theory. Building on this, he proposed his hypothesis as an extension of the theory, stating:

> Cohesion is higher where the student physician's value orientations to patients are bureaucratic and those of the student nurse are non-bureaucratic than where there is any other permutation of such orientations (Turk, 1963, p. 30).

Statistically significant findings supporting this hypothesis make up the bulk of this nine-page journal article. This report demonstrates that space limitations in journals do not preclude the identification of the relevance of the problem to theory.

The choice of terms used in a project provides further opportunity to relate the research to concepts previously shown to be useful in symbolizing phenomena under investigation by scientists exploring related areas of reality. When concepts are used that have been previously described and validated through research, the investigator benefits by the meanings that have already accrued to the selected terminology. The researcher who consistently prefers operational definitions, or terms defined independently for each project, isolates his work from that of others.

There are, of course, occasions when no appropriate concepts have been previously developed and the investigator is forced to define his terms independently. Such a lack of useful concepts occurs often in a new and developing body of theory. This absence of suitable terms often obtains in nursing research today; however, unless the nurse investigator has a rich empirical basis for creating a new term or defining a common term idiosyncratically, concepts from nursing literature or from one of the related basic or applied sciences will usually serve to make the findings of a project of greater general meaning and application than a new term.

The appropriateness of the design of a project is determined by the problem and sub-problems under investigation rather than by its relationship to theory. Whether any particular method is apt to be more useful than another in building general theory often depends on the stage of development of that body of knowledge. Descriptive research, such as is encountered in historical studies, surveys, compilations of biostatistics, and series of case studies, may be very useful in providing facts for the formulation of classification systems in young sciences. Experimental design will usually be more appropriate in testing theories; however, even an evaluated demonstration may constitute a practical test of theory. Obviously, if the project is to contribute to knowledge, practical or theoretical, it must be carried out meticulously; its methods should meet the criteria of scientific research. It is in the analysis of data that the investigator most frequently contributes to the body of knowledge or misses his greatest opportunity to do so. The products of his research are of two orders: findings and generalizations; both may contribute to theory. If his project was set up to test a theory, his findings, positive or negative, will support the theory or require its revision. If, however, the investigator is able to go past the reporting of sheer numerical facts to seek possible associations among the findings, make thoughtful guesses at implications, compare his results with those of other investigators, logically extend relationships to other variables and situations, and relate his findings to theories, he may create an important hypothesis that constitutes a leap into a new dimension of theory.

The ability to think creatively differentiates the scientist from the research technologist. Most investigators will fall into the second classification and will make their contribution through careful reporting of reliable findings; but we are dependent on the creative thinkers for the development of a science. Bronowski has stated well the relationship of the scientist to the creation of a science:

> No scientific theory is a collection of fact. . . . All science is the search for unity in hidden likenesses. . . . The scientist looks for order in the appearance of nature by exploring such likenesses. For order does not display itself; if it can be said to be there at all, it is not there for the mere looking. There is no way of pointing a finger or a camera at it, order must be discovered and, in a deep sense, it must be created (Bronowski, 1955, pp. 23–24).

Thus a research project that contributes to nursing theory can be identified through certain characteristics of its report, such as, an aim to pursue knowledge for its own sake, the statement of the relationship of the problem to research and nursing literature, the use of established meaningful terms, the association of findings to the work of others, and the logical but creative exposition of implications and further hypotheses for testing.

Summary

Judging from the histories of the development of other sciences, we may expect an orderly body of nursing knowledge to develop more rapidly and soundly if nursing theory grows out of research. To avoid being diverted by the armchair theorists, the traditionalists, or the unscientific empiricists, we in nursing are dependent on our nurse investigators, not only to conduct research with impeccable and appropriate methodology, but also to provide us with a growing body of scientific knowledge. It is hoped that there will be more rapid development of nursing theory through research in the future as more nurse investigators are prepared for the role of the scientist whose primary concern is building a body of valid knowledge. Only as concepts and principles from nursing theory are enunciated and tested can there be generalizations to solve the practical problems of nursing practice, to provide the content of nursing education, and to form the basis for further research.

References

Abdellah, F.G., & Levine, E. (1957). Developing a measure of patient and personnel satisfaction with nursing care. *Nursing Research, 3,* 100–108.

Abdellah, F.G., & Levine, E. (1958). Effect of nurse staffing on satisfactions with nursing care. *Hospital Monograph Series No. 4.* Chicago: American Hospital Association.

Bowen, R.G., Rich, R., & Schlotfeldt, R.M. (1961). Effects of organized instruction for patients with the diagnosis of diabetes mellitus. *Nursing Research, 10,* 151–159.

Boyle, R.A. (1960). *A study of student nurse perception of patient attitudes* (U.S. Health Service Publication No. 769). Washington, DC: U.S. Government Printing Office.

Bronowski, J. (1959). *Science and human values.* New York: Harper.

Dumas, R., Pelletier, I., & Dye, M. (1963). Validating a theory of nursing practice. *American Journal of Nursing, 63,* 52–59.

Dumas, R., & Leonard, R.C. (1963). The effect of nursing on the incidence of postoperative vomiting. *Nursing Research, 12,* 12–15.

Goode, W.J., & Hatt, P.K. (1952). *Methods in social research.* New York: McGraw-Hill.

Greenwood, E. (1955). Social science and social work: A theory of their relationship. *Social Service Review, 29,* 20–33.

Heidgerken, L.E. (1962). Nursing research—its role in research activities in nursing. *Nursing Research, 11,* 140–143.

McGhee, A. (1961). *The patient's attitude to nursing care.* Edinburgh: E. and S. Livingstone.

New York State Nurses' Association. (1961). *Our mutual interest—the patient.* A Report of the Second Joint Conference of the Hospital Association of New York State and the New York State Nurses' Association at Arden House, Harriman, New York, December 13–15, 1961. Albany, NY: Author.

Orlando, I.J. (1961). *The dynamic nurse-patient relationship.* New York: G.P. Putnam's Sons.

Rogers, M.E. (1961). *Educational revolution in nursing.* New York: MacMillan.

Treloar, A.E. (1961). Dilemmas in nursing. In *Dilemmas in nursing, Proceedings of the Fourth Annual Western Conference on Nursing Education.* Boulder, CO: Western Council on Higher Education for Nursing.

Turk, H. (1963). Social cohesion through variant values; evidence from medical role relations. *American Sociological Review, 28*, 28–37.

Verhonick, P.J. (1961). Decubitus ulcer observations measured objectively. *Nursing Research, 10*, 211–214.

Whiting, J.F., et al. (1958). *The nurse-patient relationship and the healing process* (A progress report to the American Nurses' Foundation, June 1955–December 1957). Pittsburgh: Veterans Administration Hospital.

Williams, M.E. (1960). The patient profile. *Nursing Research, 9*, 122–128.

The Author Comments

A quarter of a century ago, the American Nurses' Association founded the American Nurses' Foundation, a tax-exempt organization through which the nursing profession and its friends could promote research to augment the body of scientifically determined knowledge essential as a basis for nursing practice, service, and education. Between August 1961 and February 1964, I served as nursing research consultant at the Foundation. With the guidance of Dr. Clara Hardin, the agency's executive director, I visited many schools of nursing, primarily in colleges and universities, and departments of nursing services in hospitals and other nursing institutions. In each situation, I met with groups of nurses to identify research efforts in progress and to stimulate and encourage new research projects.

Back in New York City, in the office at 10 Columbus Circle (where all nursing organizations were then located), our search for and review of nursing research reports was aided greatly by Dr. Lucille Notter, editor of *Nursing Research*. The field work, literature review, and consultations with agencies that funded and supported research revealed diverse efforts, most seeking solutions to specific patient care problems (often in circumscribed settings) or describing nurses' characteristics and behaviors.

As a student of sociology and the history of its development as a behavioral science, I was familiar with the growth of theories. I knew that a theoretical base of science not deeply rooted in scientifically conducted research could suffer from erroneous fabrication by armchair theorists or could misdirect practitioners and educators who were utilizing faulty knowledge.

This article was prepared specifically for publication in *Nursing Research* as a guide to beginning nurse researchers. Discussions with Dr. Notter helped me clarify and enlarge my ideas. The article's purpose was to make explicit the need for relating nursing research efforts to a shared body of knowledge and to point out ways in which this could be done.

The section "Concept Validation Through Research" specified how various research efforts contributed to the then-evolving nursing concept of "patient-centered care," regardless of whether or not each researcher was aware of his or her contribution. The steps of a research project outlined in "Assessing the Theoretical Framework of a Research Project" point out how a researcher at each phase of work can relate the research effort to the existing concepts and relationships of phenomena as described in the existing body of theory.

—MYRTLE IRENE BROWN

Chapter 3

Towards Development of Nursing Practice Theory

Florence S. Wald

Robert C. Leonard

How shall nursing develop a scientific body of knowledge basic to nursing practice? Several approaches have been used to develop such knowledge, but all of these approaches have tried to develop nursing knowledge by applying "the basic sciences" to problems of nursing care. The central contention of this paper is that there has been a failure to use the empirical approach of building knowledge directly from systematic study of nursing experience. Therefore, we wish to describe the differences between nursing theory as applied theory and nursing theory based on hypotheses developed from an examination of actual clinical nursing practice.

The Fallacy of Nursing as an Applied Science

The historical evolution of the nursing profession determined what nurses sought as a scientific base for their practice, and during the first phase of development nursing knowledge has been inextricably linked with the growth of medical knowledge. Medicine began to elaborate its scientific base in the second part of the 19th century, when clinicians recognized the relationship between tissue changes (microscopic and macroscopic) and the processes of disease. Pathologists, histologists, bacteriologists, and biochemists systematically studied the relationships between the changes in tissues, the clinical symptoms, and the effects of treatment used. Their findings were used, in turn, by nurses to determine nursing procedures and nursing treatments—techniques for asepsis, treatments for bed sores, management of cardiac patients, infant feedings to name but a few.

In the early part of the twentieth century nursing also turned to the profession of education for its scien-

About the Authors

FLORENCE S. WALD is retired and lives in Connecticut near Yale University, where she studied, taught, and practiced nursing for more than 40 years. After receiving a M.N. degree from the Yale University School of Nursing in 1941, she worked as a visiting nurse in New York City, then as a research assistant in the Surgical Metabolism Unit of the College of Physicians and Surgeons. She later returned to Yale, receiving a M.S. in 1956 and serving as the School of Nursing's Dean from 1958 to 1968. She resigned from that position to study the care of terminally ill cancer patients and to help found the first hospice in the United States.

When asked about her long and active career in nursing, Ms. Wald replied "Direct clinical care fires me in a way that teaching and administration never have. Discovering new concepts developed by others or from my own experiences—such as Ida Orlando's nurse-patient relationship, Virginia Henderson's definition of nursing, or Cicely Saunders' focus on the patient/family and my own conceptualization of a hospice service for the terminally ill—charge me and inspire me. It's thrilling to see how many articles written by Yale University faculty and students are included in this volume. We worked very hard, argued vociferously, but I think we headed in the right direction. I thought that then and I still believe it now."

ROBERT C. LEONARD is a sociologist on the faculty of the University of Arizona, a position he has held for more than 25 years. During the 1960s, as an Assistant Professor at Yale's School of Nursing, he helped develop a research training program that resulted in six funded research grants, about 60 papers and articles, and six books by faculty and students of the School of Nursing. Since leaving Yale, his interest in nursing theory has continued. He co-authored a text, *Behavioral Science and Nursing Theory*, (St. Louis: C. V. Mosby, 1983), which won a Book-of-the-Year award from the American Nurses' Association. In 1987, he served as a consultant to the National Institute of Preventive and Social Medicine, Bangladesh, under sponsorship of the World Health Organization.

Dr. Leonard studied sociology at the University of California, Berkeley (M.A., 1958) and the University of Oregon, Eugene (Ph.D., 1962). Before becoming involved in nursing theory, he had a previous career in electronic engineering, about which he comments "This gave me a perspective on the relation between abstract basic science and everyday practical applications, which influenced my thinking about basic social science and nursing practice."

When asked about his collaboration with nurses, Dr. Leonard responded "The nurses I have worked with have been intelligent, hardworking, and humane. To me, a major satisfaction of nursing research is its potential usefulness."

Another perspective on Dr. Leonard's work in nursing comes from his co-author, Florence Wald, who was Dean of the School of Nursing at the time this article was written. She comments "Robert Leonard made an enormous contribution in all our research work. He was selfless, generous, open-minded, and very clear-headed. He put himself into a vulnerable position by holding joint appointments in Yale's Department of Sociology and School of Nursing. He never shortchanged the School of Nursing, even though the Sociology Department did not fully appreciate his contribution to nursing research!"

tific underpinnings.[1] As a part of this liaison, nursing researchers adopted the methods and aims of educational research, but these methods failed to provide nursing with knowledge basic to its practice. Whatever the merit of this vast body or research for guiding nursing educators, from the outset it proved to be of little use for guiding clinical nursing practice.[2]

In the 1930s and early 1940s nurses turned to another field—industrial management. During these years industry was studying production flow, time and motion, and the utilization of personnel. These studies were viewed as being potentially applicable to nursing because they might provide answers to the problem of the mushrooming hospital complex manned with an increasingly inadequate professional staff. However, the limitations of educational and administrative studies has become increasingly recognized in recent years (Henderson, 1957; McManus, 1961a, 1961b; Schlotfeldt, 1960; Simmons & Henderson, 1964).

In its recent stage of development, nursing has attempted to develop an alliance between nursing and the physical and social sciences, but the nature of this alliance has remained elusive. For many years nurse educators have urged that social and biological science content be included in the nurse's basic education, in order to "integrate" relevant ideas from these disciplines into the basic nursing curriculum. In the 1950's a frantic search for "basic concepts" was begun by individuals and groups (Nordmark & Rohweder, 1959; Simmons & Henderson, 1964).[3] The problems encountered in these "integration" projects, and by this approach in general, may be linked to the difficulty nurses had in finding an answer to three questions: First, "What is nursing?"[4] Second, "Which principles from other disciplines appear relevant to nursing as defined?" and third, "Which of these principles prove relevant when tested?"

Nurses have expressed much concern for finding scientific principles applicable to nursing, but they have shown little concern for the selecting out of principles which are not applicable. In the first place, no matter how much acceptance they may have within the other discipline, in the nursing situation such principles may very well prove to be invalid, or inappropriate. For example, biological science principles may be invalid when applied to nursing because the nurse deals with people in a social situation—not with animals in a laboratory. A second pitfall is that the nurse may put undue weight on a "general principle" which in reality proves relatively untested and hence unreliable.[5] The proper clinical testing of principles—especially those in the social sciences—has been retarded by a lack of knowledge about sound clinical experimental designs. But there is an even more fundamental fallacy in establishing principles of nursing practice through the "application" of principles borrowed from so-called "basic" disciplines. This approach assumes that principles for practice actually can be imported

---

[1] On the one hand, the link between nursing and education seems difficult to explain. However, it will be remembered that as nurses attempted to attain professional status, the first step they took was to prepare better teachers of nursing. The professional leaders in nursing and the universities to which they turned both believed this could best be accomplished in schools of education, and the school which became most influential in the early years was Teachers College, Columbia University, where a pattern of advanced education was established.

[2] Interestingly enough, the educating profession and the nursing profession have an important characteristic in common—both professions strive to create changes in human beings—and therefore, they might well study which activities of practice produce these changes and why. It is starting to review research done by both these professions and realize, on the one hand, how little educators have done to study the effect of one particular kind of teaching on student learning as compared with another, and on the other hand, how little nurses have done to study the effect of one particular kind of nursing on patient welfare as compared with another. James B. Conant (1963) notes this need for the teaching profession in the chapter on "Theory and Practice in Teaching" in *The Education of American Teachers* (New York: McGraw Hill, 1963).

---

[3] The group effort has been documented in the West where intermural conferences of various schools have been held under the auspices of WICHE for the purpose of finding content in various fields of nursing.

[4] The failure to answer this first question results in the kind of confusion about what nursing expects of behavioral science expressed by Sheldon (1963). It should be understood that this is not a research question, but rather a policy issue to be settled by discussion and decision by nurses.

[5] It is interesting to note that this is as true for social work, law, medicine, or engineering as it is for nursing. Social workers, like nurses, have a "tendency to treat assumptive or hypothetical knowledge as if it had been thoroughly tested and validated" (Bisno, 1960).

from these other disciplines. Alvin Gouldner warns that:

> The applied social sciences cannot be fruitfully regarded as springing Athena-like from the furrowed brow of the pure disciplines. Any metaphor which conceives of applied social science as the offspring, and of the basic disciplines as parents, is misleading (Gouldner, 1956, p. 169).

This author goes on to strongly reject "the standard view" that:

> The development of the applied social sciences requires no special planning and theoretical analyses . . . have no distinctive problems and that, with the maturation of the basic disciplines all that will be required is to transfer their developments, like carrying bones from an old graveyard to a new one (Gouldner, 1956, p. 169).

This is as true for nursing as it is for the other practices.

Nevertheless, nurses have spent the past ten years in a pursuit of nursing knowledge through the untested application of principles from the "pure" discipline. They have consulted with social scientists, asked social scientists to do research for them, and have undertaken doctoral study in the social sciences. As a result, nursing problems are being rephrased as social science questions rather than questions of practice, and nurses are studying nurses. As Henderson (1956) so pungently put it, no other discipline studies the workers rather than the work. Why have nurses studied nurses and not nursing? Since the "pure" scientist, whose help was sought, was trained to pursue his own discipline and was not trained to help others with *their* problems, it might have been expected that he would help nurses to develop his discipline rather than nursing practice.

This approach by the "pure" scientist is justified by viewing nursing strictly as an "applied" discipline but it has confused the nurses as well as the scientists trying to approach nursing questions. As Gouldner says:

> The applied social scientist . . . must be trained and prepared to make his own theoretical innovations, (or) . . . his work may be in some ways impeded . . . by the pure scientist (Gouldner, 1956, p. 169).

In the present state of the behavioral sciences and nursing, we doubt that the integration of relevant basic sciences into clinical nursing is a viable means of building nursing theory. An alternative that has been overlooked is to begin with practical nursing experience and develop concepts from an analysis of that clinical experience, rather than to try to make borrowed concepts fit. This alternative was used by psychoanalysis and, more recently, by social work.[6] In developing its own theories, nursing would become an independent "discipline" in its own right. In freeing themselves from the burden of looking only for applications of the "basic" sciences in their practice, nurses would at the same time take on the responsibility of developing their own science. This calls for the development of nursing practice theory.

Characteristics of Research Methods for Practice Science Contrasted With Methods for Descriptive Science

The important point to be understood is that there is an essential difference between the study of professional practice and the "basic" scientist's practice of his academic discipline.[7] Of course, there are similarities, the practitioner-scientist and the basic scientist both are committed to scientific rules of evidence and must observe the same steps of systematic inquiry. Exploratory observations are made, an hypothesis is derived and a way of testing the hypothesis is developed. Both kinds of study involve measurement of the variable and require sound sampling techniques and statistical analysis. Progress in both kinds of science is signaled by the accumulation of ever more general and increasingly well tested propositions. However, the difference lies in

---

[6] Gouldner points out that "the most successful of the applied psychologies"—psychoanalysis—did not start with academic psychology. Freud often stressed that his theory grew out of his own clinical experience (Gouldner, 1956, p. 169).

[7] This comparison is adapted from Greenwood, E. (1961). The practice of science and the science of practice. In W.G. Bennis, K.D. Benne, & R. Chin (Eds.), *The planning of change.* New York: Holt.

the selection of variables for study and the kind of hypotheses that are entertained. In other words, the difference is in the kind of theory they are testing.

The purpose of the practitioner-scientist is to systematically study ways to achieve changes. In the case of nursing, the aim is to study the way the nurse achieves changes in patients' responses to illness, to hospitalization, to the medical regimen, and changes in the patient's ability to utilize health measures. In other words, prescriptions for professional practice must be in cause-and-effect terms. This means that the theories developed by nurse-researchers must be causal theories. The "pure" scientist is free to include causal propositions in his theory or to leave them out, although in fact most sciences seem to strive for causal theories. Practice theory is not only limited to causal hypotheses but is further restricted to the use of causal variables that can be manipulated by the practitioner.

As an example of these differences in approach, we can look at the question of pain in human beings. The physiologists ask, "Are there substances in human inflammatory exudate and plasma which are in themselves pain producing: that is, how is this pain caused?" (Armstrong et al., 1957, p. 350). Hardy, Wolff, and Goodell ask, "Do different body areas have dissimilar levels of threshold for the sensation of pricking pain—that is, how is the pain experienced?" (Hardy, Wolff, & Goodell, 1952, p. 425). Or, to turn to the social scientist, Zoborowski looks at people from different ethnic subcultures and asks, "Do people in different cultures respond differently to pain?" (Zoborowski, 1952, p. 16).

On the other hand, the practitioner asks a different kind of question in approaching the same phenomenon. Gammon and Starr asked, "How can we *relieve* pain? By using counter-irritants? Which are the most effective?" (Gammon & Starr, 1941, p. 13). Tinterow asks, "Can hypnosis relieve the pain heretofore considered 'intractable'?" (Tinterow, 1960, p. 30). Bochnak asks, "Does the request for pain medication really mean the patient has 'pain'? Will the patient be more relieved, with or without medication, if the nurse ap-

proaches him in an exploratory, deliberative way?" (Bochnak, 1961–1962, p. 5).

It is important to note that the basic disciplines can learn from practice theory. The Tinterow study on hypnosis provides the psychologist with information about how pain is perceived and levels of consciousness. Bochnak's experiment tests sociological hypotheses about dyadic interaction.

The reverse is also true. The developer of practice theory has much to learn from physiological and psychological theories of pain developed by other disciplines. Indeed, this is precisely the path taken by Crowley (1962) and other members of the University of California at Los Angeles faculty in assembling all the theories of pain, which they then planned to relate to nursing practice. If this book leaves us dissatisfied, it is not because we doubt the usefulness of attempting to relate these theories from other disciplines to nursing practice. Rather, the next two steps—the building of a coherent practice theory and its clinical test—have not yet been taken.

Characteristics of Practice Theory Compared With Characteristics of Descriptive Theory

Any scientific theory, whether a theory of practice or not, begins with concepts naming classes of events in nature, and with questions or even hypotheses about how these concepts relate to each other. These concepts and hypotheses may come from anywhere, but we are proposing that for the building of nursing practice theory they should come in part from actual nursing experience[8] and that they must be tested by actual nursing experience.

Research not geared to improving professional practice may be limited to strictly descriptive proposi-

---

[8] To reiterate, the most popular common and prestigeful source is to borrow them from certain established academic disciplines regarded as "basic" sciences.

tions, but a practice theory must contain causal hypotheses. For example, the anthropologist William Caudill (1952), in describing the culture of a psychiatric hospital, discovered that the staff and the patients form two separate subcultures and that the two subcultures have a limited amount of communication with one another. This finding is interesting to nurses, and no doubt makes a contribution to anthropology. Yet it does not provide explicit prescriptions for nursing practice. At almost the same time, a nurse, Gwen Tudor Will (1952), looked at the same phenomenon—lack of communication between staff and patients—in a similar situation, a small private psychiatric hospital. Her research could not end with simple description—she went on to ask how the degenerative cycle of "mutual withdrawal" of patient and staff could be broken. She found that the withdrawn "asocial" patient responded to a different nursing approach. She concluded that if the nurse does not withdraw, but moves toward the patient, the patient's behavior will change and the communication deadlock can be broken. In these two approaches, the social scientist described the existing patterns of organization in the setting, while the nurse manipulated variables to see what effect she would achieve. Because of her purpose as a professional, she was interested not only in what the present situation was like, but also *how* to change it. Out of this case study came a causal hypothesis about the effect of nursing activity on the patient which can be incorporated into nursing practice theory.[9]

Barriers to Research of Practice Theory in Nursing

There are a number of particular problems which have impeded nurses in devising theories of practice through research.

---

[9] It should be pointed out that we are not using the word "theory" with the connotation that it contains only "proven facts." Will's hypothesis would need considerably more testing—preferably in well controlled clinical experimentation—before we should incorporate it into theory with a degree of confidence.

Problems in Preparing the Research Attitude

One characteristic essential to any researcher is independence in thought, yet traditionally, the nurse's role has been passive rather than creative. It is usual that the doctor diagnoses and prescribes while the nurse carries out his orders. This pattern of relationship is antithetical to the nurse scientist who must observe for herself and devise ways of acting. Therefore, if nurses are to develop as scientists they must learn new patterns of action and establish relationships with their colleagues whether these colleagues be doctor or social scientist or biological scientist. Nurses once depended on the doctor; they now might depend on these other disciplines rather than using their own powers of observation and their own intellect. While development of nursing practice theory can benefit from a close relationship with scientists, the relationship must be one of mutual give-and-take, and nurses must strive to develop independence in thought. Traditional subordination to the medical practitioner is probably reinforced by the fact that nursing is almost wholly a woman's profession. (In our European culture the woman is dependent.)

Another issue which makes matters worse is that the subordinate role of nurses is reinforced when they begin to work with the nonpracticing academic disciplines, the so-called "basic disciplines," since these disciplines have a tendency to be snobbish and to regard the practicing professions as "merely" applied fields too deviant from academic standards to be respectable. This makes intelligent collaboration with nurse-researchers difficult. Nurses tend to accept this evaluation. Typically they do not see themselves as a potentially rich source of information, of value to nursing as well as to other sciences. After all, nurses have more experience with people in sickness than any other professional group and have their observational skills highly developed.

An attitude essential to research is to question, yet much of the experience of the nurse practitioner works against development of a research attitude. Nurses are pressed to act before they have tested and validated practice. In face of the urgent and constant demand for action nurse educators have had to recommend nursing practices on the basis of untested assumptions and our theories tend to be rationalizations for existing practices which become entrenched. Pressure for the nurse to act—not to stop and think—is very real. It comes to the would-be nurse scientist from her colleagues in the hospitals, both nurses and doctors as well as from herself, as she sees the difficult situations which exist in hospitals and which immediately endanger patients' comfort and health. Further, the practitioner is trained to think in absolutes, while in sharp contrast the practitioner-researcher must live in eternal uncertainty about those same absolutes by which the practitioner justifies his actions.

Practitioner training stressing that one must not make a mistake encourages a feeling of personal infallibility and cultivates blindness to one's mistakes. Yet it is by analyzing one's mistakes that one learns how to improve practice. This desire for certitude and the concomitant reluctance to avoid examining one's own practice produces basic barriers to learning the research attitude by practitioners. Be they nurses, doctors, and social workers, they have a difficult time accepting the idea of an hypothesis and an even harder time accepting the experimental tests of the hypothetical principles of practice. This is revealed in medicine, for example, in the too frequent neglect of control groups. Practitioners appear to be shocked at the proposition that research can only disprove hypotheses—and that a fact is never "proven."

The Scientist Must Generalize

Another basic problem we have felt is that nurses are taught to treat patients as individuals. This is good practice, but it means they don't learn to generalize. Therefore, it is strange to them to make the empirical generalizations which are a necessary first step in developing a coherent scientific theory of practice and which research *requires*.[10] Medical knowledge and research consists of generalizations (about bodily function and

malfunction) and similarly nursing knowledge and research must consist of generalizations (about nurse-patient relationships, patient's reactions to illness and treatment, and nurse's reaction to the nursing situation). But however appropriate concentration on the individual case may be for the practitioner, it is impossible for the researcher. If they are to do research, nurses must learn to make this shift in orientation.

Problems in Skill in Research Methods

Lack of appropriate research methodology is a barrier to the kind of research necessary for developing empirical generalizations upon which to base nursing practice theory. By "methodology" we mean here not only specific technology but the basic metascientific underpinnings that established disciplines have accumulated in their traditions. One problem is simply asking the right kinds of questions. Practicing nurses who know what the problems are do not have, for the reasons just pointed out, the orientation and training necessary to study these problems. To begin with, one must ask researchable questions. It is not sufficient to have a "problem," although that is the beginning. The problem must be stated in a way which permits its scientific investigation. Nurses do not ordinarily learn to ask researchable questions. Thus even when they are sympathetic to research, they tend to set unattainable research objectives. Examples of such questions are: How can nursing be made more effective? Why does the nursing staff have such low morale? What can we do about the nursing shortage? What is the nurse's role? No amount of research can answer such questions as they stand! Before research can begin, we must propose specific answers to these questions. Their research can test these "hypotheses." Our experience suggests that one reason collaborative research with social scientists often answers questions that are mostly of interest to the social scientist is because the nurse has not clarified the problem enough for herself before-hand. And the social scientist does not have the background, nor the interest, to clarify the nursing problem.

In developing clinical nursing research, nurses will often be faced with a choice between precision and

---

[10] cf. Greenwood 1961, pp. 79–80.

acceptability of their findings according to standards developed for other fields and relevance to nursing practice. If nursing theory is to develop, nurses must have the courage to use a rough tool which is more relevant than a widely accepted tool which is not well suited to nursing research. This does not call for lowering standards of rigor, but rather for raising standards of relevance. At the same time, nurses must develop research methods where they do not exist.

Conclusion

We feel that the development of nursing knowledge will be sound and quick once the empirical approach to building knowledge is recognized and used in nursing research. The empirical approach we hold is not only respectable, it is essential.

References

Armstrong, D., et al. (1957). Pain-producing substances in human inflammatory exudates and plasma. *Journal of Physiology, 135,* 350–370.

Bisno, H. (1960). *The use of social science content in social work education.* Working paper for UNESCO meeting, July 1960.

Bochnak, M.A. (1961). *The effect of an automatic and deliberative process of nursing activity on the relief of patients' pain; a clinical experiment.* Unpublished master's report, Yale University School of Nursing, New Haven, CT.

Bochnak, M.A., et al. (1962). Comparison of two types of nursing activity on the relief of pain. In *Innovations in nurse-patient relationships: Automatic or reasoned nurse actions* (Clinical Papers No. 6.). New York: American Nurses' Association.

Caudill, W., et al. (1952). Social structure and interaction processes on a psychiatric ward. *Journal of Orthopsychiatry, 22,* 314–334.

Crowley, D.M. (1962). *Pain and its alleviation.* Los Angeles: University of California School of Nursing.

Gammon, G., & Starr, I. (1941). Studies on the relief of pain by counter-irritation. *Journal of Clinical Investigation, 20,* 13–20.

Greenwood, E. (1961). The practice of science and the science of practice. In W.G. Bennis, K.D. Benne, & R. Chin (Eds.). *The planning of change.* New York: Holt.

Gouldner, A.W. (1956). Explorations in applied social science. *Soc. Problems, 3,* 169–181.

Hardy, J.D., et al. (1952). Pricking pain threshold in different body areas. *Proceedings for the Society in Experimental Biological Medicine, 80,* 425–427.

Henderson, V.A. (1956). Research in nursing practice—when? *Nursing Research, 4,* 99.

Henderson, V.A. (1957), An overview of nursing research. *Nursing Research, 6,* 61–71.

McManus, R.L. (1961a) Nursing research—its evolution. *American Journal of Nursing, 61,* 76–79.

McManus, R.L. (1961b). Today and tomorrow in nursing research. *America Journal of Nursing, 61,* 68–71.

Nordmark, M.T., & Rohweder, A.W. (1959). *Science principles applied to nursing.* Philadelphia: J.B. Lippincott.

Schlotfeldt, R.M. (1960). Reflections on nursing research. *American Journal of Nursing, 60,* 492–494.

Sheldon, E. (1963). The use of behavioral sciences in nursing: An opinion. *Nursing Research, 12,* 150.

Simmons, L.W., & Henderson, V.A. (1964). *Research in nursing.* New York: Appleton-Century-Crofts.

Tinterow, M.M. (1960). The use of hypnoanalgesia in the relief of intractable pain. *American Surgeon, 26,* 30–34.

Will, G.T. (1952). A sociopsychiatric nursing approach to intervention in a problem of mutual withdrawal on a mental hospital ward. *Psychiatry, 15,* 193–217.

Zoborowski, M. (1952). Cultural components on response to pain. *Journal of Sociologic Issues, 8*(4), 16–30.

The Authors Comment

The idea for this paper was conceived by Robert Leonard after we had worked together and separately with other School of Nursing faculty. It was a position paper that grew out of our experiences in teaching nurse students who were candidates for a Master's degree in Nursing Science and out of our attempts to gain support for research that faculty wanted to undertake. At this time, a researcher was expected to state a hypothesis and design the study to demonstrate correlation between variables. We saw the need for exploratory, descriptive, and hypothesis-searching studies as precursors, such as the Gwen Tudor Will study done in 1952. Virginia Henderson's exhaustive literature search had identified the paucity of such studies and the need for them.

Donna Dier's work, first as a student and later as a colleague, arose during the process of conceptualization. The Yale philosophers Patricia James and James Dickoff, also School of Nursing faculty members, elaborated their work on this base. P.J. Wooldridge, Lucy Conant, and Ernestine Widenbach, authors of other articles included in this book, also took part in the development of nursing theory from this base.

The development of nursing theory led to research that described, explored, sought, and tested relationships of patients' needs and eventually tested hypotheses. Unfortunately (in my view), other nurses went on to elaborate concepts of the nursing process that are so complex and overdesigned that while they may serve as academic exercises, they are of little use to the clinician.

FLORENCE S. WALD

This short paper could be seen as simply advising nurses to do their own thinking—or "theorizing," to use a more pompous word. It was written at a time when a lot of money was being spent on projects that were supposed to "integrate basic concepts" into nursing. These concepts were to be borrowed from the supposedly more "basic" disciplines, such as physiology and sociology. We were busy developing a research program testing the effects (on patients) of variations in nurse-patient interactions in specific clinical settings. Whether or not this research fit with existing theories in other disciplines was subordinated. Instead, our criterion of importance was the fit with actual problems faced by nurses in everyday practice. It seemed necessary to point out that this did not mean abandoning theory, but instead promoted building theory by generalizing from specific nursing experiences rather than by applying generalities developed elsewhere.

Of course, this is a two-way street—or can be. In fact, aspects of the theory we were working with were similar to George Herbert Mead's social psychology called "symbolic interactionism." My own current work on a theory of sociosomatics is embedded in symbolic interactionism, but at the same time I would never have moved toward studying the links between society and body without the nursing research experience represented by this article.

—ROBERT C. LEONARD

Chapter 4

Toward a Clearer Understanding of the Concept of Nursing Theory

Lorraine Olszewski Walker

This article is written in a spirit of friendly criticism by one who has at some time held most of the views below. The criticisms offered are given in the hope that they will encourage more vigorous and frequent dialogue among nursing theorists.

Within nursing the terms "nursing theory," "nursing science," "nursing practice theory," and "nursing knowledge" appear to be used as syntactically and semantically equivalent. There appears to be no critical attempt to determine the exact relations among these terms.[1] However, even a superficial analysis would seem to indicate a hierarchical set of relations among these terms where "nursing knowledge" refers to the most general domain followed by "nursing theory" which in turn would seem to catch up both "nursing science" and "nursing practice theory." These relations might be illustrated as follows:

1. "nursing knowledge"
1.1. "nursing theory"
1.1.1. "nursing science"
1.1.2. "nursing practice theory"

However helpful this initial ordering of terms on the basis of their generality may be, it does not mark out the meaning of the terms in question. To accomplish this further task, the analysis done by Maccia (1968a, 1968b) with respect to educational theory would appear to be relevant. Building on and modifying the notion of praxiology explicated by Kotarbinski (1964) as the general theory of efficient action, Maccia has provided an analysis of the modes of discourse pertinent to a study of education. She asks the question, What is education? which is the organizing problem in a study of education, but which is also an ambiguous question. She then interprets this central question as a generic question in the study of education which may be answered by three different forms of inquiry: 1)

---

[1] This claim is based on a content analysis reported by L. Walker (1971) in *Nursing as a discipline.* Unpublished doctoral dissertation, Indiana University, Bloomington.

About the Author

LORRAINE OLSZEWSKI WALKER is currently the Luci B. Johnson Centennial Professor of Nursing at the University of Texas at Austin. Dr. Walker has taught at the University of Texas since 1971. A midwesterner for many years, Dr. Walker received her nursing diploma from Holy Cross Central School of Nursing and B.S.N. from the University of Dayton in Dayton, Ohio. She is also a graduate of Indiana University, Bloomington, Indiana, earning a M.S. in Nursing Education in 1965 and an Ed.D. degree in 1971.

Dr. Walker has worked as a staff nurse and has held faculty appointments at Purdue University and the University of Hawaii. A Fellow in the American Academy of Nursing, she has written many scholarly articles and cowrote (with Kay C. Avant) a book, *Strategies for Theory Construction in Nursing* (New York: Appleton-Century-Crofts, 1983).

Dr. Walker has found that research and theory development in nursing have provided her with great professional satisfaction. Her current focus is on theory and research in parent-infant nursing.

What occurs in the educational process, that is, scientific inquiry; 2) What is effective education, that is, praxiological inquiry; and 3) What is worthwhile education, that is, philosophic inquiry. These three modes of inquiry constitute in toto the basis for an answer to the organizing question, What is education?

The scientific mode of inquiry provides a description and explanation of what occurs in a given state-of-affairs, for example, the process of education. The praxiological mode provides a description and explanation of what constitutes effective practices in a given practical endeavor, for example, the lore of medical practice, but is not merely a summation of practices. Perry (1971) has further characterized praxiological knowledge as "knowledge of fixed, general relations between means and ends, as well as between practices and other practices (where a practice is a single related set of means and ends), independent of whether these practices are actual, and independent of whether they are worthwhile." In the philosophic mode a description and explanation is provided of what constitutes worthy means and ends for a given endeavor.

Using the term "nursology" to mark off the study of nursing from the process of nursing, one may similarly differentiate the discourse of nursology by applying Maccia's (1968a, 1968b) categories of analysis. Using the generic question for the field of nursology, What is nursing? this may be analyzed into three subquestions:

What is occurring in nursing? (scientific mode)
What is effective nursing? (praxiological mode)
What is worthwhile nursing? (philosophic mode)

Taking the descriptive definition of "nursing" formulated by Walker (1971) where "nursing = Df one or more persons caring for the physical and mental well-being of one or more persons with an actual or potential health problem within a setting" (chap. 2), one may further demarcate nursing in terms of four subsets: 1) persons providing care, 2) persons with health problems receiving care, 3) the environment in which care is given, and 4) an end-state, well-being. The leading question in a science of nursing, that is, What is occurring in nursing? may be seen then as constituting four subquestions dealing with the characterization of and relations among those providing care, those receiving care, the environment of care, and the end-state. Similarly, these four subsets of variables may be used to deal with the characterization of effective nursing and of worthwhile states of nursing. It is important to note that though, for instance, science of nursing may facilitate the development of praxiology of nursing, each of these three modes of discourse represents essentially nonintegrated or independent theories of nursing.

Nursing Theory: A Labyrinth of Attributes

Theory in a practice (or practical) discipline has been called many things in the nursing literature. To some it is "applied" and to others, "basic," by some it is characterized as "unique" while by others it is seen as "derived and synthesized from other disciplines." It is called "prescriptive," "normative," "situation-producing," and "scientific." Some see it as "theoretical," and still others as a body of practical directives. Certainly this myriad of attributes seems to indicate that the concept of a theory of nursing is a troublesome one. Since the intention here is not to provide a historical review of all that has been said to date about the concept of a theory of nursing, but rather to indicate some of the parameters of an adequate characterization of theory of nursing, selective commentary will be made with regard to the following: 1) How useful is the term "practice theory?" 2) May the science of nursing be most adequately characterized as basic or applied in nature? 3) How does the philosophy of nursing as characterized above differ from other uses in the nursing literature? How useful is "holism" in nursing theory?

Practice Theory

Practice theory is typically seen in the nursing literature as having the function to "prescribe the activities of the practitioner" (Conant, 1967b). What appears to be meant by this use of the term "practice theory" is sets of principles or directives for practice. This seems to be the sense intended by Dickoff and James (1968) and Greenwood (1961). In a second sense, "practice theory" might also be used as a synonym for "praxiology" as Maccia has used this term to connote the knowledge of practices. This, in fact, appears to be the sense intended by Wald and Leonard (1964) who characterize the task of those who develop practice theory as the systematic study of "ways to achieve change," and that used by Wooldridge, Skipper, and Leonard (1968). The first use of "practice theory" described above seems to represent an odd use of the term "theory" for "theory" is typically employed in the context of systematic description and explanation. Terms such as "policy," "procedure," or "principle" are typically used in referring to an action-oriented endeavor. Thus, the use of "practice theory" (or "theory of practice") in referring to principles of action, or other forms

of directives for practice probably serves to cloud what is being meant in such a case. (Perhaps the term "theory" entered the context of practice because of a relatively unrefined and polar conception of the relation between theory and practice. Hence what was not the doing was the theory.) Whatever is impetus for the notion of practice theory as directives, the use seems inappropriate and, in fact, serves to confuse the distinction between praxiology and directives for it as applied to both. As alternate terms, "principles of practice," "directives," or "practices" may be more appropriate.

In conclusion, in one sense "practice theory" may be taken as a synonym for "praxiology." In the second sense, as principles of practice, it is a misnomer and does not comprise part of a theory of nursing. In view of this last conclusion, what is then to be made of principles of practice? In this writer's view, principles of practice would seem to constitute part of the practical aspect of nursing knowledge where the latter is used loosely to refer to the practical, as well as theoretical, language of a given domain. More will be said of the practical aspect of nursing later.

Nursing Science: Basic or Applied?

The contention over whether a science of nursing represents a basic or an applied science is plagued by confusion in that the notion of an applied science appears itself to be an ambiguous one (Crowley, 1968; Folta, 1968). The problem with "applied science" seems to be that what is being applied and how it is being applied are unclear: 1) Are the theories and concepts of basic sciences, for example, psychology and physiology, merely being selectively taken and organized to form a collection of knowledges useful in bringing nurses to some scientific understanding of nursing; or 2) Are the concepts and methods of basic sciences being used in the actual inquiry into the nursing process? or 3) Is some body of scientific knowledge (either from a parent science or a distinctive nursing science) being utilized in the solution of actual problems of practice? The first two of these three alternatives seem to represent the most interesting possibilities as to the meaning of the claim that nursing is an applied science. The third alternative is of interest merely to note that this is probably not an important meaning of the notion of nursing as an applied science for every science would be applied, in some degree, in this sense. Furthermore, this third meaning may merely represent an unclear expression of the idea of a praxiology of nursing.

As indicated, in the first sense of an applied science, nursing knowledge is seen as a conglomeration of knowledge taken from the basic sciences, and in the second, as an intentional focusing of the basic sciences on certain endeavors in nursing to which the basic sciences have some pertinence. Notice that in the first of these notions the nursing process itself is not treated as an unknown to be described and explained; it seems to be assumed that it is understandable or deducible from the sciences as they stand. However, such a set of deductions which describes and explains nursing process has not been made. In the second view, an aspect of nursing may or may not be the focus of the study. For example, a sociologist might check out some general hypothesis about authoritarian behavior in the context of the nurse-patient-doctor triad, or he might attempt to characterize the nurse-patient relationship as a goal-directed system. This last example seems to hit the heart of the controversy: although nursing process is being characterized, it is being done in terms of a sociological concept and is being tested by sociological methods. Some would claim this to be basic nursing science, others that it is applied because the methods and concepts from a basic and autonomous discipline are being applied to the study of nursing. Thus, at least part of the controversy is reduced to the question of whether there is anything distinctive or unique about this kind of study of nursing. To restate the controversy, how may the study of nursing be considered a basic science if it has no distinctive methods or concepts to be employed and, therefore, merely "borrows" portions of the basic sciences.

With regard to the claim that using borrowed concepts and methods in characterizing nursing process negates the possibility of an autonomous science of nursing, and hence the status of basic science, probably the requirement being set here is too stringent. First it

overlooks that borrowed terms must be worked into a new conceptual set, and hence become new concepts although the terms remain the same. In addition, methods may also need to be altered when they are introduced into a new context. Therefore, "borrowing" may not be the simple affair that some conceive it to be. Perhaps in nursing the sin of being borrowed would be less severely chastised if the use made of what was borrowed were more sophisticated. To date, borrowed terms, for example, "stress" and "equilibrium," have not been placed into the sophisticated formalizations of more awe-inducing disciplines (Johnson, 1959). Hence, the criticism of borrowed concepts and methods may be due to a shortcoming of their use.

Thus far in the study of nursing process the claim that nursing cannot be an autonomous science, and hence not a basic science, because of the use it must make of other disciplines seems at least temporarily dispelled. It would appear that the scientific study of nursing need not be conceived as an applied science in either of the two important senses examined here for two reasons: 1) at this point, nursing seems to be a genuine unknown which will not be satisfactorily explained by taking portions of the basic sciences as they stand, and 2) introduction of terms and methods from the basic disciplines into the study of nursing requires that these terms and methods must fit into the task of describing and explaining nursing.

Philosophy of Nursing

It is important to note the common assumption that the ultimate values in the health professions are generally clearly understood and undebatable—the goal is the preservation of life and the professions may proceed uncritically to accomplish this goal dealing only with questions of means. This assumption is ill-grounded for two reasons. First, the meaning of the goal of the health professions may become quite vague and ambiguous when it is applied to classes of events. Several conflicting interpretations may arise; for example, preserving life may be interpreted either as preserving cellular life only or as preserving a level of life characterized by consciousness and goal setting. Thus, the clarification of the ultimate goal may become a subject of inquiry within the health professions. Second, even if the meaning of the goal is sufficiently clear to permit choices between alternate courses of action, for example, the choice of preservation of cellular life, it still remains reasonable to ask if the goal taken as desired is really desirable. This question belongs squarely within the range of questions dealing with the philosophy of nursing as this has been characterized here—the goal of the health professions is not simply given, but is taken, and may be subjected to philosophic inquiry. Consequently, it seems that the health professions, and specifically nursing, engage not only in means questions, that is praxiology, but also in questions about ends or goals. Results of the study of such questions ultimately will comprise the content of the philosophic study of nursing which at present is largely undeveloped.

Another assumption that may have retarded the development of a philosophy of nursing is the belief that a philosophic theory of nursing is unnecessary because the nursing profession already has a code of ethics to deal with the matter of the right conduct of nurses. This view, while correctly noting the existence of a nursing code of ethics, overlooks what will be called here the problem of the justification of the code. This problem brings to light the fact that a code of ethics represents conclusions from some line of reasoning which may not necessarily be included with the formal statement of conclusions.[2] Only with the conclusions reached are accompanied by pertinent empirical knowledge of the worthwhileness of the ideas for nursing, may the statements embodying the ideas be said to be justified. A code of ethics then becomes a product of a more fundamental set of statements, that is, a philosophy of nursing.

At this point, it may be noted that there are many kinds of things in the nursing literature called a "phi-

losophy of nursing," none of which typically approximates the characterizations set forth here. Several of these uses will be sorted out. First, "philosophy of nursing" may be used to refer to personal decisions about the aim and/or desirable methods of nursing. This seems to be the sense in which it is used by Johnson (1966) and Kreuter (1957). "Philosophy of nursing" is also used to refer to general policies, aims, and value commitments of particular nursing education and service institutions. This seems to be the use made by Sand (1955) and Elliott (1961). A fourth sense of "philosophy of nursing" seems to refer to a personal world view frequently including a view of human nature and the place of nursing, a sort of "nursing metaphysics." Rogers (1961) uses it in this way, although she does not call her view a philosophy of nursing. A fifth kind of "philosophy of nursing" is seen in statements of one's personal beliefs and attitudes toward one's profession. This is the sense in which it has been employed by Potter (1961), Olszewski (1965), and Wiedenbach (1964).

There remains one more sense of "philosophy of nursing"—one that has not been adequately dealt with —the philosophic approach which through analysis formulates criteria for adequate theorizing about nursing process, that is, a meta-theoretical or meta-nursological approach. This paper constitutes an endeavor in this last sense.

Holism and the Nature of Nursing Theory

One of the most prominent beliefs with regard to a theory of nursing is that the only truly valid theory of nursing is one which catches up the "whole man." Any theory which treats man, the patient, as a set of elements or variables is a falsification of the phenomenon, man, who exists as a complex, but unitary event. Nurses interact with patients as whole persons, so adequate theory for nursing must also catch up this wholeness. Thus, the perspectives of physiology, psychology, or sociology taken by themselves are always incomplete and falsifying of the event, man, in his totality. Variations of this view have been expressed by Ellis (1968) and Rogers (1963) among others. There are several

---

[2] The moral force of a code of ethics is not merely derived from the fact that a majority of the members of a given professional association voted in its favor unless a very positivistic notion toward moral knowledge is taken.

things correct about this view, as well as several things which seem clearly troublesome.

Where this view is really just a way of making nursing practitioners more sensitive to the multiple relationships among the nursing environment, the illness, the patient's motivation to recovery, the patient's family, et cetera, then the notion of "holism" functions as a slogan to encourage nurses to be sensitive to a wide range of cues related to a patient's well-being. As such, holism is innocuous.

As a methodological caveat to be on the watch constantly for overlooked factors and relations which affect the complex event of illness and health in humans, holism is a prudential reminder, and serves to encourage openness to previously unnoticed relations between variables in the health-illness context. Taken in this manner, holism serves to enhance the quality of both theorizing and practicing in nursing.

Holism may also be taken to mean that theory about man in the health-illness context is adequate only when all aspects of man are caught up in the theory. In this regard Rogers (1963) seems to have taken the position that since man occurs as a complex unitary phenomenon, characterizations of this phenomenon must be of comparable complexity and unity. Therefore, adequate theoretical understanding of man may only be portrayed, it seems, by a complete integration of all the sciences relevant to the study of man. Other than asking for more than science may now give, Rogers seems to be committing a fundamental mistake with regard to the nature of theory. Adequate theory to Rogers seems to be represented by a sort of photographic-like reproduction of reality. Thus, theory must mirror every aspect of man to catch up his full nature. The error committed seems to be in confusing the two kinds of understanding. While scientific theories provide understanding in the sense of providing conceptualizations under which particular instances may be brought for study, they do not provide the sort of understanding one gets from having experienced a particular event. This is roughly to distinguish the description of soup from the taste of soup (Rudner, 1967). In calling for a fully integrated and comprehensive theory of man and his environment, Rogers seems to have erred in grasp-

ing the kind of understanding science provides. She seems to have asked a science of nursing to convey the taste of human nature.

Perhaps part of the impetus behind the call for the integration of the sciences related to man that has occurred in the nursing literature associated with holism comes from a misunderstanding of what that integration would require. In one sense, at least, integration of the sciences would require that the terms and laws of distinct theories be reduced to terms and laws of other theories, for example, the reduction of physiology to chemistry. It is difficult, however, to determine exactly to which sense of "integration" this notion of holism refers. A trivial sense of integration might be achieved by simply grouping together all laws from the natural sciences which relate to man. This would represent a compilation, though, and not an integration of the laws, for the latter would require that logical links be made between these laws. Such links would presumably be difficult to establish, though, because such statements may not be clearly understood when removed from the conceptual structure in which they were developed (Schwab, 1964).

The call for holism, then, is not clear in its meaning, and is certainly troublesome in the last sense discussed. Although nothing conclusive will be said of holism here, it seems prudent to treat the notion as one whose meaning is vague and ambiguous.

Practical Knowledge of Nursing

Since the central purpose of this paper is to develop greater clarity about the notion of a theory of nursing, the practical aspect of nursing knowledge is included here to sort out this aspect of nursing knowledge from the theoretical, but not to explicate fully the nature of the practical. Whereas theoretical knowledge of nursing provides knowledge about the nursing process, practical knowledge of nursing roughly forms the rules for carrying out that process. Practical knowledge of nursing would seem to take two principal forms: principles and procedures. Taken together principles and procedures would seem to be analogous to what Price has called "rules for teaching activities" (Price, 1963, p.

24). "Principles" as used here signify imperatives, in the most general sense, and in the more particular sense, rules for the effective and moral doing of nursing. "Procedures," while also signifying a form of rule for the doing of nursing, designate the concrete sequence of operations necessary to bring about a particular state-of-affairs, for example, procedures for "cracking" oxygen tanks, procedures for opening sterile packs, and procedures for reducing anxiety in children during hospital admission. Principles, in turn, are more general than procedures and do not necessarily imply one specific set of operations. Hence, several alternate procedures might be explained by appeal to a common principle.[3]

Principles of nursing may be further differentiated according to the function they play within the conduct of nursing. Four general classes of nursing principles are outlined below. These categories while not completely mutually exclusive, are not reducible to one another.

1. Prudential rules—those related to the cautious and safe practice of nursing; that is, "Always give priority to the observation and care of critical patients." "Do not forewarn young children of minor painful procedures until they are imminent." "Never turn your back on an infant lying on an unenclosed surface."
2. Therapeutic rules—those related to the general form of treatment for certain health problems; that is, "Administer oxygen to patients who become cyanotic until they may be evaluated by a physician." "Massage the postpartal uterine fundus if it becomes flaccid."
3. Ideological rules—those related to the manner of desirable nursing practice; that is, "Treat the sick with tender loving care." "Respect the patient's privacy." "Do not divulge privileged communications."
4. "Logistics" or mechanical or procedural rules—those related to the manner of sequencing events, that is, "In-

crease the pressure within a closed container before withdrawing fluid from it." "Establish rapport with a patient before asking personal questions." "Take baseline data before administering medications and treatments to patients."

On inspection it appears that there is a particularly close relation between logistics rules and fully developed statements of a procedure. However, these two notions appear to be conceptually independent for while a logistics rule provides a guide to the sequencing of operations, it does not itself indicate the specific operations which are to be performed.

Some might raise the question, Do these principles and/or procedures constitute the "theory" of nursing pertinent to practice in a manner analogous to the way that scientific, praxiological, and philosophic theory constitute the theory pertinent to description and explanation? While this analogy may be helpful, it is inherently problematic, for it treats the notion of theory too loosely. Where "theory" is used in a highly refined sense as in science, the answer to the question would be "no" for two reasons. A theory may be differentiated from other forms of knowledge by, among other things: 1) the nature of the terms used, and 2) the character of its internal relations. The terms within a theory are "systematically related," that is, logically related, such that deductions from certain fundamental statements to other derived statements become possible (Rudner, 1967). The nature of the terms within a theory are general, and thus form an organizational scheme for describing and explaining certain recurrent existential states-of-affairs. However, the practical knowledge of nursing fails to meet these conditions of logical organization and generality.

With regard to the first condition, logical organization, the practical knowledge of nursing, that is the principles and procedures, do not manifest the logical relations which tie together statements within a theory. This would appear to be true for several reasons. First, the feasibility of nursing procedures is bound to particular time-place contexts, that is, procedures presume certain available technologies, certain cultural contexts, and certain immediate physical facilities. Such contingencies could not be caught up in the more abstract

---

[3] It seems important to note here that principles as rules for nursing are not to be confused with another frequent use of this term in nursing literature in which principles are equated with scientific laws and theories and statistical empirical generalizations. This latter use encompasses indicative statements from the sciences and may also frequently be called "facts" in the nursing literature; however, this use refers to propositions and is in contrast to the general imperative nature of a practical body of knowledge being characterized here. This distinction is not meant to disclaim the many links between such general propositional knowledge and the general principles of nursing, but is made to avoid collapsing the two senses into one.

principles from which would be deduced the more concrete practices; this is in effect to say that principles do not imply procedures. Second, even among only the principles themselves, the hope of reducing these to a deductive system based on some fundamental principle, such as "Always be prepared," seems unlikely, for to have a guiding function in practice, the content of principles must at least specify general conditions for their applicability and suggest a general class of actions. Both of these, however, would not seem to be implicit in a very abstract fundamental principle, such as "Always be prepared."

With regard to the condition of generality, practical knowledge of nursing fails to meet this condition for some of the same reasons as above that is, while procedures and principles may be stated in general form, procedures are always context bound, and the principles from which these spring find their full meaning only as they are related to a myriad of conditions of practice; implicit in the meaning of a principle is an infinite number of qualifications which are embedded in its use in action. These aspects of a principle are not learned from its general form, but are learned by relating the principle to events. Thus, while principles may be stated in a general form this generality is not like, it seems the generality of universal propositions such as scientific laws.

If, however, one chooses to speak very loosely of "theory" as merely the language of a given field of endeavor, then in this sense principles and procedures may be seen as the "theory" of the practice. Such loose use of the term "theory" would seem to have little to commend it, however, for it blurs the differences between the scientific, praxiological, and philosophic study of nursing and the principles and procedures for carrying out the nursing process.

The Relationship Between Theory and Practice

One more set of concerns related to the notion of a theory of nursing remains to be considered: the relationship between theory and practice. Many of the mis-conceptions about this problem area seem to stem from a failure to observe some of the distinctions mentioned in the last section. First among these is the notion that verification in practice of the efficacy of a principle or procedure is a direct verification of aspects of the theory on which the principle or procedure is based, that is, that practice tests theory. Thus, if a particular procedure or principle does not bring about the expected results in practice, then this is seen as a disconfirmation of the theoretical concerns on which the former is based. However, Merton and Lerner (1961) have argued that the predictions generated from scientific theories are based on the assumption that all things being equal, if X, then Y. However, in the throes of practice, as opposed to the tightly controlled conditions of research testing, the assumption that all other factors are held constant and equal is very difficult to defend. Hence, the failure to achieve a given change based on a given set of theoretical statements does not in itself warrant the rejection of the theory, but rather the questioning of the assumptions about the technology and conditions under which the change was attempted. In other words, the conditions for rejection of a theory are much more stringent than those which everyday practice can provide. This certainly should not be taken to mean that qualified researchers may not adequately test theory through clinical research, but rather that practitioners in the midst of practice are more than likely not in a position to provide the conditions necessary for adequately testing a theory.

A second and related notion which seems misguided is that of seeing the observation of the clinical practice of nursing as a well-spring for theory development (Conant, 1967a, 1967b; Ellis, 1969; Dickoff et al., 1968a, 1968b; Dickoff & James, 1968). This notion seems to be based on either of two errors: the collapsing of praxiology with principles and procedures of nursing into some vague notion of "theory" which simultaneously explains, as well as directs practice, and on a notion of theory development as a Baconian kind of induction in which categories arise from data and observation. The epistemological inadequacy of this latter notion has already been dealt with by others (Maccia, 1964). The difficulties with the former, that is, the collapsing of praxiology with principles and procedures, has largely gone unrecognized and perhaps results from a failure to distinguish between nursology (theoretical knowledge) and the practical knowledge of nursing that guides the practice of nursing. Consider the confusion about theory in this passage from Dickoff and James (1968), who fail to make the distinction between the two aspects of nursing knowledge:

> The major contention here is that all theory exists finally for the sake of practice (since in a sense every lower level of theory exists for the next higher level and the highest level exists for practice) and that nursing theory must be theory at the highest level since the nursing aim is practice or else nursing is no longer a profession as distinct from some mere academic discipline (Dickoff & James, 1968, p. 199).

In failing to sort out the theoretical aspect of nursing from the practical as two distinct and legitimate endeavors, the former is made to serve the more narrow and immediate purposes of the latter.

A confusion closely related to the notion that theory develops in practice is the failure to sort out the development of theory from the development of nursing practices. Ellis (1969), for instance, has characterized practitioners as theorists in selecting and restructuring theories from the basic sciences relevant to nursing care, in qualifying the conditions under which such general statements apply, and also in the testing out of theories in actual practice. From this Ellis seems to equate the critical and deliberate use of theory with the development of theory, that is, being a theorist. However, these two sets of activities are clearly distinct since they are governed by different sets of norms. The norms or canons that govern development of a good theory—explanatory power, simplicity, consistency—are not the same norms that govern the application or use of theory—feasibility, cost, risk. It would seem apparent that there are two related, but distinct activities that cast the doer in two distinct roles. What Ellis has seen as theoretical activities on the part of practitioners seems more accurately to consist in the development of adequate nursing practices, not the development of ade-

quate nursing theory. Ellis had quite accurately seen that developing adequate nursing practices, for example, setting out the conditions under which patients should be encouraged to verbalize, is not a mere deduction from theory. Application of a generalization to practice requires: 1) the selection of a norm (not in the statistical sense) or end to be achieved, 2) the discrimination of the conditions of practice under which a given theoretical generalization is instrumental in achieving that end, and 3) the adoption of a technology that has been worked out, or may be worked out, by means of which the end may be realized. Particularly two and three are very significant aspects of the application of theory to practice, but they do not themselves comprise theory development. It may be worthwhile to note here that although the practitioner as the developer of nursing practices may have some implicit methods which he follows in developing practices, this is not the same as claiming that he operates on an implicit nursing theory. If such methods as are used by practitioners as developers of practices could be made explicit, this would probably constitute a methodology of nursing practice development, and not a theory of nursing. Such a methodology would be a guide to nursing practice development, but would not consist in an explanation of nursing process.

One final difficulty arising from the relation between theory and practice is that of the logical relation theory to principles and procedures, or nursing practices. While Abdellah and Levine (1965) claim that nursing practices are derived from the basic sciences, the nature of this derivation remains problematic. The relation of theoretical knowledge to practices has been carefully examined in the educational literature particularly with regard to the bearings of philosophy on practices. Burns has argued that the relation between philosophy and educational practices cannot be precisely explained. "What we do know is that the connection between philosophy and educational practice cannot be explained or formalized in terms of strictly logical implication, nor in terms of material implication" (Burns, 1962, p. 62). Similarly, Newsome noted that "theory has no direct reference and no formal implication for practice" (Newsome, 1964, p. 37). Guttchen also concluded that "the question of how philosophy guides practice is still open" (Guttchen 1966, p. 134). Clearly, the force of these conclusions seems equally germane to the problem of the relation of theory to practice in nursing. At this point, the most that may be said of this problem area is that its resolution represents an unknown. Hence, claims that certain nursing practices are logically derived from particular theoretical bodies of knowledge would seem to be either false or based on a tacit methodology which has yet to be explicated.

Summary

In an attempt to develop greater clarity about the notion of the concept, nursing theory, this paper discusses current concepts as reflected in the literature. Following an explanation of the author's proposal of a tripartite approach to the development of nursing theory, troublesome and conflicting notions about theory in nursing are examined and distinctions between practical and theoretical knowledge and between theory and practice are discussed.

References

Abdellah, F.G., & Levine, E. (1965). Better patient care through nursing research. *International Journal of Nursing Studies, 2,* 1–12.

Burns, H.W. (1962). Logic of the educational implication. *Educational Theory, 12,* 63.

Conant, L.H. (1967a). Search for resolution of existing problems in nursing. *Nursing Research, 16,* 114–117.

Conant, L.H. (1967b). Closing the practice-theory gap. *Nursing Outlook, 15,* 37–39.

Crowley, D.M. (1968). Perspectives of pure science. *Nursing Research, 17,* 497–498.

Dickoff, J. et al. (1968a). Theory in a practice discipline: 1. Practice-oriented theory. *Nursing Research, 17,* 415–435.

Dickoff, J. et al. (1968b). Theory in a practice discipline: 2. Practice-oriented research. *Nursing Research, 17,* 545–554.

Dickoff, J., & James, P. (1968). A theory of theories: A position paper. *Nursing Research, 17,* 197–203.

Elliot, F.E. (1961). Philosophy and curriculum. *Canadian Nurse, 57,* 35.

Ellis, R. (1968). Characteristics of significant theories. *Nursing Research, 17,* 217–222.

Ellis, R. (1969). Practitioner as theorist. *American Journal of Nursing, 69,* 1434–1438.

Folta, J.R. (1968). Perspectives of an applied scientist. *Nursing Research, 17,* 502–505.

Greenwood, E. (1961). Practice of science and the science of practice. In W.G. Bennis et al. (Eds.). *The planning of change.* New York: Holt, Rinehart and Winston.

Guttchen, R.S. (1966). Quest for necessity. *Educational Theory, 16,* 134.

Johnson, D.E. (1959). Nature of a science of nursing. *Nursing Outlook, 7,* 291–294.

Johnson, D.E. (1966). A philosophy of nursing. In B. Bullough & V. Bullough (Eds.). *Issues in nursing* (pp. 145–151). New York: Springer.

Kotarbinski, T. (1964). *Praxiology: An introduction to the sciences of efficient action* (Olgierd Wojasiewicz, Trans.). New York: Pergamon Press.

Kreuter, F.R. (1957). What is good nursing care? *Nursing Outlook, 5,* 302–304.

Maccia, E.S. (1964). Retroduction; a way of theorizing through models. In *Communicaciones libres.* Memorias del XIII Congreso Internacional de Filosofia (pp. 545–562). Mexico, D.F.: Universidad Nacional Autonoma de Mexico.

Maccia, E.S. (1968a). Development of theory in the curriculum field. *Samplings, 1,* 5–6.

Maccia, E.S. (1968b). *Methodology of educational inquiry.* Unpublished manuscript. Indiana University, Bloomington, IN.

Merton, R.F., & Lerner, D. (1961). Social scientists and research policy. In W.G. Bennis et al. (Eds.). *The planning of change.* New York: Holt, Rinehart and Winston.

Newsome, G.L. (1964). In what sense is theory a guide to practice in education? *Educational Theory, 14,* 37.

Olszewski, L. (1965). Philosophy of nursing care. *Nursing Forum, 4*(4), 32–35.

Perry, J.F. (1971). Praxiology of education. In *Philosophy of Education; 1971. Proceedings of the Twenty-Seventh Annual Meeting of the Philosophy of Education Society.*

Potter, T. (1961). Philosophy of nursing. *Canadian Nurse, 57,* 741.

Price, K. (1963). Discipline in teaching: In its study and in its theory. In J. Walton & J.L. Kuethe (Eds.). *Discipline of education.* Madison, WI: University of Wisconsin Press.

Rogers, M.E. (1961). *Educational revolution in nursing.* New York: Macmillan.

Rogers, M.E. (1963). Some comments on the theoretical basis of nursing practice. *Nursing Science, 1,* 11–13.

Rudner, R.S. (1967). *Philosophy of social science.* Englewood Cliffs, NJ: Prentice-Hall.

Sand, O. (1955). *Curriculum study of basic nursing education.* New York: Putnam.

Schwab, J.F. (1964). Problems, topics, and issues. In S. Edam

(Ed.). *Education and the structure of knowledge*. Chicago: Rand McNally.

Wald, F.S., & Leonard, R.C. (1964). Towards development of nursing practice theory. *Nursing Research, 13*, 309–313.

Walker, L.O. (1971). *Nursing as a discipline*. Unpublished doctoral dissertation, Indiana University, Bloomington.

Wiedenbach, E. (1964). *Clinical nursing*. New York: Springer.

Wooldridge, P.J., Skipper, J.K., & Leonard, R.C. (1968). *Behavioral science, social practice, and the nursing profession*. Cleveland: Press of Case Western Reserve University.

Bibliography

Abdellah, F.G. (1969). Nature of nursing science. *Nursing Research, 18*, 390–393.

Brown, M.I. (1964). Research in the development of nursing theory. *Nursing Research, 13*, 109–112.

Cleary, F. (1971). Theoretical model: Its potential for adaptation to nursing. *Image, 4*(1), 14–20.

Ellison, M.D., et al. (1965). Uses of behavioral sciences in nursing: Further comment. *Nursing Research, 14*, 71–72.

Gunter, L.M. (1962). Notes on a theoretical framework for nursing research. *Nursing Research, 11*, 219–222.

Harris, I.M. (1971). Theory building in nursing: A review of literature. *Image, 4*(1), 6–10.

Jacobson, M. (1971). Qualitative data as a potential source of theory in nursing. *Image, 4*(1), 10–14.

Johnson, D.E. (1968). Theory in nursing; borrowed and unique. *Nursing Research, 17*, 206–209.

Kaufman, M. (1958). *Identification of theoretical bases for nursing practice*. Los Angeles: School of Education, University of California.

King, I. (1964). Nursing theory in problems and prospect. *Nursing Science, 2*, 394–403.

Kotarbinski, T. (1962). Praxiological sentences and how they are proved. In E. Nagel, et al. (Eds.). *Logic, Methodology and Philosophy of Science: Proceedings of the International Congress of Logic-methodology and Philosophy of Science*, 1960 (pp. 211–223). Stanford, CA.: Stanford University Press.

Mathwig, G. (1971). Nursing science: The theoretical core of nursing knowledge. *Image, 4*(1), 20–23.

McKay, R.P. (1965). *Process of theory development in nursing*. New York: Columbia University Teachers College.

McKay, R.P. (1969). Theories, models, and systems for nursing. *Nursing Research, 18*, 393–400.

Moore, M.A. (1968). Nursing: A scientific discipline? *Nursing Forum, 7*(4), 340–348.

Norris, C.M. (1964). Toward a science of nursing: A method for developing unique content in nursing. *Nursing Forum, 3*, 10–45.

Putnam, P.A. (1965). Conceptual approach to nursing theory. *Nursing Science, 3*, 430–442.

Rogers, M.E. (1963). Building a strong educational foundation. *American Journal of Nursing, 63*, 94–95.

Rogers, M.E. (1970). *Introduction to the theoretical basis of nursing*. Philadelphia: F.A. Davis.

Sarosi, G.M. (1965). On the nature of nursing and the phenomenon of man's health. *Nursing Science, 3*, 298–306.

Sasmor, J.L. (1968). Toward developing theory in nursing. *Nursing Forum, 7*(2), 190–200.

Walker, L.O. (1968). Every patient is unique. *Nursing Outlook, 16*, 39.

Wiedenbach, E. (1970). Nurses' wisdom in nursing theory. *American Journal of Nursing, 70*, 1057–1062

The Author Comments

This article was written as an outgrowth of my doctoral study in philosophy of education at Indiana University. As a nurse pursuing doctoral work in a discipline other than nursing, I was struck by the difficulty of merging what I had learned about the philosophy of science with literature about nursing theory. The goal of this article was to integrate philosophical modes of thought with what I then saw as burning issues pertinent to the substance and structure of nursing theory. Then and now, I am indebted to Rose P. McKay, now deceased, for the illumination provided to me by her dissertation, *Process of Theory Development in Nursing* (1965). She grasped the complexity of nursing theory long before I did.

—LORRAINE O. WALKER

Reaction to Walker's Article

Rosemary Ellis

In discussions of nursing theory, it is common to find confusion arising between those who are speaking of *a* theory of nursing and those who are speaking about the multiple theories or conceptualizations that must implicitly underlie many nursing practices. I believe such confusion is reflected in Walker's comments about my articles on theory. I have never written with reference to *a* theory of nursing. I have addressed myself to the theories underlying nursing practices and to various theories which might hold promise for improving the production of the phenomenon of nursing with patients. My remarks have never been intended to apply to *a* theory of nursing and should not be read as applying to *a* theory of nursing. I must apologize if I have failed to make this clear in the past. It should also be made clear that my goal has not been to develop *a* theory of nursing practice. My goal has been to get nurses to make explicit the foundations from which they operate, to make explicit the orientation and organization of ideas and facts that produce what Walker

terms *principles of nursing*. My goal is to get nurses to question and test these orienting frameworks or foundations. Development of the various theoretical bases underlying nursing principles is the order of theory development with which my articles have been concerned, not the development of *a* theory of nursing.

Walker is correct in indicating that the clinical practice situation does not provide the control for a final test of theory. It does, however, offer opportunity to question *why* a theory is not supported and so offer opportunity for possible recognition of important variables or relationships not hitherto specified in a particular theory. Further, the astute professional practitioner in nursing may be a source for identification and recognition of patterns or relationships in illness or health behavior that may lead to hypotheses amenable to scientific testing.

Verification of the efficacy of a principle of which Walker speaks is but one aspect for study of principles. One ought also to study *why* principles work or fail to

About the Author

ROSEMARY ELLIS was born in Berkeley, California. She lived and worked in the midwest for more than 30 years until her death in 1987. Dr. Ellis received an A.B. degree in Economics and a B.S. in Nursing from the University of California, Berkeley-San Francisco, followed by a M.A. in Nursing Education and a Ph.D. in Human Development from the University of Chicago. At the time of her death she was a Professor of Nursing, a position she held at Case Western Reserve University, since 1964. Before that, she taught at the University of Chicago, worked as a head nurse in California, and served as a Lieutenant in the Army Nurse Corps during World War II.

A member of the American Nurses' Association since 1944, Dr. Ellis also was affiliated with several other professional organizations, including the American Association for the Advancement of Science and the American Association for Nursing History. Dr. Ellis authored or co-authored more than 30 articles, book chapters, and other scholarly works, including four in the *Japanese Journal of Nursing Research*.

When asked about her major satisfactions from nursing, Dr. Ellis replied ". . .learning about life-styles, beliefs, and resources of so many diverse people I have met as patients and feeling I have made a critical difference in the lives of a number of patients and some students." As for the future of nursing, she commented "Imperative questions we must ask are: How should nursing be described as a discipline or field of inquiry? What methods of inquiry can produce the rationalized humanistic knowledge required for nursing practice?".

work. *Why* they work or don't is quite distinct from whether they work or don't. The knowledge to explain *why* may be as important as tests of efficacy. Often the *why* currently is in the form of theory not carefully tested. There is need for theory development at this level as well as at the level of a concept of nursing theory.

The Author Comments

These comments were solicited by Lucille Notter, Editor of *Nursing Research*, as a response to those ideas that Walker criticized in her article. To my knowledge, it was the first time that an editor sought to evoke dialogue between writers *before* publication of a criticizing article.

—ROSEMARY ELLIS

Meta-Theories of Nursing: A Commentary on Dr. Walker's Article

Powhatan J. Wooldridge

One problem with meta-theoretical discussions, and indeed with philosophical and theoretical discussions in general, is that one tends to categorize rigidly that which is actually a matter of degree. This problem was brought to mind by Lorraine Walker's characterization of "the practical knowledge of nursing" as nontheoretic because it "fails to meet these conditions of logical organization and generality."

First, as the author notes, principles of practice *are* generalizations. And they seem to hold much the same relationship to specific procedures as general praxiological theories hold to the relationship between specific means and ends, as general "scientific" theories (in Walker's sense) hold to specific descriptive statements, and as general philosophic theories hold to specific statements of worth. Nor do the "infinite number of qualifications" embedded in the use in action of a general principle appear to differ in kind from the qualifications embedded in the application of a general scientific law to the explanation, prediction, or manipulation of real world phenomena. Second, while the author is correct in arguing that the logical interrelation of principles of nursing practice is not very well articulated, this is also true of existing praxiological, scientific, and philosophical theories of nursing—and of most theories in the social and behavioral sciences as well. And certainly *some* integration exists in the form of hierarchical ordering of principles according to their importance, and in the form of general principles which recommend certain combinations of procedures and contraindicate others. This sort of integration does not appear to be different in kind from the sort of integration achieved by nursing philosophy on the one hand, or by nursing science and praxiology on the other.

It appears to me that Maccia's typology of forms of inquiry (on which Walker's analysis is based) tends to be potentially confusing because it implicitly employs two quite different criteria for classification, and it fails to exhaust the logical possibilities or to clarify the similarities between the types listed.

About the Author

POWHATAN J. WOOLDRIDGE lives in Buffalo, New York, and is an Associate Professor of Nursing at the State University of New York at Buffalo, where he teaches graduate level courses in statistics, research, and theoretical inference and serves as a research consultant to the faculty. Dr. Wooldridge has been on the faculty at SUNY—Buffalo since 1979. He has also held faculty appointments at the University of Rochester, University of Waterloo (Ontario), University of Iowa, Case Western Reserve University, Yale University, and the University of Arkansas.

Dr. Wooldridge has studied physics, mathematics, and sociology, receiving degrees in the three disciplines. He began his education at the University of Chicago (B.A.) and then continued study at the University of Florida at Gainesville (B.S., M.A.). In 1965, he received a Ph.D. in Sociology at Yale University. Along with his work in nursing, Dr. Wooldridge has maintained an active professional career in sociology through teaching, writing, and research.

When asked about personal activities that relate to his professional perspective, Dr. Wooldridge replied "I enjoy playing tournament bridge and hold the rank of 'Life Master' from the American Contract Bridge League. Playing tournament bridge involves the development and testing of general strategies and principles through direct practice application. Unlike much of my professional work, however, it provides direct and immediate feedback on the success or failure of my efforts in the form of tournament results. I find that very gratifying."

About his work in nursing and with nurses, Dr. Wooldridge had these comments: "One major satisfaction in working with nurses is the opportunity to help develop and test applications of social and behavioral theories to the improvement of health care delivery. Another is the ability to test one's theories directly through clinical trials, rather than indirectly through survey research. I believe that there are health care applications of behavioral science theory that rank in potential importance with those of the physical sciences. Nursing has a central role in doing the research necessary to develop theoretical principles and then actually to put the principles into practice. A crucial component in this process is the development of the analytical skills needed to assess the weight of research evidence in support of specific theoretical interpretations. Much of what I have written and taught has been directed to this end."

First, Maccia's "scientific" and "praxiological" modes of inquiry are based on empirical investigations; whereas the "philosophic" mode of inquiry is based on assertions of value. In this respect, the scientific and the praxiological modes of inquiry differ more from the philosophic mode of inquiry than from each other. This suggests that perhaps they ought to be considered subtypes of a single mode, rather than separate modes of inquiry. Second, the typology makes no provision for a type of theory based *both* on the results of empirical investigation *and* on assertions of value. Such theories might be termed "ideological." and nursing principles (as Walker defines them) might well be general propositions in such a theory. The fourth logical possibility would be a mode of inquiry based *neither* on the use of empirical investigation *nor* or assertions of value. This category would seem to be limited to purely formal theories, all of whose basic propositions or axioms are arbitrarily assumed rather than asserted or empirically demonstrated (for example, mathematical theories).

This analysis suggests the following typology of theories in terms of their modes of validation:

Criteria for the Validation of Fundamental Propositions		Proposed Theoretical Type	Walker's Terminology
Empirical Investigation	Assertions of Value		
Yes	No	scientific	scientific, praxiological
No	Yes	ideational	philosophical
Yes	Yes	ideological	principles (nontheoretic)
No	No	formal	—

As applied to nursing, this typology differs from that suggested by Walker in two major respects. First, it treats both "what is occurring in nursing?" and "what is effective nursing?" as scientific questions. Second, it treats "what is appropriate nursing?" as corresponding to a distinct mode of inquiry (ideological inquiry) and suggests that Walker's "principles" of nursing might well be thought of as propositions or laws of ideological theory.

The classification of questions of "what is occurring in nursing" and "what is effective nursing" as belonging to the same general mode of inquiry should not suggest that I think the distinction between them is unimportant. On the contrary, although inquiry into "what is occurring in nursing" may be of considerable interest to a nurse, I have argued elsewhere that such theory is not properly regarded as nursing theory at all. Such "theories about nursing" are nursing theories only in the sense that nurses are the subject matter to be investigated (Wooldridge, Skipper, & Leonard, 1968). They are no more "nursing theories" than inquiry into "what is occurring in biology?" is biological theory. It is practice theories of nursing (that is: praxiological theories) that are the special province of nursing science in the sense that they comprise a special body of scientific knowledge which the nursing profession has a unique responsibility to investigate and develop.

In a sense, the ideological mode of inquiry is a stepchild of the praxiological mode and the philosophical mode in that it has no unique logic of verification of its own. The development and formalization of such ideological theories depend, therefore, on the prior development and formalization of practice (praxiological) theories and ideational (philosophic) theories. This increases the difficulty of developing integrated theoretical structure in this area; since nursing principles are subject not only to scientific uncertainties about the reliability and validity of substantive inference, but also to moral and metaphysical uncertainties which attend the weighing of one value against another. In spite of the difficulties involved, however, this theoretical area would seem to be crucial, since it is most closely related to practice.

In light of the above discussion, Walker's conclusion that the relation of theory to practice in nursing is "unknown" seems unduly pessimistic. And it encourages the fallacious notion that theory-building is an ivory tower exercise with little practical utility. The confusion seems to come once again from treating matters of degree in absolutist terms.

First, Walker's argument that practice does not test theory is an overstatement. True, the conditions of practice reduce the validity of practice outcomes as a test of praxiological theories, but they do not negate them entirely. Nor is even the most rigorously controlled research entirely free from "questioning of the assumptions about the technology and conditions under which the change was attempted." In other words, completely valid tests of theories don't exist; we make do as best we can with whatever empirical evidence we can get—and the results of practice constitute one source of such empirical evidence. Walker is quite right in pointing out the need for caution in interpreting such evidence and the need to collect better evidence whenever possible; but this caveat should be extended to include all empirical evidence (including "rigorously controlled research") according to the degree to which other interpretations of the evidence are possible.

Second, while Walker is right in asserting that nursing practices cannot be shown to be entirely and explicitly "logically derived from particular theoretical bodies of knowledge," it is also true 1) that nursing practice is guided by principles and procedures that can be considered theoretical in their own right, and 2) that such ideological theories are strongly influenced by the development of scientific and ideational theories. The degree to which nursing practices are explicitly based on scientific and ideational theories is closely related to the extent to which nursing practice has become "rationalized" (Wooldridge et al., 1968). The important point here is not the difference in terminology, but the explicit recognition that the validity of empirical evidence in support of a theory and the linkage between practice and theory are matters of degree, not of kind.

Insofar as Walker defines her terms clearly, there

is no meta-theoretical basis for arguing with the terms she chooses. However, it seems to me that there are several ways in which Walker's terminology is potentially misleading to the casual reader. For example, the distinction between "praxiological" and "scientific" modes of inquiry suggests that praxiological theories are not "scientific." This might falsely suggest that praxiological theories do not depend on scientific empirical research for verification. Similarly, the use of the term "practical" in Walker's characterization of principles and procedures as "practical knowledge" in contrast to "theoretical" knowledge might contribute to the common misconception that theoretical knowledge and development is not a practical activity. (I would argue that it is only through theoretical development that major increases in nursing effectiveness and efficiency are possible). Also the use of "principles" to refer to abstract general imperatives may be confusing, since the term is commonly used to refer to a general proposition in the praxiological mode of inquiry, as in "the principle of aesepsis,"—or even to refer to theoretical propositions in general, as in "the principles of economics." I believe that the term "guidelines" (or perhaps "technical norms") is therefore somewhat to be preferred (Wooldridge, Skipper, & Leonard, 1968, pp. 14–21).

I offer this commentary in the spirit of contributing to the "vigorous and frequent dialogue among nursing theorists" which Walker wishes to encourage. Terminology aside, I found more points of agreement than I found differences between our approaches to the conceptualization of nursing theory; and I found her article to be both stimulating and important.

Reference

Wooldridge, P.J., Skipper, J.K., & Leonard, R.C. (1968). *Behavioral science, social practice, and the nursing profession*. Cleveland: Case Western Reserve University Press.

The Author Comments

I taught at the Yale School of Nursing from 1963 to 1965, where I participated in a large number of formal and informal discussions concerning the nature of nursing theory and research. Yale was an exciting place to be at that time, with Robert Leonard, Florence Wald, James Dickoff, Patricia James, Ernestine Wiedenbach, and Lucy Conant (all contributors to this book) on the faculty. In retrospect, I believe that we all had a sense of being participants in what T.S. Kuhn (1970) refers to as a "scientific revolution," in which new paradigms (models) for nursing research and theory building were being formulated. Although my next academic position (at Case Western Reserve University) was in the Department of Sociology, my contacts with nurse scientists working toward doctoral degrees continued to stimulate my interest in these issues, and I co-authored (with R.C. Leonard and J.K. Skipper, Jr.) the book to which Walker refers in her article–*Behavioral Science, Social Practice, and the Nursing Profession* (Case Western Reserve University Press, 1968).

When asked to comment on Walker's article by Lucille Notter, editor of *Nursing Research*, I was teaching at the University of Iowa. At the time, Ada Jacox was working on her article, "Theory Construction in Nursing: An Overview" (see Chapter 33 of this book), and we exchanged comments on each other's papers. As I recall, I generally liked Walker's article and was pleased to see someone else writing explicitly about meta-theory, but I felt that my (and my co-authors') meta-theoretical position had been referred to in a way that was somewhat oversimplified and perhaps misleading.

My co-authors and I (none of whom were nurses) had consciously tried to avoid making any value assertions of our own about "what is worthwhile nursing." However, we had attempted to describe the value systems of nurses as they related to "appropriate nursing goals" and "appropriate nursing means." We had also discussed "what is occurring in nursing" as it related to "typical frameworks for the provision of care." These two issues (both scientific) were then used as a background for our discussion of how to formulate nursing theory propositions in a way that would maximize their relevance to "what is effective nursing." These theoretical propositions about effective nursing were to be stated in objective terms so that they would be subject to empirical verification. In other words, we recommended that theoretical propositions in practice theory be value-free in formulation and testing, but value-relevant in their implications.

The values to which nursing practice theory was to be made relevant were nursing values concerning the importance of goals and the suitability of means. These value issues were conceptualized as transitory aspects of the social structure, which could nevertheless be determined at any given time by the scientific study of the nursing profession. This was quite different from practice theory as defined by Dickoff and James (and criticized by Walker), since Dickoff and James explicitly incorporated value elements in formulating their theoretical propositions. In terms of the typology I proposed in my commentary, Dickoff and James were using an *ideological* approach to the question "what is effective nursing," whereas my co-authors and I were using a *scientific* approach.

In using the terms "ideational" and "ideological" to refer to the two types of nursing theory in my typology, I may have erred by selecting terms that were more familiar to sociologists than to nurses, since neither term ever caught on. In my most recent work, *Behavioral Science and Nursing Theory* (St. Louis: C.V. Mosby, 1983), I used the term "philosophical" (as Walker did) for theories that depend solely on value assertions for validation, and the term "prescriptive" for theories that depend both on value assertions and empirical research. I have also refined and restated the meta-theoretical principles for constructing theories in what Walker and Maccia refer to as the "praxiological" mode of inquiry as follows:

1. That practice theory should be stated in such a way that the assumed cause-effect relationship between the means and the goal(s) can be empirically tested.
2. That practice theory should focus on causal agencies that are manipulable by the practitioner, on effects that are deemed relevant to evaluating the achievement of practice goals, and on those contingent conditions that are applicable to practice situations.
3. That practice theories developed by a given profession should focus on means for which that profession can assume autonomous prescriptive authority, both through direct manipulation of practice and through the structuring of practice guidelines.

In addition to these meta-theoretical principles, I have recently examined in some detail the issues related to (a) designing research to maximize its relevance to "praxiological" theory (Wooldridge, Leonard, & Skipper, 1978), and (b) analyzing the internal and external validity of research in the context of its relevance to praxiological theory (Wooldridge, Schmitt, Skipper, & Leonard, 1983). Nursing knowledge in the psychosocial area needs to be systematically organized in terms of general principles of practice and tested through clinical trials. Overly broad theory at a level of abstraction too high to permit testing needs to be emphasized *less,* and "middle range" theories that are well grounded both in nursing practice and nursing research need to be developed.

—POWHATAN J. WOOLDRIDGE

REFERENCES

Kuhn, T.S. (1970). *The structure of scientific revolutions* (2nd ed.). Chicago: University of Chicago Press.

Wooldridge, P.J., Leonard, R.C., & Skipper, J.K. (1978). *Methods of clinical experimentation to improve patient care.* St. Louis: C.V. Mosby.

Wooldridge, P.J., Schmitt, M.H., Skipper, J.K., & Leonard, R.C. (1983). *Behavioral science and nursing theory.* St. Louis: C.V. Mosby.

Wooldridge, P.J., Skipper, J.K., & Leonard, R.C. (1968). *Behavioral science, social practice, and the nursing profession.* Cleveland: Case Western Reserve University Press.

Obfuscation or Clarification: A Reaction to Walker's Concept of Nursing Theory

Jeannette R. Folta

For generations nurses have entered into an argumentative dialogue about the definition, function, purpose, means, goals, utilitarianism, and uniqueness of nursing as though "it" were a unitary phenomenon. The seeking of the precise "it" has neither automatically "self-destructed" nor have the problems become less intense through intellectual or scientific endeavors. As a matter of fact, the seeking of the precise but elusive "it" has created and developed new dilemmas currently disguised within scholarly works which utilize a sophisticated linguistic system that both obfuscates and adumbrates the issues.

Concern is now focused on arguments about whether theories in nursing should be theories of nursing, for nursing, or in nursing, or whether nursing theory should be considered as opposed to, say, biological theory in nursing (Norris, 1969–1970). Such arguments are more grammatical than real. Prepositional phrases describing nursing theory as theories of, for, or in nursing place nursing as the object of theory; adjec-tive phrases such as nursing theory place nursing as the qualifier, and possessional phrases make nursing or others the owners of the theory. The latter cannot be the case as no discipline is sole possessor even of its own knowledge. Knowledge, to quote a song, "belongs to everyone." Distinctions between these phrases, it seems to me, are not crucial to the definition of the concept of nursing theory, although they may serve to articulate the approach or goal of any given theoretician. One must be wary lest the issue itself serve to hinder rather than expedite the development of theory.

As a result of a combination of at least two characteristics of the behavior of nurses, coupled with the current stage of development of the nursing profession, discussions of nursing theory have led to more rather than less confusion regarding its nature and direction. A case in point is the article "Toward a Clearer Understanding of the Concept of Nursing Theory" by Lorraine O. Walker, which appeared in the September-October 1971 issue of *Nursing Research*.

About the Author

JEANNETTE R. FOLTA is a member of the faculty at the University of Vermont, where she has been teaching since 1969. Currently she is Professor and Chairperson of the Department of Sociology. Dr. Folta also has held faculty appointments at Boston University and the University of California—San Francisco, and has spent a summer as a visiting professor at the University of Alberta, Edmonton, Canada.

Dr. Folta is a graduate of Burbank Hospital School of Nursing in Fitchburg, Massachusetts. She received a B.S. in Psychiatric Nursing from Boston University (1959) and a Ph.D. in Sociology and Nursing from the University of Washington in 1963.

Dr. Folta has long been active in both nursing and sociology; she describes her professional work as a "dual career." Recent work has focused on research in the areas of death and dying and African studies. From September, 1983 to August, 1984 she was in Zimbabwe, Africa, with Edith Deck collecting information for their current research on "Black African Women: Loss and Change," a study of widows and mothers who lost children through death in the Communal Lands of Zimbabwe.

In addition to her teaching and administrative duties, Dr. Folta keeps busy with an active schedule of speaking, writing, and involvement in professional organizations. Dr. Folta is a member of the American Nurses' Association, is a Fellow in the American Sociological Association, and in 1978, was elected a Fellow in the American Academy of Nursing. Currently she is preparing a text on *The Interpersonal Process of Grief* and a series of articles based on the research done in Zimbabwe.

The first characteristic of the behavior of nurses is the variety of role behaviors engaged in under the rubric of nursing. While all registered nurses wish to be identified as nurses, their behavior ranges from "technical patient care" to "professional nursing care"; from teaching, administration, and research, to theory development. This series of different types of behavior engaged in by nurses makes it confusing, if not impossible, to deal with the notion of developing a single unified theory of nursing. The fact that not all nurses engage in patient care is one of the prime problems in attempting to clarify the concept of nursing theory.

Another characteristic of the behavior of nurses is that most who are engaged in research and/or theory development are educated in the scientific world and tend to view the world from the empirical and/or neo-positivistic tenets of philosophy. Yet nursing is, in practice, if not in philosophy, an art and science based on the pragmatic utilitarian philosophy of applied knowledge. The gap between these philosophies is vast. All the empirical positivistic knowledge nursing may develop may be interesting and even informative but it will not in the long run produce sufficient theoretical knowledge necessary for quality nursing because differ-

ent kinds of nursing behavior require their own philosophical justification and theories.

Nursing is at a new stage of development. While recognizing clinical practice as its stated reason for being, nursing has generally accepted research as an integral aspect of its professional development. This acceptance, while not without its own problems, has led the profession to a new degree of sophistication and prestige. Most research has been of the theory-testing nature with little concern from whence came the theories. Now nursing appears ready to move to the stage of developing its own theories and consequently the issue of nursing theory is of increasing importance in today's scene. Perhaps a degree of security within the profession in its ability to conduct its own research is a factor moving nursing in the direction of positing the development of nursing theory as a value which is seen as both necessary and desirable. The pinnacle of scientific disciplines is the development of theory and nursing is moving toward this pinnacle.

The confusion within our minds, our verbiage, and our endeavors regarding the nature of nursing theory can be cleared only by increasing our breadth of knowledge of philosophy, accepting *sine qua non* the variety of nursing behaviors within the profession, and allowing creativity to determine the direction of this development. To achieve this requires time to be spent in intensive discussion and debate of a wide variety of philosophical positions from which nurses may develop theory that will ultimately improve all aspects of the profession. Thus, I welcomed the opportunity provided by the editors of *Nursing Research* to enter into the dialogue about nursing theory via Lorraine Walker's article.

Dr. Walker's article contributes generously to the pursuit of an intellectual debate on the concept of theory but it does little to clarify for this author the muliplicity of issues involved in developing a "clearer understanding of the concept of nursing theory." Perhaps it is the result of her attempt to cover too many topics in too little space that leads to inadequate analysis and apparent contradictions. Or, the confusion may be related to the frequent change in purposes stated throughout her paper which include:

1. To encourage vigorous and frequent dialogue (Walker, 1971, p. 428)
2. To indicate the parameters of an "adequate characterization of theory of nursing" (Walker, 1971, p. 429)
3. To formulate criteria for adequate theorizing about nursing process, that is, a meta-theoretical or meta-nursological approach (Walker, 1971, p. 431)
4. "To develop greater clarity about the notion of a theory of nursing" (Walker, 1971, p. 432).

Yet another factor contributing to the confusion is her indeterminate use of the term "theory" and the difficulty posed by a lack of clear statement of when the term "theory" is being utilized within her own definition of theory and when she is using the term as others have used it.

It would, of course, be impossible to give consideration to all of the multiplicity of issues raised by Walker. Many volumes have been written on some of these issues; therefore, I shall limit my discussion to a few perceived salient issues. These are the following:

1. The notion of mode of inquiry
2. The concept of holism
3. Nursing practice—goal versus means.

Modes of Inquiry

Walker appears to beg the very question central to her paper: to clarify the concept of nursing theory. She proposes that there are three forms of inquiry (surely there are more!): the scientific, or what is occurring in nursing; the praxiological, or what is effective practice; and the philosophical, or what is worthwhile nursing. There are several problems inherent in her discussion of the relationship of these modes to nursing theory. First, she initially states that the three modes "represent essentially nonintegrated or independent theories of nursing" (Walker, 1971, p. 429). This implies that all three modes of inquiry constitute theory, yet in her later attempts to differentiate each, she implies only the scientific mode is theory and the other two modes nontheories. Secondly, she posits that they are independent and they are not. There appears to be a basic misunderstanding about the implications of these three distinctions. That is, one cannot develop theory (as explanation) *ex nilo*. It must be developed within an empirical context, if one is to use her definition of theory. Thus, the distinction between the scientific, the praxiological, and the philosophical mode is not unintegrated theories but theory versus criteria (effective and worthwhile). What is effective implies criteria as does what is worthwhile, yet the author never elucidates these criteria, their independence from each other, nor does she specify how she has determined a lack of interaction between the criteria. Praxiology, for example, has obvious content of scientific explanation but this issue is neither explored nor analyzed. Instead, the author adumbrates other writers who have talked about this issue.

Another distinction Walker later implies about the three modes is that among current practice (scientific), proposed (effective) practice (praxis), and ideal practice (valued in terms of goals). This distinction ignores the fact that proposed or effective practice has to be scientifically validated before it can be introduced as such into current practice; therefore, the distinction is bogus. You cannot develop a set of proposed, "effective" practices until they have been sufficiently introduced into practice so that one can determine whether or not they are going to produce the effective result they are supposed to produce. Thus, there is confusion in the stated division between praxiology and the scientific mode.

When the author talks of a philosophy of nursing, she appears to be talking about ideal practice. Here she introduces the notion that behavior in this instance is an activity that is valued in terms of its goals and distinguishes between goals and means. Hence, philosophy becomes the goals and practice the means. This adds to the confusion, for ideal practice is something that does not exist; therefore, the notion of applying theory to ideal practice does not fit into her definition of theory. She defines theory as explanation but does not recognize the fact that one cannot explain what does not exist.

Holism: Some Reservations

Having now added to the confusion in a step toward a clearer understanding of the concept of nursing theory, let us turn to Dr. Walker's treatment of the philosophical concept of holism (not to be confused with Wholeism)[1] and its relationship to theory. While on the one hand concluding the notion to be "one whose meaning is vague and ambiguous," she states (though it is unclear whether this is her idea or representative of the holists), "any theory which treats man, the patient, as a set of elements or variables is a falsification of the phenomenon, man, who exists as a complex, but unitary event" (Walker, 1971, p. 431). This poses an interesting problem: Since all knowledge and theories of man are incomplete in that they deal only with select elements or variables (and this includes scientific knowledge), one must conclude, if Walker's premise is true, that all knowledge and theories of man are a falsification of man. This is obviously not the case. Existing theories may be incomplete and not fulfill the notions of holism but that neither necessarily implies inaccuracy nor falsification; it may simply imply inadequacy. Only the most global theory could attempt to encom-

pass all the variables plus the "more than the sum of the parts" contained in this notion. Global theory of this nature, were it possible, probably would be overly cumbersome or overly reductionist.

Another problem with the holistic view is the notion of man as a "unitary event" rather than as a unit. As Dubin points out, "for purposes of any scientific theory we need to distinguish between a unit and an event. . . . The reason for distinguishing between a unit and an event is twofold: 1) We want to distinguish certain types of historical explanation from theory, and 2) We want to dispose of the nagging problem of the uniqueness of all things at each point in time" (Dubin, 1969, p. 32). He goes on to state that an event is a singular occurrence and an explanation of that occurrence is not applicable in explaining another event. If we were to accept his notion that theory is "concerned with modeling the processes and outcomes of particular units interacting in systems, whenever these systems exist and under all conditions of their existence" (Dubin, 1969, p. 33), the notion of man as an event rather than unit would prohibit the development of a theory of man and reduce us to a series of historical explanations.

Further, the notion of theory as scientific, analytic, and deductive precludes the development of a theory of holism. Holism is synthetic, that is, made out of pure substances (variables, elements, et cetera) in combination and creating something new (greater than the sum of the parts). Thus, there is confusion created by an implied desire to explain a synthetic man with an analytic theory. Did this phenomenon occur because synthesis, as Mauksch points out, awaits its "full recognition as an autonomous science-using process which requires its own conceptual scheme, its own criteria of rigor and its own methodological system" (Mauksch, 1969, p. 155)?

Nursing Practice: Goal or Means

Some of the confusion in the usage of the term theory in nursing may be related to the consideration of nursing practice as the goal or means of the profession. For some, nursing is considered primarily as a profession

---

[1] *Wholeism* refers to man as the sum of his parts, and *holism* refers to man as greater than the sum of his parts.

with clinical practice as its goal. This view is characterized by a plea for a return to the bedside. In contrast, others take the position that nursing is or should be primarily a science with clinical practice as its means, that is, practice to be used to generate and/or test theory. This issue raises the question of whether one can contribute to the practice and not the science of nursing or vice versa. However, nursing is both practice and science. The separation of practice from science (or theory) is a chicken-egg dilemma. It is in fact artificial, for after all the chicken is merely the egg's way of reproducing itself.

The profession of nursing needs both practice and science as they constitute parts of the same system: patient care. Yet Walker appears to want to both separate theory and practice and yet relate them to each other. She sees errors in the notion of practice as a means to the development and testing of theory yet qualifies this position under certain circumstances as she implies practice is the means—if utilized by "qualified researchers."

Walker states that there are two errors in the notion that clinical practice of nursing may be a "wellspring for theory development." These errors include: "the collapsing of praxiology with principles and procedures of nursing into some vague notion of 'theory' which simultaneously explains, as well as directs practice, and on a notion of theory development as a Baconian kind of induction in which categories arise from data and observation" (Walker, 1971, p. 433). She dismisses the latter by saying someone else already dealt with this matter (Maccia) and ignores authors such as Glaser and Strauss (1967), who have well documented the utility, need, and strategies for theory induced or arising from data and observation.

Perhaps a more critical side of this issue lies at the heart of theory testing. Walker states it is an error to think practice tests theory because in practice as opposed to research one cannot "hold all other factors constant and equal." She concludes from this— "hence, the failure to achieve a given change based on a given set of theoretical statements does not *in itself* warrant the rejection of the theory, but rather the questioning of the assumptions about the technology and

conditions under which the change was attempted" (Walker, 1971, p. 433). Perhaps the key words are "in itself." If so, one has to agree, yet there seems a bit of magic afoot, that is, if the end result does not occur, it must be we performed incorrectly. Further, she implies, only "qualified researchers" may test theory in clinical areas yet no criteria are established for "qualified researchers."

Summary

The dialogue has begun. Many issues were initiated by Walker, a few were examined, none was resolved. Whatever the position taken on the issues, one must acknowledge that the term theory is currently in vogue and symbolic of prestige. Not to use the term is to be out of step in an increasingly sophisticated world. Often to use the term enables one to engage in erudite but unproductive academic fights, for truth has it we all theorize but few are theoreticians, and as Walker points out, there is a difference. The symbolism of prestige accorded the term theory may create serious problems as common usage can serve to obfuscate a clear understanding of the concept of nursing theory and could easily lead to unfruitful arguments about the definition and criteria for theory while the actual work of theory construction lies dormant and fades away.

Nursing is on the threshold of an exciting venture into new domains of knowledge and application. Currently nursing consists of a perspective and a body of knowledge which provides guidelines rather than models. Nursing is challenged to construct and implement appropriate, useful (praxis), and worthwhile (philosophical) responses to its problems, namely to develop theories. To assume theory can only be scientific and analytic is to severely restrict not the definition ("theory is a coherent group of general propositions used as principles of explanation for a class of phenomena") but rather the scope of inquiry. Nursing is a profession and as such is synthetic, rather than simply deduced from "borrowed sciences" in that it selects relevant variables, theory, and knowledge and orders them in unique patterns in light of a professionally established hierarchy of relevance, appropriateness, and social value. As a synthetic perhaps it can lead the way toward developing theories from synthesis rather than analysis.

References

Dubin, R. (1969). *Theory building*. New York: Free Press.

Glaser, B.J., & Strauss, A.L. (1967). *Discovery of grounded theory: Strategies for qualitative research*. Chicago: Aldine.

Mauksch, I.O. (1969). Summary. In C. Norris (Ed.). *Proceedings of the Second Nursing Theory Conference*, University of Kansas. Kansas City, KA: Department of Nursing Education, University of Kansas Medical Center.

Norris, C. (Ed.). (1969-1970). *Proceedings of First, Second, and Third Nursing Theory Conferences*. Kansas City, KA: Department of Nursing Education, University of Kansas Medical Center.

Walker, L.O. (1971). Toward a clearer understanding of the concept of nursing theory. *Nursing Research, 20*, 428–435.

The Author Comments

The late 1960s to the early 1970s was a time of intense excitement and struggle in the areas of both nursing research and theory. While few were participating in the struggle, the atmosphere was challenging and electrifying. Catherine Norris' Nursing Theory Conference, held at the University of Kansas in 1969, set the stage that caught many of us up in a whirlwind of activity that was to transform our practice through theory development. I had the opportunity to participate in that early conference and it transformed my own thinking.

It was in this atmosphere that Lucille Notter took a bold step in invoking critique and dialogue among scholars around an as-yet unpublished article on theory. An unusual step–but then Lucille Notter is an unusual person. Creative and innovative, she was an early champion of nursing research and theory development, recognizing the importance of critique in the development of knowledge and science and foreseeing nursing's rightful place in that struggle. The issue was no longer whether we should participate in research and theory development, but rather how best to contribute and to whom we are accountable in the implementation of this new knowledge.

Thus it was a distinct pleasure and honor to be invited by Lucille Notter to participate in an open, written dialogue with other scholars around Lorraine Walker's very important article.

—JEANNETTE R. FOLTA

Clarity to What End?

James Dickoff
Patricia James

Responding in the spirit of Walker's friendly criticism, we shall offer specific points and questions highly critical in nature. This mode, though negative, is a compliment to the clarity of Walker's article. The article is forthright in its espousal of some of the views we deem generally covertly held by nurses. We find these views detrimental to any attempt by nurses to deal with theory so as to use theory to make a difference to nursing practice. With no attempt to patronize the author by softening our response, we enumerate some reactions. Our comments are directed to the paragraphs of the article.

Paragraphs 1–2

Is dialogue enough? Is more dialogue what is needed? Compare our coming article in the volume, edited by Verhonick, to be published by Little, Brown; the volume is entitled *Theories Basic to Research*. There we put the question as to whether talking and deprecating have not been overdone by would-be nursing theorists. Emphasis on conception or theory in relation to the amelioration of practice or instruction is perhaps more to the point than attempts "to determine the exact relations among these terms"—namely, "nursing theory," "nursing science," "nursing practice theory," and "nursing knowledge."

Paragraph 2

The impractical bias of the hierarchy set forth in paragraph two is evident. Since nursing practice theory is but a part of nursing science, which is but a part of nursing theory, which in turn is but a part of nursing knowledge, pretty clearly nursing practice is not the primordial interest of nursing, according to Walker. This strikes us as a very alarming admission.

About the Authors

JAMES DICKOFF is Professor and Chair of the Department of Philosophy at Kent State University, Kent, Ohio. He has been teaching at Kent State since 1970, when he joined the faculty after a 10-year appointment at Yale University. Dr. Dickoff was born in St. Louis, Missouri. He studied philosophy at Washington University, receiving a B.A. in 1954, and continued his study of philosophy at Yale, receiving a M.A. in 1958 and a Ph.D in 1962.

Dr. Dickoff maintains a full schedule of teaching, speaking, consulting, and writing about nursing and various other subjects. He also finds time to pursue other interests, particularly music. He comments "Music is at once the most sensuous and intellectual of the arts, where a great complexity of 'immediacy' is managed by the intellect without ignoring individual emotional response."

As a philosopher who has worked with nurses for more than 20 years–and who, as he says, has "persistently been there"–Dr. Dickoff has a unique, thought-provoking, and often controversial perspective on nursing. When asked about nursing's future, he replied "Would there were in the current intellectual development of nursing more guard against adopting a stance parallel to the stance of reaction promulgated at the 1815 Congress of Vienna, where the leadership of Europe attempted to turn back the clock by restoring pre-revolutionary institutions as the governing modes of life."

PATRICIA JAMES is a Professor of Philosophy at Kent State University in Kent, Ohio. A graduate of the University of Detroit, she received a B.S. in Mathematics in 1955. She was a Fullbright Scholar in Louvain, Belgium, from 1955 to 1956, then returned to the United States to study at Yale University, where she received a M.A. in 1958 and a Ph.D. in 1962. She remained at Yale as a faculty member in the Department of Philosophy until accepting her current appointment at Kent State in 1970. Along with her position at Kent State, she has been a Visiting Professor at the Oregon Health Sciences University School of Nursing since 1982.

Dr. James has been collaborating with Dr. Dickoff in areas of scholarly knowledge and thought since they first met at Yale. Together, they have written more than 25 papers and presented at numerous conferences. Besides their work in nursing, they have written and spoken to audiences on education and health care ethics. Dr. James is particularly interested in concepts as they bear on action, especially with regard to the Enlightenment, Pragmatism, and Continental Thought as it relates to Pragmatism. She comments that her work with nurses has provided interaction basic to rethinking theory and concept, which leads toward output germane to an audience extending beyond nurses.

When asked about the future of nursing, Dr. James responded with two questions: "Will nurses realize—before they lose it to others—the opportunity and leadership they have or could have in the endeavor of humanizing doing? When will nursing realize its potential as *the* basic discipline of a service-oriented world?"

Paragraph 3

The appeal to Maccia and educational theory is but one more attempt to shove the dimensions of nursing into a conceptual framework articulated for a different purpose—specifically here, education. That, for example, the patient stands in a more nearly client relation to nurses than does a pupil to teachers may be highly pertinent for nursing practice. Moreover, that philosophic inquiry is limited to the question of what is worthwhile as opposed to what is effective (praxiological inquiry) or what is the case (scientific inquiry) is hardly an unquestioned stance in philosophy or philosophy of education—the domain of Maccia's inquiry. Yet nurse-like, Walker takes as dogmatic this starting position which begs the question at issue in discussing what nursing theory is or should be to make any difference to nursing practice. Not irrelevant is the fact that Walker makes these discoveries or suggestions about nursing in the course of doing a doctoral dissertation in the School of Education at Indiana. And is Maccia perhaps the director? These apparently *ad feminam* remarks are anything but idiosyncratically directed. What percentage of nursing research and speculation is done under just such external-to-nursing demands, constraints, or encouragements?

Paragraph 4

Despite a footnote to Perry that gives the aura of authority to what constitutes praxiological inquiry, again neither the scientific, the praxiological, nor philosophic inquiry is necessarily defined as suggested by Walker, echoing Maccia. To think that there is a fixed definition —to be discovered—of scientific inquiry, for example, is a naive view of conceptualization. This view, held by many even outside of nursing, is, moreover, in part responsible within nursing for some of the endless research and talk attempting to define exactly not only what nursing theory is but also what nursing is.

Paragraph 5

We are told that nursology is the study of nursing as opposed to the process of nursing. Two questions arise: In terms of what discipline is this distinction made? Secondly, is reflective thought about nursing not an essential feature of the process of nursing?

In our view, any definition can be proposed, and the definition is good if it suits the purpose for which the definition is made. But did Walker note that according to her definition of nursing the activity of a policeman, the activity of a teacher, a mother, a father, a football coach, et cetera, qualifies as nursing? Similarly, to distinguish four aspects (probably poorly named as "subsets") is all to the good if the distinction fulfills the purpose intended. But did Walker note, for example, that the end state (her fourth subset) is not necessarily always for nursing well-being? What of nursing terminally ill persons? Or of prolonging unduly the life of a medically indigent elderly person? Or of a badly deformed newborn? Similarly, some conception of the patient (the receiver of care) as providing some of his own care is already a relevant notion in rehabilitation nursing and probably highly relevant to most all nursing situations. These examples of too much broadness

and too much narrowness in concept, a broadness and narrowness perhaps overlooked by the proposer, strike us as representative of a prevalent tendency among nurses cutting their teeth on theory.

In contrast to an overemphasis in calling for exact, univocal, and universal definitions of terms is the careless use of a term such as "subset"—a fairly technical term in set theory or group theory. Is Walker using the term technically? Pretty obviously not, and her usage probably makes no trouble. But when she talks of "four subsets of variables" more room for trouble emerges, since "variable" is so elaborately used a term, with careful definition for some and a careless usage for others.

Paragraph 6

What is the standard in terms of which the adequacy of a characterization of nursing theory is to be given? Is it in terms of the Walker-Perry-Maccia demarcation? If so, what justifies that demarcation? If not, what is the standard and what justifies it? Note that "useful" and "most adequately characterized" are value characterizations and hence this inquiry is a philosophic one in terms of the Walker-Perry-Maccia demarcation. But even given that demarcation, note that the word "worthwhile" is itself a value term and, moreover, an empty term if that for which the worthwhileness is in question be not specified.

Paragraph 7

Conant and Greenwood may speak for themselves. But for our part, what is meant by practice theory is not just "sets of principles or directives for practice." Our conception of theory and of practice theory suggests that practice theory has, structurally speaking, three basic ingredients: goal-content, prescription, and the survey list. Most generously to Walker, we might note that her reading perhaps captures part of the sense of the prescription-ingredient. But, it grossly misses the fairly articulate suggestions we have made—even in the article she herself quotes—with respect to the highly more elaborate structure of a theory capable of being a good practice theory in the sense of being a conceptual framework that might if employed make a difference to nursing practice. Where the confusion lies here is perhaps less patent than Walker suggests.

Paragraph 8

A quiet disclaimer to the view that neither what occurs in nursing nor what is worthwhile for nursing are appropriate parts of practice theory for nursing.

Paragraph 9

Some thinkers, including us, do not take it as a *reductio ad absurdum* that perhaps all sciences are applied sciences.

Paragraph 10

To describe or to explain—what constitutes these maneuvers of inquiry? Would a nursing description of a patient's condition, for example, be exactly like a physician's, a social worker's, or a theologian's description or explanation? This question is meant to point out that describing and explaining are far less antiseptic activities than is sometimes realized by those discussing "scientific inquiry" and by those trying to make a neat and clean distinction between basic and applied sciences.

Might nursing's basicness be related to its aim rather than to its concepts or methods, whether idiosyncratic or borrowed?

Paragraph 11

Why is borrowing a sin—however unsophisticated? Once output for nursing practice becomes a relevant measure of the goodness of theorizing for nursing rather than some notion of originality or contribution to a "body of knowledge for a learned discipline"—as one nursing leader phrases the matter—this foolish emphasis on idiosyncrasy in concept, method, or definition can perhaps be abandoned for concerns more useful to nursing practice. Walker's apology for nursing's borrowings does not escape the edge of these remarks.

Paragraph 13

If the philosophic study of nursing—even given the definition of philosophic inquiry used by Walker-Perry-Maccia—is, as indicated by Walker at the end of paragraph five, nonintegrated with and independent of the scientific or praxiological inquiry into nursing, what bearing will this philosophic inquiry have on nursing practice or process? Or even on praxiological inquiry for nursing? For example, note that Walker talks of cellular life or the life of consciousness and goal setting; it is not at all obvious that she can entertain the notion that nursing might function to hasten desired death. Not just ambiguity but genuine differences in value orientation—some of them radically different from the habitual voiced pieties of those in the health professions—may be pertinent not only to the philosophy of nursing, as demarcated by Walker, but also to the very process of nursing and its study.

Paragraph 14

What makes statements "more fundamental" and hence, "philosophic"? What justifies those more fundamental statements? Or do they function as do footnotes—as ways to place the burden of justification externally to the speaker or situation in question? The relation of a mouthed or voted-on code of ethics to the hoofed and headed "values" of practicing professionals is a crucial question, we claim, for anyone interested not just in "justifying" or seeing as holy the nursing angels of mercy but in seriously enabling professionals to practice in the light of, and for the procurement of ends deemed by them worth their professional effort or investment. Philosophy—whether done before the fact to get on with the practical show or after the fact to justify verbally some practical or conceptual position—is an ascetic or luxury commodity. Other views of philosophy exist. We as philosophers, let alone as persons interested in nursing theory for the sake of nursing practice, hold such a differing view as do such philosophers as Plato, Hume, Dewey, and Wittgenstein.

Paragraph 15

One of the senses of "philosophy of nursing" missed by Walker in her enumeration is our irreverent and controversial notion that for most instances—or too many—in nursing literature or conversation, "philosophy of nursing" is very nearly synonymous with "religion of nursing." The notion that a philosophy is not a personal credo but is or should be, from a practical point of view, a less idiosyncratic stance is gaining some acceptance. Our paper "Beliefs and Values" in this journal, deals very directly with this point. Our recent controversial exchange with our co-author and colleague Ernestine Wiedenbach centers on this matter and indicates both the controversialness of the issue and the difficulty of quiet exchange with respect to matters so intimate, fundamental, and "sacred."

Paragraph 16

Walker's meta-theoretical approach to philosophy of nursing brings up two questions: 1) In terms of what will she justify the criteria as she assesses the adequacy of theorizing about nursing process? 2) How will she know when she has "adequately dealt with" this sense of "philosophy of nursing"? Will she take happy output for nursing practice as her measure—as we would suggest? If not, why not? If not, what? And why *that* what?

Paragraphs 17–22

Walker's discussion of "holism" is rather peculiar as a claimed metatheoretical approach. Her attack is not on the structure of the theory or its mode of production or validation but rather on the subject-matter-scope of the theory. "Holism" is noted to be vague and ambiguous; would Walker hold that any concept is without at least a measure of vagueness and ambiguity? The view that language is, or should be, or could be exact is one of the naif assumptions imported into nursing perhaps by nurses dealing with equally naif social or natural scientists or even philosophers. Since Plato, and markedly in

the 20th century Wittgenstein, has emerged the realization that language is a much more living tool than is suggested by the outlook on language that links a given word to just one clear and exact meaning and sees any variation only as inexactness or misuse. Compare our forthcoming article mentioned above.

Paragraph 23

The central purpose of Walker's paper is to "develop a greater clarity about the notion of a theory of nursing." Why is that a worthwhile purpose? Some would say, "Clarity is not enough." Others, "that clarity is not possible, especially at the outset." Our version of these purposely mocking questions is this: What are you going to do with the clarity after you get it? How many years longer should we try for such clarity? Compare again our last-cited paper.

What makes a "doing of nursing" effective or moral?

Are all procedures thoroughly specific with respect to concrete sequence of operations? Highly dubious. Compare, for example, the step included in many procedures, so called, to "clean and return the equipment after use."

To whom are the principles as imperatives directed? And what is the source and binding force of the injunction? How do they differ from doctor's orders?

Paragraph 30

The reference to Rudner to justify that within a theory terms are "'systematically related,' that is, logically related such that deduction from certain fundamental statements to other derived statements become possible," is another example of use of reference to one "authority" to give the impression of a generally held view of theory or, more basically, to suggest that a view is justified if you can find someone else who says it. The hypothetical-deductive model of theory is but one among even the relatively received notions of theory. Moreover, some theorists of theory (notably us) have persisted in making the suggestion that: 1) with respect to systematicness, many relations are possible other than just the linear consequential order of deducibility from initial axioms; and 2) logical order is not identical with such relatively trivial consequential order. Specifically our claim is that for practice theory as opposed to merely predictive theory the systematic interrelation is a coherency relation and not merely a linear consequential relation, and that, moreover, the elements systematically related are not homogeneous in kind.

Compare "Theory in a Practice Discipline," written by Ernestine Wiedenbach and us and cited by Walker as references 33 and 34. The technique for argument used by Walker is a much used one but nonetheless questionable for being widely appealed to: The technique cites a definition of, say, "theory," on authority or without further justification and then discredits or questions all other proposed definitions of, say, "theory," by pointing out that they are not the definition here given.

Paragraph 31

Another clue to the essentially impractical orientation of Walker is her willingness to invest in theory—at least to bother to talk about it—though she sees no possibility of incorporating into theory feasibility considerations for nursing nor of producing (according to the demands of her espoused model of theory) a deductive system for nursing.

Paragraph 32

What makes the general the general? Walker seems to have a notion of generality as an absolute rather than seeing it as relative to the more specific.

Paragraph 33

This paragraph argues explicitly in the mode we have just pointed out (under Paragraph 30): Other notions of theory are to be discarded or to be uncommended since the usages do not conform to the distinctions the paper sets down between scientific, praxiological, and philosophic inquiries and between these inquiries as three kinds of independent and unintegrated theories, on the one hand, and principles and procedures for carrying out nursing process, on the other hand.

Paragraph 34

Consider these words: "Practitioners in the midst of practice are more than likely not in a position to provide the conditions necessary for adequately testing a theory." *Of what possible use for practice is a theory that is validated with respect to something other than practice?* The particularization of this point we have urged repeatedly in our attempts to put the proper scorn on the well-nigh universal research procedure of regarding as "validated" some hypothesis about, say, nursing admissions, when the research was done by a "nurse" without service commitments and with no obligations beyond admitting patients chosen for her sample. We could add examples *ad nauseam* from the literature of nursing research. This kind of complaint, which we first sensed from objections to research urged by Ernestine Wiedenbach, is no objection in principle to research, but is a striking point against the methodological correctness of foolish attempts to generalize to "nursing" the findings made by artificial staff members under artificial conditions—artificial with respect to virtually all "existential states of affairs" in nursing.

Paragraph 35

Walker credits us, among others, with the misguided notion of seeing "the observation of clinical practice of nursing as a well spring for theory development." The misdirection is credited to one of two errors. First, to collapsing the distinctions urged in this paper of Walker's. We have already spoken to the inconclusiveness of this mode of arguing. That our views differ from those given here does not necessarily justify our views, but such mere difference is hardly conclusive grounds for rejection—unless, of course, the grounds of this paper are without question. The second source of error is credited to reliance on "a Baconian kind of induction" for theory development. How ironic, for Bacon (Cp. Book II of the *New Organon,* especially the second half) is hardly the one who thinks the categories arise from data and observation. Bacon emphasizes (as we pointed out in the paper done with Wiedenbach and cited by Walker at this point) both the need for "first vintage"—a recognized leap beyond the data to attempt characterization of the "latent process and latent configuration" of the phenomenon in question. Bacon emphasizes also the use of Polychrest instances as especially useful for developing hypotheses for testing for fruit (usefulness) if not for light. 'Polychrest instances' is a poetic name for gratuitously occurring occasions for nightwatch on nature as provided not by artificial settings and contrivances but by the practical products embodying the features under study (windmills and power; bridges and principles of support, et cetera).

That Walker does not realize that if Maccia represents Baconian induction as described here, then Maccia should read Bacon again is another example of the problem nurses face in moving in new areas where they must depend on others but have in themselves inadequate bases for assessing the adequacy of those on whom they depend.

We are cited as failing to make the distinction between theoretic knowledge and practical knowledge in nursing. Our "failure" is a very purposeful and persistently made attempt to discredit the propriety of such a distinction; our attempt is to show that such a distinction leads to a kind of theorizing that will never make a difference to nursing practice. Our suggestion needs evaluating not with respect to its difference from certain classical views of theory or practice theory or its difference from the Perry-Maccia-Walker distinctions but in terms of whether or not theory produced and regarded according to our conception does or does not make a positively practical difference to nursing practice. Have nurses any business indulging themselves in the luxury of theory unless theory can make such a difference? Our view is that they do not.

The Authors Comment

Appreciating Walker as an Early Reaction to Dickoff/James on Theory

Differences on Theory

We can give an introductory summary of our 1985 look at our 1971 comments on Walker in terms of four comments that highlight significant differences in the Dickoff/James position and what we call here a "Walker-like" position on theory.

1. *Dickoff/James difference on theory as purposeful and not inadvertent.* The Dickoff/James proposal concerning the levels of theory differs from other views of theory; the difference is significant and intentional. It was not an oversight on our part nor an unintentional failure to meet someone else's standard view as to what theory is. Walker fails to appreciate the difference as intentional.
2. *Differences on theory traced to differences in conception of nursing activity.* The Walker view on theory, the view that Walker expounds and seems to espouse, has many contemporary variants. A Walker-like view embodies a deprecating stance toward concepts as guides to action. Such a deprecating stance differs significantly from the Dickoff/James stance and is perhaps the root difference between a Walker-like view of theory and our notion of theory. In giving to concepts only a limited potential for guiding action, Walker-like views fail to appreciate that thought and thoughtfulness—both products and guides of which are concepts—are the prime tools of a practitioner. A Walker-like view of theory results in an oversimplified view of nursing activity. In this approach to theory, nursing activity fails to qualify as what we characterize as "complexly considerate thoughtful doing." Our stance is that what is at issue ultimately in these differing views about *theory* is differing views about the very nature of *nursing activity.* If nursing activity is to be complexly considerate thoughtful doing

rather than merely any lesser kind of activity, then nursing theory needs to be conceived of as situation-producing theory in the Dickoff/James sense.

3. *The more than only speculative origin of the Dickoff/James theory difference.* A Dickoff/James approach to theory and the resulting Dickoff/James concept of theory differs significantly from a Walker-like approach and view of theory in part because of our experience within nursing. That "experience" was shaped in part by our notions of "the expert" and of "inquiry" and in part by our good fortune in being associated with strong and intelligent nurses. As we recount in the comments to the symposium articles (see Chapter 8), we worked with nurses in the Yale encounter and we worked with them on *specific* problems. We did not come as experts with a specific construct or well-specified content that if adopted would be the solution to the current troubling difficulty. Quite the contrary. Our interaction with nurses was a mutual or joint inquiry into problems rather than being two kinds of experts (nursing experts and philosophy experts) exchanging information (nursing information and philosophy information). It is true that we had philosophic information at our fingertips and that the nurses were informed about the various areas of nursing. But, in general, it was not thought that a piece of philosophic or nursing information would solve the problem at hand. An inquiry was needed. In shaping that inquiry, we as philosophers brought to bear a philosophic perspective, and the nurses contributed a nursing perspective. (Often what constituted the distinctively philosophic or nursing perspective became more clearly outlined in the course of the actual exchange rather than standing out, well demarcated, at the beginning of the inquiry.) Though the particularities of the inquiry depended upon the particularities of the persons and their backgrounds, still the "dialectic" was other than an exchange of information: *Thought was brought to bear on a problem.* (Happily, this kind of fruitful interaction still continues—most recently at Oregon Health Sciences University under the deanship of Carol Lindeman, where we have had repeated occasions for exchange with faculty as we functioned there as lecturers, consultants, or visiting faculty.) In other words, our "experience" with nurses has been in the form of a mutual inquiry with nurses pressed with some practical commitment. So it is not surprising that we came to realize that the purpose of theory in a practice discipline is to provide for action.

4. *Appreciation of Walker as an early warning sign of misapprehension of or resistance to the Dickoff/ James theory difference.* Our fourth summarizing comment here, rather than highlighting a significant difference between Walker's and our conceptions of theory, relates our comments on Walker to our later thought. In recent work, we have developed a technique that we call FLIPRAC—*fast lane intensive post-ritual appreciation and critique.* This is not the place to elaborate on the details and purpose of that technique. Mention of FLIPRAC pertains to our response to Walker this way: The clarity article was emphatic on critique, less emphatic on appreciation; today we would emphasize both poles equally. The great virtue of Walker's article was its courageous press to articulate a position distinctively enough to allow it to be grasped, understood, and appreciated for what it is—and hence to be subject to criticism. The move to such overtness is a risk-taking venture whose virtue is often underpraised. Our point-by-point critical comments on the Walker view implied such an appreciation but neglected to express it overtly.

Techniques Dickoff/James Employed in Their Critique of Walker

Our mode of criticism of Walker was a detailed enumeration of questionable points. This approach required that we seriously encounter Walker's position, that we—in our terminology—appreciate her position. The critical items one by one and as a totality brought to light two objectionable features of the Walker view: (1) concepts are underutilized as guides to nursing actions, and (2) the theoretical-practical distinction as it functions in Walker is an *imperious distinction,* a distinction presumed to be an absolute standard as though it had been settled once and for all in a specific way. Any questioning of the distinction or of the specification of the distinction is taken as an error—without further reflection.

The critique of Walker is an early version of a technique we now call "dissonance reading." To read a nursing text for dissonance is to bring to light the warring tendencies within it. Statements made in one part are dissonant with those made elsewhere in the text. The parts do not cohere; they fall apart, oppose or contradict one another. The unstableness of such texts stems, in our diagnosis, from the clash of opposing tendencies within nursing itself, tendencies alive within the individual nurse and surfacing in the text through the creation of non-fits or opposing statements. In general, we have diagnosed that conflicts or clashes of wills within nursing are ultimately the sources of these dissonances. We have called these the "will to nursing" (the drive to give nursing care to a person in need), the "will to research" (the drive to create a validated knowledge base for nursing through the use of inquiry), and the "will to professionalization" (the determination to achieve an appropriately recognized social status for a profession of nursing). We call them opposing wills because often in trying to reach their respective goals, one attempt thwarts or nullifies or makes more difficult the others. These ultimate "wills" appear in many guises, but these guises are, in our analysis, different manifestations of these three fundamental wills. In Walker we detected dissonances stemming from (1) the mouthing of docented knowledge as gospel, from (2) the failure to take seriously that nursing is a practice and as a practice its conceptualization would differ in part from the kinds of conceptualizations used in nonpractice contexts, and from (3) the desire to meet standards set by those external to nursing.

Our critique, though highly critical, was not an attack on Walker as a person. The approach was one of depersonalization: we focused on her *words,* her text, as articulating a representative thought-pattern emerging in nursing as nursing moved into the academy. We might add that the thought-pattern is not, we think, peculiar to nursing, but surfaces in any practice discipline as it attempts to intellectualize—"professionalize" is the more nearly usual jargon—its doings or service. So Walker is more than a representative of a stance in nursing. Her position signals an outlook often found in any practice discipline as it attempts to professionalize itself; and so, our appreciation of Walker goes far beyond merely criticizing Walker. In two senses, then, our critique of Walker is a depersonalized one. Rereading our comments to Walker, we sense their pertinence to many much later and even current pieces relating nursing theory to nursing practice.

Nor was our critique a patronizing one. We attended closely to Walker's words, trying to grip her position in its details. We did not practice selective focus on a single spot or on an isolated passage or two; we did not indulge in a gross dismissal or glib acceptance of a vague whole. Instead, we weighed her words and considered them in the light of our exchanges within nursing. (Note that this critique and our interaction with nurses predates the more recent excursion of philosophers into "the practical," a movement itself not wholly untinged by a deprecating patronization.)

Today we would say that our critique was flawed in its oversubtlety. A quotable broadside probably would have been more effective, but it too would have missed the end we were trying to achieve. Our itemized persistence with details was designed to provoke in the reader *a reflective questioning* of the Walker position. It is not clear to us whether that occurred; at any rate, it never occurred in any markedly visible printed exchange. The current nursing scene is still marked by various restatements of a Walker-like position without any obvious awareness of the critique already offered; see, for example, the Beckstrand articles in Chapter 50 of this book, the Chinn and Jacobs text *Theory and Nursing: A Systematic Approach* (St. Louis: C.V. Mosby, 1983), and the nursing-science stance supplemented by the APE (aesthetic, personal, ethical) view of, say, Fawcett or other Carper followers.

Our response to Walker did not include an *explicit* reflection on the position we advocated. Could we be charged then with having been dogmatic? Probably not, since from the beginning we had called for and offered a pattern of an *empirical test* of our conception of practice theory—a test of feasibility, coherency, and palatability. *Our position has not yet been genuinely read or encountered.* Because it is different, it is not consumed, taken in, assimilated. (Ironically, though the occasion for setting forth our theory of theories was our association with nursing, a test of that conception is, in a sense, being broached in the work of a physician. Dr. Gary Benfield is attempting a conceptualization of neonatology in terms of a practice-theory structure.)

Nursing—A Parasite On or A Development of the Academy?

Two basic questions faced nursing as it moved into the academy: (1) What is nursing going to teach nursing majors that is uniquely nursing? (2) What marks a nursing faculty as a scholarly faculty contributing to the advancement of the discipline of nursing and so worthy to be a faculty of the academy? The answers that emerged were these: nursing teaches its undergraduates nursing knowledge, some part of which includes nursing theory; nursing faculty are authentic university faculty because they advance the discipline of nursing by doing nursing research. These answers are not objectionable because they are vacuous. Who, after all, would advocate vice over virtue? So, let us ask instead. (1) What sort of "thing" is nursing knowledge, or nursing theory, or nursing science? (2) How is nursing research generated and what is the logic of the resulting inquiry or research? These questions provoke differing and controversial responses.

A Walker-like approach says in effect that the intellectual tools the academy has already forged are sufficient to answer these questions: In short, (1) nursing knowledge, theory, or science is at best just plain old predictive theory; (2) nursing research is in the same genre as, say, sociology research and is governed by that kind of logic. In contrast, we (Dickoff/James) say that extant tools are not wholly satisfactory: (1) Nursing theory is not exhausted in terms of predictive theory—nursing as a service, as an activity, requires conceptions to guide activity, and the structure of such conception differs from the structure of predictive theory, though predictive theory is one of the resources called on within nursing theory. (2) Both the problems that nursing research investigates and the validation tests employed by nursing research must bring to bear considerations that do not arise in nonpractice disciplines such as, say, sociology. Consequently, the tests need to employ a logic that goes beyond that commonly used in disciplines that do not aim to bring into existence situations of a specified kind—in short, nonpractice disciplines. We see nursing's move into the academy as an opportunity to enlarge the intellectual tools of the academy—an enhancement of the academy—whereas Walker et al. seem to see the move as nothing more than nursing's appropriation of tools already present in the academy.

Walker's and current Walker-like views on the theory question—Fawcett, Beckstrand, Chinn, and Jacobs—are in our eyes the results of "docented knowledge," the products of "docented knowledge" rather than being the results of engaged or living thought. ("Docented knowledge" is knowledge we have been taught or that we have gleaned from secondary sources. It is knowledge we are not quite at home with.) In explaining a piece of docented knowledge to others we betray ourselves. We say things that to a discerning eye show we have at best a relatively superficial grasp of the matter we are discussing—however much we can itemize selected particulars or test others on selected particulars. We all pass through the stage of docented knowledge; it is often a step on the way to genuine understanding or mastery. But human beings are not above "putting on airs." (Didn't the precocious ones wrap themselves in the finery of knowledge, dropping learned phrases here and there to impress their auditors, to exhibit their learnedness and so show themselves worthy of intellectual acceptance? The seventeenth century phenomenon of preciocité is probably a version of docented knowledge.) Nursing's move into the academy—and the paraded move to professionalization—is marked by a similar determination to be "worthy." "Before I retire I am determined that nursing shall be recognized as a learned discipline" is a pronouncement we have heard from more than one prominent leader in the nursing field.

The move to make nursing learned often becomes a move to disassociate nursing from its practice: We—the academic nurses—are the learned ones; the others are just service givers. (Ada Sue Hinshaw in her 1983 WICHEN keynote on images for nursing spoke as though academic nursing should get "them" to follow a certain image; practicing nurses were regarded not as image-makers but rather as those on whom an image should be imposed.) The academics are concerned with intellectual matters; the service nurses, with practice. Research and theory are in the province of the learned; doing is the concern of the others. This split is even more destructive and unwholesome than the chasm between physicians and nurses. The contempt that the one party feels for the other is harmful enough, but that is only a small part of the harm wrought by the split. Far more telling and harmful is the outlook such a split occasions in its advocates: Nursing science, nursing theory, nursing research can be generated by academic nurses independent of practice considerations as seen by practitioners. Nursing science, nursing theory, and nursing research become self-contained realms distinct from nursing practice. Though nursing science, nursing theory, and nursing research may speak to one another, nursing practice has nothing to say to them, and insofar as the three realms communicate with nursing practice, the communication is a one-way transmission of truth—a bringing of the message to Garcia.

Walker and other like thinkers fail, in our eyes, to appreciate that nursing is more than a learned discipline, and is also a service or practice. Any view of theory that does not allow nursing to be conceptualized as a doing—a complexly considerate, thoughtful doing—fails to meet the needs of nursing. The question is whether nursing is to be distorted (disfigured) to fit into the academy or whether the academy is to be enlarged to meet the needs of nursing as a practice discipline. Is doing to become thoughtful and complexly considerate? Or is it to be left to the whim and happenstance of the moment? A Walker-like approach makes nursing a parasite on the academy; we find the incorporation of nursing into the academy a potential for the development of the academy.

—JAMES DICKOFF AND PATRICIA JAMES

Rejoinder to Commentary: Toward a Clearer Understanding of the Concept of Nursing Theory

Lorraine Olszewski Walker

The September-October 1971 issue of *Nursing Research* contained an article by Lorraine Olszewski Walker entitled "Toward a Clearer Understanding of the Concept of Nursing Theory" (pp. 428–435). Comments on Dr. Walker's article were invited for the purpose of encouraging further dialogue on the concept of nursing theory, and reactions were published in the November-December 1971 issue (pp. 493–502). Commenting were Rosemary Ellis. "Reaction to Walker's Article"; Powhatan J. Wooldridge, "Metatheories of Nursing: A Reaction to Dr. Walker's Article"; Jeannette R. Folta, "Obfuscation or Clarification: A Reaction to Walker's Concept of Nursing Theory"; and James Dickoff and Patricia James, "Clarity to What End?" Doctor Walker's response to these discussions develops further thoughts on nursing theory.

Because the focus of each of the four commentaries on "Toward a Clearer Understanding of the Concept of Nursing Theory" was largely nonoverlapping, the response below will deal with each commentary separately.

"Reaction to Walker's Article" by Rosemary Ellis

Ellis' commentary was helpful in more precisely interpreting her writings. From her commentary, presumably we would both agree that her work is directed at the critical development of adequate nursing practices, including all three activities outlined earlier as involved in applying a generalization to practice: 1) the selection of an end to be achieved, 2) the discrimination of the conditions of practice under which a given theoretical generalization is instrumental in achieving that end, and 3) the development and/or adoption of a particular set of means, including in some cases specific technological devices, which are indicated by the generalization (Walker, 1971, p. 433). Further, *critical* development of nursing practices might also require that 1) the end selected be shown to be desirable, 2) the generalization being applied be clear in meaning and have some reasonable degree of empirical confirmation and 3) the means utilized be shown to be superior to any alternate means which are feasible.

"Meta-Theories of Nursing: A Reaction to Dr. Walker's Article" by Powhatan J. Wooldridge

Wooldridge's rejection of the position that practical knowledge of nursing—that is, principles of nursing—is nontheoretical formed a persistent strand throughout his commentary. While I concede that principles of nursing may be general in much the same way as are scientific propositions, the problem of the logical organization of principles into a theoretic system is more than a contextual one (i.e., that it has not been successfully done to date). The more cutting concern with regard to the logical organization of principles seems to be this: What is the method of integration? Even if some sort of hierarchy between principles may be demonstrated, this in itself does not indicate how that hierarchy has been established. Is it merely that some principles are more general than others? Is it that some principles logically entail others? Or is there some other variety of interrelationship? Until these questions can be answered the systemization of practical knowledge seems to be, at best, a hypothesis.

Wooldridge's espousal of the theoretical nature of practical knowledge recurred in his proposed typology of theories based on their mode of validation. From this typology, he generated the category of ideological theory within which principles of nursing might constitute the propositions. Ideological theory is seen as "based *both* on the results of empirical investigation *and* on assertions of value" (Wooldridge, 1971, p. 494). However, then it is noted "In a sense, the ideological mode of inquiry is a stepchild of the praxiological mode and the philosophic mode in that it has no unique logic of verification of its own. The development and formalization of such ideological theories depend, there-

fore, on the prior development and formalization of practice (praxiological) theories and ideational (philosophic) theories" (Wooldridge, 1971, p. 495). While noting the difficulties involved in developing ideological theory, Wooldridge stated ". . .this theoretical area would seem to be crucial, since it is most closely related to practice" (Wooldridge, 1971, p. 495). Presumably, then, ideological theory tells what ought to be done in practice based on certain desired outcomes and certain praxiological statements. In effect, however, this characterization of ideological theory would seem to render it nontheoretic. First, it appears not to be a mode of inquiry, but rather the application of extant knowledge to produce certain outcomes. Second, it appears not to be a unique mode of theorizing in that its propositions may be warranted only through appeal to other underlying propositions within other theories.

While it will be conceded to Wooldridge that the differences in the support given to a theory on the basis of observation in practice and on the basis of controlled research is a matter of degree, this would seem to be a rather critical difference in degree.

Finally, inasmuch as Wooldridge's commentary contained a serious effort to establish some consonance in meaning between his work and mine, it represented an effort aimed at overcoming mere verbal differences in order to deal with genuine theoretical disputes.

"Obfuscation or Clarification: A Reaction to Walker's Concept of Nursing Theory" by Jeannette R. Folta

In reading Folta's commentary, something seems to have misfired. I was unable to recall or find where she found the implication that praxiology and philosophy of nursing were nontheories. I was also unable to find where the implication was made that the three modes of discourse (science, praxiology, and philosophy of nursing) might be distinguished according to "current practice (scientific), proposed (effective) practice (praxis), and ideal practice (valued in terms of goals)" (Folta, 1971, p. 497). Thus, no response can be made here.

With regard to holism, it is perhaps a fault of my style of writing that the belief in "holism" was attributed to me by Folta. Where she quoted this view from "Toward a Clearer Understanding of the Concept of Nursing Theory," I was merely attempting to report what the view meant to others. I did not intend to give the impression that I saw holism (i.e., the belief that theory must mirror the full complexity and unity of the event studied to be adequate) as a criterion for adequate theory of nursing.

The relation of theory to practice also seemed to need further clarification. Let it be made clear what concrete claims I would uphold:

1. Practitioners, no matter how close they may be to the nursing data, are in an unlikely position to produce theory.
2. Some researchers may have idiosyncratic traits which make them more likely to see relationships or to generate ideas when in the practice context. (Some may do these things better in the library or in the pub!)
3. Qualified researchers—that is, those who have studied and mastered the content and method of research techniques in nursing or a related discipline—are much more likely to be able to test hypotheses in the practice context without mistakes, such as sampling biases, than are nurse practitioners without such background.

Looking at the relation of theory to practice from a more theoretical perspective, the characterization of theory development as a process of induction from data appears to be inadequate on two counts. First, it fails to account for the selecting principles that in effect render the data to the category of data. Second, it has a missing link between observing data and putting forth conceptualizations which organize data (Peirce, 1958). This epistemological rejection of induction as a characterization of theory generation is different from the denial that some researchers may be able to theorize better in the midst of "data." The first is a philosophic matter, the second an empirical one.

"Clarity to What End?" by James Dickoff and Patricia James

Some introductory remarks seem pertinent in responding to the Dickoff and James commentary. Although

"Toward a Clearer Understanding of the Concept of Nursing Theory" perhaps lacks some of the messianic zeal of the writings on nursing theory of Dickoff and James, the difference is deliberate. It seems that, indeed, we are operating on different principles. The primary purpose of "Toward a Clearer Understanding of the Concept of Nursing Theory" was to clarify certain concepts in the discourse related to nursing theory, and only secondarily did it attempt to affect any patterns of action with regard to the conduct of nursing research and nursing theory development. My purpose was, therefore, declaratory in that the aim was a lucid exposition of some problems within nursing discourse related to nursing theory. Dickoff and James, in contrast, appeared to have a program to sell—one not only aimed at changing the content of linguistic behavior dealing with nursing theory, but also aimed primarily at changing the method and content of nursing research and nursing theory. Where Dickoff and James in effect chose to legislate through their programmatic exposition of theory, I chose to describe in order that others might make their choices about the content and method of nursing research and nursing theory, hopefully with a clearer understanding of the language they use to describe and guide their activities. Where I have spoken critically of certain practices related to nursing theory, it has been because these appeared to be based upon certain inadequate conceptions about nursing theory.

Dickoff and James see the Walker approach to discourse about nursing theory as defective in that it is "detrimental to any attempt by nurses to deal with theory so as to use theory to make a difference to nursing practice" (Dickoff & James, 1971, p. 499). By defining theory broadly, Dickoff and James considered that the proper relevance of theory to practice was made. However, integral to their broad definition of a theory as "a conceptual system or framework invented to some purpose" (Dickoff & James, 1968, p. 198), was the contention "that all theory exists finally for the sake of practice (since in a sense every lower level theory exists for the next higher level and the highest level exists for practice) and that nursing theory must be theory at the highest level since either the nursing aim is practice or else nursing is no longer a profession as distinct from some mere academic discipline" (Dickoff & James, 1968, p. 199).

While Dickoff and James have argued in a compelling manner, their argument seems to contain several defects. First, by arguing for the continuity between theory and practice, they have collapsed two distinct activities into the notion of nursing theory, that is, the activity of theory development and the activities of practice development. Second, in arguing that all theory exists for the sake of practice, they have failed to differentiate between the practice of nursing and the practice of nursology (see Walker, 1971, p. 428, for a definition of "nursology"), and have also failed to note that while in a sense theory exists for the sake of practice, in another sense it does not.

The argument has already been made for the distinct natures of theory development and practice development (Walker, 1971, pp. 433—434). With regard to the notion that theory exists for the sake of practice, the most immediate practice for which theory would exist would appear to be the practice of nursology itself, in that the manifest purpose of theory is the description and explanation of a set of events taken by that discipline as problematic. In addition, while the end of theoretical inquiry, that is, nursing theory, may become in turn a means to nursing practice development, the instrumental nature of nursing theory in the practice context does not warrant the short-circuiting of the end of inquiry by tying it to nursing practice. Such a short-circuiting is not warranted, for it would seem to jeopardize the goal of inquiry by tying it to immediate practical payoff, and thus block the development of a more adequate product of inquiry whose practical relevance might not be obvious to the more theoretically naive.[1] This would seem to be the risk taken when Dickoff and

James chose "output for nursing practice" as the "relevant measure of the goodness of theorizing" (Dickoff & James, 1971, p. 500).

In contrast, I would argue that the end of theoretical inquiry is the development of a theory which adequately describes and explains nursing process and consequently provides understanding of that process. This is *not* at all to say that such a theory would be irrelevant to practice development, but merely to say that practice development is not the appropriate norm for judging the adequacy of theory as such.

Dickoff and James have asked on what basis the Walker conceptualization of adequate theorizing about nursing is justified. The criteria which have been taken as appropriate are 1) the greater clarity and precision rendered to the concept of nursing theory, and 2) the consistency of the conceptualization with notions of theory in the more well-established sciences. Since my goal was to clarify certain concepts in nursing discourse and not to promote a programmatic conception of nursing theory, the norms were those dealing with the quality of analysis, and not the quality of practical outcomes.

One of the fundamental failures cited of the Dickoff-James conceptualization of nursing theory in the original article was its failure to distinguish between the theoretical and practical knowledge of nursing. Their commentary reaffirmed that "such a distinction leads to a kind of theorizing that will never make a difference to nursing practice" (Dickoff & James, 1971, p. 502). Their claim seems to be unwarranted. There appears to be no reason why distinguishing between theoretical and practical knowledge would in itself make incompatible the application of nursing theory to the development of new or more adequate nursing practices. In fact, distinguishing between these two kinds of nursing knowledge might serve to promote the development of each by clarifying to nurses the task in which they are engaging and the norms which are appropriate.

While I cannot formulate a logic for proceeding error-free from a nursing theory to the development of

---

[1] That the relevance of theory to practice may not seem obvious at first glance may not indicate a fault with theory, but rather a fault with the person.

specific practices, some analysis in this area has been carried out in the initial article on nursing theory and in this rejoinder in the response to Ellis above. That science, praxiology, and philosophy of nursing are characterized as nonintegrated theories (i.e., not logically intertwined theoretical systems) does not indicate that they are irrelevant to nursing practice as Dickoff and James have charged; statements from these theories may be combined to provide guides to nursing practice.

The criticism of the broadness of the proposed definition of nursing was warranted in that a portion of the definition was inadvertently omitted during the preparation of the manuscript. The definition (Walker, 1971, p. 429) should have read:

> Nursing = $_{Df}$ One or more expert persons caring for the physical and/or mental well-being of one or more other persons with an actual or potential health problem within a setting.

I am indebted to Dickoff and James for pointing out the potential for conflict between the goals of mental and physical well-being, as in the case of the terminally ill. Thus the definition above has been modified so that both mental and/or physical well-being are sought. No norms are laid out in the definition for establishing the preeminence of mental or physical well-being over each other, as the definition was intended to be descriptive in nature.[2] Questions dealing with such value determinations are seen as more properly occurring within the context of philosophy of nursing.

Dickoff and James found the discussion of "holism" peculiar within the context of a paper which purported to be meta-theoretical. However, inasmuch as holism has been suggested by some as a criterion for adequate nursing theory, an examination of this concept seemed appropriate (Ellis, 1968; Rogers, 1963; Spring, 1969). The examination of holism was not a quest for the one true meaning of the concept. It was rather an attempt to point out the ambiguity of the term so that issues surrounding its several uses might be examined independently and the confusion resulting from the failure to dissociate the different meanings of the term might be dissipated.

While Dickoff and James hold views different from this author on the adequacy of induction as a method of theory development and on the appropriate context and method for the testing of hypotheses about nursing process, our most fundamental difference occurs in the evaluation we made of attempts to clarify a body of discourse. Dickoff and James' implication of the abortive nature of analysis in producing advances in theory development seems essentially to mislead, for it presumes that attempts at clarifying discourse are incompatible with attempts to develop theory. While it is true that analysis does not produce theory, it also seems false to assert that analysis precludes theorizing. I would hold that attempts to improve the clarity of a body of discourse are appropriate as long as that discourse continues to evince signs of confusion which vitiate the purpose of the discourse.

Concluding Remarks

As Folta stated in her reaction, "The dialogue has begun." I am deeply indebted to the respondents who took the time and thought to respond to "Toward a Clearer Understanding of the Concept of Nursing Theory." Let us hope that the dialogue will continue and lead to a more mature body of metanursological thought which can not only bring understanding, but also contribute to the smooth development of nursing theory.

References

Dickoff, J., & James, P. (1968). A theory of theories: A position paper. *Nursing Research, 17,* 197–203.

Dickoff, J., & James, P. (1971). Clarity to what end? *Nursing Reasearch, 20,* 499–502.

Ellis, R. (1968). Characteristics of significant theories. *Nursing Research, 17,* 217–222.

---

[2] The discussion of the need for a descriptive definition of nursing to mark off the parameters of nursing as a field of study is developed in Walker, L. O. (1971). *Nursing as a discipline.* Unpublished doctoral thesis, Indiana University, Bloomington.

Ellis, R. (1971). Reaction to Walker's article. *Nursing Research, 20*, 493–494.

Folta, J.R. (1971). Obfuscation or clarification: A reaction to Walker's concept of nursing theory. *Nursing Research, 20*, 496–499.

Peirce, C.S. (1958). In P. Wiener (Ed.). *Values in a universe of chance; selected writings of Charles S. Peirce.* New York: Doubleday Anchor.

Rogers, M.E. (1963). Some comments on the theoretical basis of nursing practice. *Nursing Science, 1*, 11–13.

Spring, F. E. (1969). *Man: A holistic conception for nursing (Pilot project final report).* Cleveland: Francis Payne Bolton School of Nursing, Case Western Reserve University.

Walker, L. O. (1971). Toward a clearer understanding of the concept of nursing theory. *Nursing Research, 20*, 428–435.

Wooldridge, P.J. (1971). Meta-theories of nursing: A commentary on Dr. Walker's article. *Nursing Research, 20*, 494–495.

The Author Comments

Prior to receiving the page proofs of the commentaries published in the November-December (1971) issue of *Nursing Research*, I did not know that the editor, Lucille Notter, had invited criticism of my article, "Toward a Clearer Understanding of the Concept of Nursing Theory." After a temporary shock, I was pleased that the article had provoked so much interest and asked Dr. Notter if I might publish a rejoinder. She agreed and I began to try to clarify my initial ideas and rebut the criticisms. I was surprised to find how much I enjoyed the chance to seriously interact (in print) with others about such an esoteric topic. It was a peak experience, and I thank Lucille Notter for having made it possible. I hope that nurses reading these articles from the three issues of *Nursing Research* (September-October, 1971 through January-February, 1972) can catch the excitement and energy we all experienced in those early struggles to understand the theoretical base for nursing.

—LORRAINE O. WALKER

Chapter 5

Theory, Practice, and Research in Perspective

Lorraine Olszewski Walker

Attempting to place theory, practice, and research in perspective is no small task! Although many nurses act as if theory, practice, and research are totally independent activities, it is uncommon to find someone who actually admits to holding such a belief. Instead, the more usual pattern is to find numerous affirmations of the intimate relations that prevail between and among theory, practice, and research. Thus, theory leads to research; research leads to practice; and so on the pious chants go. Today, I invite you to look with me beyond the rhetoric and incantations to see whether relations do exist, and if so, to attempt to make these more precise.

In a nutshell, I would like to look in serial fashion at the relationships that obtain, or do not obtain, between theory and practice, practice and research, and research and practice. I will do this sometimes from a philosophic perspective and sometimes from a practical perspective. I will attempt to indicate which viewpoint I am using in order that you may be tuned in to what game I am playing and what rules I am following. In addition, if there are any germane conceptual gaps or issues pertinent to theory, practice, or research, I will try to work these in throughout the paper.

Theory and Practice

Let us turn first to a consideration of theory and practice. One of the problems in trying to reach any agreement on how these two concepts interact is that "theory" has a wide range of meanings in nursing literature and is frequently defined in a broader way than in the basic sciences. Both of these factors leave one with a rather amorphous conception of what "theory" means in nursing. Simply for purposes of illustration, let us look at what Ellis said about theory, since she is one of the writers who has taken the time to clarify her notion:

This paper was presented at the American Nurses' Association Ninth Nursing Research Conference, San Antonio, Texas, March 21–23, 1973. Reprinted by permission of the author.

By "theory" I mean a coherent hypothesis, or set of hypotheses, or a concept, forming a general framework for undertaking something. Theory means a conceptual structure built for a purpose. For nursing, that purpose is practice. (Ellis, 1969, p. 1434)

Contrast this notion of theory with one put forth by Rudner: "A theory is a systematically related set of statements, including some lawlike generalizations, that is empirically testable" (Rudner, 1966, p. 10). Noticeably absent from Rudner's definition is any mention of to what purpose theorizing is aimed. Presumably, this is because in the sciences theory is implicitly aimed at description, explanation, and prediction—as it is these purposes with which the game of science concerns itself. In comparing these two uses of "theory," it seems clear that Ellis will let more count as theory than Rudner. While Rudner counts as theory systematically related (i.e., deductively related) sets of statements, Ellis will accept hypotheses, which presumably will take the form of statements, as well as individual concepts as long as these serve to form a "general framework for undertaking something" (Ellis, 1969, p. 1434). The openness of Ellis's description of theory would seem to allow metaphors, models, and other heuristic conceptions to be counted as theory. In addition to its broadness, Ellis's notion of theory in the field of nursing seems to have another difficulty. In pointing out that in nursing, theory is for the purpose of practice, Ellis seems to overlook the possibility that in nursing, theory may have the same aim as in any other science, i.e., to describe, explain, and make predictions about events occurring in the universe of discourse of the theorist.

I would like temporarily to skirt the issue of whether theory in nursing is for the sake of practice or for the sake of description and explanation, i.e., understanding, and merely indicate that within this presentation I am opting for a tighter use of "theory" more in line with its conventional use in the sciences.

Now, on to the relationship of theory and practice. Several commonly held beliefs in this area need to be examined: (1) that theory guides practice, (2) that practice is a source of theory, and (3) that practice tests theory. Let us start with the idea that theory guides

practice. It is the nature of the guidance that seems to be problematic. Dickoff and James (1968), for instance, have seen theory as prescribing actions to be performed to bring about certain goals. Theory guides in this viewpoint by literally telling one what to do. However, Dickoff and James belong to the set that use the notion of theory in a broader way than is intended in this presentation. Thus, their notion of the relation of theory to practice needs to be pushed back one step to what they have called "descriptive theory." How then does descriptive theory guide practice? Or, to put it in Dickoff and James's terms, how does descriptive theory guide the development of situation-producing theory? In my estimate, the mechanism for moving from descriptive theory to situation-producing theory has never been made adequately clear. Simply describing the components of situation-producing theory does not explain how one moves from the theoretical level to the practical level.

Ellis also has contributed some insights into other complexities involved in explaining how theory guides practice in nursing:

. . . The practitioner cannot just select from a rack of ready-to-wear theories, because the knowledges and theories as we find them in the basic sciences are insufficient for practice. Instead, nursing practice requires that she structure converging, and sometimes conflicting, facts from many fields which produce knowledge about human beings. (Ellis, 1969, p. 1434)

Further, because we attempt to nurse the individual, general theories cannot suffice. General theories of human behavior describe the typical or the norm, not the exception or the individual. Or sometimes, they describe the extremes and not the middle range.

As one moves from general theories about human behavior to those relevant to all of the helping professions, and then to those relevant to patient behavior, there is need for an increasing number of conditional statements. What applies is shaped by the context, roles, and, for patients, the physical status that presents.

Related to this is the fact that the professional can encounter conflicting theories, with each supported by some evidence. If she is to take some action she must choose a theory, either consciously or not, for her action is not independent of history; it stems from some framework.

The practitioner who follows a practice based on theory must appraise and criticize the theory if she follows it in nursing patients. She must weigh the risks and benefits in a manner not required of the scholar who theorizes about a phenomenon in the specific or in general, but who does not treat the individual. (Ellis, 1969, pp. 1434–1435)

And finally, Ellis says:

It is the professional practitioner who is able to criticize the theory in use, and determine its value for directing actions to achieve defined outcomes. In this she is not only a *user* of theory, but she may be a *modifier* as well. She is also a *chooser* of theory. (Ellis, 1969, p. 1435)

Although I disagree with Ellis as to whether practitioners are generally able to do the things she asks, her description of the dilemmas involved in moving from theory to practice are quite accurate. Ellis surely highlights that moving from theory to practice is not a passive affair like ironing an appliqué on a pillow case. Whoever the middle man is between theory and practice, he is not only a user, but also a chooser and a decision-maker. This would seem to hold true both for theories used from the "basic" sciences, as well as for so-called nursing theories, for the latter might be just as conflicting and abstract as the former.

In order to deal with the dilemma that theory guides practice on the one hand, and on the other hand is frequently inappropriate or inconclusive for guiding practice, I would like to present a conception that I have found helpful. This is the conception that the theory-practice relationship is mediated through a process of practice development in which generalizations are fitted into contextual circumstances. Practice development stands as a distinct activity between theorizing and practicing. Let us look at each of these activities separately for a moment.

The end product of theorizing is a body of statements taken to be true on the basis of evidence. These statements are typically highly general in nature and hold true when all extraneous contextual factors are held constant.

Practicing, as Ellis (1969) has pointed out, is not only dealing with the individual, but dealing with him or her in a context. There are thus lots of pertinent client variables, context variables, as well as practitioner variables. In addition, there is a need to operationalize theory in terms of some particular set of techniques, and perhaps hardware, before it may be "applied" to practice. To use the words of E.S. Maccia, who introduced me to the concept of practice development, ". . . in order for . . . [theory] to be the source of practicing power it must be in a useful form . . ." (Maccia, 1968, p.25).

Practice development is a complex affair that requires knowledge of a wide range of things. Let me list several: (1) an understanding of theories relevant to the particular area of practice with which one is working, (2) knowledge of significant contextual factors that might affect the outcome of practices developed, and (3) an understanding of materials and resources that might have potential use in a particular set of practices. In addition to these kinds of knowledge, practice development would seem to require that mystical thing called "creativity." This is because these knowledges do not spell out any one concrete piece of hardware or techniques, but leave application an open-ended process. You cannot logically deduce a Skinner-box from theory! Consequently, from one developer to another, there may be subtle and sometimes striking differences in practices developed for a particular clinical situation. Some of these differences would also be accounted for through different theoretical bases used, different materials selected, and differing estimates of what constitute significant contextual factors.

Before moving away from this idea, I would like to note that theorizing or theory development, practice development, and clinical practicing are three distinct activities because they are governed by different sets of norms and different goals. Theorizing is aimed at providing understandings and is guided by norms that facilitate explanation, that is, simplicity, explanatory power, fruitfulness, consistency, and so on. Practice development is aimed at facilitating clinical practice so it is governed by such norms as cost, feasibility, and effectiveness in bringing about desired outcomes. Clinical practicing is aimed at aiding particular clients with needs as they are identified. Let me hasten to point out that although the activities are distinct in nature, this does not preclude that some individual might be involved in each of the activities in fairly close sequence; the difficulty with being involved simultaneously with theorizing, developing practices, and practicing is not a logical one, but a practical one!

One related issue that I would like to spend a few moments on is the idea that theory exists for the sake of practice. To quote Dickoff and James:

> The major contention here is that all theory exists finally for the sake of practice . . . and that nursing theory must be theory at the highest level since the nursing aim is practice or else nursing is no longer a profession as distinct from some mere academic discipline. (Dickoff & James, 1968, p. 199)

Inasmuch as in this case Dickoff and James are addressing themselves not only to situation-producing theory, but also to descriptive theory, they are articulating a view commonly expressed in the nursing literature. Inasmuch as I presume that this view addressed itself to theory in the tighter sense I have opted for here, the issue goes beyond a merely verbal disagreement about what theory is. In response to the view, it seems that the most immediate practice for which theory would exist would be the practice of theorizing itself, in that the manifest purpose of theory is the description and explanation of a set of events, taken by a discipline as problematic. In addition, while the end of theoretical inquiry may become in turn a means to practice development, the instrumental nature of theory in the practice context does not warrant the short-circuiting of the end of theoretical inquiry by tying it to practice. Such a short-circuiting is not warranted, for it would seem to jeopardize the goal of inquiry by tying it to immediate practical payoff, and thus block the development of a more adequate product of inquiry whose practical relevances might not be obvious at the moment. This would seem to be the risk taken when Dickoff and James choose "output for nursing practice" as the "relevant measure of the goodness of theorizing" (Dickoff & James, 1971, p. 500). In contrast, I would argue that the end of theoretical in-

quiry is the development of a theory that adequately describes and explains the events taken by the theorist as problematic, and consequently provides understanding of these events. This is not at all to say that such a theory would be irrelevant to practice development, but merely to say that practice development is not the appropriate norm for judging the adequacy of theory as such.

Practice as a Source of Nursing Theory

Now let us turn to the second belief about the theory-practice relationship: that practice is a source of nursing theory. Conant, for instance, has said, "Theory helps determine practice, but practice is itself essential in developing theoretical concepts in nursing" (Conant, 1967, p. 37). Wald and Leonard have said the following:

> In the present state of the behavioral sciences and nursing, we doubt that the integration of relevant basic sciences into clinical nursing is a viable means of building nursing theory. An alternate that has been overlooked is to begin with practical nursing experiences and develop concepts from an analysis of that clinical experience, rather than to try and make borrowed concepts fit. (Wald & Leonard, 1964, p. 310)

Claims of this nature may be placed in the larger context of questions related to the logic of discovery. By logic of discovery I mean, roughly, methods for developing new hypotheses and theories. This is to be contrasted with the logic of justification, which deals with the canons followed in substantiating theories and hypotheses by the use of empirical evidence. The most common conception of a logic of discovery in nursing seems to fall into the category of induction. However, Hempel has noted:

> There are . . . no generally applicable rules for induction by which hypotheses and theories can be mechanically derived or inferred from empirical data. The transition from data to theory requires creative imagination.

Scientific hypotheses and theories are not derived from observed facts, but *invented* in order to account for them. (Hempel, 1966, p. 15)

Induction, as a proposed method of discovery, has the added *logical* difficulties of failing to account for the selecting principles that, in effect, render data to the category of data. Also, it does not account for the move from merely observing data to putting forth conceptualizations that organize data. This logical rejection of induction as a method of discovery is not to be confused, however, with the fact that some people do, *in fact,* theorize better in the midst of data. Such empirical observation that some theorists produce when confronted with data only, in my estimation, sets out their personal conditions for creativity and does not support induction as a logic of discovery. Nor would the fact that some theorists report that they theorize by induction warrant the assumption that they therefore have reasoned to their discoveries in this manner.

From whence, one may ask then, do these insights come? One suggestion put forth by Peirce and further explicated by Maccia is the notion of retroduction. This is not simply another name for induction, but postulates that in addition to being confronted with data, the inquirer adopt "a point of view that would resolve the wonder arising from pondering phenomena or objects" (Peirce, 1958, p. 14). Maccia has explicated retroduction in terms of the use of models to develop theory. In attempting to conceptualize a given set of events, the inquirer uses a model as the point of view for developing theory. The model acts much as an analogy in that the model is represented in the theory although it is not the same as the theory (Maccia, 1963). The repertoire of models available to a theorist is, of course, limited by experience and the ability to exploit that experience. A classic example in point is Kekule's (1890) dream of the circle of snakes, which led him to hypothesize the structure of benzene. The use of retroduction as a method of theory development does not guarantee, however, that the theory developed will correspond to subsequent evidence used to test it. Unfortunately, there is no theorizing without risk. Sometimes the risks produce great successes, other times, glaring failures.

Practice as a Test of Theory

The third view about the theory-practice relationship asserts that practice tests theory. One difficulty with this view is that it is never clear which ballpark one is in when someone puts forth this view because of the ambiguity of the term "theory." Since the use of "theory" in this presentation has been delimited, the statement that practice tests theory will be examined from that viewpoint of "theory." Note further that I am taking this statement to mean that practice itself is the test of theory, and not clinical research done in practice settings.

The difficulties with this view are in general more practical than logical. They seem to fall into two categories: *credibility* problems and *feasibility* problems. The credibility problems are largely due to being able to know and being able to control what happens in the practice context. Thus, one may be uncertain as to what has transpired in the clinical situation when one is not present and how what happened may affect outcomes obtained. The problems of control are certainly also perplexing. Extraneous events may affect the amount of manipulation of variables a practitioner is able to achieve, unanticipated and anticipated confounding variables may not be controllable, and biases may unwittingly enter in both in terms of the population sampling and the practitioner. The outcome of all these control problems is a rather questionable basis from which to attempt to confirm or disprove theory!

Feasibility problems relate essentially to the impinging priorities and lack of resources that limit the ease with which a practitioner may conduct any test of theory where the primary commitment is to practice. Simple availability of time to carefully carry out a test in practice may be prohibiting. Also, the resources for carrying out the test may not be given in the practice setting. There is also the question of which practitioners are expected to do this testing of theory: associate degree or diploma graduates? baccalaureate graduates? clinical specialists?

I do not mean to give the impression of a hard and fast line between testing theory in practice as opposed to in clinical research in a practice setting, for surely credibility and feasibility problems may limit clinical research, too. The differences are more a matter of degree, but that degree of difference would appear to be a critical one from the perspective of quality of results.

Theory and Research

It would seem appropriate at this point to shift our focus to the relationship between theory and research. Writing on the nature of scientific progress, Causey has said:

> At any given time in a certain field of study . . . there is a stock of well-confirmed and generally-accepted beliefs which I will call the "knowledge" of the field at that time. Some of this knowledge is of particular facts. . . . Some of this knowledge is in the form of general laws. . . . Moreover, it is mistaken to think that this knowledge consists only of descriptions of what is directly observable. . . . For instance, we know the atomic mass of the neutron is 1.00892 ± 0.000003, but this is not known simply by direct observation. (Causey, 1969, p. 22)

The other arm of a field of study is the understanding it offers of the body of knowledge. This understanding is provided by "theory going beyond the body of knowledge" (Causey, 1969, p. 25). In a field such as nursing, knowledge is gained by research, and to some degree, practice. Understanding is gained by theory. A science develops through progress on both of these fronts. Causey further explains the relationship between knowledge and understanding.

> For short periods of time the one can increase without increase of the other, but the two interact in such a way that, if there is not eventually a dual development, then science will begin to stagnate. Fortunately, the invention of a bold new theory points the direction towards new experiments which can lead to increase of knowledge. Conversely, the discovery of new knowledge presents us with new facts and laws to explain, and thus encourages us to develop our current theories further and perhaps to invent new theories. (Causey, 1969, p. 25)

Picking up this thread of the interaction between theory and research in nursing, Brown has said:

> If nurse researchers are to meet the challenge of building a body of nursing theory, we who conduct, promote, support and use nursing research must add new criteria in the analysis and criticism of our own and others' investigatory efforts. Of each research project, we should ask: In what ways and to what extent is this investigation linked to theory? What contribution does this investigation make to a scientific body of knowledge? Is the theoretical framework from one of the basic sciences, an applied science, or, more specifically, nursing theory? (Brown, 1964, p. 111).

In addition to research providing interesting facts to be explained, and theory offering understanding of these facts, research and theory interact in terms of the justification or confirmation of theory. This interaction falls under the old saw that research tests theory. In the confirmation of theory, events that the theory would predict are looked at through a wide range of means that vary among fields of study.

There are two other ways in which theory and research may interact. One of these is in the use of research for the induction of theory. The difficulties with induction from a philosophical point of view have already been treated above in the consideration of induction of theory from practice, so I will not repeat them here except to say that the same difficulties obtain.

The other remaining use of research in relation to theory is in the evaluation of practices based on theory. This is perhaps a less orthodox use of the term "research," and some simply might prefer to call it "evaluation" instead, or perhaps "applied research." The name is not so important as the concept of using systematic ways to evaluate the efficacy of practices developed. Interestingly, in my readings of the nursing literature, research is often seen as contributing to practice through making evaluations of practices developed. Practice itself may also contribute to this evaluation by the questioning of unevaluated practices that have become entrenched in practice. In this respect, nursing is not alone in having inadequately exploited the use of systematic ways to evaluate practices. Feinstein, for instance, has spoken to this problem in the field of medicine. He says:

There are controversies about such routine daily problems as the best way to treat a cold, set a fracture, relieve a backache or deliver a baby. And there are controversies about such major dilemmas as the optimal management of diabetes mellitus, the diet, drugs, or surgery to be used for peptic ulcer, the desirability of rigorous treatment for essential hypertension, the value of anticoagulants in myocardial or cerebral infarctions and the choices of radical surgery vs. simple surgery vs. radiotherapy vs. chemotherapy for cancer. A thoughtful physician who seeks documented data, logical analysis and validated proof to support the various claims in these therapeutic controversies cannot find the evidence. (Feinstein, 1970, p. 849)

There is little consolation in knowing that nursing and medicine are soul mates in this respect.

I would like to close by saying: Let us remain clearheaded in recognizing the distinctions between theory, practice development, practice, and research; yet let us also maximize the contributions that each of these may make to the other.

References

Brown, M.I. (1964). Research in the development of nursing theory: The importance of a theoretical framework in nursing research. *Nursing Research, 13,* 109–112.

Causey, R.L. (1969). Scientific progress. *Texas Engineering and Science Magazine, 6*(1), 22–29.

Conant, L. H. (1967). Closing the practice-theory gap. *Nursing Outlook, 15,* 37–39.

Dickoff, J., & James, P. (1968). A theory of theories: A position paper. *Nursing Research, 17,* 197–203.

Dickoff, J., & James, P. (1971). Clarity to what end? *Nursing Research, 20,* 499–502.

Ellis, R. (1969). The practitioner as theorist. *American Journal of Nursing, 69,* 1434–1438.

Feinstein, A. (1970). What kind of basic science for clinical medicine? *New England Journal of Medicine, 283,* 847–852.

Hempel, C.G. (1966). *Philosophy of natural science.* Englewood Cliffs, NJ: Prentice-Hall.

Kekule, A. (1890). Address before the German Chemical Society. In *Berichte der deutschen chemischen gesellschaft, 23,* 1302.

Maccia, E.S. (1963). Models and the meaning of 'retroduction.' *Construction of Educational Theory Models* (Cooperative Research Project Report No. 1632). Columbus, OH: The Ohio State University.

Maccia, E.S. (1968). *Methodology of educational inquiry.* Unpublished manuscript, Indiana University, Bloomington.

Pierce, C.S. (1958). In P.W. Weiner (Ed.). *Values in a universe of chance.* New York: Doubleday.

Rudner, R.S. (1966). *Philosophy of social science.* Englewood Cliffs, NJ: Prentice-Hall.

Wald, F.S., & Leonard, R.C. (1964). Towards development of nursing practice theory. *Nursing Research, 13,* 309–313.

The Author Comments

This address was given in response to an invitation to present the opening paper at the Ninth Nursing Research Conference held by the American Nurses' Association. (The Council of Nurse Researchers was an outgrowth of this final research conference.) The ideas captured in this presentation are ideas that I still deal with today as a practicing nurse scientist. Basically, the ideas embodied in the presentation boil down to the recognition that there is no quick, easy road to building the nursing science needed for informed nursing practice. What is required is a "good" idea, courage to follow that idea, and then, simply, the discipline to methodically refine and test the idea. This holds true for me whether I am working on a theoretical piece, a research project, or a clinical intervention. Probably the best integration of these three perspectives is in the actual conceptualizing and clinical testing of nursing interventions. Even there though, I find that one must be aware and responsive to the unique "semantics" and "syntax" of theory, research, and practice respectively.

—LORRAINE O. WALKER

Chapter 6

Nursing's Theoretical Evolution

Margaret A. Newman

The need for knowledge which is specific to nursing has been recognized since the beginning of modern nursing. Florence Nightingale wrote:

> I believe . . . that the very elements of nursing are all but unknown . . . are as little understood for the well as for the sick. The same laws of health or of nursing, for they are in reality the same, obtain among the well as among the sick. (Nightingale, 1859, p. 6)

The elements which Nightingale identified and attempted to explicate focused on the environment, nourishment, and observation of the patient and on the interpersonal relationship between the nurse and the patient. Even then, participants in nursing confused knowledge of pathology with knowledge of the laws of health. In her attempt to clear up the confusion, Nightingale explained:

> Pathology teaches the harm that disease has done. But it teaches nothing more. We know nothing of the princi-ple of health, the positive of which pathology is the negative. . . .

> It is often thought that medicine is the curative process. It is no such thing; medicine is the surgery of functions, as surgery proper is that of limbs and organs. Neither can do anything but remove obstructions. . . . Surgery removes the bullet out of the limb, which is an obstruction to cure, but nature heals the wound. So it is with medicine; the function of an organ becomes obstructed; medicine, so far as we know, assists nature to remove the obstruction, but does nothing more. And what nursing has to do, in either case, is to put the patient in the best condition for nature to act upon him. (Nightingale, 1859, p. 74)

Although over a hundred years ago our charge was clear, the direction we have taken in search for nursing knowledge has led us at times away from our responsibility. Only within the past decade have we begun to discover the kinds of information that will assist us in establishing optimal health for man, in sickness and in health.

About the Author

MARGARET A. NEWMAN was born in Memphis, Tennessee, and currently resides in St. Paul, Minnesota. A Professor in the School of Nursing at the University of Minnesota, Dr. Newman has been teaching nursing for more than 25 years; previous faculty appointments include the Pennsylvania State University, New York University, and the University of Tennessee. Dr. Newman has earned three degrees in nursing: B.S.N. from the University of Tennessee (1962); M.S from the University of California, San Francisco (1964); and a Ph.D. in Nursing Science and Rehabilitation Nursing from New York University (1971).

Dr. Newman has always enjoyed mathematics, music, dancing, and art. These interests have influenced her thinking in relation to pattern, movement, time, space, and consciousness. This thinking is reflected in her theory of health, which she has been developing and refining over the past two decades. This theory was introduced in her 1979 book, *Theory Development in Nursing* (Philadelphia: F.A. Davis) and later elaborated more fully in her 1986 book, *Health as Expanding Consciousness* (St. Louis: C.V. Mosby). A chapter on the application of the theory to family health appeared in *Family Health: A Theoretical Approach to Nursing Care* (New York: John Wiley & Sons, 1983). She is currently conducting research on pattern recognition and its application to practice. Asked about her satisfactions in nursing, Dr. Newman commented, "I have always enjoyed the contemplation of the infinite complexity of the human being and questions regarding the meaning of life, health. . ."

In addition to her work in the area of theory development, Dr. Newman is actively involved in other aspects of the nursing profession. She is a Fellow in the American Academy of Nursing and a member of the Nursing Theory Think Tank, and was active on the Nurse Theorist Task Force of the North American Nursing Diagnosis Association. She has been a reviewer for a number of scholarly journals and continues to serve on the review panels for *Advances in Nursing Science* and *Nursing Science Quarterly*. She also serves as a consultant to educators, practitioners, and graduate students throughout the United States and parts of Canada and in various other countries, including New Zealand and Finland.

Historical Development

Throughout most of the past century, the approach to nursing was based largely on medical knowledge. Nurses, taught by physicians, were instructed in what physicians thought they needed to know to carry out the medical regimen for the patient. Even the advent of university education for nurses did not change the approach, for curriculums were organized by medical specialty areas. To some extent, this organizational focus persists today.

Another approach to nursing knowledge has been pursuit of the educational process and method. The earliest opportunities for nurses to pursue graduate education were provided by schools of education. The nursing leaders who were prepared in this way thought that the key to improving the quality of nursing care was in improving nursing education (McManus, 1961). Consequently, the research these nurses pursued related primarily to educational and, to some extent, administrative problems in nursing.

Along with the increase in the number of collegiate programs in the early fifties came a growing awareness on the part of nursing faculty of the need for scientifically based knowledge specific to the nursing process. A major step in directing the attention of nurses to research was accomplished with the publication of the first issue of *Nursing Research* in 1952. One of the purposes of this journal, as stated in the first issue, has been to stimulate research in nursing.

An overview of the categories of research and concerns reported in *Nursing Research* during the past 20 years suggests the trends of nursing's theoretical evolution. (Frequencies reported are based on the major articles of the journal and the first-named author.) The magazine's expansion from an original three-times-a-year publication to its bimonthly status has been accompanied by change both in the quantity of research published and in its content and quality. For example, during the early period, the number of studies that emphasized the role and characteristics of nurses comprised approximately 32 percent of the articles. At the same time, studies relating to the nursing process and the behavior of man accounted for only about 12 percent. Since 1968, although the number of studies emphasizing the functions and characteristics of nurses continued at approximately 24 percent, the number relating to nursing process and the behavior of man has risen to approximately 36 percent.

The change in types of contributors to *Nursing Research* through the years is also indicative of the changes that have taken place in theory development. Whereas 36 percent of the contributors in the 1952–58 period were non-nurses and 26 percent were nurses with doctorates, only 16 percent of the contributors since 1968 have been non-nurses and the proportion of articles contributed by nurses with doctorates has risen to 49 percent.

The large proportion of non-nurse contributors during the early period may explain the bulk of studies on functions and characteristics of nurses. During those years nurses tended to turn to social scientists for help in studying nursing. This approach resulted in restatement of nursing problems as social science questions, with nurses studying nurses, rather than nursing. Wald and Leonard point out that the "pure" scientist was trained to pursue his own discipline and "it might have been expected that he would help nurses develop his discipline rather than nursing practice" (Wald & Leonard, 1964, p. 309).

Approaches to Nursing Theory

Concern about nursing theory, which began to become evident in the early sixties, has received considerable attention since 1968. During this period, three main approaches to the discovery of nursing theory emerged: (1) the "borrowing" of theory from other disciplines with an intent to integrate it into a science of nursing; (2) an analysis of nursing practice situations in search of the theoretical underpinnings; and (3) the creation of a conceptual system from which theories could be derived.

Theory From Other Disciplines

Since 1962, when the federal government started funding the nurse-scientist program to enable nurses to study in other disciplines for the purpose of relating their theory to nursing, the number of nurses who have received doctorates has increased considerably. In exercising the diligence necessary to attain competence in these other disciplines, however, nurses who pursued this type of research preparation have been confronted with a problem in maintaining an intimate relationship with nursing. Although many theories from other disciplines are relevant to nursing, the testing of these theories within the framework of another discipline relates the data more clearly to that discipline than to nursing.

Dorothy Johnson has said that knowledge from the basic sciences is relevant to nursing but that the knowledge needed for nursing practice is incomplete until "we learn to ask . . . nursing questions about events in nature of specific concern to us" (Johnson, 1968, p. 206). One of the purposes of encouraging nurses to obtain research preparation in related disciplines was to provide a means for enlarging the research potential of nursing faculties. Since this purpose has been accomplished to some extent, supporters of this approach to the development of nursing theory are now beginning to recommend the development of doctoral programs in nursing, with the accompanying emphasis on research of nursing questions (U.S. Health Manpower Education Bureau, 1971).

Practice Theory

The second approach, that of analyzing nursing practice in search of conceptual relationships, has gained support since 1968. Wald and Leonard (1964) exhorted nurses to direct their attention toward building knowledge directly from a systematic study of nursing experience. They asserted that nursing is a professional practice rather than an academic discipline and that the purpose of a practitioner-scientist is to study ways to achieve changes—changes in patients' responses to such experience as hospitalization or other health measures. They believed that theory of this type could best be derived from and tested in the actual nursing arena.

One of the problems inherent in an analysis of the nursing situation is the lack of agreement on answers to such questions as: What is nursing? What is the specialized role of the nurse? Only three years ago, at a conference organized for the purpose of synthesizing a theory of nursing, the participants, who were considered leaders in theory development, found these questions stumbling blocks to the advancement of theory basic to nursing (Norris, 1969).

Most recently, in a critique of current nursing theory, Walker begins her discussion with what she considers "the leading question in a science of nursing, that is, What is occurring in nursing?" (Walker, 1971, p. 428). After a century of asking ourselves that question, we are still not much closer to our goal of nursing theory.

A Conceptual System

Much of the confusion about what we should be studying was eliminated, in my opinion, when Rogers (1964) identified the phenomenon which is the center of nursing's purpose: *man.* It sounds simple, yet many a graduate student will attest to the difficulty of reorganizing one's thinking about man in order to consider him a unified being and not as a composite of organs and systems and various psycho-social components. The clear-cut delineation of man as the focus of nursing gave direction for the development of theory that is not just relevant to nursing, but basic to nursing.

Thus, a conceptual framework of nursing theory was born. Confident in her designation of man as the phenomenon which is the focus of nursing's purpose, Rogers reviewed the available literature in an effort to identify basic assumptions regarding man and determined that the following statements could be accepted as true:

• Man is a unified whole possessing his own integrity and manifesting characteristics more than and different from the sum of his parts (wholeness) (Rogers, 1970, pp. 46–47).

• Man and environment are continuously exchanging matter and energy with one another (open system) (Rogers, 1970, p. 54).
• The life process evolves irreversibly and unidirectionally along the space-time continuum (unidirectionality) (Rogers, 1970, p. 59).
• Pattern and organization identify man and reflect his innovative wholeness (pattern and organization) (Rogers, 1970, p. 65).
• Man is characterized by the capacity for abstraction and imagery, language and thought, sensation and emotion (sentience) (Rogers, 1970, p. 73).

On the basis of these assumptions, she proceeded to synthesize a conceptual model of man and from there to formulate some general principles from which theories of man can be derived and tested. The relationship of Rogers' conceptual system to data is shown on Figure 6-1.

Hempel, in emphasizing the importance of developing a system of concepts from which general explanatory and predictive principles can be formulated, points out that "science is ultimately intended to systematize the data of our experience. . . ." (Hempel, 1952, p. 21). He perceives a scientific theory as similar to a complex spatial network: the concepts represented by the knots and the unifying principles represented by the strings. Using this network, the scientist can pro-

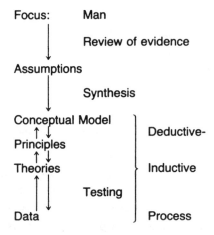

Figure 6-1   *Relationship of Conceptual System to Data*

ceed back and forth in the system to observable data and thereby expand the explanatory power of the system.

Other theorists in nursing have called for a conceptual system from which nursing theory can be derived (Batey, 1971; Brown, 1964). King (1971) has recently proposed four ideas as the conceptual base of the dimensions of nursing: social systems, health, perception, and interpersonal relations. She agrees that the basic abstraction of nursing is the phenomenon of man and his world. The selection of her conceptual base is rooted in her belief that "nurses, in the performance of their roles and responsibilities, assist individuals and groups in society to attain, maintain, and restore health." More specifically, "man functions in *social systems* through *interpersonal relationships* in terms of his *perceptions* which influence his life and *health*" (King, 1971, pp. 21–22). Although on the surface King's system may appear to be quite different from that proposed by Rogers, comparison of statements from the two positions reveals a certain amount of congruity (see Table 6-1).

The principles and postulates identified by Rogers and the premises formulated by King indicate that there

Table 6-1
Comparison of Excerpts From Rogers' (1970) *An Introduction to the Theoretical Basis of Nursing,* and King's (1971) *Toward a Theory of Nursing*

Rogers	King
The principle of reciprocity: The human field and the environmental field are continuously interacting with one another. The relationship . . . is one of constant mutual interaction and mutual change (pp. 96–97). Basic assumption: Man and environment are continuously exchanging matter and energy with one another (p. 54). The principle of synchrony: Change in the human field depends only upon the state of the human field and the simultaneous state of the environmental field at any given point in space-time (p. 98).	The dynamic life process of man involves a constant restructuring of the real world. The transactions . . . that occur in human interactions are an exchange of energy and information within the persons involved (intrapersonal) and between the individual and the environment (interpersonal) (pp. 87–88). . . . thus action results from factors in the situation and in the individual at any point in time (p. 88).
Man is a unified whole possessing his own integrity and manifesting characteristics that are more than different from the sum of his parts (p. 47). The human field possesses its own identifiable wholeness . . . it maintains identity in its everchanging but omnipresent patterning (pp. 90–91).	Man as a composite of mind and body reacts as a total organism to his experiences which are viewed as a flow of events in time (p. 88).
Helicy: . . . the life process evolves unidirectionally in sequential stages . . . is a function of continuous innovative change growing out of the mutual interaction of man and environment along a spiraling longitudinal axis bound in space-time (pp. 99–101).	Time is an irreversible process in the life cycle . . . (p. 88).
Man is characterized by the capacity for abstraction and imagery, language and thought, sensation and emotion (p. 73).	Man is a social being. Through language man has found a symbolic way of communicating his thoughts, actions, customs, and beliefs over time (p. 88).

The principles and postulates identified by Rogers and the premises formulated by King indicate that there is some agreement in the evolving theoretical framework from which hypotheses are being derived and tested and the data therefrom are fed back into the system. The comparisons are by no means complete, either for these two theorists or for other nursing theorists whose formulations may provide additional elaboration of the system. The examples are selected to illustrate that a conceptual system of nursing focused on man is evolving similarly in the minds of nursing theorists and does provide meaningful direction for research. As Rogers (1970) has said, "The science of nursing aims to provide a body of abstract knowledge growing out of scientific research and logical analysis and capable of being translated into nursing practice" (p. 86).

is some agreement in the evolving theoretical frame-work from which hypotheses are being derived and tested and the data therefrom are fed back into the system. The comparisons are by no means complete, either for these two theorists or for other nursing theorists whose formulations may provide additional elaboration of the system. The examples are selected to illustrate that a conceptual system of nursing focused on man is evolving similarly in the minds of nursing theorists and does provide meaningful direction for research. As Rogers has said, "the science of nursing aims to provide a body of abstract knowledge growing out of scientific research and logical analysis and capable of being translated into nursing practice" (Rogers, 1970, p. 86).

The fruitfulness of this conceptual approach to theory development is borne out by the research which has been conceived from ideas based on the wholeness of man's constant interaction with his environment. A series of studies of the effect of the stimulation of total body movement on man have resulted in an evolving theory of movement or motion (Earle, 1969; Neal, 1968; Porter, 1971). Other studies are beginning to outline characteristics of man's spatial and temporal awareness and have implications for his continuous reciprocal interactions with his environment (Felton, 1970; Newman, 1972; Rodgers, 1971; Schlochter, 1971).

Continued exploration of patterns of stimulation are introducing evidence regarding man's capacity for maintaining his pattern in an ever-changing environment. Again, these examples are only a few of the rapidly growing number of studies designed to test the theory of man, with the ultimate purpose of identifying laws regulating this continuous interaction of man and his environment. Knowledge of such laws would then guide nursing practitioners in their goal which is, in essence, to help man achieve his maximum health potential.

Theory of Theories

Proponents of practice theory assert that theory for a profession must go beyond merely describing, explain-

ing, and predicting a particular phenomenon. Dickoff and James (1968) have described four levels of theory: (1) factor-isolating theory (classification); (2) factor-relating theories (situation-depicting); (3) situation-relating theories (predictive); and (4) situation-producing theories (prescriptive). Theory, they assert, must provide conceptualization intended to guide the shaping of reality to a profession's purpose. Situation-producing theory, they believe, incorporates the other three levels of theory and, in addition, prescribes the desired outcome of a situation and the activities necessary to produce that outcome. Inherent in this approach is the assumption that the "desired" outcome can be identified.

Nursing is referred to, from time to time, as a learned profession, an applied science, and a practice discipline—somehow with the connotation that these terms have different meanings. Each of the terms, however, has two components: one which indicates the rigors of scientific inquiry, and another which implies a commitment to service. The development of theory for nursing, therefore, is likely to proceed at more than one level of generalization. At present, nursing theorists are working primarily at the descriptive and predictive levels, but the possibility of a prescriptive level exists.

There now appears to be consensus among nursing theorists that nursing is concerned with assisting man to maintain optimal health throughout his life process. There is also some agreement regarding the conceptual framework of nursing. Whether the theory evolves inductively from ideas conceived in clinical practice or deductively from broad generalizations within the theoretical framework does not seem particularly important. What is important is that the nursing investigator determine the relationship of her study question to the overall conceptual system in nursing and thus expand and elaborate the system by the testing of theories that have derived from it.

Validation of Theory

One of the problems we face in nursing is the need for more valid methods of measuring the variables of our research if we are to learn anything about the reality of the world in which we live. The rigidly controlled experimental studies necessary for baseline studies do not adequately explain the totality of man's interaction with his environment. Field work studies, on the other hand may be of equally questionable validity. If the phenomenon of man's interaction with his environment is to be described, explained, and predicted in such a way that it is applicable to man in his environment, we must continue to seek new methods of measurement.

On the Threshold

Nursing is coming of age. We have established a viable conceptual system—one that provides us with clear, relevant guidelines for theory building and research. We are no longer overly concerned with ourselves as nurses. Concerned with the phenomenon of man, we are beginning to understand man. We no longer are completely dependent on other disciplines for the knowledge of our practice, but neither are we completely independent. We are beginning to realize our own potential for discovering a particular kind of knowledge that is relevant to other disciplines and essential to nursing. The problem of the past has been the dearth of nursing knowledge. The problem of the future will be the acceleration of that knowledge.

References

Batey, M.V. (1971). Conceptualizing the research process. *Nursing Research, 20*, 296–301.

Brown, M.I. (1964). Research in the development of nursing theory. *Nursing Research, 13*, 109–112.

Dickoff, J., & James, P. (1968). A theory of theories: A position paper. *Nursing Research, 17*, 197–203.

Earle, A. (1969). *The effect of supplementary postnatal kinesthetic stimulation on the developmental behavior of the normal female newborn.* Unpublished doctoral dissertation, New York University, New York.

Felton, G. (1970). Effect of time cycle change on blood pressure and temperature in young women. *Nursing Research, 19*, 48–58.

Hempel, C.G. (1952). *Fundamentals of concept formation in empirical science.* Chicago: University of Chicago Press.

Johnson, D.E. (1968). Theory in nursing: Borrowed and unique. *Nursing Research, 17*, 206–209.

King, I.M. (1971). *Toward a theory of nursing.* New York: John Wiley & Sons.

McManus, R.L. (1961). Nursing research—its evolution. *American Journal of Nursing, 61*, 76–79.

Neal, M.V. (1968). Vestibular stimulation and the developmental behavior of the small premature infant. *Nursing Research Report 3*, 3–5.

Newman, M.A. (1972). Time estimation in relation to gait tempo. *Perceptual and Motor Skills, 34*, 354–366.

Nightingale, F. (1859). *Notes on nursing: What it is, and what it is not.* London: Harrison and Sons.

Norris, C.M. (Ed.) (1969). *Proceedings of the First Nursing Theory Conference.* Kansas City, KA: Department of Nursing Education, University of Kansas Medical Center.

Porter, L.S. (1971). Physical-physiological activity and infants growth and development. *American Nurses' Association Seventh Nursing Research Conference.* New York: American Nurses' Association.

Rodgers, J.A. (1971). *The relationship between sociability and personal space preference among college students in the morning and in the afternoon.* Unpublished doctoral dissertation, New York University, New York.

Rogers, M.E. (1964). *Reveille in nursing.* Philadelphia: F.A. Davis.

Rogers, M.E. (1970). *An introduction to the theoretical basis of nursing.* Philadelphia: F.A. Davis.

Schlochter, L. (1971). *The relation between anxiety, perceived body and personal space and actual body space among young female adults.* Unpublished doctoral dissertation, New York University, New York.

Wald, F.S., & Leonard, R.C. (1964). Towards development of nursing practice theory. *Nursing Research, 13*, 309–313.

Walker, L.O. (1971). Toward a clearer understanding of the concept of nursing theory. *Nursing Research, 20*, 428–435.

U.S. Health Manpower Education Bureau. (1971). *Future directions of doctoral education for nurses.* Report of conference held in Bethesda, Md. (DHEW Publication No. NIH 72–82) Washington, DC: U.S. Government Printing Office.

Reactions

"Theory Development," *Nursing Outlook, 20*(10), 630.

. . . Margaret A. Newman's article "Nursing's Theoretical Evolution" is excellent in that she has succinctly identified the highlights in the historical development of nursing theory. Her discussion of three main approaches to discovery of nursing theory should be helpful to graduate faculty and students.

I agree wholeheartedly that there is more "congruity between the King and the Rogers theoretical systems." It is my hope these and other theoretical systems in nursing are widely tested through research during the next decade.

IMOGENE M. KING
Professor, School of Nursing
Ohio State University
Columbus, Ohio

The Author Comments

This article was my first attempt to make sense of what seemed, at that time, to be rather disparate activities of nurse researchers and theorists. I was responsible for a new doctoral seminar on nursing science at New York University. I felt a need for nursing to get its act together for presentation to the students. The conclusions that emerged as I wrote the article surprised me as much as anybody and I was pleased to see the rather orderly progress we were making. It began to dawn on me that nursing was on the frontier of knowledge about the life process and health within a new paradigm of pattern and relatedness. Updates on my thoughts on the emergence of nursing science can be found in the following chapters: "A Continuing Revolution: A History of Nursing Science" in N.L. Chaska (Ed.), *The Nursing Profession: A Time to Speak* (New York: McGraw-Hill, 1983); "Nursing's Emerging Paradigm: The Diagnosis of Pattern" in A.M. McLane (Ed.), *Classification of Nursing Diagnoses* (St. Louis: C.V. Mosby, 1987); and "Nursing Paradigms and Realities" in N.L. Chaska (Ed.), *The Nursing Profession: Turning Points* (St. Louis: C.V. Mosby, 1990). Currently, I am collaborating with Marilyn Sime and Sheila Corcoran-Perry on an article elaborating the focus of the discipline of nursing.

One other note: In rereading this article, I am painfully aware of the masculine orientation of the language. At the time it was written 20 years ago, I was not as enlightened as I am now.

—MARGARET A. NEWMAN

Chapter 7

Perspectives on Nursing Theory

Margaret E. Hardy

In recent years, the discipline of nursing has invested considerable time and effort in developing knowledge about theories, models and conceptual frameworks in order to direct nursing practice and establish the boundaries of its knowledge. Nursing conferences, journals and graduate curricula reflect this interest and concern. Nurses are now asking: What is nursing theory? What theory can nurses use? What is a theory as opposed to a conceptual framework? Although some of us may at times be dissatisfied and impatient at the speed with which these questions are being answered, we can perhaps gain a better understanding of theory development by looking at the total process objectively. Furthermore, the evaluation of nursing theory may be more appropriate and useful if the evaluator is aware of the stages of scientific development.

Stages of Scientific Development

Paradigms and Preparadigms

The dissent and confusion about "what is theory" and "what is nursing theory" may be typical of the early stages of scientific development in any discipline. Kuhn (1970), in *The Structure of Scientific Revolutions*, presents a fascinating thesis on the development of scientific knowledge; some of his points may shed considerable light on nursing's present concern with theory. Kuhn points out that the early stage of scientific development, the preparadigm stage, is characterized by divergent schools of thought which, although addressing the same range of phenomena, usually describe and interpret these phenomena in different ways. Nursing appears to be now in this preparadigm stage.

From Advances in Nursing Science, *October 1978, 1(1), 27–48. Copyright © 1978, by Aspen Systems Corporation.*
Reprinted with permission of Aspen Systems Corporation.

About the Author

MARGARET E. HARDY writes: "My citizenship is Canadian. I imagine that my orientation toward knowledge and university education probably reflect my Canadian values, unbeknownst to me. I was born in Alberta, spent most of my growing-up years in Ottawa, and went to the University of British Columbia in Vancouver to study for my B.S.N. I loved Vancouver—the culture and the general outlook on life. My nursing class was an extremely close-knit group. To the frustration of faculty, typically we were often more interested in the social aspects of university life than the academic, and oddly enough more concerned about the psychosocial problems of patients and their families we were confronted with than was usually considered part of the nursing domain.

I was a public health nurse in Vancouver for several years and enjoyed the independence as well as the responsibility for people in 'my area.' In particular, I enjoyed the community mental health aspect of the work. This work involved case finding at schools and in the community and subsequently, on the basis of an interdisciplinary team evaluation and recommendations, working with these families with socio-emotional (and often economic) problems. Usually the family work was initiated because the youngsters were having problems at school and it was thought the problems were related to their family situation.

My husband and I moved to Seattle to pursue graduate education and were there for 8 years. I was studying at the University of Washington, where I received a M.A. in Community Mental Health Nursing with a minor in Sociology (1965) and a Ph.D. in Sociology (1971). Our weekly trip to the mountains for hiking or skiing (depending on the season) and sailing on Puget Sound counterbalanced the frustration and inactivity of graduate work. This type of outdoor experience tended to provide a great deal of 'think time' in a very special context and probably contributed to the development of my philosophical interests. My husband was in the Physiology department, and the graduate students in that department were a very cohesive group. My early interest and belief in good science was continually reinforced by my friends in this group. I also became very aware of scientific activities in physiology as being quite different from those in sociology. The Sociology Department was strong in research methodology and quantitative analysis. In the Physiology Department, research involved specimens, equipment, computers, and scientists; the department was always busy. In the Sociology Department, work was not evident on a day-to-day basis, as much of the work was done at home. The excitement of doing science was visible only in the Physiology Department.

In 1972, I joined the faculty at Boston University, with a joint appointment in Nursing and Sociology. In the late 1980s, I accepted a faculty position at the University of Rhode Island. My summer mountain hiking, tennis, and bicycling are still survival hobbies. My use of a word processor and home computer is another survival strategy when working with limited support staff and confronted with massive amounts of knowledge that need to be systematized and updated.

My major satisfaction in 'doing' nursing is being involved in the psychosocial aspects of health/illness and doing group work. In the academic setting, I enjoy working with both master's and doctoral students in a seminar or another independent learning situation. I also enjoy doing research and working with data. Currently, I miss not having ongoing contact with a clinical setting and with patients.

In addition to my interest in theory, research, social, and psychological aspects of sociology, medical sociology, and organization, I am interested in feminist knowledge, women and health, sociology of knowledge, and computers. I have worked in the theoretical area of social exchange and am now interested in combining this approach with symbolic interaction. I keep current by involvement in the profession at many levels, including activities in professional sociological organizations, the Nursing Theory Think Tank, Boston Association for Theory Development in Nursing, and the American Academy of Nursing, as well as serving on the editorial boards of *Advances in Nursing Science* and *The International Journal of Women and Health*."

Kuhn challenges the commonly held belief that scientific knowledge advances through slow and steady increments; he proposes that while accumulation of knowledge plays a major role in the advances of scientific knowledge, progress occurs as a result of scientific revolution. Kuhn's model of the development of scientific knowledge may be represented as given in Figure 7-1. In each revolution, a prevailing paradigm with its associated theories, concepts and research methods is overthrown when anomalies in the accumulating data cannot be accounted for. Then a new paradigm with its own theories, concepts and methods, which more fully accounts for the anomalies, replaces the prevailing paradigm. If a paradigm is to prevail in a discipline, it must attract an enduring group of adherents away from competing scientific orientations, and it must be sufficiently open-ended to leave all sorts of scientific problems to solve.

The paradigm of interest in this article is the *metaparadigm.* This is a gestalt or total world view within a discipline; it provides a map which guides the scientist through the vast, generally incomprehensible world. It gives focus to scientific endeavor which would not be present if scientists were to explore randomly.

The metaparadigm is the broadest consensus within a discipline. It provides the general parameters of the field and gives scientists a broad orientation from which to work. A more restricted type of paradigm is the *exemplar.* This paradigm is more concrete and specific than a metaparadigm. A discipline may have several exemplar paradigms which direct the activities of scientists. For example, in the field of social psychology scientists may group according to their agreement on the model of human nature: noble (Maslow), hedonist (Skinner) and cognator (Mead). This discussion of the metaparadigm and the exemplar paradigm will make the reader aware that the two types of paradigms exist, differentiated primarily on their level of abstraction;

a metaparadigm may subsume several exemplar paradigms.

In summary, the metaparadigm or prevailing paradigm in a discipline presents a general orientation or total world view that holds the commitment and consensus of the scientists in a particular discipline. In general the paradigm: (1) is accepted by most members of the discipline, (2) serves as a way of organizing perceptions, (3) defines what entities are of interest, (4) tells the scientists where to find these entities, (5) tells them what to expect and (6) tells how to study them (i.e., the research methods available).

What do paradigms have to do with nursing theory? Kuhn's (1970) discussion of paradigms suggests that the metaparadigm and the exemplar paradigm are endorsed by a discipline and its subgroups because of their scientific-empirical support. The existence of a prevailing paradigm facilities the normal work of science. Research is purposeful, orderly and raises few unanswerable questions.

When a dominant paradigm does not exist, a discipline may be in a crisis situation characterized by competing paradigms or it may be in a *preparadigm* stage with different, ill-defined perspectives that are heatedly argued and defended. In the preparadigm stage of a discipline, there is little agreement among its scientists as to what entities are of particular concern, where to locate these entities or how to study them. Such is the status of nursing today, with energy going into attempts to justify one of several embryonic paradigms rather that into purposeful, orderly research. Confusion prevails as to what exactly nursing should be studying; the research that is conducted is often poorly focused and unsystematic.

Kuhn's theory of paradigms and scientific revolution suggests that the development and evaluation of knowledge in nursing may proceed at a very slow pace, not because nurse-scientists lack the necessary ability to

Paradigm₁ $\longrightarrow$ Normal Science $\longrightarrow$ Anomalies $\longrightarrow$ Crisis $\longrightarrow$ Revolution $\longrightarrow$ Paradigm₂

Figure 7-1 *Process of Scientific Revolutions*

develop empirically-based scientific knowledge but because so much time is being devoted to justifying the various preparadigms. Until there is a prevailing paradigm and exemplar paradigms to give focus to the thinking and work of nurse-scientists, knowledge in nursing will develop slowly and somewhat haphazardly. This leaves the practicing nurse in a difficult position of deciding what knowledge is usable and how it should be evaluated for use.

Nursing as a Preparadigm Science

If Kuhn's conception of science is correct and if nursing is indeed in the preparadigm stage, then the time spent in defending one of the existing nursing conceptualizations (Riehl & Roy, 1974), the present concern with conceptual frameworks, models, theory construction and research methods are all part of an evolutionary process that other disciplines have either experienced already or have yet to face. Although this period of theory development in a discipline is characterized by ambiguity and uncertainty, nurse-scientists can help build the knowledge base that will help formulate an acceptable paradigm. They can do this by being well informed in a substantive area and participating actively in both theory construction and research. Nursing cannot decree that a specific paradigm will be adopted; the adoption of a paradigm will be based on its scientific credence and its potential for advancing scientific knowledge is nursing.

The preparadigm stage of science is one of confusion and frustration, with much dispute over theory, research and frequent factional power struggles. Nurse-scientists who realize this may be able to raise themselves above the battleground and focus their efforts and skills on developing sound nursing knowledge. Their work to solve very specific nursing-care problems may contribute significantly to developing exemplar paradigms and a predominant paradigm in nursing. The predominant nursing paradigm, when developed, will make it possible for other nurses to define more clearly their own "turf" or subject matter. While working on knowledge for practice, nurse-scientists must at present tolerate loosely constructed theoretical notions.

This preparadigm stage of nursing science is difficult not only for those developing theory and research but also for those attempting to evaluate and use nursing knowledge.

The Development of Theory

The Nature of Theory

Before addressing the question of theory evaluation, the term theory must be defined. In common usage, the meaning of theory ranges from a hunch or a speculative explanation to a body of established knowledge. Kaplan (1964), in *The Conduct of Inquiry,* elaborates on the process of theorizing, suggesting that theory formation may well be the most important and distinctive attribute of human being. He does not perceive theorizing as a process removed from experience as opposed to brute fact.

In science, the term *theory* refers to a set of verified, interrelated concepts and statements that are testable. In his discussion of the human ability to develop scientific theory, Kaplan says:

> In the reconstructed logic, . . . theory will appear as the device for interpreting, criticizing, and unifying established laws, modifying them to fit data unanticipated in their formulation, and guiding the enterprise of discovering new and more powerful generalizations. To engage in theorizing means not just to learn by experience but to take thought about what is there to be learned. (Kaplan, 1964, p. 295)

Nurses will do well to remember the vital part that experience plays in theorizing.

Since a theory is a validated body of knowledge about some aspect of reality, it is appropriate that in developing theory nurses should concern themselves with identifying aspects of reality they wish to focus on, developing relevant theory and evaluating the soundness of the knowledge they develop. The scientist, in developing theory, looks for lawful relationships, patterns or regularities in the empirical world. Such relationships between concepts, sets facts or variables are carefully studied in order to identify conditions that modify or alter the original relationship.

Few "theories" in nursing or related disciplines are sufficiently well developed to permit specification of both lawful relationships and the condition under which these relationships vary. One possibility is behavior modification theory, which expresses a lawful relationship between specified behavior and reinforcement. Furthermore, this relationship may alter according to the type of reinforcement schedule employed.

Relationship Between Theory and Practice

Kaplan stresses the interrelatedness of theory and experience. In nursing, scientists and practicing nurses are frequently out of touch with one another. The nurse-scientist is a thinker unconcerned with the practice setting, while the practitioner is a provider of nursing care and is sometimes referred to as a technician. But it is from the practice setting that the nurse-scientist should derive ideas, and it is for the nurse in the clinical setting that ideas are developed. If the nurse-scientist is to be the major developer of theoretical knowledge, the practitioner must be in a position to provide the nurse-scientists with research-worthy problems and, at the same time, must be able to evaluate the knowledge generated for its soundness and applicability. A similar symbiosis has been highly successful in other fields. For instance, the theoretical physicist develops ideas and the engineer applies those ideas for the practical benefit of human beings.

Nursing has a mandate from society to use its specialized body of knowledge and skills for the betterment of humans. The mandate implies that knowledge and skills must grow in such a way as to keep up with the changing health goals of society. Furthermore, nursing must regulate its own practice, control the qualifications of its practitioners and implement *newly developed knowledge*.

The majority of nurses are clearly "doers" or practitioners. However, the discipline must also include scientists dedicated to generating knowledge. These scientists must be committed to finding things out, to obtaining an understanding and explanation of phenomena in their world and to identifying means for controlling significant phenomena. Nursing practice and nursing science, as pointed out earlier, are not antithetical; each depends on the other. It is important that theory be useful and encompass significant concepts and conditions that can be applied and favorably altered in the clinical setting.

Drawing on Work in Other Disciplines

Nursing draws on theories and knowledge from the disciplines of psychology, sociology and physiology. This is entirely legitimate; there is no reason for nurse-scientists to spend years of hard work duplicating knowledge that already exists but is housed in other disciplines. However, theory from another discipline must first be empirically validated to determine if its generalizations are applicable to nursing and its particular problems and needs. For example, generalizations from cognitive dissonance theory should be assessed to see if they can be used by nurses in practice settings; it is conceivable and, in fact likely, that modifications will first be necessary.

A large number of hours has been expended by social scientists in developing empirically based theoretical frameworks on role and social exchange. If nurses and nurse-scientists wish to employ these two sets of knowledge, they will need to determine how, when and where the concepts and empirical generalizations are applicable. In making this evaluation, they are likely to identify conditions unique to nursing practice which alter the social scientists' generalizations; they may also find they need to expand the original theory.

Types of Theory: Grand Versus Circumscribed

If the discipline of nursing is indeed in the preparadigm stage, consideration must be made for the level of theory development. Given a set of criteria for evaluating theory, the evaluator must make a decision as to what can be considered to be theory. A body of knowledge which is in the preparadigm stage cannot be evaluated as rigorously as a theory, nor can formulations which are "grand theories" or philosophies about nursing. They provide neither solid nor practical foundations for nursing practice; they are difficult to evaluate for their scientific value.

A theory in the early stage of development is characterized by discursive presentation and descriptive accounts or anecdotal reports to illustrate and support its claims. The theoretical terms are usually vague and ill defined, and their meaning may be close to everyday language. A paradigm at this embryonic stage is very readable and provides a perspective rather than a set of interrelated theoretical statements. This type of formulation *lacks empirical support*; the empirical illustrations accompanying it are not tests of the theoretical perspective.

This type of formulation, the "grand theory" or "general orientation," is aimed at explaining the totality of behavior (Merton, 1957). Grand theories tend to use vague terminology, leave the relationships between terms unclear and provide formulations that cannot be tested. Examples of grand theory might be Parsons's theory of Social Systems, Rogers's (1970) formulations of nursing theory, crisis theory, and some of the stress formulations. All present unique ways of looking at reality, but their ill-defined terms and questionable linkages between concepts make them impossible to put into operation and test empirically—and testability of a theory is one of the most important conditions a formulation must meet (Gibbs, 1972).

In addressing the problem of grand theories, Merton (1957) makes a plea for scientists to move into the study of partial theories. Since this plea, social scientists seem to have been successful in developing and testing partial or circumscribed theories. These circumscribed formulations may become exemplar paradigms; the move from grand formulations to circumscribed theory may take a discipline from a preparadigm stage to a paradigm stage with exemplar paradigms.

Circumscribed theories focus on selective aspects of behavior such as communication, social exchange, role behavior and self-consistency. In time, these formulations may lead to explication of theoretical terms and hypotheses which can be tested by carefully designed studies. The cumulative research and resulting theory is sound. Of the paradigms developed, one may eventually predominate, several may combine into a new paradigm which will address a larger part of reality, and several may coexist as exemplar paradigms.

The circumscribed theories on which scientists focus may seem irrelevant and unimportant when compared to the complex day-to-day problems confronted by nurses. Yet nurses must recognize that such complex problems cannot be solved quickly—as is evident in the enormous number of hours this country has spent trying to determine what cancer is and how it develops. Complicated scientific problems usually must be broken down into smaller, more manageable parts and tackled one by one. The scientific process for developing knowledge is slow, but it is the only sure one we have.

The norms that guide scientific activities seem to be universal; they are not specific to a discipline or country (Hardy, 1978). These norms include the need for public discourse on knowledge; the need for establishing the validity of scientific work; the need for critical assessment of both theory and research; and the need for empirical, objective work which can be replicated by others. It is in a milieu influenced by these norms that knowledge is generated and theory is developed; thus the outcome of the scientific process, the scientist's major goal, is achieved. If theory application is to contribute to the advancement of knowledge and to the professional code of ethics, nurse-scientists must adhere to these norms when developing knowledge.

Evaluation of Theory

Scientists have a variety of criteria for assessing knowledge. They examine their theories for explanatory and predictive power, for parsimony, generality, scope and abstractness (Hage, 1972; Hardy, 1978). For nurse-scientists, there is also a subset of criteria relating to the application of a particular theory in clinical practice. The following questions might be asked for such a theory: Is it internally consistent or *logically adequate*? How sound is its *empirical support*? Does the theory present concepts and conditions which the nurse can actually *modify*? Can the theory be used in bringing about *major, favorable changes*?

Logical Adequacy (Diagramming)

Since a theory is a set of interrelated concepts and theoretical statements, its structure can be analyzed for internal consistency or logic (Hardy, 1978; Rudner, 1966). This involves examining the syntax of the theory rather than its content. If the structure is inconsistent or illogical, then empirical testing may not provide a test of the theory itself but only of unrelated or loosely related hypotheses.

One method for examining a theory's internal consistency involves identifying all the major theoretical terms. These may include constructs, concepts, operational definitions or referents. Once identified, each term can be represented by a symbol. Use of symbols serves to decrease the evaluator's bias and thus lessens the likelihood that substantive meaning will be attributed to the theory when it is not present.

The next step is to identify the relationships or linkages between terms. The linkages are usually expressed as follows: direction, type of relationship (positive or negative) and form of relationship (Hage, 1972). Symbols are used to signify the linkages; if the theory does not specify a linkage, this will become obvious as the structure of the theory is diagrammed.

To illustrate this process, consider the statement "high role conflict experienced by a person results in less communication with coworkers" and the statement "frequent communication with coworkers is associated with job satisfaction." The structure of these two statements would then be as shown in Figure 7-2. Diagramming these statements shows clearly that there are no contradictions in the specified linkages, and that there is no link specified between role conflict and satisfaction. This type of diagramming makes it possible to identify gaps, contradictions and overlaps. Linkages between constructs, concepts and operational definitions can also be diagrammed. (See Figure 7-3.) Diagramming a theoretical formulation will clearly show whether the hypothesis to be tested flows logically from the more abstract theoretical statements.

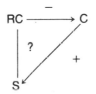

RC = role conflict
C = communication
S = satisfaction
+ = positive linkage
− = negative linkage
? = unspecified linkage

Figure 7-2 *Typical Linkage Diagram*

Empirical Adequacy

Empirical validity is perhaps the single most important criterion for evaluating a theory which is to be applied in a practice setting. However, a theory cannot be empirically valid if it is logically inadequate. Many theories are proposed but only a few are testable. Unfortunately, it is all too easy to select a theory which seems plausible or fits our own belief system and then use it in teaching students and working with patients. Among others, popular theories which have such questionable empirical support are psychoanalytic theory, crisis intervention theory and Erikson's theory of developmental crisis.

Assessment of Empirical Support

Assessing the empirical support for a theory is a rigorous but exciting puzzle-solving activity which involves several independent but closely related steps. Suppose an individual is planning to go to a major theoretical work and attempt to identify the key theoretical terms and the linkages between them. This process is identical to the processes used in determining the internal consistency of the theory, and a linkage diagram is used. When the individual has diagrammed the theory and identified predictions and hypotheses, it is necessary to examine the empirical support which actually exists. This requires going to the literature and identifying related studies.

After the pertinent studies have been reviewed, they may be classified according to the strength of their

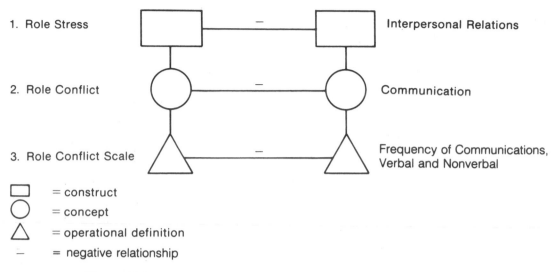

1. Role Stress

Interpersonal Relations

2. Role Conflict

Communication

3. Role Conflict Scale

Frequency of Communications,
Verbal and Nonverbal

☐ = construct
○ = concept
△ = operational definition
— = negative relationship

Figure 7-3 *Linkage Diagram Showing Relationships Between Terms**

research methodology and the empirical support given to the hypotheses tested. Care must be taken in judging which studies represent valid empirical tests of the theory. Case studies, anecdotal reports or descriptions of processes presented in discursive accounts of the theory do not constitute empirical tests. Such accounts are generally presented to give the reader the feeling that the theory is plausible and congruent with life events. This type of material may, however, be used to assess the theory's potential scope and generality.

It should not be forgotten that researchers usually have vested interests in their studies and may have introduced biases that alter the interpretation of the findings. During the critical reading, a study's hypotheses and their empirical referents may be diagrammed, as may the empirical relationship found between the concepts. The congruence between theoretical predictions and empirical outcomes can then be readily assessed in a relatively objective manner.

Factors to Consider

In evaluating research, possible changes in meaning of terms and concepts should be kept in mind. For example, in the literature of the 1950s on therapeutic communication theory, the concept of negative feedback may have been defined as derogatory (negative) communication, while in the 1970s, negative feedback has been redefined to mean any communication that alters (increases or decreases) the communication of the other person.

In analyzing a theory and its empirical support, it is necessary to determine that the hypotheses tested are clearly deduced from the theory. If they are not, the research is not testing that theory. In examining theoretical terms and their corresponding operational definitions, one's immediate concern is with the validity of the operational definitions. A theory may be logically sound—the hypotheses may follow clearly from it and be stated in a form that can be confirmed or rejected—but if the operational definitions do not reflect the meaning of the theoretical concepts, the research is not really addressing the theory and results will have limited or no bearing on it.

To complete the assessment, the entire body of relevant studies must be evaluated in terms of the extent to which it supports the theory, or some part of the theory. This assessment should result in a decision as to whether empirical support is sufficient to warrant the theory's application. The absolute necessity for determining the empirical adequacy of a theory cannot be overemphasized. If nurses are taught "theories" that have little or no empirical support, the nursing care interventions based on such "theories" may have deleterious effects on clients who believe in the nurse's skill, expertise and competence. And indeed there has been a tendency to base nursing actions on tradition, intuition and conceptual frameworks which seem sound but have not been empirically tested. Though they may be creative and may give nurses a sense of security in what they do, these sources of knowledge remain in the realm of myth and nonscientific knowledge.

For example, even if a conceptual framework for crisis intervention makes intuitive sense to a nurse, using it as a basis of action when it does not have sound empirical support is a serious error in judgment and one that has considerable ethical implications. There is a need to develop and use empirically sound scientific knowledge if nursing is to retain its reputation as a profession. And the process of evaluating a theory empirically should be shared with students since they, as practicing nurses, should carry out this same process for the remainder of their nursing careers.

Usefulness and Significance

Since nursing is an applied profession, it follows that relevant theories are those which nurses may use in the clinical setting. After a theory has been identified as having internal consistency and strong empirical support, can it actually be put to use by a nurse? The theory is *useful* to the degree that the practitioner is able to control, alter or manipulate the major variables and conditions specified by the theory to realize some desired outcome. Knowing multiple sclerosis is caused by a virus that lies dormant in a person for 30 years does not provide nurses with a basis for immediate intervention. On the other hand, the awareness of the empirical association between smoking and both lung cancer and heart disease allows the nurse to manipulate variables that can decrease the occurrence and severity of these diseases. Here theoretical knowledge is useful. Inhaling carcinogens from cigarettes is an activity over which the nurse can exert some influence, either through per-

suading individual patients not to smoke or by assisting in more general public education efforts.

Related to the usefulness of a theory is its *significance*. Given two theories which are internally consistent, have strong empirical support and encompass variables that the nurse is able to modify, what else should influence the choice of which theory to use? Assuming that both are focused on the same nursing problem, presumably the nurse would act on the one which would bring about the *strongest, most favorable outcome*. Take, for example, psychoanalytic theory and behavioral modification theory, both of which may address the problem of obesity. Although one theory addresses the childhood origins of obesity and the other the environmental factors influencing overeating, both can be used to assist patients to lose weight. However, behavior modification appears to bring about more major and enduring changes in eating habits. In this example, no comparison is being made of the internal consistency of empirical support of the two theories; the point is to illustrate the efficacy of one theory over another in achieving desired behavioral outcomes.

Nursing as a health profession and as a scientific discipline has come a long way, but it still has much to achieve. As a discipline, it needs to struggle through and beyond the preparadigm stage of scientific development. This will entail challenges and risks, but the process should help create a corps of nurse-scientists able to develop knowledge which reflects sensitivity to problems in clinical practice, and a corps of their clinical counterparts capable of evaluating and using this knowledge.

References

Gibbs, J. (1972). *Sociological theory construction.* Hinsdale, IL: Dryden Press.

Hage, J. (1972). *Techniques and problems of theory construction in sociology.* New York: John Wiley & Sons.

Hardy, M. (1978). Perspectives on theory. In M. Hardy & M. Conway (Eds.). *Role theory: Perspectives for health professionals.* New York: Appleton-Century-Crofts.

Kaplan, A. (1964). *The conduct of inquiry.* New York: Chandler Press.

Kuhn, T. (1970). *The structure of scientific revolutions* (2nd ed.). Chicago: University of Chicago Press.

Merton, R. (1957). The bearing of sociological theory on empirical research. In R. Merton (Ed.). *Social theory and social structure.* New York: Free Press.

Riehl, J., & Roy, C. (1974). *Conceptual models for nursing practice.* New York: Appleton-Century-Crofts.

Rogers, M.E. (1970). *An introduction to the theoretical basis of nursing.* Philadelphia: F.A. Davis.

Rudner, R. (1966). *Philosophy of social science.* Englewood Cliffs, NJ: Prentice-Hall.

Reactions

Advances in Nursing Science, 1(3), viii–ix.

To the Editor:

. . . I would like to have Margaret Hardy's explanation, description, or definition of paradigm as a concept before she gives us examples of two classes of paradigms. Incidentally, I found her article most thought provoking and significant. . . .

BETTY D. PEARSON, R.N., Ph.D.
Associate Dean
Graduate Program in Nursing
School of Nursing
The University of Wisconsin
Milwaukee, Wisconsin

Response: *Advances in Nursing Science, 2*(3), viii–x.

To the Editor:

This letter is in response to Dr. Betty Pearson's letter. . . . Kuhn's term "paradigm" is central to my article "Perspectives on Nursing Theory" (*Advances in Nursing Science, 1*(1), 37–48). The term paradigm has been used frequently and with a wide variety of meanings by Kuhn (1962, 1970) as he developed his ideas on the growth of scientific knowledge. Although the term paradigm is central to his work, he left it undefined. He does say that the established usage of the term—meaning model or pattern—is not his usage (Kuhn, 1972, p. 23).

Masterman (1970), in an analysis of Kuhn's original work in 1962, identifies paradigm as being used in at least 21 different senses. Masterman clusters these 21 different meanings of paradigm into three groups. One of these, the metaphysical or metaparadigm, is the only type of paradigm that Kuhn's philosophical critics have referred to (Masterman, 1970, p. 65) and it is the type of paradigm central to my ANS 1:1 article. From this article I would like to quote what I consider to be a general definition of a metaphysical or metaparadigm.

> The . . . metaparadigm . . . is a gestalt or total world view within a discipline; it provides a map which guides the scientist through the vast, generally incomprehensible world. It gives focus to scientific endeavor . . . . The metaparadigm is the broadest consensus within a discipline. It provides the general parameters of the field and gives scientists a broad orientation from which to work. (Hardy, 1978, p. 38)

This definition of paradigm as a gestalt, cognitive orientation or general perspective that has broad consensus within a discipline is based on several descriptive phrases used by Kuhn. Here I will cite phrases referring to the gestalt nature of paradigm. In a recent paper (Hardy, 1979), I focus on the significance of a paradigm having consensus within a discipline. Kuhn (1962), for example, refers to paradigm as a set of beliefs, as a successful metaphysical speculation, as a standard, as a way of seeing, as an organizing principle overriding perception itself, as a map, and as something that determines a large area of reality. Masterman points out that Kuhn's metaparadigm is neither "basic theory" nor a "general metaphysical viewpoint" (Masterman, 1970, p. 61). The metaparadigm is far broader than scientific theory and is prior to it. It is an idealogic, philosophic, and cognitive entity that has gained the consensus of scientists in a discipline.

In response to Dr. Pearson's request, I have gone to considerable length in quoting both Kuhn and Masterman. I have done so because philosophy is not my field of specialization and those with more expertise in this area may make different inferences than I, and secondly, because I think that the meaning of metaparadigm is not easy to grasp, particularly for those of us who are heavily steeped in the tradition of scientific theory, hypothesis testing, and research. Finally, I think it is an important concept for those of us in nursing who are attempting to identify nursing knowledge as opposed to knowledge in the basic and social sciences.

MARGARET E. HARDY, Ph.D.
Boston, Massachusetts

REFERENCES

Hardy, M.E. (1978). Perspectives on nursing theory. *Advances in Nursing Science, 1*, 37–48.

Hardy, M.E. (1979, April). *Paradigms as tools for structuring the professional science of nursing.* Paper presented at the 1979 Rozella M. Schlotfeldt Lectureship, Case Western Reserve University, Cleveland.

Kuhn, T. (1962). *The structure of scientific revolutions.* Chicago: University of Chicago Press.

Kuhn, T. (1970). *The structure of scientific revolutions* (2nd ed.). Chicago: University of Chicago Press.

Masterman, M. (1970). The nature of paradigm. In I. Lakatos & A. Musgrave (Eds.). *Criticism and the growth of knowledge.* London: Cambridge Press.

The Author Comments

I started to teach the two doctoral-level theory courses at Boston University around the mid-1970s and used Kuhn's *The Structure of Scientific Revolutions* in the second course. Some of Kuhn's ideas seemed to provide a context for understanding the confusion that existed in the minds of the students. The nature of nursing doctoral programs, courses, and examinations relative to other disciplines made sense if the notion of preparadigm was introduced as an explanatory idea. The "nursing theories" became more comprehensible when considered within the same framework. The notion that science is a developmental process and that doctoral education is going to reflect the state of development seemed plausible and comprehensible to students. They were very excited about the readings—many "aha!" experiences occurred in class as we explored Kuhn's ideas.

By coincidence, I had a phone call immediately following the above class, asking whether I would be interested in participating in a NLN program on theory. Still on a "high" from the class discussions, I volunteered to talk on the topic of metaparadigms. Later, I was asked by Peggy Chinn whether the paper could be published in the first issue of *Advances in Nursing Science*.

I think it is germane to note that I find my thinking and idea generation stimulated by teaching. I find student seminars exciting—many of my ideas and the direction my ideas take come from needs and questions of students, during preparation for class, and, of course, during class itself. I find graduate seminars a very exciting forum for idea identification and development. I am still not a professor who can pull out last year's class folder and teach on the basis of last year's notes. I find I have to become actively engaged in reading and thinking about, at a minimum, the very same material assigned to students. This is a time-consuming process, but well worth it. It is the reworking of class material that takes me into new related readings and keeps me actively thinking. I find the ideas of students insightful and very stimulating.

I still have a strong aversion to "unprepared" professors who focus primarily on "group process." I have a strong commitment to create a challenge and a climate for learning graduate-level thinking and for scholarship among nursing students. I frequently say to the master's-level students in my role theory course that I am never certain whether "watered-down" books, abbreviated bibliographies, and page-limited assignments reflect a belief that nurses cannot deal with actual scientific knowledge per se, a belief that women either cannot handle and make use of this knowledge or will not be in the workplace long enough to invest in their learning on a level with males, or a belief that knowledge in the social sciences is well established and easy to acquire. In any case, the individual nurse and the nursing profession likely will be severely handicapped in the health science marketplace by such quasi-graduate level education.

—MARGARET E. HARDY

REFERENCES

Kuhn, T. (1962). *The structure of scientific revolutions.* Chicago: University of Chicago Press.

Kuhn, T. (1970). *The structure of scientific revolutions* (2nd ed.). Chicago: University of Chicago Press.

Unit Two

Nursing Theory: Philosophical Considerations

Unit One was presented as a map with a series of landmarks to guide one in the study of nursing theory. The first landmark, presented in Unit Two, is that of philosophy. This theme will be continued throughout the book with the following landmarks presented in subsequent units: Unit Three—science; Unit Four—structure; Unit Five—practice; and finally, Unit Six—research.

Nurses have always been concerned with the importance of philosophical thinking. Nightingale certainly presents a cogent view of philosophy, tempered by her ever-present pragmatism. In this Unit, eight articles are included that touch on various aspects of philosophical thinking that has occurred in nursing.

Chapter 8, "A Theory of Theories: A Position Paper" by James Dickoff and Patricia James was first presented at the nursing theory symposium held at Case Western Reserve University in 1967. Dickoff and James, philosophers, discussed the type of theory that would be important for a practical discipline such as nursing.

Chapter 9, "Theory in Nursing: Borrowed and Unique" by Dorothy E. Johnson was also a presentation at the Case Western Reserve theory symposium. Johnson presents a clear view of the hazards of borrowed theory and the need for developing a unique nursing perspective to nuture the discipline.

Chapter 10, "ReVisions in Knowledge Development: A Passion for Substance" by Afaf Meleis and Chapter 11, "Structuring the Nursing Knowledge System: A Typology of Four Domains" by Hesook Suzie Kim provide two perspectives on the type of knowledge that can be generated within nursing. Meleis argues for substance and depth in nursing knowledge and Kim provides an interesting counter-point, suggesting a model for the organization of the knowledge thus generated.

Chapter 12, "Philosophical Sources of Nursing Theory" by Barbara Sarter analyzes the roots of nursing theory as presented in the work of four contemporary nursing theorists. This type of analysis is essential to understand where nursing theory comes from in order that it can be used appropriately in practice, education, and research.

Chapter 13, "Theoretical Thinking in Nursing: Problems and Prospects" by Hesook Suzie Kim presents an international influence on nursing theory—Kim acknowledges that many of the ideas she presents took hold during a sabbatical in Oslo, Norway. Likewise, Chapter 15, "Nursing Values and Science: Toward a Science Philosophy" by Susan Gortner also evolved during the author's time abroad. Gortner acknowledges the important influences her international colleagues have had on her thinking. These two articles are representative of the exciting trend in nursing toward a more international focus.

Finally, Chapter 14, "Nursing Theorizing as an Ethical Endeavor" by Pamela G. Reed links the important concept of ethics to nursing theory. Certainly ethical thinking in nursing has always been acknowledged as valuable and important; Reed makes the linkage between this endeavor and theoretical thinking explicit.

It is interesting to note that there is a twenty year gap between the first two chapters in this unit and the remaining eight. This is not to suggest that for twenty years nurses did not think or write about philosophical issues. Throughout this book there are thoughtful essays on all manner of philosophical thinking. But it seems that in recent years, nurse scholars have turned their attention, once again, to the same important philosophical issues that are imperative for the discipline. This unit brings together some of the more diverse and some of the more recent thoughts of scholars that have appeared in the nursing literature of late, as well as some of the very earliest ideas that were presented.

Chapter 8

A Theory of Theories:
A Position Paper

James Dickoff
Patricia James

This paper takes a position on two important issues: first, on the issue of what a theory is; then, on the issue of what a nursing theory should be. Even more fundamentally, the position is taken that the difficulty in identifying and developing nursing theory stems in part from a conceptual muddle as to what theory is in any of its manifestations and also from the tendency in nursing, as in any discipline or individual, to grasp any structural security—even one that vitiates the basic purpose of the individual or discipline—rather than to rest without security or even to bravely fumble toward a more significant security.

The Position in Four Theses

The position taken can be seen in outline through four theses:

1. Theory is a conceptual system or framework invented to some purpose; and as the purpose varies so too must vary the structure and complexity of the system.

2. Professional purpose requires a commitment beyond mere understanding or describing.
3. Significant nursing theory must be theory at the highest level—namely, so-called situation-producing theory.
4. A profession or practice discipline has built-in advantages that facilitate theory development for that discipline.

These four theses will be elaborated and then the third thesis—that significant nursing theory must be theory at the highest level, must be situation-producing theory—will be presented as the thesis most central to the position taken.

What is Theory?

In some nebulous way we all know what theory is. But if we want to deal with theory at close quarters—if we want to develop, criticize, or use theory—then a more explicit awareness or agreement is needed as to what is meant by theory, at least within the context of any given discussion. Our claim is that a real advance in clarity and potential usefulness is made if we view theory in this perspective: A theory is a conceptual system or framework invented to some purpose.

To emphasize theory as a *conceptual* device is to urge careful discrimination of theories and theoretical entities from things or reality, on the one hand, and from the inarticulate and incommunicable mental awareness, on the other hand. Theory is essentially verbalizable and hence communicable; but theory is a structuring proposed as a guide, control, or shaper of reality, and is not itself reality. Things, situations, matters of fact, histories—all these are to be distinguished from conceptual entities that are or go to make up theories. Entities on the conceptual or theoretic level are *concepts, propositions, laws,* and *sets of propositions* (and sometimes the linguistic expression of these conceptual entities). The question of the relation to reality of theoretical entities either in isolation or as systematically interrelated is the question of validation for theories. But, as we will urge later, no such simple-minded notion as isomorphism or mirroring exhausts or even helps much with the question of this relation—particularly in the higher reaches of theory.

Ontologically, then, theory is an entity at the conceptual level. But what is the structure of this "conceptual entity"? Practically speaking, no concept in isolation and rarely any proposition or law in isolation is deemed a theory, though strictly speaking even such single-element systems might be proposed as theories. Speaking most generally, a theory is a *conceptual system or framework.* That is, a theory is a set of elements in interrelation. All elements of a theory are at the conceptual level, but theories vary according to the number of elements, the characteristic kind and complexity of the elements, and the kind of relation holding between or among the theory's elements or ingredients. The factor (or concept) is the simplest element; a proposition or law is a certain relation among concepts. Theory at one level might be a coordinate set of factors or a co-ordinate set of propositions. But theory at its highest level has elements that are not merely coordinate, elements that differ from one another in level of complexity and even some elements that contain whole theories as elements.

A theory, then, is a conceptual system—but a conceptual system invented to some purpose. To emphasize that theory is invented rather than found in, or discovered in, or abstracted from, reality calls attention not only to the conceptual status of theory but also to the necessity for imagination and risk-taking in the proposing of a theory. Reality is not prefactored; and even more obviously, no relation among factors comes automatically noted or automatically labeled.

Although theory is no mere picture of reality, neither is theory an invention that is a mere fancy. Rather, theory is a conceptual system invented to some purpose. And a good theory—or, in perhaps more familiar terms, a true or valid theory—is a theory that in fact fulfills the purpose for which it was proposed or invented. As the purpose of the theory varies, the structure or level of the theory varies—and so also will vary the mode of validating and even of proposing the theory. Theory whose purpose is prediction is the most familiar kind of theory, and the most developed methodology is that for testing the "goodness" of such a theory (or at least of the component elements of such a theory). But the position is taken here that important types of theory are presupposed by predictive theory and that moreover a more sophisticated kind of theory exists within which predictive theory functions as an element of an element of the theory. Nursing theory is of this elaborate kind.

What is a Professional Purpose?

To consider what kind of theory is needed for a professional discipline requires articulating professional purpose. A true professional, as opposed to a mere academic, is action-oriented rather than a professional spectator or commentator. But unlike a mere technician, a professional is a doer who shapes reality rather than a doer who merely tends the cogs of reality according to prescribed patterns. A true professional—as opposed to a mere visionary—shapes reality according to an articulate purpose and in the light of means conceptualized in relation not only to purpose, but also to existing reality. In short, a professional cannot just watch, cannot just do, and cannot just hope or dream.

The position taken here is that a theory for a profession or practice discipline must provide for more than mere understanding or "describing" or even predicting reality and must provide conceptualization specially intended to guide the shaping of reality to that profession's professional purpose.

What Would Constitute a Nursing Theory?

If nursing is a profession, then, the position taken here is that nursing must have an action orientation that aims to shape reality— not in a hit-or-miss manner, but rather through a conception of ends as well as means. This conception of ends and means is based somehow on conceptual awareness deemed adequate to take into account reality in its structure, course, and potential. A proper nursing theory, then, would be a conceptual system invented to serve the requisite purpose. Given the purpose, quite clearly the desired conceptual apparatus is necessarily more elaborate than any merely predictive theory. The position taken here is that nursing theory must be theory at the fourth or highest level—namely, situation-producing theory. Situation-producing theory is called fourth-level theory because it presupposes the existence of three prior levels of theory, whereas predictive theory is a kind of third-level theory.

Situation-producing theory is deemed the highest level of theory because each of the other levels exists in part at least to allow or provide basis for the next level of theory. But situation-producing theory is not as such developed for the sake of producing a theory of more elaborate structural level, but rather for producing or shaping of reality according to the situation-producing theory's conception. In plainer terms, situation-producing theory is produced to guide action to the production of reality. The major contention here is that all theory exists finally for the sake of practice (because in a sense every lower level of theory exists for the next-highest level and the highest level exists for practice), and that nursing theory must be theory at the highest level (because either the nursing aim is practice or else nursing is no longer a profession distinct from a mere academic discipline).

How Could Nursing as a Profession or Practice Discipline Hope to Produce so Sophisticated a Theory?

On the surface, it seems unreasonable to expect that a discipline newly dedicated to producing its own theory should have the capacity to produce a theory whose structural sophistication is necessarily greater than the sophistication of, say, physics, psychology, or biochemistry. But the position taken here is that nursing—like any practice discipline—has certain built-in advantages that could, if properly exploited, facilitate theory development within the discipline. As one level of theory presupposes another, so theorizing itself presupposes prior nontheoretical awareness (and prior activity other than theorizing). The privileged and habitual intercourse with empirical reality carried on in a practice discipline—often within the bounds of rote-like or carefully specified procedures—is a rich source of such preconceptual awareness. In the terms of "the father of empiricism," Francis Bacon, nursing or any profession is richly endowed with so-called "polychrest instances" —i.e., without artifice, a "night watch" can be taken on highly complex phenomena and patterns of behavior and other changes.[1]

Not only is there a privileged and nonartificial field of observation at any present instance but also —thanks to the unity and history of the profession —there is a fund of practical wisdom passed on now often by word of mouth or apprenticeship. This wisdom could, if properly viewed, be precipitated and surveyed with keener scrutiny not just as a guide to the immediate practice of the scrutinizing individuals but for the sake of being put into more communicable, more stable, more generalized, and hence more amendable form. Nursing not only is rich in nonthetic awareness (because its "professionals" engage habitually in practice and so encounter reality at least nonconceptually), but also possesses certain regularized patterns of behavior which are inherited and persistent over time—a built-in body of accepted practice, if not a body of knowledge in some other

---

[1] Bacon. *New organon* Book II, especially Aphorisms 50 and 41.

sense. That is, nursing has at the very least some awareness of the basis from which a constructive criticism should start. Moreover, not all this "basic wisdom" remains at the preconceptual level. Within nursing practice and tradition there is a certain abundance of written sources—among these the lowly or mighty procedure books—which could constitute a veritable gold mine of "incipient theory," recoverable and refineable given appropriate tools, energies, and aims.

In the pursuit of a scientific body of knowledge, nursing or any profession must be on guard against the two-fold temptation: 1) on the one hand, of a too quick contempt for anything already possessed or developed before the newest phase within the profession, or developed without or independently of skills newly acquired and hard won by current leaders in the profession; and 2) on the other hand, the temptation of embracing seemingly safe procedures from any other discipline, without very critical scrutiny of what those procedures have done for that discipline, let alone what they might do for nursing.

What must be admitted is the complexity and difficulty of producing a nursing theory in accordance with the position taken here. The temptation will be to do something easier, even though perhaps useless to nursing; to do something less novel and more in keeping with rigid stereotypes of researchers and theorists in natural and social sciences; to do what will make an acceptable doctoral thesis, whether or not useful to nursing; or to do what is fundable, whether or not useful to nursing. These temptations may be difficult to resist. But recognizing that, by succumbing, you sell your birthright as a nurse may give you the impetus and energy to: 1) entertain the proposed notion of theory with the burden of its detail; 2) persist in nursing inquiry despite the allurements of smoother sailing and quicker payoff in status and funds to be found in repetition or imitation of inquiry in a more academic discipline; and 3) exploit the advantages, history, and special peculiarities of nursing toward an appropriate bias within nursing inquiry.

Nursing Theory as Situation-Producing Theory

Let's sketch out what we take to be the levels of theory and some of the distinctive features of theory at each level. We but sketch these levels and features here for two reasons. First of all, too much detail here on these matters would move the focus away from the four-thesis position taken by this paper. A more detailed consideration of these matters is offered in a paper basic to this discussion entitled "Theory in a Practice Discipline," written by us with Ernestine Wiedenbach and to be published in a forthcoming issue of *Nursing Research*.[2] Secondly, the task of the present paper is in part to create the need for that more detailed consideration. Unless there is some awareness of the practical import of seeing the relation of professional purpose to the mode of theorizing, exploring in depth levels and structure of theory could constitute just one or more academic distraction for nursing. The point here is to emphasize the structure of fourth-level or situation-producing theory, so as to render somewhat more concrete the kind of structure we deem any viable nursing theory should have. Without initial awareness of the needed structure of theory, it is hard to see how any progress can be made in assessing any purported theory as to its adequacy or in deciding: 1) where work is already done, 2) where work must be done, and 3) how to guide in economical and feasible ways the time, energies, and talents at nursing's disposal so that the inquiry made will neither founder in despair nor constitute a mere status search or distraction.

The Kinds or Levels of Theory

A severe limitation in many current notions of theory stems from the oversimple view that takes as theory only sets of causal laws, so that the only conceptual systems regarded as theories are those that allow prediction on their bases. We have suggested that we can profitably see as theory conceptual frameworks which

---

[2] Ed. note: See chapters 46 and 53 in this volume. Cp. especially the sections on "What is Theory?" and "What is Nursing Theory?"

allow something less than prediction (for example, theories of classification or more simply systems or even conventions for naming or marking off significant elements) as well as conceptual frameworks that go beyond mere prediction.

It seems to us that careful attention to the structure of predictive theory suggests three things: 1) predictive theory presupposes the prior existence of more elementary types of theory; 2) predictive theory is not the only kind of theory dealing essentially with relations conceived as between states of affairs; and 3) there is a type of theory which presupposes and builds on theories at the level of relations between states of affairs.

The point of emphasis here is that in addition to factor-isolating and depicting theories (presupposed by predictive theories) and to predictive or causal theories (including what we elsewhere call promoting or inhibiting theories), there does or could exist another kind of theory that presupposes and builds on these other levels of theory. This fourth-level of theory can be called prescriptive theory, goal-incorporating theory, or perhaps most graphically, situation-producing theory. Situation producing theories are not satisfied to conceptualize factors, factor relations, or situation relations, but go on to attempt conceptualization of desired situations as well as conceptualizing the prescription under which an agent or practitioner must act in order to bring about situations of the kind conceived as desirable in the conception of the goal.

In "Theory in a Practice Discipline" (section on "The Four Levels of Theory"), the lands of theories are charted thus:

I. Factor-isolating theories
II. Factor-relating theories (situation depicting theories)
III. Situation-relating theories
   A. Predictive theories
   B. Promoting or inhibiting theories
IV. Situation-producing theories (prescriptive theories)

Situation-Producing Theory

A theory is here viewed as a conceptual framework invented to some purpose, and since the purpose of a situation-producing theory is to allow for the production of situations of a desired kind, the three essential ingredients of a situation-producing theory are: 1) goal-content specified as aim for activity, 2) prescriptions for activity to realize the goal-content, and 3) a survey list to serve as a supplement to present prescription and as preparation for future prescription for activity toward the goal-content. The goal-content specifies features of situations to be produced. The prescriptions give directives for activity productive of such situations. The survey list calls attention to those aspects of activity and to those theories at whatever level deemed by the theorist relevant to the production of desired situations but not (or not yet) explicitly of fully incorporated into goal-content or prescriptions.

We suggest that six aspects of activity fruitful to highlight as well as to use to organize a theory's survey list are these:

1. Agency
2. Patiency
3. Framework
4. Terminus
5. Procedure
6. Dynamics

In "Theory in a Practice Discipline" these ingredients and organization of situation-producing theory are charted as follows:

Ingredients of a Situation-producing Theory
   Goal content
   Prescriptions
   Survey list (organized, e.g., as follows)

1. Agency (explored, e.g., with respect to)
   a. Dimensions of the aspect (here agency) deemed especially relevant
     (1) External resources of agents
     (2) Internal resources of agents
     (3) Factors of agency proposed as significant in the statement of the theory or for acting under the theory
   b. Theories from other disciplines (at whatever level) deemed relevant
2. Patiency
   a. Relevant dimensions or realities
   b. Relevant theories

3. Framework
   a. Relevant dimensions or realities
   b. Relevant theories
4. Terminus
   a. Relevant dimensions or realities
   b. Relevant theories
5. Procedure
   a. Relevant dimensions or realities
   b. Relevant theories
6. Dynamics
   a. Relevant dimensions or realities
   b. Relevant theories

The Structure of Nursing Theory

Our contention is that any practice-minded nursing theory must be a theory at the situation-producing level. Looking at the ingredients typical of a situation-producing theory and at a survey list organized along the suggested dimensions is a first step toward rendering the contention plausible. Once initial plausibility is granted, the further investment of energy in the articulation of such theory becomes less academic and moves us one step closer to seeing whether practice bears out the contention.

What is the point of calling attention to goal, prescription, and survey list as essential ingredients of any nursing theory in a context where we are emphasizing the explicit conceptual nature of theory and the practical orientation of theory for any professional discipline? Emphasizing goal as a theoretical entity has three advantages: we dare or dein to become articulate about the explicit features of what we desire to produce; secondly, we see goals as giving explicit practical direction rather than merely emotional tone; and thirdly, we see the essential and respectable function of professional bias in the formulation of a practice theory. That is, goals become speakable—and hence communicable and alterable, functional, and finally viewable as professional rather than personal prejudices.

Calling attention to prescription as an essential ingredient of nursing theory, first of all, stresses the extra-academic features of a professional and of his situation-producing theory. Demand for prescriptions toward the realization of stated goals furnishes not only a stimulation to practical thought but also an antidote to

the "beautiful soul" syndrome of the self-righteous reformer who won't sully ideals in any interplay with demands of practice. More specifically, a call for prescriptions constitutes a demand for bringing into the practical realm—in terms of real personnel and circumstances—the ideally desirable.

Presence of the survey list is a healthy reminder that the basis of professional judgment is incredibly complex and probably at no time fully articulate rather than something mysterious, ineffable, or inborn. The suggested six-fold organizational pattern for the survey list gives at least one mode of rendering more manageable the admittedly wide, rich, and deep scope of nursing activity. Any suggested patterning would provide an initial basis of exploration or command of this scope. The six-fold analysis suggested—along the dimensions of agency, patiency, framework, terminus, procedure, and dynamics—brings the mind to bear on certain features of nursing which though perhaps noted dumbly in practice are often unnoted in theory or actively repressed from theory.

Considering *agency*—or who or what performs the activity—could be useful in at least bringing up for theoretical consideration the practical value of considering as agents of nursing activity not just registered nurses but also other professionals and nonprofessionals who might be directed or exploited to contribute to realization of a nursing goal. Shouldn't a nursing theory take theoretical account of the proper function of at least, say, licensed practical nurses and aides? And is the sick person ever an agent?

With similar generality, considering the aspect of *patiency* (who or what is the recipient of the activity) makes us realize that even if we consider only the registered nurse as agent her activity is received or "suffered" by many others in addition to the sick "patient." And realizing that sometimes inanimate things such as charts or machines "receive" a registered nurse's activity might broaden the conception of both agent and patient not just beyond the registered nurse and the sick but also to include things other than persons. But what's the purpose of so irreverent an extension of agent and patient? Perhaps this: seeing their analogy to inanimate things may increase the theoretical sensitivity to the limits of elasticity and of repertoire and to the need for upkeep and fuel-input not only for immediate service but also for any long-range expectation of serviceability.

Attending to *framework* makes less plausible the insistence on registered-nurse-sick-patient dyad functioning in isolation as the sole focal point of a viable nursing theory. Part of professional purpose may in fact be to support or maintain not only the "patient" but also the profession and its supporting institutions. Practice would never deny this; why does theory not note it?

Emphasis on the aspect of *terminus* (what is the end point of the activity?) calls for not recipes for service but apt characterizations of practical units of work. Conceiving these practical units might stimulate articulation of alternative modes of realization. But perhaps more importantly, considering terminus calls attention to the function of the mode of conceptualizing activity as a possible contributor to the ease of doing or receiving the activity in question.

Giving explicit status to the *procedure* aspect of activity requires attending to the safety, economy, and controlled performance that constitute some of the virtues of rote, ritual, and policy and seeing procedures as distinct from terminus demands an attempt at integrating appropriate detail with appropriately sensed direction.

Focusing on *dynamics* (what is the energy source for the activity?) brings up for specific consideration such aspects as psychological input and makes discussable in theoretical terms the question of the appropriate place of, say, motivation other than service motivation in the rendering of professional services. Moreover, the very multiplicity of the noted dimensions makes evident the need to consider in theory as well as in practice the mutual interaction of these dimensions and their relation to prescription and to goal.

Given this general notion of nursing theory as a situation-producing theory with the three characteristic ingredients and with the survey list ingredients organized along the lines of the six distinguished aspects of activity, now it might be proper to ask where particular theories of biology, psychology, and sociology, to name a few, would fit within a nursing theory. Any one of these theories—or some specific part of any one of them—might (considering only structural demands) be a cited theory under any heading of the nursing theory survey list. More generally, a nursing theory is a situation-producing theory which presupposes the existence of many lower level theories. Natural and social science theories are likely to be important contributors for these lower level theories of prediction, correlation, and terminology. But to say that nursing science or theory is merely applied biology, or applied psychology, or applied anything is misleading if it makes us overlook that conceptualization at a very sophisticated level constitutes the integration of the so-called pure sciences into nursing theory. These theories are building blocks, so to speak, in the mansion of nursing theory. This remark is not meant to demean the importance of these supporting theories, but to call attention to the mighty labor needed to exploit these basic sciences intelligently toward the nursing function.

This Theory of Theories— Its Novelty and Its Viability: An Immodest Proposal

Novelty alone is no reason to accept a theory or anything else. To the timid or conservative the tinge of novelty may in fact be reason sufficient to reject any proposal. Nonetheless, for two special reasons we point out what are the novel aspects of the position offered here. First of all, to label as inappropriate—before it appears—a rejection of the position offered on the mere grounds that the position differs from certain currently theories of theory. This reason for rejection, though inappropriate, is the more likely to appear the more recently acquired is the awareness of other theories of theory and the more pain spent in acquiring that awareness. Secondly, to emphasize that no apology is made for the novelty—quite the contrary.

The first point of novelty to be urged is the contention that nursing or any so-called applied theory is more, rather than less, conceptually sophisticated than are so-called "pure" theories. To exclude the possibility of specific conceptual guidance in the attempts to put to use descriptive theories of reality is to confuse the present state of theory production with the theoretic possibilities for theory production. This remark leads to the main point of novelty claimed. We suggest that proposing a theory of theories that sees theory as a conceptual system invented to some purpose—when seen in its full consequences—has revolutionary possibilities. The proposal allows at last for theory to be viewed as a proper tool to man even in his role of providing himself with purpose. But how is the novel related to the old? As Einstein's theory of relativity is to the Newtonian physicist, so is our theory of theories to the, shall we say, classical theories of theory. The theories of Hempel, Carnap, Toulmin, Nagel, and so on, are special cases of the broader theory proposed here; these earlier views are not wrong so much as they are overly restrictive, concentrating only on one kind of theory without backing up to inquire as to theoretic activity itself and without seeing that one kind of theory—predictive-in relation to other possible kinds.[3]

The theory of theories offered here may be novel; but is it correct? To answer this question requires answering whether or not the proposed position constitutes a fruitful view of theory. It is important to realize that—whether the domain be nursing or theory—the theory of that domain must be invented rather than

"discovered" from a hidden store of truth or "abstracted" somehow from the real. But consulting empirical reality is an important way of assessing fruitfulness. Reality may be so consulted by carefully controlled experiments with all action on the basis of the questioned theory postponed until research results are in and interpreted. But sometimes action cannot and should not wait on such niceties: the face validity, so to speak, of a theory or hypothesis may be sufficient to lead us to the acceptance of a conceptual framework as a tentative guide to action, with the resolution to note the results of following the guide so as to be prepared for needed amendments or to be sure of knowing how to repeat the happily followed path. For—as will be clear in our remarks on research—sometimes time, money, or energy demands make research narrowly defined too costly a mode of reassurance. And more importantly, there are some things about which we seek reassurance but for which research narrowly conceived can never be justly expected to constitute a reliable guide.

---

[3] For example: Hempel, C.G. (1952). Fundamentals of concept formation in empirical science. In O. Neurath, et al. (Eds.), *International encyclopedia of unified science,* Vol. 2, No. 7. Chicago: University of Chicago Press.; Hemple, C.G. (1966). *Philosophy of natural science.* New York: Prentice-Hall.; Carnap, R. (1956). Methodological character of theoretical concepts. In H. Feigl & M. Scriven (Eds.). *Minnesota studies in philosophy of science, Vol. 1: Foundations of science and the concepts of psychology and psychoanalysis,* Minneapolis: University of Minnesota Press.; Toulmin, S.E. (1953). *Philosophy of science,* London: Hutchinson.; Nagel, E. (1961). *Structure of science.* New York: Harcourt, Brace, Jovanovich.

The Authors Comment

The Symposium Invitation

Probably through the aegis of Dean Florence Wald of the Yale School of Nursing, who was familiar with details of our work with the faculty and students of the Yale Masters Program in Nursing, we were invited to participate in the 1968 Case Western Reserve University Symposium on Theory Development in Nursing. As young philosophy faculty at Yale, we had been invited in 1962 to teach logic to the nursing faculty, interested then in doing research in nursing. Our first effort was directed at introducing them to the techniques of symbolic and traditional logic. We soon saw, however, that the need was broader than for what formal and traditional logic had to offer, however useful the *logic* might be. Our attention gradually moved to *conceptions* for nursing and then to *theory* for nursing.

Week by week, we as philosophers interacted with strong and strongly self-respecting people (faculty and selected graduate students) who were open to the possibility of "genuine" novelty—including new thoughts—unhampered by disciplinary restraints or budgetary or workload pressures. It is worth emphasizing that our conception of theory for nursing was not the imposition of a notion borrowed either from philosophy or from some other discipline outside nursing. Quite the contrary; our conception of theory for nursing *evolved from our interaction with nurses.* It was fashioned in response to two things: (1) our philosophically educated awareness and enthusiasm for possibilities of concepts as guides for action and (2) our intensive work with nurses involved in enhancing nursing research, nursing practice, and nursing education by developing the conceptual dimension of nursing.

Orlando's *Dynamic Nurse-Patient Relationship* (New York: Putnam, 1961) was newly in print when we began our work with the nurses. Yale nursing faculty had watched the progress of that work, and that work pretty clearly constituted a moving on from Peplau's *Interpersonal Relations in Nursing* (New York: Putnam, 1952), which was already in print. As we recall, there were not many calling these "theory" books in those earlier days but there was an eagerness for conceptual advances, whatever they might have been called.

Weekly workshops with faculty members were devoted to work on close analysis of extant nursing-practice measures, to work on extant nursing procedures (as written), and to attempts to spell out observation sheets for use in systematic nursing observation prior to actual nursing measurement within the field. Note, then, that our earliest conceptual work in nursing envisioned interconnected concerns of nursing education, nursing service, and nursing research.

From the prolonged interaction of these two poles—the nursing pole aware of nursing richness and nursing needs, and the conceptual pole aware from philosophy of the resources and limits of concepts as such—the conception of theory for a practice discipline evolved. Joyce Semradek (later at the University of North Carolina, Chapel Hill, and currently at Oregon Health Sciences University) is the one person who worked with us in virtually every aspect of our Yale involvement and with whom we have had an uninterrupted—if sometimes intermittent—exchange for over 20 years now on matters of conception for nursing (see Dickoff, James, & Semradek, 1975a, 1975b). Ernestine Wiedenbach is another who was with us in virtually every one of our earliest endeavors with nursing at Yale.

Note that it was in an atmosphere concerned about *action possibilities for nursing* that the notion of a theory for a practice discipline emerged. There was not yet (at least at Yale) any of what later emerged as preoccupation with the professionalization of nursing or with the development of nursing theory as a response to the call for professionalization of nursing. (See our 1975 paper in the Verhonick volume for a sense of our thoughts then on nursing theory and our concerns for nursing theory in its developments.)

Six Benchmarks for Nursing Theory and Its Development

In the give-and-take of interaction at Yale, several benchmarks emerged:

1. Nursing is a practice, and *as practice* could be enhanced by the more vigorous use of conceptual guidance.
2. As *intentional action,* nursing calls for conceptual guidance beyond concepts enabling prediction and other descriptive conceptions.
3. Even if predictive theory existed in all the areas and in all the specificity needed by nursing, such predictive theory would not exhaust the conceptions needed to guide a practitioner in giving nursing service.
4. It is to be expected that nursing seen as action constituting a service would change and alter over time; a nursing theory, then, should not be looked upon as an atemporal "truth"—as perhaps a predictive theory in physics should be.

These four reference points give rise to two others concerned with the development of nursing theory:

5. Nursing practice predates both research findings and explicit attempts at theory building in nursing; hence, articulation of extant conceptions in nursing practice would be a more promising and economical starting place for theorizing in nursing than would be the stance of claimed ignorance, which

demands that nursing theory be built up from research findings purposely isolated somehow from the ongoing complexities of nursing practice reality. (In Bacon's terms from the *New Organon,* Book II, Aphorism 50, nursing practice serves as a "polycrest instance" or "instance of general use" for developing nursing theory.)

6. Extant nursing practice is not necessarily good nor as good as it might be. Similarly, no conception articulated for nursing—whether articulated from a stimulus in nursing practice or articulated on the basis of some other theory, practice, or reality—is necessarily good or as good as it might be. What's more, the passage of time may have made a previously "good" theory or conception less than good. Testing or otherwise developing nursing theory, then, calls for a continuous interplay between, on the one hand, practice guided by conception and, on the other hand, reflective or inventive conception that takes into account—along with whatever else—both the concepts that are guiding practice and the results of practice guided by those concepts.

These six benchmarks constitute standards of adequacy for proposed nursing theories and their developments.

Distinctive Features of the Dickoff/James Conception of Practice Theory

Our conception of theory was a purposive and innovative move—a reconception of theory itself. We have emphasized that this move was prompted by our interaction with a practice discipline (nursing) casting about from its position within the academy for "nursing concepts." We were physically and persistently there, interacting with nurses in their attempts at, in their search for, conceptualizations adequate to the needs of nursing. We characterized what was going on as a search for theory, as an unrecognized need for a theory suitably complex to be taken as a guide to activity within a practice discipline. The nurses did not characterize the need that way, did not put the "need" into terms of theory. No wonder. Other accounts of theory that were in the air at that time—often social science versions of somewhat attenuated logical positivist explications of theory in the physical sciences—did not yet recognize a need that we came to see could be supplied for nursing and other practice disciplines. In fact, the then-going or prevalent theories of theory did not take much account of nursing or any other practice discipline when formulating a view of theory. In the eyes of such theories of theory, such "practice disciplines" were mundane, outside the scope of thought and thoughtfulness, at best mere "applications" of thought or science, with that application left to whim, chance, "expertise"—or whatever—of any given practitioner at any given moment in any given situation. (A view, we might add, unfortunately too much alive today within some of "professionalized" nursing.)

Originally our workshops and discussions at Yale with nurses were about this or that specific nursing concept. Eventually we responded to a sensed lack of a *pattern or unification* of concepts to meet the needs of nursing. Responded how? With the suggestion that theory, were it suitably reconceived with adequate complexity and unity, could still countenance as theories those "things" already commonly so called, but could also include possibilities heretofore excluded.

Our proposed reconceptualization tried, then, to allow for the *kinds* of concepts a practice discipline such as nursing required in order to exist—that is, in order to practice. What is required are *concepts adequate to guide actions.* What's more, the conceptions should *be guides in the shaping or producing of reality to desired ends*, not just guides in reacting to or controlling reality. The phrase "adequate to guide action" carries a great deal of weight. What we wanted that phrase to express is made clearer by several realizations: the very *structure* of practice theory we articulated, situation-producing theory (with its particular ingredients and particular relations to other levels of theory), *is proposed as an "organizer"* or unification focus of practice theory. Our intent was further clarified by our insistence that any particular practice theory *needed to be subject to empirical test, including a test in practice.* Still further, we insisted that *practice theory was constituted*—at whatever level of theory—*by concepts that can guide activity in its very responsiveness to the particulars* surrounding the existential activity. Such concepts need, for their suitable use, to be used with an awareness that the concepts are to be regarded as more than only a compendium of past awareness and with an awareness that current input may call for deviation from the letter of the conception taken as guide. This last "insistence" we see better now as the notion that concepts need to be taken with a "procedural bent"; that concepts that can serve as guides to action have this kind of "meaning". (Dickoff & James, 1984a, 1984b).

Talking in the abstract and without reference to the specificities of the structure of practice theory is difficult. Let us rather say, more grossly perhaps, that an early realization in our move toward practice theory was this: conceptions are needed to guide practice more than predictions or other merely descriptive conceptions. *Predictions—or any other descriptive concepts—without the presumption of goal do not serve as conceptual guides to action*—however much such conceptions *inform* a person. What's more, *there is no need to leave goal as merely presumption of theory.* We reject the "empeasanting" of practice that treats goals and values as unconceived—and, as some go so far as to say, inconceivable—backgrounds of habits, custom, or the lived-world of some community. Goals can be articulated as ingredients of theory, and the theory can—with the goal incorporated explicitly—be subject to empirical testing. The further complexities that surround a goal and a prediction also need articulation within the theory. There should be some conceptual guide to what complexities need to be taken into account in applying any conception.

The three big issues we saw in relation to practice theory are *(1) response to complexity, (2) articulated goal, and (3) a demand for empirical testing.* Additionally, we saw that *even naming*—the inventing or finding and then tagging of significant wholes, units, factors in such a fashion as to make them graspable, discriminable, or somehow noticeable and manageable within the demands of action—*should count as theorizing.* (See how Rosemary T. McCarthy realized this function of names in her 1972 study, which involved recasting nursing action in the postoperative recovery room by applying a conception that allowed the suitable *early* discrimination of postop patients—a discrimination made on the basis of likelihood of voiding relatively soon postoperatively.)

Notice that for us a theory is not a natural entity; theory as such is a man-made entity, not a pre-set essence. The man-made conception of theory abroad prior to the 1960s was needlessly restrictive. In short, *ours is a purposeful but not gratuitous nor merely speculative reconception of theory.* We offered what a practice discipline needed in order to practice with concepts as guides to activity. What we conceived is what can be called situation-producing theory, practice theory, theory for practice disciplines.

It might be noted that just as our work in the 1960s offered a re-conceptualizing of theory, so some of our current work constitutes a re-conceptualizing of concepts themselves, where theory is but one of the kinds of conception (Dickoff & James, 1984b).

The Philosophic Distinctiveness of Dickoff and James in Their Work With Nurses

Why were we as philosophers able to work fruitfully with nurses? At Yale we, not wholly dim, found ourselves with intelligent and open-minded nurses. The Yale nurses were, for the most part, alive to new possibilities. Many had the courage for new thought—as we have remarked. What's more, being at Yale one almost automatically regards oneself as among the happy few at the Battle of Agincourt well before the broader world knows the significance of the battle being fought. But the Yale *esprit* is by no means the whole story.

In the early 1960s, the thought of philosophers working with nurses still provoked condescending smiles, despite the fact that Socrates characterized himself as a midwife. Philosophy is often taken to be grand and esoteric speculation having no direct bearing on practical life, let alone on something so intimately practical as nursing. As one philosopher dramatically announced to us, "I deny categorically that philosophy is at all concerned with practical matters. That is a debasing of philosophy." The glory of philosophy, it is sometimes said, is its very uselessness. Philosophy bakes no bread, it alters nothing, it is just the attempt to understand. Understand what? Oh, life, the whole of things. To see life steady and to see it whole, to see things under the aspect of eternity, to view things as God must, seeing the whole understandingly—*that* is philosophy.

We were not taken in by that elitist notion that was then and even today is so popular in the academy—though the scarcity of jobs for professional philosophers is eroding the once highly prevalent prejudice. We were not taken in, perhaps because we had read the "profound" thinkers. Yale philosophy in the late 1950s had not succumbed to only analytic philosophy, and we read thinkers rather than only secondary sources about thinkers. A churl might say that it was us who were unenlightened or obstinate in interpreting great philosophers—including Plato—as holding that philosophy was more than impotent speculation that made no difference to anything save perhaps one's smugness or peace of mind.

Let us return to our question as to why we as philosophers were able to work fruitfully with nurses. Obstinance and unenlightenment on our part we reject as answers. And something more than openness, intelligence, and Yale *esprit* is required as an explanation. In simple fact, it was probably our philosophic interest and particular training in philosophy that was the catalyst enabling our work with nurses. As philosophers, our interest centered on "concepts as they mattered for action." Within philosophy we had concentrated on normative philosophy, including ethics but especially logic; even in the more speculative parts of philosophy we gravitated to problems of action-oriented thought, Dewey's notion of intelligence as being problem oriented, emphasizing an appeal to thought, feeling, and action as inputs for cognitive advance; the admonishment of William James that "concepts are what we go back to experience with; what help us notice differences" and that theory is *not* "a transcript of reality"; Plato's conception of the enhancement of mere know-how by conceptual guidance; Northrop's delineation of contrasts in conception on the basis of whether they did or did not integrate value considerations—all these were prominent background influences that helped shape our conception of theory for practice disciplines. Both Aristotle's fourfold causal analysis and his analysis of action, as well as Bacon's alert to the function of practice as a stimulus to more explanatory "scientific" concepts, were also formative factors. Still another factor germane in our invention of the notion of practice theory was our training and work in formal logic, where a system (of formal logic) is proposed and then measured for fit with the intended interpretation of the system (and where it is common-place that more than one "system" or "theory" might "fit").

Retrograde Motion in the Current Theory Scene?

There is currently a move to stress the existence of nursing science: just as there exists the science of physics and the science of chemistry, so it is claimed there exists—or is about to exist—a nursing science. The point of putting forth nursing science is to say that nursing predictions have been established by empirical research (or that there are nursing explanations). In the early 1960s, it was thought that nursing science alone was sufficient for nursing to carry out its practice, i.e., if we have nursing science, then nursing practice will be scientific. For the most part, the advocates of nursing science still saw no need for practice theory. Today those who advocate nursing science are a bit more enlightened. Unlike their predecessors of the early 1960s, they realize something more is needed for a nurse to nurse than only nursing science.

Current attempts—Fawcett-like or Beckstrand-like—in some dimensions follow Carper. These attempts try to limit (or accept a limit on) scientific theory in such a fashion that great expanses of conception beyond the so-called scientific are called for within nursing. But these expanses are relegated to a realm of the untested or the tested but apparently "nonscientifically." We purposely refer to as APE (*a*esthetic, *p*ersonal, *e*thical) the current characterization of those "other" conceptual realms to emphasize that we see as *retrograde motion* the reversion to a notion of theory that does not demand strenuous empirical tests for these other conceptions; does not demand a conception of the integration of various "domains" through concepts adequate in complexity but still adequate in unification so that they can be concepts to guide action. (Such current views are, in our eyes, just current versions of a Walker-like position which we criticized in 1971 in our "Clarity" response to Walker—see this volume, Chapter 4.)

—JAMES DICKOFF AND PATRICIA JAMES

REFERENCES

Dickoff, J., & James, P. (1985). Theory development in nursing. In P.J. Verhonick (Ed.). *Nursing research: Vol. I.* Boston: Little, Brown.

Dickoff, J., & James, P. (1984a). Towards a cultivated but decisive pluralism for nursing. In M. McGee (Ed.). *Theoretical pluralism in nursing science.* Ottawa, Canada: University of Ottawa Press.

Dickoff, J., & James, P. (1984b, January). *Conceptual trends, conceptual needs, prospects for a fit.* Paper presented at the 2nd Annual Meeting of the Society for Research in Nursing Education, San Francisco.

Dickoff, J., James, P., & Semradek, J. (1975a). 8-4 research part I: A stance for nursing research—tenacity or inquiry? *Nursing Research, 24,* 84–88.

Dickoff, J., James, P., & Semradek, J. (1975b). 8-4 research part II: Designing nursing research—eight points of encounter. *Nursing Research, 24,* 164–176.

McCarthy, R.T. (1972). A practice theory of nursing care. *Nursing Research, 21,* 406–410.

Chapter 9

Theory in Nursing: Borrowed and Unique

Dorothy E. Johnson

It is extremely hazardous to attempt to differentiate between borrowed and unique theory in nursing. It is hazardous first of all because the man-made, more or less arbitrary divisions between the sciences are neither firm nor constant. It appears there is an essential unity in knowledge, corresponding to a unity in nature, which defies established boundaries, and continuously presses for the larger, more cohesive view. Moreover, knowledge does not innately "belong" to any field of science. It is not exactly happenstance that a given bit of knowledge is discovered by one discipline rather than another, but the fact of discovery does not confer the right of ownership. Viewed in this light, borrowed and unique have no real permanence, nor any real meaning.

It does seem important to accept the risks involved for several reasons. Most scientific fields do have reasonably clear and established boundaries, despite what I have just said. This enables us to anticipate what can be expected from the disciplines on which nursing draws, and permits our concentration on problems about which we are not so likely to gain understanding through the work of other disciplines. Differentiation may also help to dispel the notions either that nursing depends entirely upon the findings of the pure sciences for application in practice, or that nursing depends upon these sciences not at all. Finally, and most importantly, examination of the question, what is borrowed and what is unique, may help to clarify nursing's appropriate place and focus in theory development.

As a working definition, I have defined borrowed theory as that knowledge which is developed in the main by other disciplines and is drawn upon by nursing. Unique theory is defined as that knowledge derived from the observation of phenomena and the asking of questions unlike those which characterize other disciplines. The question of borrowed and unique will be considered by employing two related, but somewhat different perspectives. The first inquires into the nature of the knowledge required for nursing practice

About the Author

DOROTHY E. JOHNSON grew up in Savannah, Georgia, and has spent most of her life in the south and on the west coast. Ms. Johnson received a B.S.N. from Vanderbilt University in Nashville and a M.P.H. from Harvard University School of Public Health in 1948. She began her teaching career at Vanderbilt University and in 1949 accepted a faculty appointment at the University of California at Los Angeles, where she taught until her retirement in 1977. She now makes her home in Key Largo, Florida.

About nursing, Ms. Johnson comments "I have always been an avid reader, with a particular interest in the history of ideas and science. Florence Nightingale's *Notes On Nursing* had a profound influence on my thinking about nursing.

The intellectual growth of students and their subsequent achievements have been, I suppose, my major source of satisfaction, in nursing. Another source of satisfaction, however, has come from observing the growth of nursing as a professional and scientific discipline and from the feeling that I may have contributed in some small measure to that growth. Because today's generation of nurses contains the largest number of well-educated, thoughtful, and committed people in our history, the future cannot help but be full of promise for further advancement."

and the availability of that knowledge. The second considers the problem of nursing's objects in scientific investigation.

The Nature of Knowledge Required

The knowledge required for practice in nursing can be conceived as consisting of three parts, each composed of a general type of knowledge. These classifications are admittedly rough, with blurring and overlapping of boundaries and some fuzziness in description quite apparent. Despite these problems and the oversimplification inherent in this classification scheme, such a division seems reasonable and analytically useful.

The first part, or type, might be called knowledge of order. An essential assumption of the scientific perspective is that there is order in nature and that this order can be discovered and understood. By order in nature it is meant there are regularities in the arrangements and sequences which underlie and govern the relations of physical, biological, and social objects and events. Out of this order and its discovery and verification have emerged the laws, concepts and theories of scientific knowledge. Knowledge of order for our purposes refers to that knowledge which describes and explains the "normal" state of man and the "natural" scheme of things.[1]

The second type of knowledge is that of disorder. Reference here is to knowledge about such phenomena as wars, riots, earthquakes, disease, and the like. The label disorder for such events is a misnomer of course, for what seems to be disorder must in some sense represent order or the phenomena observed would not be sufficiently durable or repetitious to be amenable to study. The label is useful, if not entirely accurate, in classifying that knowledge which helps us to understand those events which pose a threat to the well-being or survival of the individual or society, or which are deemed undesirable for some other reason.

Knowledge of control is the third type. This is knowledge which allows us to prescribe a course of action which, when executed, changes the sequence of events in desired ways and toward specified outcomes. Knowledge of this kind goes beyond prediction in the sense in which that term is often used in science, al-

---

[1] "Normal" and "natural" are placed in quotes here to indicate that the problems in the use of these words are recognized. So, too, is the difficulty with respect to values and order recognized. No assumption is being made either that the order characterizing objects and events is invariant, or that the order discovered and described is necessarily socially valued. Discussion of these subjects, no matter how significant, is beyond the scope of this paper, however, since it would not fundamentally influence the point being made.

though prediction is clearly involved. For example, the course of events under certain conditions may be predicted even though the knowledge needed to change that course of events and to achieve different, specified outcomes may not be available. It is the difference between knowing that the disorganized tissue growth we call cancer often leads to death, and knowing what can be done to avert such a "natural" outcome. Knowledge of control represents what others have called for as prescriptive theory (Greenwood, 1961; Wald & Leonard, 1964).

Clearly knowledge coming under each of these three general types is basic to the practice of nursing. The maintenance of order is society's general charge to all of the health professions. To maintain order, the practitioner must know order, for this is her ultimate goal. She must know disorder, for this she must recognize in its actuality or in its potentiality. And she must know control either to prevent disorder or to convert disorder into order. But what specific knowledge is needed under these three general types, and is it available?

Knowledge of order has been the distinctive focus of what are called the basic sciences, and knowledge of this kind represents to a considerable degree all that has been learned through the scientific method about man and his universe. The biological and behavioral sciences, each from its own perspective and through its focus on particular objects and events, have provided knowledge which helps us to understand biological man, psychological man, and social man. There are deficiencies in this knowledge to be sure, and there is unquestionably much more to be learned from each of these several perspectives, but a solid base for understanding is available. Even more importantly, from nursing's perspective, there are hopeful signs of coalescing scientific interests in the study of man. It does not seem too much to anticipate that a unified theory of human behavior may eventually emerge through the work of the several basic sciences concerned.

I believe that nursing is concerned with man as an organized and integrated whole and this is the specific knowledge of order we require. Obviously knowledge

of this kind and at this level is not now available to us. Until such time as the basic sciences develop this knowledge, as I am sure they will, we must "make do" by collating and synthesizing to the extent possible the findings of several fields. While nurse scientists may, and some undoubtedly will, contribute to the general knowledge of order in man, it seems to me this is now, and will continue to be borrowed knowledge.

Knowledge of disorder has not been in the past a major interest of the basic sciences despite continuing attention on the part of some scientists and periodic concern in some disciplines. The knowledge accumulated by these disciplines is comparatively small in amount and it is generally restricted, as one would expect, to such knowledge as the perspectives of these disciplines would suggest. It includes, for example, knowledge about various forms of social deviance, personality defects, and malfunction in physiological processes. Although it is quite likely that the basic sciences will continue to add, and perhaps increasingly, to our knowledge of social disorders, psychological disorders, biochemical disorders, physiological disorders, and the like, one may question the likelihood of investigation by these disciplines into phenomena of concern to nursing or from a perspective useful to nursing.

Medicine can be used to illustrate the point. Medicine is not concerned per se with biochemical disorders, or physiological disorders, or physical disorders, but with another class of biological disorders, an overriding class called disease, which may and often does involve all of these underlying disorders. The phenomena studied and the questions asked by the basic sciences simply do not yield the knowledge needed by medicine to understand disease. Although the knowledge of disorder produced by the basic sciences in these areas is exceedingly useful, it is and will continue to be qualitatively insufficient for a profession which must have a more holistic perspective in examining more pervasive phenomena. To acquire the knowledge needed to fulfill its societal responsibilities, medicine has been studying the causes and nature of disease for years.

Nursing must ask: With which of all the possible

classes of disorder are we concerned? Is it biological disorder in general, or disease in particular, in which we are interested? Are we concerned with psychological disorders or social disorders, or with selected subclasses of these general classes? Or, would some other classification scheme better suit our need to isolate the specific kind of disorder with which it is our primary responsibility to deal? What questions must we ask about the phenomena so isolated to yield the knowledge we require? Unless the answers to the questions on phenomena and perspective are the same as those in one or more of the basic sciences or in medicine, then the knowledge of disorder we require is probably not now available, nor likely to be made available. In this area we very probably must develop our own theory.

Since knowledge of control stems from and thus is directly related to knowledge of disorder, it is premature to raise the question of the availability of control knowledge until questions on knowledge of disorder are answered. It may be noted, however, that in general, the basic scientist is more inclined to study what is, than to be concerned about what might be. This is not entirely true of course, for there are many social and natural scientists working in "applied" fields who are vitally concerned with control.

The Objects of Scientific Investigation

The unanswered questions in the preceding discussion and its "iffy" quality are directly related to a continuing problem in the field. It has become almost trite to say that nursing is ill-defined as a field of practice. Not so commonly noted but equally significant is the fact that nursing is equally ill-defined as a field of inquiry and in the eyes of some the boundaries of the field are essentially unlimited. These stark facts constitute a most serious obstacle to our future professional and scientific development. We cannot know with certainty what specific knowledge is required for practice until we know with reasonable clarity toward what end that knowledge is to be used. Nor can we know with certainty the proper objects of investigation and the appro-

priate questions to ask until we know with reasonable surety the area of our primary responsibility to patients.

Many individuals in nursing have thought and continue to think that the question: What is nursing? is an improper, or at least an unnecessary question. Nothing could be further from the truth. In its answer, we will find our boundaries as a professional and a scientific discipline. Some have suggested that it is a policy question to be answered primarily by nurses (Ellison, Diers, & Leonard, 1965). Difficult as it would be to achieve consensus on such a question as policy, it would not be enough. In the end the boundaries of the field will have to be established in concert with the society we serve. That society will grant a monopoly of judgment for an area of original responsibility only when there is proof that we have acquired the knowledge needed to solve problems of social significance.

All of this makes it sound as if nursing is in a vicious circle with no way out. In my opinion the way out can come through research, and this takes us to consideration of the second perspective referred to earlier. If there is an area for study and theory development unique to nursing, it will evolve only through the study of phenomena and the asking of questions in a way that is not characteristic of any other discipline. This not because it is the "thing to do," but because only in this way will we acquire the knowledge we need for practice. As is true in other disciplines, these will be man-made boundaries, but they may be less arbitrary because they stem from our responsibilities to society.

The determination of what phenomena to study and what questions to ask will not be easy. It will require a fresh and creative approach to the consideration of alternatives, and an originality expected only of the most outstanding scientists in other disciplines. Obviously, originality must be tempered by reason, and reason by the objective characteristics of the world of practice; but only originality will take us away from the well-worn paths we have been following. If we continue to observe behavior from the perspective of sociology, anthropology, or psychology, if we continue to study disease with the aim of elucidating etiologies, properties, or life cycle, or if we continue to inquire into biological functioning or malfunction, we will be serving the cause of science but not necessarily the cause of nursing.

It must be obvious by now that I am personally convinced that there is an area of study and theory development unique to nursing. It is equally obvious that I do not know with certainty what this area is. While my faith is strong, my ability to isolate and articulate what I consider to be the proper phenomena and perspective is limited. On traditional and logical grounds, I believe the phenomena with which nursing is concerned come under the general class of behavioral disorders. These are not disorders of a social, interpersonal, or intrapersonal nature, but rather behavioral *system* disorders. By this I mean the patterned and repetitive ways of behaving that characterize the life of man can be conceived as forming an organized and integrated whole made up of interrelated and interdependent parts. This system, or total way of behaving, is determined by—as well as regulated and controlled by—many biological, psychological, and social factors. Certain conditions must be met if this system and its subsystems are to grow and survive. If these conditions are not met, or if a breakdown in regulatory and control mechanisms occurs, malfunction becomes apparent in problems manifested in part by disorganized or erratic behavior. These problems represent disorders of the behavioral system.

This conceptualization is comparable in many respects to that of man as a biological system and disease as a biological system disorders. Just as medicine is interested in the etiologies, properties, course and prognosis of biological system disorders, nursing must be interested in the etiologies, properties, course, and prognosis of behavioral system disorders. Just as medicine is interested in a multiplicity of variables, acting in complicated ways, associated with the onset, course, and prognosis of biological system disorders, so too nursing must be interested in many of the same kind of variables for their influence in behavioral system disorder. Just as medicine is interested in discovering the means of control of disease, so must nursing be interested in the means of control of behavioral system disorders.

These personal thoughts are offered primarily as a stimulus to further thinking about nursing's objects in scientific investigation. They represent only a beginning, and they may in the end prove to be practically useless, theoretically unsound, or professionally inappropriate. They do illustrate, I think, the possibility, if not the need, for considering alternatives in answering our questions about the uniqueness of theory in nursing.

Summary

The contribution of the basic sciences to the knowledge that underlies nursing practice cannot be denied, and we can and will do much in the years ahead to test and extend the theories of these disciplines. On the other hand, the body of knowledge needed for nursing practice will be incomplete, I believe, until we learn to ask what I would call nursing questions about events in nature of specific concern to us because we are committed to their management. This is not because of default by the basic sciences, nor because no other discipline could not (or indeed might not at some future time) ask these same questions of these particular events. It is because the knowledge is needed for practice, we need it, and we need it in the here and now. There may well be a long period of fumbling before consensus on our boundaries is reached through investigation and a sound beginning in theory development for nursing practice is made, but I believe it will come.

There are two thoughts from Walter Orr Roberts that I would like to leave with you. Speaking of the social sciences, he stated something that applies equally well to nursing:

> In the sciences that deal with man's interactions, we still have unburned witches to deal with. There are many wrong turns ahead in these sciences—but it is an essential of science to blunder down some of these wrong

turns, to develop and test wrong hypotheses. That is the way we get ahead. The social sciences must not be thrown down the drain because of some of the essential blundering that will make real progress possible (Roberts, 1967, p.3).

Roberts further stated:

To be what we can be, we must first and foremost know what we want to be. (Roberts, 1967, p. 3).

References

Ellison, M.D. Diers, D., & Leonard, R.C. (1965). The uses of the behavioral sciences in nursing: Further comment. *Nursing Research, 14,* 71–72.

Greenwood, E. (1961). Practice of science and the science of practice. In W.G. Bennis et al. (Eds.). *The planning of change.* New York: Holt, Rinehart and Winston.

Roberts, W.O. (1967). Science, a wellspring of our discontent. *American Science, 55,* 3–14

Wald, F.S., & Leonard, R.C. (1964). Towards development of nursing practice theory. *Nursing Research, 13,* 309–313.

The Author Comments

As I recall, the planners of this conference asked participants to simply discuss theory development in nursing. This was nearly 10 years after publication of my earliest relevant papers, and in the interim I had continued to speak and write about the need to develop the scientific basics for nursing practice. It was probably for this reason that I was invited to participate, and I was pleased to be included in such a distinguished group to share my thoughts on the subject.

In the years preceding the symposium, discussions about nursing theory had gradually become more widespread, particularly among academicians, as the number of nurses completing work for higher degrees had increased. Such discussions were still perceived by the large majority of nurses as belonging only to the ivory tower and of little practical value. Even among those holding higher degrees and positions of leadership in nursing, there was considerable controversy about nursing's goal in patient care and the appropriate scientific focus for the field. In this group, however, it was not a question of the need for nursing science, but rather of what the nature of that science might be. In bringing together for the first time a group of participants with diverse viewpoints on the subject, the symposium was indeed a landmark in the evolution of nursing.

—DOROTHY E. JOHNSON

Chapter 10

ReVisions in Knowledge Development: A Passion for Substance

Afaf Ibrahim Meleis

Members of the nursing community have been engaged in numerous debates, some of which are related to the roles of holism and particularism in the care of clients and in the development of nursing knowledge. Others center on most and least congruent methodologies for nursing research. These healthy debates have played a significant role in invigorating the discipline of nursing. If they continue without special attention to nursing's substance, however, they may detract from its knowledge development. By refocusing the debates on substance, that is, on the major phenomena and theoretical propositions considered central to nursing, progress in the development of nursing knowledge will be enhanced. Other reVisions include coopting some existing methods in knowledge development that are congruent with feminist approaches and not limited to certain strata of populations or certain nations, thus highlighting international nursing as an arena for the generation of gender-sensitive and culture-sensitive theories. Finally, the commitment to reVisions in knowledge development means a personal commitment of nursing scholars to health care in general and to the discipline of nursing in particular.

Visions

Visions about nursing by those who dared to dream helped make nursing a full-fledged and acceptable profession. The visions ranged from hopes, in the early days, for some kind of education for a new breed of workers called nurses, to better and higher types of education as the profession progressed, better and more efficient use of nurses and nurses' time as nursing became established, to current visions of autonomy and self-governance as the profession comes of age. Past visions dictated the kinds of discourse and the types of questions that nurses engaged in answering for decades. Some of these visions were realized and some dissipated in thin air. Others continued to be illusive or were merely mirages. Those that have been realized,

About the Author

AFAF IBRAHIM MELEIS was born in Alexandria, Egypt, and received a B.S. in nursing from the University of Alexandria in 1961. She moved to the United States in 1962, where she matriculated at the University of California Los Angeles (UCLA), receiving a M.S. in Nursing (1964), a M.A. in Sociology (1966), and a Ph.D. in Sociology (1968). After teaching at UCLA for 5 years, Dr. Meleis then joined the faculty at the University of California San Francisco (UCSF) in 1971. She is currently a Professor in the Department of Mental Health, Community, and Administrative Nursing at UCSF.

An internationally recognized scholar and researcher, Dr. Meleis notes that reaching out internationally has been a particular source of satisfaction in nursing. In 1985, her book *Theoretical Nursing: Development and Progress* (Philadelphia: J.B. Lippincott) was published. Currently, Dr. Meleis is developing a coherent conceptualization of the relationship between transitions and health, as well as studying women's health in developing countries. Dr. Meleis notes that "women are a significant link to the health care of other members of a family, the key to infant and child mortality rates and to understanding the level of development in societies. Yet they have been among the underserved around the world."

When asked about the future, Dr. Meleis commented "I hope that we are moving into a more collaborative and interdisciplinary approach to providing health care. If so, then theories of the future will help to achieve the goals of health for all in the year 2000."

made room for new visions. Only these visions were more specifically related to the primary business of nursing. In Florence Nightingale's words, the primary business of nursing was "putting the patient in the best condition for nature to act upon him." In today's terms, it is articulated by the ANA's Social Policy Statement (ANA, 1980): to understand people's perceptions and people's and the environment's responses to health and illness situations in order to maximize healing potential, decrease suffering, and enhance well-being. Those who envisioned the essence of the business of nursing also helped to articulate ways in which to bring about those outcomes that are the heart of the business of nursing. The range of nursing therapeutics includes modifying people's responses, changing their environments, enhancing their awareness, or helping them to find new meanings in the events they encounter or the responses they experience to such life processes as birth, death, health, and illness.

Visions about the business of nursing helped to identify a core of central concepts and a core of central shared assumptions (Flaskerud & Halloran, 1980; Meleis, 1986; Yura & Torres, 1975). Whereas there may be a beginning consensus on the domain assumptions, concepts, and central questions, ongoing healthy debates remain about the most appropriate ways of "knowing"—that is, nursing units of analysis and nursing methodologies. It is time to reflect on where our theorists, metatheorists, and scientists should place their energy; it is time for some reVisions of our visions regarding knowledge development. These reVisions are developed with the premise that the acquisition and use of knowledge in nursing evolves from practice, and that it is through the integration of theory, research, and practice that meaningful theories will emerge.

ReVisions

ReVision 1: A Passion for Substance

Debates are healthy processes for understanding diverse viewpoints, for resolving issues, or for stimulating more discourse. They can be a sign of maturity in a discipline and a sign of growth and development. Such debates can take an ontological form, that is, discussing whether or not the interpretive or critical philosophies are congruent with the mission of the discipline of nursing. They also can be substantive debates grounded in the domain's concepts and key questions. The results of such debates may be compromise, resolution, synthesis, understanding, or polarization.

Nursing has had a historical tendency toward polarization and dichotomies. For example, recruitment patterns used to focus on white, middle-class females (rather than a broader spectrum of the population) and the either/or tendency in educational routes (diploma or baccalaureate degree). Another example is the early "either/or" roles required of nurses and women in many countries, such as either being married or becoming a professional—that is, opting for a mothering role or that of a career woman.

When one reviews the history of theory development in nursing in the United States, one can observe other indications of such dichotomies. When the metatheorists in nursing were speaking of theory as a product of tested and verified hypotheses and statements, a group of visionary theorists were developing conceptualizations of nursing that were images of coherent wholes, not particularly based on research findings. Each group adhered to a different philosophical view of science, although they both shared a complementary vision of knowledge development; however, the relationship between the two visions appeared more dichotomous than complementary.

Some of these polarities still exist and may keep the debates going, emphasizing the dichotomized nature of nursing knowledge development. I would like to propose two ways to deal with these polarities that may further facilitate knowledge development in nursing. The first strategy is to focus the debates, the critiques, and the discussions on the nursing domain, that is, on the business of nursing. The second strategy is to consider polarities not as either/or, not with a "versus" in between, but rather with an "and" between the polarities; in other words, learn how to live with our paradoxes.

Let me first address the strategy of focusing debates on the business of nursing. The focus for dialogues and debates in other disciplines may at times be more epistemological and ontological than substantive. The intent of these debates is to replace older, more established beliefs with another set of assumptions and a methodology that is more congruent with the current goals of the discipline. These sciences range from such well-established ones such as physics to those still vying for scientific recognition, such as sociology and psychology. In each of these sciences the methodological debates occur after the more substantive debates, therefore allowing for cumulative knowledge development within the disciplines. Not nursing!

The discipline of nursing has undergone a very unique path toward its knowledge development, one which proceeded from debates about the structure of its knowledge rather than its substance. These debates ranged from whether or not there is nursing theory and whether or not we should be or are capable of developing nursing theories to whether the methodological goals should be set by the positivist demons or phenomenological angels. Other debates included whether the discipline should use quantitative or qualitative research, a Cartesian or hermeneutic approach, basic or applied science, and feminist or traditional methodology. As healthy as the debates may be, they could have diverted the scientific community's energy from its more cogent task—that of developing knowledge related to the disciplines's central questions, which is the business of nursing. I am not proposing that we should halt all epistemological debates or ontological discourses. I am merely suggesting that if these debates were more focused and related to domain questions and domain concepts, they would offer a more constructive potential for the development of nursing knowledge. The difference is in the degree of emphasis on process and substance and in the goals of the debates. A debate that is focused on whether phenomenology or hermeneutics is the more congruent philosophy for the development of knowledge in nursing or for nursing practice would be more constructive if it focused on one of the domain questions in nursing as well. For example, a research program focused on the patterns of responses of immigrant clients to health-illness transitions, their patterns of coping with health transitions that are superimposed on geographic transitions, and the most effective nursing therapeutics could be pursued using different ontological beliefs and methodological approaches. The questions then would be: Which approach tends to lead to more cogent questions? Which philosophical premises may increase and enhance understanding of these questions, and which provide the more cogent answers for the development of future knowledge and for the care of these clients? *What I am proposing here is revising our passion for methodology, for science, and for philosophy.* Let us have a similar *passion* for *substance,* for the *business of nursing.* A passion for the knowledge itself, and not how we get the knowledge.

The second proposed strategy for facilitating knowledge development is to cast new meanings on some of the dualities in the domain and to consider their complementary nature. Two of these dualities, particularism and holism and received and perceived views, have been selected for discussion here.

Particularism and Holism

Particularism and holism have been used by nurse theorists as frameworks in developing concepts regarding the nursing client and therapeutics. Kim defines holistic perception and conception of an object or a situation "as having meanings as a totality" (Kim, 1983, p. 15). This is in contrast to perceiving and conceptualizing the situation or object in terms of individual parts that are selected for study. Nurses have used both perspectives interchangeably and according to the goals of a particular analysis. Clinicians may have a focus on a particular critical behavior, and researchers may have to isolate one subsystem for the sake of study and analysis. Though our analytical stance is one of viewing the nursing client as a unitary human being and as a whole human being, the limited availability of research strategies congruent with such ontology may curtail further knowledge development. Viewing the particular cannot be rejected outright, and a unitary approach cannot be wholly adopted until we are able to resolve the issue of availability of research methods and designs to represent both. To adopt *both* particularism and holism allows for temporary acceptance of the limitations in existing modes of inquiry, but it does not preclude the need for the future development of other modes more congruent with the emerging shared ontological beliefs (Meleis, 1986).

Received and Perceived Views

A received view in theory development is one that is derived through the consideration of logically deduced and verified propositions. It is a view that promotes cause and effect relationships and promotes prediction as its goal and explanation as an outcome of prediction. It promotes objectivity, control of biases, value-free theories, and a view of reality as the one truth that is based on sensory data. A received view derives its premises from an empirical positivistic philosophy. Studies that are geared toward meticulous, observation-based data, with attention focused on control and prediction, and where a careful reduction into operationalized units is the goal, are considered empirical positivist studies. The findings of these studies then, become the bases for theories.

In contrast, a perceived view allows a more fluid view of theory; one that is based on the interpretations of the researcher as well as those of the research subjects. It allows for the biases of the researcher to be articulated and not avoided, disclaims value-free science, and promotes the contextual explanation of phenomena. It also allows for attempting to see the world through the glasses of the subjects and for modifications and reinterpretations through a discourse involving both subjects and researchers.

Some researchers in nursing have promoted the received view. Clinicians, on the other hand, tended to base their clinical work on ontological beliefs derived from phenomenological and interpretive philosophies. Perhaps not totally cognizant of their philosophical beliefs, some nurses published clinical descriptive studies that considered perceptions and interpretations that are personal and clinical.

It has been proposed (Allen, 1985; Baer, 1979; Carper, 1978; Chinn, 1985; Meleis, 1985a) that both perspectives are useful for the development of nursing knowledge. More important, a substantive discourse and debate focused on the nursing domain could help specify which components and questions within the domain of nursing are more amenable to and congruent with which ontological beliefs and selected philosophical modes of inquiry.

ReVision 2: Gender-Sensitive Knowledge

The scientific enterprises in many disciplines have reflected a masculine culture, bias, and ideology. Women and their traditional female values have been conspicuously invisible. Many a discipline has become poignantly aware of the imbalance, and measures have been taken to correct it. The shift and change is slow, but at least there is a movement in the right direction.

Nursing's literature is beginning to reflect these universal concerns and criticisms. In fact, knowledge development in nursing has been specifically criticized for its lack of utilization of feminist methodology. While attempts are being made to raise the consciousness of the discipline's scientists and clinicians, we may also be getting on another bandwagon that may deflect needed energy that should go into the *business* of nursing. By carefully considering our own nursing heritage, we may reconsider the foundation for this criticism.

The overwhelming majority of nurses are women, and therefore, in comparison to other disciplines, women have been able to rise, hold, and maintain prominent positions within nursing. Experiences of women have also been at the center of nursing subject matter in such areas of investigation as nurses' perceptions of their roles, women's roles, and the experience of mothering and of birthing, among others. Feminist methods such as description, contextuality, multiple approaches to data gathering, subjectivity, consideration of the perception of clients, and gender as a variable (Roberts, 1981) have been used in the practice of nursing. But it is true that these methods have been less utilized in nursing research because this research has been more influenced by an ideology and a definition of science limited to objective, observable, and verifiable reality. What is needed, perhaps, is a rediscovery of some of the strategies used by our clinicians in developing theories and a co-opting of these strategies for use by researchers and theoreticians.

Feminist approaches are also manifest when a discipline is concerned with women's issues and experiences. Though a good number of the studies in nursing related to women maintain an image of women subjects within the structure of the family, more recently the focus of nursing studies of women's health has changed to other concerns. It is most encouraging to witness the emergence of interest in topics that are significant to women, which have received limited attention by members of other disciplines. Examples are numerous. They include hot flashes during menopause (Voda, 1985); rape and processes of recovery (Holmstrom & Burgess, 1978); osteoporosis during menopause (McPherson, 1985); patterns of social support and seeking help in battering situations (Limandri, 1985; McKenna, 1985); and patterns of support of chronically ill lesbian women (Browne, 1985). All of the above are representative of this shifting trend.

Although I definitely subscribe to feminist theories, I prefer the term *gender-sensitive* for its broader meaning. Gender sensitivity does not translate only to sensitivity regarding sex differences. Gender-sensitive knowledge is based on removing the barriers that exist between the subject matter and the researcher, between the subject and the researcher, and between the practice and the research roles (Stacey & Thorne, 1985). It is knowledge that evolves through a deliberate attempt at allowing research subjects to be active participants in the research process, to be involved in a process of interpretation of their experiences, and, when needed, to be a part of the process of definition and redefinition of the meaning of these experiences. Therefore, gender-sensitive knowledge considers the sex of the researcher, the sex of the subject, and the context of the research encounter. Gender-sensitive theories that evolve to describe, explain, predict, and prescribe nursing phenomena have the potential to provide and maintain a sense of the whole—therefore being more congruent with ontological beliefs in nursing.

In examining our nursing heritage, we may be able to discern those conditions that are congruent with gender-sensitive knowledge, as well as significant for the continuous development of nursing knowledge central to its practices. What I am proposing here is to articulate some of the conditions inherent in the domain of nursing that could continue to augment the knowledge development process. I adhere to the position that theories help in identifying levels of knowl-

edge development in a discipline. Theories help in articulating research questions, the answers to which lend
support to early hunches or shed new light by stimulating further questions (Carper, 1978; Tilden & Tilden,
1985).

Three considerations are proposed here that
should be made whenever knowledge is developed in
nursing, and that emerge when different philosophies
are considered. I am proposing that these considerations become the cornerstones in our substantive debates or in our selection of the inquiry modes we use in
our research. They are the considerations that may help
us explicate the meaning of contextuality when viewing phenomena in nursing. They are necessary, but not
sufficient, conditions in the development of nursing
theories.

Experiences

Nursing practice encompasses care provided by
one human being to another. Both people come to the
situation with various life experiences. Nursing practice is also the arena from which nurses describe phenomena and discover relationships between phenomena. These phenomena represent the bases on which
theories are developed. Therefore, it is proposed that
the experiences of nurses and clients be considered and
accounted for in nursing theories in order to enhance
their descriptive and explanatory power, as well as
their scope and utility.

Utilizing experience in developing theory is not
new for nurses. For example, the experience of nurses
in providing nursing care was the impetus for one of
Nightingale's first theoretical formulations in 1860.
(Kopf, 1978). More recently, nursing's concern with
the lived experience of clients has been discussed by
many authors, for example, Oiler (1986).

Patients' experiences are no less significant for
knowledge development. Their responses take a different meaning when placed in the context of past life
experiences.

Perceptions

Nurses have demonstrated their concern with
"perceptions" and their belief in the centrality of

client's views in clinical, research, and theoretical writing. Perceptions have been discussed, for example, in
several existing nursing theories (King, 1981; Orlando,
1961). Patients' perceptions have been considered a
central variable in nursing theory and in numerous
research projects as well (Dracup & Breu, 1978) and
emerge historically as a central property of many of the
variables that have been explored in nursing. Examples
of such perceptual variables include: locus of control,
perceptions of premenstrual symptoms, and perceptions of health care and family interactions. Therefore,
it is proposed that when we engage in knowledge development in nursing through research or theory building,
a nursing perspective requires the inclusion of perception as a central property.

Meanings

Nurses deal with responses of clients and environments. The meanings of these responses are different
when viewed by people with different sociocultural
and health care experiences. Personal meanings attached to health and illness responses and situations
influence the nursing assessment and subsequently the
intervention. Personal meanings are understood in the
nursing situation within the context of societal and
cultural meanings. Meanings attributed to multiple realities create the context for the understanding of
responses.

ReVision 3: Global Approach

To achieve a range of perceptions, experiences, and
meanings, a mandate for international collaboration
emerges as a third significant ReVision. The United
States is a nation that has been built of immigrants and
refugees. It is also a nation that is looked upon by other
nations as one that provides assistance and support.
Nurses are at the hub of these expectations. Our commitment to health has significant social value and therefore can have a global impact if we follow a systematic,
conscious, and global approach to nursing knowledge
development. If those of us whose research and theory
interests correspond with interests of nurse theoreticians and researchers in other countries collaborate,

reciprocate, debate, and exchange ideas, we could develop broader theories that will help us understand, explain, and predict a wide range of human responses and develop more effective therapeutic approaches.

Focusing our approach on global knowledge development in nursing is possible if we utilize the domain perspective to guide our collaborative interests (Meleis, 1985b). This could be achieved through the establishment of data banks for global research and theory in nursing. Each theorist and researcher would be expected to identify an area of investigation that requires a global approach to enter in the bank. International researchers and theoreticians interested in the development of global theories would select one of these areas of investigation to guide their work. The results could provide nursing with more powerful theories for understanding human responses and more theoretical options for nursing therapeutics. This represents only one approach to global theories; others may be developed on smaller scales and through other networks. The ReVision of a global approach is a commitment to nursing knowledge development in areas of global concern, while maintaining a domain focus.

ReVision 4: Joy and Engagement in Knowledge Development

Knowledge development in nursing should not only be focused on the subject matter of the discipline, but should also consider the qualities of the researchers and theoreticians of the discipline. If we accept the premise of the significance of perception, experience, and meanings, then a concern for the theoretician and/or researchers arises. Intuition, reflection, and dialogue are three important tools for knowledge development. Taking time to develop these tools either formally or informally has the potential of enhancing the joy inherent in developing theories.

Dr. Evelyn Fox Keller, a mathematician and a humanist, said it best. If scientific inquiry is "serious in its commitment to the most reliable and fullest description of the natural world, then [it] requires the full use of *all* our talents and available pathways to knowledge, and not only those that have historically been labeled mas-

culine. Feelings, identification with nature, even love, in principle (if not always in practice) as available to men as to women, have a necessary as well as productive place in the pursuit of science" (Keller, 1985, p. 96). When knowledge development takes a personal meaning, there is a potential for renewed commitment and for zest and joy in the process. It makes the process of knowledge development less mechanical and more humanistic, an appropriate endeavor for dealing with nursing as a human science.

The Path to ReVisions: Guideposts

There are some markers on the reVisions' path. Three areas of accountability are signs that we are on the right road: (1) accountability to the domain of nursing; (2) accountability to humanity; and (3) accountability to ourselves.

Accountability to the Domain of Nursing

An area of investigation becomes meaningful for the general development of nursing knowledge if we go beyond the simple task of answering research questions. Throughout the research process, from conceptualization to interpretation, we can ask how an isolated research project is related to the domain of nursing. Answers to this question may help in revising components of the domain, shedding some light on one of its concepts, understanding its questions and its goals, or explaining the relationships within it. The centrality of the questions to the domain should be periodically questioned. In other words, we should be dealing with questions that have some domain relevance or significance. To have domain significance is different from, but unrelated to, clinical significance. Clinically significant issues may be of concern for the immediate resolution of issues, such as those surrounding the identification of self-care needs of patients receiving high doses of chemotherapy. A question that has domain significance on the other hand, such as patterns and processes inherent in immigration transition, emerges out of interest in the relationships among transition, culture, and human processes related to health; such as question will eventually, although perhaps not immediately, have an impact on clinical nursing.

Asking the following sorts of questions may help to indicate accountability to the domain of nursing:

• What is the relationship of one's investigation to domain assumptions, concepts, and central questions?
• Does the potential exist for theory development through cumulative investigative programs?
• Is there potential for development and use of innovative approaches to modes of inquiry that are congruent with the nature of nursing and the central tenets of its domain?
• Have conditions of contextuality such as experiences, perceptions, meaning, particularism, and holism been used?

Instead of modeling a problem with existing, more acceptable philosophical views such as the empirical positivist, phenomenological, or critical philosophies that dictate an existing mode of inquiry, new modes may be developed. We may want to consider that the area of investigation leads to the methodology rather than the reverse.

Accountability to Humanity

In our zeal for empirical precision, for fitting into the scientific arena, and for adjusting our interest to correspond with a limited definition of science, we may have investigated minutiae, replicated more minutiae, and published inconsequential findings. Nursing science has been redefined as process and not only as end result. It is not simply a collection of true statements that are valid, reliable through replication, objective in nature, and devoid of prejudices and biases. Rather, it is a human process that engages both the scientist and the subject of its study in a dialogue to help in understanding the nature of the phenomenon and in revealing its meaning to all concerned and to humanity in general. In our interpretation of the problematics of our research and of the results, I, therefore, challenge all of us to consider what difference our research makes to humanity.

The following sorts of questions may help indicate accountability to humanity:

• Have we made the connection of our research to health care in general? Have we explicated what differences our findings make to human concerns and whether or not the results are attempting to answer socially and professionally significant questions?
• Have we bridged the science-practice gap or made plans to cross the gap by publishing in clinically oriented journals and by presenting our findings to clinicians locally or nationally?
• Have we made attempts and plans to span the science-public bridge?
• Have we made attempts and plans to cross boundaries such as class, culture, and national boundaries, by making our work relevant to those other than white middle-class males and females?
• Have we gone beyond our findings to think of social policy implications?

Accountability to the Self

Having redefined science to include the biases (that is, the values and not the value judgments) of the scientist rather than attempting the unattainable task of controlling or obliterating all such biases in the process of interpreting the meaning of data, one of the challenges ahead of us is to search for the meaning of our research for ourselves. Time for reflection and time for dialogue are integral to time for the search for truth. It is by allowing time for all of these that we can establish a process of multiple truths finding. Reflection and dialogue could be and should be with self, nature, other objects, and/or our subjects.

Taking time to reflect on and discuss the meaning of a research result and how it all fits in with professional and life plans can be energizing and nurturing in further developing that area of knowledge.

Indicators of accountability to the self are the experience of a sense of joy and exhilaration that is associated with the innovation, discovery, and development of knowledge. Additional indicators are the experience of a self-initiated urge to share, discuss one's research with others, take time to brainstorm, challenge each other's ideas, and support each other's attempts at knowledge development.

Conclusion

We have traveled full circle—from rejecting a great deal about nursing practice or existing nursing knowledge (its contextuality, its qualitative methodology, its advocacy role) to accepting and cherishing nursing's heritage, its current accomplishments, and its future developments. We are learning to tolerate varying methodologies of inquiry, and to savor flexibility in living with and appreciating the paradoxes and the healthy diversity that characterize nursing's knowledge base. Diversity breeds excellence. It has become apparent that some of the clinical modes of inquiry that nurses have used for decades could be used in systematically developing nursing knowledge. To further such development, we should focus our investigations on the domain of nursing, develop gender-sensitive knowledge, use global approaches to knowledge development, and use multiple approaches to conceptualize and investigate phenomena. Experiences, perceptions, and meanings are essential considerations for theory development in nursing; however, the challenge before us is how to use these considerations in theory and research. The development of knowledge in nursing is also predicated on meeting the challenge of accountability to the domain, humanity, and self. It is time to challenge each other to think beyond current modes of thought and inquiry, but not to be immobilized by the urgent need for some innovative approaches. I challenge all in nursing to deal head on with our perpetual propensity to avoid the business of nursing by falling in love with such religions as science and philosophy. These religions are only ways and means to focus on developing the business of nursing. Let us get off the bandwagons and get on with the development of the business of nursing. Let us have a passion for substance.

References

Allen, D. (1985). Nursing research and social control: Alternative models of science that emphasize understanding and emancipation. *Image, XVII*(2), 58–64.

American Nurses' Association. (1980). *Nursing: A social policy statement*. Publication Code NP-63 35M 12/80

Baer, E.D. (1979). Philosophy provides the rationale for nursing multiple research directions. *Image, II*(3), 72–74.

Browne, S. (1985). Supportive and nonsupportive environments for the lesbian chronically ill. Unpublished dissertation, University of California at San Francisco.

Carper, B.A. (1978). Fundamental patterns of knowing in nursing. *Advances in Nursing Science, 1*(1), 13–23.

Chinn, P. L.(1985). Debunking myths in nursing theory and research. *Image, XVII*(2), 45–49.

Dracup, K. & Breu, C.S. (1978). Using nursing research findings to meet the needs of grieving spouses. *Nursing Research, 27*(4), 212–216.

Flaskerud, J.H. & Halloran, E.J. (1980). Areas of agreement in nursing theory development. *Advances in Nursing Science, 3*(1), 1–7.

Holmstrom, L. & Burgess, A W. (1978). *The victim of rape: Institutional reactions.* New York: John Wiley & Sons.

Keller, E.F. (1985). Point of view: Contending with a masculine bias in the ideals and values of science. *The Chronicle of Higher Education,* October 2, 96.

Kim, H.S. (1983). *The nature of theoretical thinking in nursing.* Norwalk, CT: Appleton-Century-Crofts.

King, I.M. (1981). *A theory for nursing: Systems, concepts, process.* New York: John Wiley & Sons.

Kopf, E.W. (1978). Florence Nightingale as statistician. *Research in Nursing and Health,1* (3), 93–103.

Limandri, B. (1985). Help-seeking behavior of battered women. Unpublished dissertation. San Francisco.

McKenna, R. (1985). Social support of battered women. Unpublished dissertation, University of California at San Francisco.

MacPherson, K.I. (1985). Osteoporosis and menopause: A feminist analysis of the social construction of a syndrome. *Advances in Nursing Science, 7*(4), 11–22.

Meleis, A.I. (1985a). *Theoretical nursing: Development and progress.* Philadelphia: J.B. Lippincott.

Meleis, A.I. (1985b). International nursing for knowledge development. *Nursing Outlook, 33*(3), 144–147.

Meleis, A I. (1986). Theory development and domain concepts. In P. Moccia (Ed.). *New approaches to theory development.* New York: National League for Nursing.

Oiler, C.J. (1986). Qualitative methods: Phenomenology. In P. Moccia (Ed.). *New approaches to theory development.* New York: National League for Nursing.

Orlando, I.J. (1961). *The dynamic nurse-patient relationship.* New York: G. P. Putnam's.

Roberts, H. (1981). *Doing feminist research.* London: Routledge and Kegan Paul.

Stacey, J., & Thorne, B. (1985). The missing feminist revolution in sociology. *Social Problems, 32*(4), 301–316.

Tilden, V. & Tilden S. (1985). The participant philosophy in nursing science. *Image: The Journal of Nursing Scholarship, 18*(3), 88–90.

Voda, A.M. (1985). Alterations of the menstrual cycle: Hormonal and mechanical. In P. Komenich et al. (Eds.). *The menstrual cycle* (2nd ed.). New York: Sperry.

Yura, H. & Torres, G. (1975). *Today's conceptual frameworks with the baccalaureate nursing programs* (NLN Pub. No. 15–1558, pp. 17–75). New York: National League for Nursing.

Response: ReVision and Passion

Peggy L. Chinn

Meleis's call for reVisions in knowledge development contains several ideas that struck a particular chord for me. Each of her proposed reVisions are critical ideas that can move our discipline in a self-chosen direction. To review her proposals, they are:

- ReVision 1: A passion for substance
- ReVision 2: Gender-sensitive knowledge
- ReVision 3: A global approach
- ReVision 4: Joy and engagement in knowledge development.

My response to these proposals focuses on ReVision 2, gender-sensitive knowledge. My own work and experience confirm Meleis's conceptualization of what gender-sensitive knowledge might be, and I concur wholeheartedly with the critical need to develop gender-sensitive knowledge. I like this terminology for labeling what "it" is or might become. The issue I would like to address, however, concerns a lack of clarity in the distinction between feminism and gender-sensitive knowledge. I am addressing this issue in a

spirit of continuing discussion, not with the intent of disagreement.

Meleis presented a critical need for gender sensitivity that is well defended. The traits of gender-sensitive knowledge, however, can also be called "feminist," and I would urge that we consider the need to embrace this identity for what we do in developing nursing knowledge. At this point in history, it is premature to make choices in language or in thinking that hold a potential for obscuring the experience and reality of women. Until women's reality and experience are well identified and valued, a view that incorporates both women and men will not be possible. The term "gender sensitive," while having many implied meanings that are valuable, also seems somewhat like an apology—a reassurance that we will, indeed, include male reality and not overly stress the reality of women. Because masculine experience is so prevalent in our thinking and so completely commands our attention, making this compromise may once again assist in our complicity with various forms of erasure of women's reality (Bright, 1982; Spender, 1982). Recognizing this reality, and its inherent dangers, is one important step toward Meleis's reVisions.

I agree with the well-stated warning that Meleis issues against jumping on a bandwagon, and I also agree that feminist ideology can often seem like just another bandwagon. In my own experience of putting feminist ideas into action, however, I have found that if it is a bandwagon, it is a profoundly difficult one to jump onto! It is for this reason that I think feminist thinking is not a simple issue, nor is it a fad. It is a revolutionary world view that values all human experience—and it is revolutionary precisely because it includes the experience of women. At this point in history, women's experience must be a central focus in order to begin to reach a point of integrating female and male experience (Chinn & Wheeler, 1985).

It very well could be that our persistent denial of our own experiences as women accounts for our persistent lack of substantive discourse, debate, and theory development in nursing. Nurses, primarily socialized to preserve the status quo and to serve the male-dominated system of health care, are well disciplined to deny their own experience. If we can begin to own more fully the essence of our experience as nurses and as women, I think that we will simultaneously begin to address each of the reVisions that Meleis has proposed.

Because feminism and nursing seem so disparate in experience, and because we have been socialized to think of ourselves and our own work as not valuable and inferior, the prevailing view in nursing has been that nursing's theoretical writings somehow fall short. In some respects they do, and I agree with some of the shortcomings that Meleis identifies—particularly in relation to a need for greater specificity and substance. For several years, though, I have been amazed at the extent to which nursing's theoretical writings hold promise for the development of substance, and the extent to which this substance indeed coincides with many of the central ideas found in feminist writings (Chinn & Wheeler, 1985). In reflecting on why this is so, it occurs to me that it is because the authors of these ideas in nursing are indeed women, and when women in nursing are in touch with their own experience it shows in their writings and ideas.

One reason we are sometimes intimidated by the ideas of feminism, and even our own best substantive ideas in nursing, is that these ideas are not consistent with the status quo. They are, indeed, revolutionary. Feminism values and endorses women, critiques male thinking, challenges patriarchal systems, and focuses on creating self-love and respect for all others and for all forms of life. Nursing can be viewed in parallel terms, as a profession that:

- values and endorses health
- critiques health-care practices that endanger health and reduce the quality of life
- challenges a health-care system that is dehumanizing
- threatens the economic imperatives of the prevailing health-care systems
- focuses on approaches to care that create individual wholeness and health based on a respect for all forms of life.

As with all ideas derived from women and women's experience, these ideas are not overly well received in the prevailing system. In fact, for centuries, women's ideas have been ridiculed, trivialized, and discounted (Daly, 1984; Spender, 1982). Many of these ideas have been ideas of nurses. Spender demonstrates how this process has occurred for centuries. If we examine Spender's notions about the ideas of women in general and mentally substitute the concepts of nursing and medicine, this is an example of what we find:

> What if this view of the world [the prevailing male view] does not match with a woman's [nurses'] own experience of herself and others? . . . To be confronted every day with the injunction to be subordinate when one does not feel subordinate, to manifest deference to males [physicians] when one does not see them as superior, to be urged to give way to men [medicine] in the name of reason when it feels most unfair, to be obliged to give consensus to male [medicine's] problems being the basis of society's [health-care systems'] problems when one believes that women's [nurses'] problems are equally, if not more, central and significant, could be to inhabit a chaotic, conflicting and confusing world (Spender, 1982, p. 6).

It is no wonder that we are sometimes frightened by what we envision. We cannot maintain the values that we derive from our experience, and continue to "make nice" in the health-care system as it now exists. What Meleis is calling for in her article is not something that will be easily put on like a suit of clothes. It takes conscious effort to learn to value our own experience and that of other women. As we do, we will develop the passion for substance that she has envisioned. Because of our experience, we will begin to create gender-sensitive knowledge, we will be led to a global perspective, and we will find not only joy and engagement, but ecstasy, in our knowledge development. We will create a massive stir, beginning within ourselves.

I believe that the shift toward Meleis's reVision is a revolution that has been rumbling, unrecognized, for a long while. It is now gathering strength, and soon, I hope, it will become our prevailing reality.

References

Bright, C. (1982). But what about the men? In M. Cruikshank (Ed.) *Lesbian Studies: Present and Future.* Old Westbury, NY: The Feminist Press.

Chinn, P.L., & Wheeler, C.E. (1985). Feminism and nursing. *Nursing Outlook, 33*(2), 74–77.

Daly, M. (1978). *Pure lust: Elemental feminist philosophy.* Boston: Beacon Press.

Spender D. (1982). *Women of ideas and what men have done to them.* Boston: Routledge and Kegan Paul.

Response: Early Morning Musings on the Passion for Substance

Nancy Fugate Woods

Meleis proposes four revisions for nursing knowledge development:

1. Developing a passion for substance in our research and theory-building efforts.
2. Generating gender-sensitive knowledge.
3. Using global approaches to knowledge development.
4. Experiencing joy and engagement in knowledge development.

I propose that the *passion for substance* is central to advancing nursing theory development. In the following response, I will illustrate how focusing on the substance of nursing knowledge can propel us, as a discipline, toward the generation of knowledge that is sensitive to the individuals, families, and populations we study; the use of strategies for knowledge development that transcend disciplinary and geographic boundaries; and the experience of joy in and love of our work. I will use experiences from an ongoing nursing research program to illustrate these points.

The Passion for Substance

There is no substitute for fascination with an important issue central to one's discipline. When that fascination occurs, it produces engrossment with ideas and a preoccupation with the topic in solitary moments, during discussions with colleagues, and in the course of conversation with members of one's social network. For the past 10 years, I have been involved in a collaborative program of research focused on women's experiences of perimenstrual symptoms that has been infused with a passion for substance. Our commitment to advancing women's health propelled us to publish the first description of the prevalence of perimenstrual symptoms among a cross section of U.S. women (Woods, Most, & Dery, 1982). Earlier studies focused on research participants who were college undergraduates, women who were seeking help for symptoms, or women institutionalized for mental illness, thus yielding a biased picture of all women's experiences. The passion that led us to study a cross section of the population of women, rather than a select subset, also influences our current work. As nurses, our ultimate concern is identifying methods to promote women's health through modifying their experience of symptoms and/or enhancing their ability to respond to symptoms.

As a basis for specifying therapeutic alternatives for women, we have explored the relationship between the social environment (stressors and supports), health-promoting or health-damaging practices (such as smoking and dietary habits), general health status, feminine socialization, and perimenstrual symptom experiences (Woods, Lentz, Mitchell, Taylor, Lee, & Barash, in progress). The passion for understanding the phenomenon has led us across disciplinary boundaries to collaboration with nutritionists, physiologists, social and behavioral scientists, and epidemiologists. We collaborate with participants as we invite them to discuss the validity of our findings, and with clinicians as we jointly generate therapeutic approaches to enhance women's well-being.

Focus on understanding the *substance*—that is, women's experience of a complex of symptoms around the time of menstruation—has demanded understanding of particulars as well as of the whole. There are some aspects of women's symptom experience that can be understood best through detailed nutritional analysis of micronutrients, such as B_6 levels. Yet, such nutritional information alone cannot provide a picture of the woman's life without reference to the social context in which she lives. Poverty as a daily reality may explain both the nutritional deficit and symptoms. Using quantitative as well as qualitative methods has broadened our understanding to include women's perceptions, experiences, and the meanings women ascribe to their symptoms. Triangulation of measures has enriched our understanding of how women view their lives and symptoms (Mitchell, 1986). Participants record their perceptions and experiences in a daily diary over a 3-month period and also participate in two interviews using standard techniques. There are both striking consistency and glaring difference across some measures, prompting lively debates within our investigator complex. This passion for substance is what ultimately builds knowledge.

Knowledge Sensitive to Human Experiences, Perceptions, and Meanings

Meleis stipulates that gender-sensitive knowledge development need not be limited to sensitivity to sex differences. Instead, she recommends that investigators explore experiences, perceptions, and meanings of phenomena within the individual's context. Indeed, the context surrounding the phenomenon of interest could be extended beyond the individual to other units of analysis, including families, communities, and cultures.

Passion for substance in nursing demands intellectual flexibility to move between the particularistic and holistic and an understanding of the connectedness of personal experiences with the molecular and macrolevels of human functioning. Our studies of perimenstrual symptoms have compelled us to consider women's experiences from their perspectives as women, to be sure. It has also demanded our sensitivity to women in the context of their cultural and social groups. For example, to extend our understanding of perimenstrual symptom experiences, we have included women from many ethnic and socioeconomic groups. We find surprising diversity in women's symptom experiences as well as in their life experiences. In our passion for substance, we have learned that cultural and social sensitivity in this effort is as important as gender sensitivity.

Strategies for Knowledge Development That Transcend Disciplinary and Geographic Boundaries

Meleis recommends that we seek international collaboration as a strategy for extending our understanding. As we follow our passions for substance, this strategy becomes a necessary part of scientific discourse. Scientific descriptions of "premenstrual syndrome" (PMS) reappeared in the 1970s, although the initial work was conducted in the 1930s. Moreover, the few published cross-cultural studies of women's perimenstrual symptoms suggest that PMS is not a universal phenomenon. Emergence of PMS in contemporary U.S. clinical literature parallels an increase in the incidence of depression among U.S. women over the past two decades, during which aspirations of women were greatly expanded and social structural supports reduced or held constant. In order to comprehend the phenomenon fully, our research has involved investigators from a variety of disciplines that support the study of biopsychosocial phenomena. Nurses, physiologists, nutritionists, and social and behavioral scientists' collaborative efforts will help us clarify to what extent perimenstrual symptoms are a product of acculturation, social milieu, health practices, general health status, reproductive system functioning, and physiologic responses to their milieu. Our passion for substance can lead us to understandings that transcend disciplinary, geographic, and temporal boundaries.

Joy and Love

It is the passion for substance, for understanding the phenomena of central concern to our discipline, that has generated the fervor necessary to sustain our effort over a decade and perhaps future decades, throughout the vagaries and vicissitudes of financial and collegial support for our love. The passion pervades our daily lives, not just at grant deadlines, but during social gatherings. It is simultaneously demanding and satisfying, difficult and joyful. Through commitment to understanding emerges a joy and love for the work, a unity between what we study, teach and practice, and a sense of coherence in our lives.

References

Mitchell, E. (1986). Multiple triangulation: A methodology for nursing science. *Advances in Nursing Science*, *8*, 18–37.

Woods, N., Lentz, M., Mitchell, E., Taylor, D., Lee, K., & Barash, N. In progress. *Perimenstrual symptoms, social environment, socialization, health practices, and health status.* Final report to the National Center for Nursing Research, USPHS.

Woods, N., Most, A., & Dery, G. (1982). Prevalence of perimenstrual symptoms. *American Journal of Public Health*, *72*(11), 1257–1264.

The Author Comments

Scholarship in nursing is measured by the extent to which we tend to develop a sense of accountability to the discipline of nursing, to humanity in general, and to ourselves. In this article, I discuss processes by which we can continue to develop our discipline of nursing while continuing to be accountable to the discipline and to those who matter most: our clients. The article reflects on four areas in nursing that concern me greatly and that continue to be the focus of my writings, my research, my teaching, and my presentations: the grounding of philosophical and theoretical debates in the substance and the core of the discipline, the role of U.S. nursing in international nursing, nursing care of minorities and disenfranchised populations, and alternative approaches to knowledge development that are more congruent with nurses and nursing.

When I wrote this article, I was beginning to feel uneasy about our continuing preoccupation with form over substance. We have had an historical propensity in nursing to debate structure, such as the appropriateness of different approaches and strategies for the development of knowledge. This historical pattern is reflected in more recent discourses debating different philosophical approaches without grounding the debates in the domain's central foci and goals—that is, the well-being of clients. Although I am a firm believer in diversity and in the initiation and continuity of healthy debates, I thought that we should pause and make sure our debates are grounded in the substance of nursing and the core of the discipline. Therefore, I proposed that substantive debates should take precedence over structural debates.

Another general tendency that has been of concern to me (as well as to others in nursing) is our tendency to trivialize our rich heritage and the fine work that nurses have accomplished over the decades. We have done that by adopting other's description of our discipline and our work. Therefore, taking into account nursing gender orientation and its historical work with stigmatized and disenfranchised populations, I have also proposed some principles that I believe to be essential to the development of nursing knowledge.

I believe, as we integrate our curricula to reflect the synthesis between philosophy, theory, research, practice and area of specialization, it will be easier for the graduates to ground structural discussions and debates with central disciplinary concerns dealing with the health and well-being of our clients. Also, I believe that nursing will be taking a major role in the development of knowledge related to the health care of minorities and stigmatized and disenfranchised populations in the U.S. and abroad.

That, in my opinion, is what scholarliness in nursing is about.

—AFAF IBRAHIM MELEIS

Chapter 11

Structuring the Nursing Knowledge System: A Typology of Four Domains

Hesook Suzie Kim

A typology divides the universe of interest so that empirical events considered to be important for the given discipline can be placed within the classification scheme. Assuming that nursing is actively involved in delineating the sphere of nursing phenomena, it is important to develop a typology that can be used to systematize research and ever-cumulating knowledge in nursing. A typology of four domains is proposed as a conceptual "map" of nursing and as a "sensitizing" scheme for further research. The typology includes the client domain, the client-nurse domain, the practice domain, and the environmental domain.

A cursory examination of the nursing literature indicates a proliferation of conceptual delineations of nursing phenomena, including those labeled as ones to be included in a nomenclature of a nursing diagnosis system. This paper suggests that the discipline of nursing science is in the midst of knowledge development focusing primarily on the problems of delineating the sphere of nursing phenomena. While a community of scientists may engage in activities at various stages of knowledge development such as that specified by Hardy (1986), for a knowledge system to be the fundamental requisite for the orderly development of knowledge it seems obvious to consider the aspect of classification and systematization. Since classification has to do with the issue of delineating and ordering the sphere of relevant concepts for a field of study, the conceptual sphere for nursing has to include those phenomena considered relevant by the community of nurse scientists and has to be based on organizational schemes that allow new inclusions of essential concepts and exclusions of the insignificant.

As Turner (1986) suggests, development of analytical schemes is an important and necessary aspect of theorizing in a discipline. A typology divides the universe of interest into an order so that explanation of an empirical event can take place within the classificatory

About the Author

HESOOK SUZIE KIM was born and raised in Seoul, Korea, and came to the United States in 1960 as an undergraduate student at Indiana University. She received a B.S. in nursing from Indiana University in 1962 and a M.S. in Nursing Education from the same institution in 1963, then pursued graduate study in Sociology at Brown University, receiving a M.A. in 1972 and Ph.D. in 1977.

Dr. Kim moved to Rhode Island in 1964. After teaching at the Roger Williams General Hospital School of Nursing for 8 years, she joined the faculty at the University of Rhode Island College of Nursing in 1973. She is currently a Professor at URI, teaching in the doctoral program.

When asked about personal satisfactions experienced in nursing, Dr. Kim replied "I have drawn most of my professional satisfaction from my interactions with students and colleagues. Graduate students have been a continuing source of stimulation for theoretical thinking in nursing. I have to say that a major satisfaction experienced in nursing was working with foreign colleagues from Norway, Japan, and Finland on collaborative nursing research projects." Looking to the future, Dr. Kim continued "I am delighted by the progress we are making in the generation of nursing knowledge. However, I think it is time for us to examine critically the nature of knowledge we are developing and assess what kinds of answers we are producing for nursing practice problems."

scheme. As I have argued earlier (Kim, 1983), an organizing framework that permits scientists to impose order on the phenomena of interest is a necessary prerequisite for developing theories and theoretical models. In this sense, the typology of domains presented here qualifies as representing what Turner calls *descriptive/sensitizing schemes*.

Turner states that descriptive/sensitizing analytic schemes are loosely assembled congeries of concepts intended only to sensitize and orient researchers to certain critical processes and to guide the development of theories; therefore, they should be flexible and provisional (Turner, 1986, p.11). Hence, at the disciplinary level (i.e., law, biology, medicine, nursing, etc.), what is required is a classification scheme through which relevant phenomena are selected and differentiated within the perspective of the discipline. Because the nursing scientist selects those phenomena and concepts of relevance for study, it is equally desirable for the nursing scientist to develop classification schemes for systematization of knowledge within the field.

Durkheim and Mauss suggested that at the turn of this century the purpose of classification systems was to "advance understanding and make intelligible the relations which exist between things" (Durkheim & Maus, 1963, p. 81). What Shapere refers to as "domains" (i.e.,

fields) are the focus at this level. He defines a scientific domain as being composed of "related items for scientific investigation," constituting a unified subject matter that poses important problem(s) for scientific investigation and having the quality of "readiness" in a scientific sense to deal with the problem the subject matter presents (Shapere, 1977, pp. 518–527). The issue of classification at this level, accordingly, has to be based on the conceptual or theoretical schema that asserts the relatedness of the items included within the unified subject matter.

Where are we then with respect to systematization of nursing knowledge? The typology of three domains proposed in earlier work (Kim, 1983) was an attempt to classify essential concepts in nursing. The nursing perspective proposed within this typology considers the universe of nursing phenomena in three separate domains: client, environment, and nursing action. Rethinking this differentiation of three domains for the larger "domain" of nursing has prompted me to consider a structure of four domains—namely, *the client domain*, *the client-nurse domain*, *the practice domain*, and *the environmental domain* (see Figure 11-1). This revision is based on separation of the original nursing action domain into two domains. This division is appropriate to conform to Shapere's (1977) criteria of

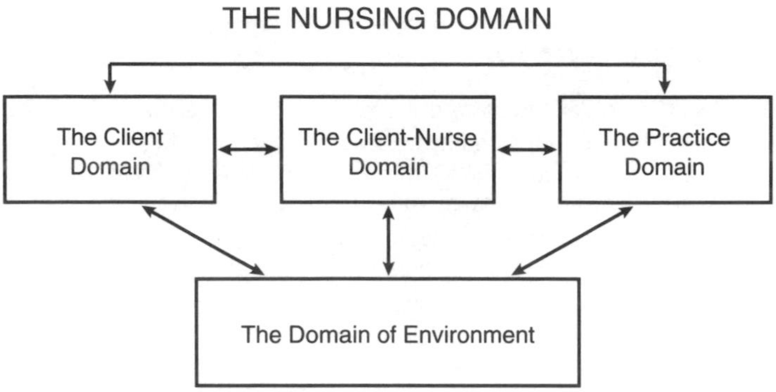

THE NURSING DOMAIN

Figure 11-1 *A typology for the nursing knowledge system.*

relatedness of items and of a unified problem for a domain. Although differentiation of the nursing "domain" into four separate domains is appropriate, the separate domains may still need to be combined into a larger domain if the larger domain poses a distinct problem that cannot be independently addressed by the subdomain solutions for the domain-based problems. Hence, for nursing we are in the first instance concerned with the problems specifically related to the four individual domains and in the second instance with the problem of the discipline, that is, the combine domains. The domains point to four spheres of the empirical world in which nursing-relevant phenomena could be located, while at the same time orienting the scientist to possible relationships. In this sense the typology of four domains is for the discipline an effort to provide a unified conception of nursing.

Four Domains: Structuring Nursing Knowledge

Figure 11-1 shows the organizational schema of the four domains in nursing as contributing to the larger *domain* of nursing. While this typology is primarily designed to orient nursing scientists to a conceptual "map" of nursing, practitioners of nursing should be able to contribute to the ultimate form of the map by examining the empirical applicability of the typology.

The Client Domain

This domain is defined as the area of epistemological concern related to the client. The emphasis is on gain-

ing knowledge about human phenomena within a nursing perspective (Kim, 1983). Kim identifies four classes of client phenomena as critical for nursing attention: (a) essential concepts, (b) developmental concepts, (c) problematic concepts, and (d) health care experiential concepts (Kim, 1983, pp. 42–45). It appears that the major thrusts for knowledge development in this domain should be oriented toward the development and testing of a nursing theory of humanity and toward the development and testing of middle-range theories that deal with particularistic phenomena in the client domain. Nursing knowledge in this domain has been the central focus both for many of the theoretical developments in nursing and for empirical testing.

There are mainly three types of scientific efforts for knowledge generation in this domain: (a) theory generation and reformulation of theoretical propositions, (b) empirical testing of middle-range theories pertinent to the explanation and prediction of client phenomena, and (c) conceptual clarification of client phenomena. The first type of effort has been evident in the works dealing with nursing's theoretical models such as those advanced by Rogers, Roy, and Orem, which provide explanatory frameworks for client phenomena. The second type of effort has been summarized partly by Barnard (1984), Denyes (1984), and Fleming (1986) for works in the area of child phenomena; by Stevenson (1984) for works in adult phenomena; and by Adams (1986) for works in aging phenomena. Women's health is emerging as an area in which several middle-range theories are being proposed, tested, and revised (see Voda & George, 1986, for example). For this type of effort, diverse theoretical models in physiology, psychology, sociology, and nursing have been empirically tested.

The third type of effort is most evident in the works associated with the nursing diagnosis conference group. Nursing diagnoses, as problematic concepts within this typology, have been accumulated without much effort devoted to developing explanatory theories. The methodology most frequently adopted for the generation of nursing diagnoses has been descriptive specification based on empirical generalizations (frequently using averaging or modal cases). The fervent movement in developing a nomenclature of nursing diagnoses is an attempt to address pragmatic needs for the identification of problematic concepts so that nursing may appear to "solve" problems of the client. While this is honorable and may be necessary, both nursing scientists and nursing practitioners have to realize that a nomenclature of nursing diagnoses that is not based on one or more explanatory, theoretical frameworks cannot contribute to the development of scientific solutions (i.e., nursing therapeutics). Nursing diag-

noses that are not developed within an explanatory framework have to be accepted only as descriptive "averages" to be used for the purpose of communication and documentation. This is not to say that descriptive generalizations are futile efforts toward theorizing in nursing.

What is needed is a development of analytic schemes for nursing diagnoses (i.e., schemes for the problematic concepts in the client domain). Future effort, then, has to be directed toward reconstructing nursing diagnoses through application in clinical settings or through development of theoretical schemes that could contribute to the nomenclature. In the meantime, nursing researchers should continue to develop instruments to measure client phenomena in order to arrive at the conceptual clarification and operational validity and reliability that are the building blocks in the testing of propositions.

An area that has not received systematic attention from nursing scientists is the study of health care experiential phenomena. Health care experiential phenomena arise from a person's experiences in receiving

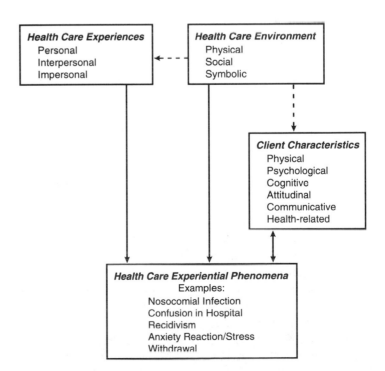

Figure 11-2 *An overall framework for studying health care experiential phenomena.*

health care. Such phenomena are the by-products of persons' involvement in the health care system and are not necessarily germane to the problems that brought the individuals to the attention of health care professionals; they may be influenced by and/or impact upon the persons' problems. The most well-studied health care experiential phenomena are nosocomial infection, recidivism, and sensory deprivation. Two types of knowledge are needed to develop nursing strategies dealing with health experiential "problems" either preventively or therapeutically: (a) causal or predictive explanations of occurrences of health care experiential phenomena, and (b) knowledge of the effects of health care experiential phenomena on an individual's health and recovery. Figure 11-2 depicts an overall framework for theoretical and empirical considerations for studying health care experiential phenomena.

As stated above, it is evident that further expansion of knowledge in this domain is needed in developing measurement tools for essential concepts in the domain and in developing and testing explanatory and predictive theories for client phenomena, taking client-based, environmental, and interactive factors as independent variables.

The Client-Nurse Domain

The client-nurse domain is defined as the area of study in nursing related to phenomena arising out of encounters between client and nurse. The client-nurse domain is an essential component of nursing's knowledge system and requires codification and investigation for systematization of tentative ideas, assumptions, propositions, and hypotheses relative to exchange phenomena. Client-nurse interaction is the major aspect of the client-nurse domain and has ramifications as both independent and dependent variables in explaining many nursing phenomena. The client-nurse domain is conceptualized to include many facets of interaction that occur between the client and nurse in the process of providing nursing care (Kim, 1983). An important perspective entails consideration of the client-nurse interaction as a medium through which nursing care and therapies are provided to clients insofar as there is hu-

man contact between the client and nurse in providing the care. Contacts between the client and nurse are occasions during which transfer and/or interchange of information, energy, and affection/humanity occur. Such contacts are the medium for delivering nursing care and for helping clients. In this sense, understanding the nature of the client-nurse interaction will enhance and improve the delivery of nursing therapies, which in turn will affect the client's status (such as general well-being, feeling states, and satisfaction) and increase the effectiveness and efficiency of nursing therapies.

Many theories of human interaction require reformulations within the nursing perspective to the extent that the dependent variables of significance in this perspective have to reside in the client. There is a need to develop and refine theories of client-nurse interaction that can be applied to influence the outcomes of nursing therapies through variations in the quality and process of client-nurse interaction. Knowledge in the areas of human and social interaction suggests that there are at least four sets of variables applicable for consideration: (a) individual actors (client and nurse), (b) social context of the interaction, (c) nature of interaction —process and property (see below), and (d) client health outcomes. Conceptual linkages among the four sets of variables are identified in Figure 11-3 as an overall conceptual framework for the client-nurse domain with an emphasis on interaction.

The first set of variables in Figure 11-3 are related to the individual actors who are participants in an interaction. Individual actors bring with them physical, psychological, cognitive, social, and ethical characteristics, including values, attitudes, abilities, and interactive patterning developed through past social experiences. Such attributes may be considered the predisposing, enabling, and hindering factors for the process and property of interaction. The interaction interactive encounters between client and nurse may be initiated, developed, or terminated in various forms according to the individual orientations the participants bring with them to interactive situations. Studies in therapeutic touch and empathy specifically suggest the

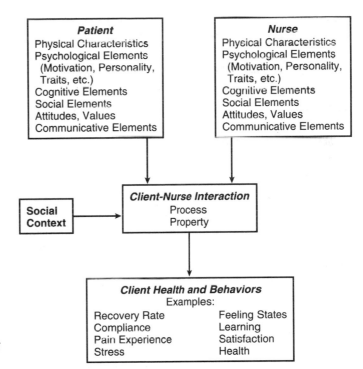

Patient	Nurse
Physical Characteristics	Physical Characteristics
Psychological Elements	Psychological Elements
(Motivation, Personality,	(Motivation, Personality,
Traits, etc.)	Traits, etc.)
Cognitive Elements	Cognitive Elements
Social Elements	Social Elements
Attitudes, Values	Attitudes, Values
Communicative Elements	Communicative Elements

Social Context

Client-Nurse Interaction
Process
Property

Client Health and Behaviors
Examples:
Recovery Rate   Feeling States
Compliance   Learning
Pain Experience   Satisfaction
Stress   Health

Figure 11-3 *Conceptual linkages among variables in client-nurse interaction.*

influence of nurses' characteristics in the client-nurse interactive process. Work in the area of stigmatization and labeling suggests also that stigmatizing or undesirable (that is, socially undesirable) facets of personal characteristics tend to influence the ways in which people react to each other's communications and the degree to which people maintain social distance from each other (see Goffman, 1963, and Scheff, 1966). These and other studies point to a need for in-depth understanding and reformulation regarding the effects of individuals' properties and characteristics on the client-nurse interaction.

The second set of variables, those related to the social context of interaction, have been studied at length in sociology. As suggested by Leonard and Bernstein (1970), the social context of interactions may not only be influential as a prerequisite condition for interactional encounters, but also may actually become a significant aspect of therapeutic communications. The study in pain management by Fagerhaugh and Strauss (1977) also suggests that the context of interaction in-

fluences the ways in which pain trajectories and patterns of interaction are developed according to the established rules of behavior, the meanings of specific communicative symbols, and the structural orientations of the context. Bogdan, Brown, and Foster (1982) indicate that the context of patient care predetermines the kinds of information that are transmitted to parents of sick children. The client-nurse interaction takes place in somewhat specialized social contexts in which the power distribution is unequal among the participants, role-prescriptions are socially well-institutionalized, and the cybernetics of control are generally preestablished. The major focus of interest for nursing for this set of variables, then, is in gaining understanding of the specific influences such social contextual factors have on the interactive processes and outcomes.

The third set of variables pertain to the interaction itself. Client-nurse interaction is considered along two dimensions: (a) the process of interaction and (b) the property (quality) of interaction. The process of interaction refers to the interactional sequence, trajectories, progression, and patterning. On the other hand, the property of interaction refers to the quality of interaction in terms of the elements of exchange (such as information, affection, support, energy, and resources) and communication types. Both as independent variables influencing the client's health outcomes and dependent variables influenced by the first two sets of variables, interaction variables in the nursing frame of reference have to be examined as a special case. While client-nurse interaction may have significant influence on nurses' well-being, the main focus of interest is the client's well-being. As suggested earlier, in meeting client needs a nurse does not simply perform actions in isolation from the client but has to perform in encounters with the client. In this sense, interaction is the most important medium through which the client's health can be influenced therapeutically and supportively.

The fourth set of variables pertain to the client's well-being. All major explanatory and predictive models in the nursing knowledge system ultimately have to deal with the client's well-being as the main dependent variable, and in so doing place the explanatory models within the nursing framework. Major dependent variables of the client's well-being within the interactive framework reported in the literature are recovery rate, compliance, coping, and information retention; however, although many findings begin to merge into a more codified set of general propositions, the literature contains many contradictory results and uncertain findings. This points to the need to refine research strategies and to reformulate theoretical rationales for specific application within a nursing framework.

While there has been a great deal of rhetorical emphasis on the importance of client-nurse interaction in the delivery of nursing care, very little has been done either in theory development or in empirical testing of the theories. There is a rich array of theoretical and empirical work accomplished in sociology and social psychology that is transferable to this nursing domain. There is a need to have an understanding of how the special nature of client-nurse interactions modifies sociological, social psychological, and communication

theories. Much work, therefore, needs to be done to revise and reformulate existing knowledge to explain and predict phenomena in the client-nurse domain.

The Practice Domain

The practice domain is conceptualized to include phenomena particular to the nurse who is engaged in delivering nursing care. The concept of practice refers to the cognitive, behavioral, and social aspects of professional actions taken by a nurse in addressing clients' problems. Phenomena in the domain of practice, however, have not been well conceptualized in the nursing literature. The effectiveness of nursing practice depends on an understanding of how nurses think, make decisions, transfer knowledge into actions, or use available knowledge (both universal and personal) in actual practice. Thus, the important phenomena that require explanation and understanding in the practice domain include, for example, the style and process of nursing care decision making, modes of transfer of knowledge into practice, variations in nursing actions, competence development, use and development of expertise in nursing practice, and the modes in which nurses resolve ethical dilemmas.

Two kinds of variables may be essential for studying phenomena in the practice domain. One is *exogenous* to the nurse and the other is *intrinsic* to the nurse. Exogenous factors for study may be distinguished into four areas: (a) organizational and structural factors of the nursing care setting; (b) culture of nursing practice including norms, ethics, conventions, and standards; (c) client-oriented factors such as nursing care requirements; and (d) spatiotemporal aspects. Intrinsic factors include personal attributes, the formation of personal knowledge systems and cognitive style, attributes developed as a result of previous experience, and professional characteristics such as attitudes, commitment, and socialization (Kim, 1983, p. 137).

Theoretical and research questions related to this domain have not been appropriately addressed in the literature, in spite of a wealth of knowledge apparent in decision sciences, operations research, cybernetics, and behavioral sciences. Much of the work summarized by

Gortner (1985) in the area of ethical inquiry with the "nurse" as the unit of analysis deals with the phenomena in this domain. There is also beginning interest in the area of decision making in nursing practice (see Corcoran, 1986; Grier, 1976; Joseph, 1985). Kramer's work (1974) on "reality shock" is an important beginning in examining professionalization as it affects the performance of nursing. Benner's work (1984) indicates a growing concern with the development of explanatory frameworks for understanding the nature of nursing practice and development of nursing expertise. An inquiry into the modes through which practicing nurses abstract the importance of certain client phenomena as opposed to other phenomena presented to them is also a critical subject for this domain.

The Environmental Domain

While this domain appears to lack the conceptual unity apparent in other domains in the typology, the concepts and phenomena of environment are important concerns to nursing. Environment of the client encompasses three variations: namely, time, space, and quality (see Kim, 1983, pp. 80–94). While the aspects of environment have to be considered primarily in the context of providing a more comprehensive understanding and explanations for the phenomena in the other three domains, it also seems appropriate and necessary for nursing scientists to test and develop theories that deal with the phenomena in the environment domain as a unity. For example, an understanding of differential distribution of health information among different family structures would be illuminating. Similarly, an explanation of the ways in which ethical concerns regarding, for example, "the right to self-determination for life and death," are developed in a society and institutionalized will be critical in understanding other phenomena such as collaborative decision making, client-nurse interaction patterns during conflict, and so on.

Much data and knowledge exist in the literature on the nature of environmental influences (physical, social, and symbolic) on morbidity, health perception, health-risk behaviors, and health care behaviors. The causal links among such variables are not obvious; however, neither do we have understandings about the mediating or cumulative processes by which environmental factors impact on our health. In addition, the conceptualization of the health care environment as problematic has been avoided for a long time through the protective attitudes of professionals. Health care settings such as the environment of the client, client-nurse interaction, and practice have to be conceptualized as having physical, social, or symbolic qualities, and such conceptualizations lead to explanations of phenomena in the client, client-nurse, and practice domains. The social environment of hospitals, measured in terms of the degree of social control, has been found to impact on patients' experiences (Baider, 1976); the impact of the symbolic milieu of patient-care units on nurses' conduct has also been noted (Crisham, 1981). Both the positive and negative influences of health care settings on patients' recovery, the process of interaction, and the nature of nursing practice have to be identified and investigated as the critical issues in the domain of environment within the nursing perspective. The phenomena of environment are important explanatory variables in enriching our understanding of the client, the client-nurse interaction, and the practice.

Conclusions

What I have presented in this paper is a status report on a revised typology of nursing science. This set of analytic schemes for nursing can be used to systematize the knowledge gained in the field of nursing and identify the gaps in the knowledge system that require scientific attention. Codification of what Turner (1986) calls "propositional schemes" within this typology of nursing science seems to be the next step, although current scientific efforts in nursing call primarily for a systematization that is provisional and concept-based rather than formalized and proposition-based. As suggested earlier, the proposed typology is tentative and requires scrutinizing as we begin to fit the phenomenal world into the classification schemes and develop theoretical understandings about the relationships among essential nursing concepts. As such, the typology is a tool for scientists to make discoveries about relationships and arrive at conjectures, hypotheses, and theories of various levels. What has become obvious to me over the years spent battling with this typology is the realization that it is based on a descriptive framework pointing toward the development of several, if not many, theories for description, explanation, and prediction in and of nursing.

References

Adams, M. (1986). Aging: Gerontological nursing research. In H. H. Werley, J.J. Fitzpatrick, & R.L. Taunton (Eds.). *Annual review of nursing research: Vol. 4.* (pp. 77–103). New York: Springer.

Baider, L. (1976). Private experience and public expectation on the cancer ward. *Omega 6,* 373–381.

Barnard, K.E. (1984). Nursing research related to infants and young children. In H.H. Werley & J.J. Fitzpatrick (Eds.), *Annual review of nursing research: Vol. 1.* (pp. 3–25). New York: Springer.

Benner, P. (1984). *From novice to expert excellence and power in clinical nursing practice.* Menlo Park, CA: Addison-Wesley.

Bogdan, R., Brown, M.A., & Foster, S.B. (1982). Be honest but not cruel: Staff/parent communication on a neonatal unit. *Human Organization, 41,* 6–16.

Corcoran, S. (1986). Task complexity and nursing expertise as factors in decision making. *Nursing Research, 35,* 107–112.

Crisham, P. (1981). Measuring moral judgment in nursing dilemmas. *Nursing Research, 30,* 104–110.

Denyes, M.J. (1984). Nursing research related to school-age children and adolescents. In H.H. Werley & J.J. Fitzpatrick (Eds.). *Annual review of nursing research: Vol. 1.* (pp. 27–53). New York: Springer.

Durkheim, E., & Mauss, M. (1963). *Primitive classification* (R. Needham, Trans.). Chicago: The University of Chicago Press.

Fagerhaugh, S.S., & Strauss, A. (1977). *Politics of pain management: Staff-patient interaction.* Menlo Park, CA: Addison-Wesley.

Fleming, J.W. (1986). Preschool children. In H.H. Werley, J.J. Fitzpatrick, & R.L. Taunton (Eds.). *Annual review of nursing research Vol. 4.* (pp. 21–54). New York: Springer.

Goffman, E. (1963). *Stigma.* Englewood Cliffs, NJ: Prentice-Hall.

Gortner, S. (1985). Ethical inquiry. In H.H. Werley & J.J. Fitzpatrick (Eds.). *Annual review of nursing research: Vol. 3.* (pp. 193–214). New York: Springer.

Grier, M. (1976). Decision making about patient care. *Nursing Research, 25,* 105–110.

Hardy, M. (1986, April). *Stages of theory development.* Paper presented at the Third Annual Nursing Science Colloquium, Boston.

Joseph, D. (1985). Sex-role stereotype, self-concept, education and experience: Do they influence decision-making? *International Journal of Nursing Studies, 22,* 21–32.

Kim, H.S. (1983). *The nature of theoretical thinking in nursing.* Norwalk, CT: Appleton-Century-Crofts.

Kramer, M. (1974). *Reality shock: Why nurses leave nursing.* St. Louis: C.V. Mosby.

Leonard, H.L., & Bernstein, A. (1970). *Patterns of human interaction.* San Francisco: Jossey-Bass.

Scheff, T.J. (1966). *Being mentally ill: A sociological theory.* Chicago: Aldine.

Shapere, D. (1977). Scientific theories and their domains. In F. Suppe (Ed.). *The structure of scientific theories* (2nd ed.) (pp. 518–599). Urbana, IL: University of Chicago Press.

Stevenson, J.S. (1984). Adulthood. In H.H. Werley & J.J. Fitzpatrick (Eds.). *Annual review of nursing research: Vol. 1.* (pp. 55–74). New York: Springer.

Turner, J.H. (1986). *The structure of sociological theory.* Chicago: Dorsey Press.

Voda, A.M., & George, T. (1986). Menopause. In H.H. Werley, J.J. Fitzpatrick, & R.L. Taunton (Eds.). *Annual review of nursing research: Vol. 4* (pp. 55–75). New York: Springer.

Response to "Structuring the Nursing Knowledge System: A Typology of Four Domains"

Ada Sue Hinshaw

Reviewing Kim's article "Structuring the Nursing Knowledge System: A Typology of Four Domains" has been an exciting and challenging endeavor. Several major issues have been raised by Dr. Kim in evolving a classification for structuring knowledge. This paper elaborates three issues: (a) relevancy of the typology to practice, (b) when to apply or utilize such typologies within the practice arena, and (c) consideration of diversity versus standardization in adopting such typologies for the discipline.

Relevancy to Practice

Developing structures, typologies, and classifications for the evolving knowledge base within the discipline is important if such knowledge is to be made specific and visible for individuals in nursing practice. The concept of descriptive/sensitizing schemes, as advanced by Turner (1986), provides a convincing argument that if either researchers or practitioners in the discipline are

to use the knowledge base, then it must be organized in such a manner as to allow for visibility and sensitization to the discipline's major themes and issues and to direct attention to certain critical processes. Through such a sensitization process, the knowledge can be used deliberately for the guidance of practice decisions and the development of theoretical explanations, as well as researchable questions. The policy statements of the discipline would reinforce Turner's arguments of the need for such structural systems. The ANA's *Directions for Nursing Research: Toward the Twenty-first Century* (1985) cites as one of the major priorities for nursing research the development of classifications specifically for nursing and client phenomena.

Because the nomenclature used is closely attuned to nomenclature used by the practicing nurse, Kim's typology of four domains would seem to be particularly relevant for the nursing discipline, especially for the guidance of practice decisions. The four domains are labeled according to constructs that are well accepted within the nursing profession (i.e., client domain, client-nurse domain, practice domain, and environmental domain). These domains are familiar and closely reflect the components cited by Fawcett (1984) as part of nursing's concerns (i.e., man, health, environment, and nurse). Thus, Kim's evolving typology is consistent with other major conceptualizations in the field in terms of its major domains and constructs. The major difference is the lack of stipulation of a goal or construct such as health, which is almost universally cited in other typologies. The question raised is: Is health a strand that permeates each of the cited domains for Kim's evolving classification rather than a major separate domain?

There are several special contributions made by Kim's particular typology which do not seem to be as evident in other classifications. These special foci of Kim's structuring of knowledge provide a helpful understanding of information and concepts for the practice arena. One clear example of the special foci is that of the health care experiential concepts under the client domain. Health care experiential concepts are defined as those phenomena that "arise from a person's experiences in receiving health care" (Kim, 1983, p. 103). Such phenomena are considered to be the outcomes or by-products of a person's involvement in the health care system, which may or may not be germane to problems that have motivated the individuals to seek health care. This section of the article, particularly well developed in Figure 2, outlines a number of the major concepts that will come under each of the larger construct headings for health care experiences, health care environment as they interact with client characteristics, and, ultimately, the health care experiential phenomena. Many of the examples cited by Kim are phenomena nursing has the capacity to influence, such as nosocomial infections, confusion, return to the hospital, anxiety reactions, and withdrawal. Thus, these particular phenomena become of interest to practitioners, due to their ability to intervene and to prevent or allay much of the effect of these types of phenomena.

The relevancy in this form of structuring knowledge for researchers in the discipline is that it makes visible the major entities and factors that need to be dealt with in evolving explanations about the relationships among and within the domains as outlined by Kim. Typologies are not by definition meant to articulate or specify these relationships, and, true to this format, Kim's structure outlines a number of important concepts but does not elaborate on relationships that may exist among them. Rather, she issues the challenge to scientists in the field to evolve explanations that will relate the concepts in the different domains in a rational and practice-relevant manner. Her challenge is well taken, and in issuing this challenge, she has proposed several broad relationships using the arrows to indicate either causal or correlational relationships. In addition to depiction of flow within each domain separately, it would have been helpful if guidance had been given relative to flow across the four domains.

Application to Practice

By its very nature, a typology of knowledge that structures concepts and principles for a discipline is continually evolving. Kim's knowledge typology is no exception. The issue raised is this: At what point in the development of a typology are the domains within the typology complete enough to be presented to practitioners in the discipline for consideration, feedback, and ultimate application in guiding practice decisions? For example, Kim's typology has two relatively undeveloped domains: environment and practice. The less developed nature of these domains is clearly acknowledged by the author. Should such domains be shared with practitioners at this point in time or should they be more completely developed through interaction with the nursing research community before release to practitioners? The opposing aspect of this issue is the value that would accrue to the typology if practitioners were able to review and provide feedback. Drawing on their experiential base, practitioners would be able to provide additional concepts and factors to be considered in domains such as environment and practice and perhaps greatly further the development of these particular domains. Thus, the very growth of the typology may depend on providing the current structure to individuals practicing nursing and on using their information and input to continue the evolution and development of the domains. Certainly such input should increase the relevancy of the typology for the practitioner in the discipline. For this process to ensue, however, nursing requires that its practitioners have a high level of sophistication in terms of handling knowledge. The practicing nurse is being asked to selectively review, critique, and use that information which is solid and ready to guide practice while selecting out the information which is new and possibly untested. The latter case calls for providing feedback on such information and carefully filtering the information in terms of its use in practice.

Diversity Versus Standardization With Nursing Typologies

The issue of diversity versus standardization in terms of the knowledge typologies for the discipline is a complex one. The dominant response to this issue changes given the subgroup involved in the discipline. The question of diversity versus standardization is not different from earlier issues raised in terms of one theory or several. The scholarly and scientific answer to this question has evolved to include the valuing of multiple theories and the comparison of their strengths and weaknesses in terms of providing explanations for the practice of nursing. Their diversity has ultimately been valued in terms of the questions provoked and the various perspectives provided for understanding constructs/concepts and relationships within nursing practice. From a practitioner's perspective, however, nursing professionals have been concerned about evolving a common standardized nomenclature and set of categories for structuring knowledge to guide practice in order to facilitate documentation of practice issues and provide a common base for communication among practitioners and other disciplines. Thus, the response to this particular issue of diversity versus standardization varies and will not be consistent across the discipline. Learning to live with this inconsistency will be an important factor. Only in this manner will the discipline be able to strive for standardization in order to guide practice-relevant considerations on one hand while promoting diversity within the scientific community in order to continue the stimulation and search for knowledge on the other.

In summary, Kim's typology or structuring of knowledge into the four domains of client, client-nurse, practice, and environment presents a new framework and possibilities for consideration of relationships among constructs and concepts. This knowledge typology provides several ways of understanding health care and, more specifically, nursing care that are extremely helpful; for example, health experiential problems within the client domain. Any typology raises recurring issues for the discipline to which we need to be sensitive. Kim's dedication to the continuing evolution of such a typology and structuring of knowledge in a way that is relevant for multiple practitioners within the nursing discipline is commendable.

References

American Nurses' Association (1985). *Directions for nursing research: Toward the twenty-first century.* Kansas City: Author.

Fawcett, J. (1984). The metaparadigm of nursing: Present status and future refinements. *Image: The Journal of Nursing Scholarship, 16*(3), 84–87.

Turner, J.H. (1986). *The structure of sociological theory* (4th ed.). Chicago: Dorsey Press.

The Author Comments

The Nature of Theoretical Thinking in Nursing, published in 1983, was organized around my initial thinking on the nature of a metaparadigm for nursing knowledge that was divided into three domains. As I began work with my graduate students and colleagues at the University of Rhode Island using this typology for organizing concepts in nursing and theories for identified nursing phenomena, it became obvious that the original domain of nursing action needed to be separated into two domains: the client-nurse domain and the practice domain. This separation is based on specifying the phenomenal fields that are distinct for analytical purposes. I believed that it was necessary to distinguish those nursing realities that are only possible in instances of client-nurse contacts from those that are embedded in the nurse in practice. Because I was not interested in revising the book solely on the basis of this revised thinking about the typology, I resorted to writing this article to present the four-domain typology. I think the ideas in the article clarify further the ways we can systematize nursing knowledge.

—HESOOK SUZIE KIM

Chapter 12

Philosophical Sources of Nursing Theory

Barbara Sarter

This article analyzes the philosophical roots of four contemporary nursing theories: Rogers' science of unitary human beings, Newman's theory of expanding consciousness, Watson's theory of caring, and Parse's theory of man-living-health. It is shown that these theories share many common philosophical views, but also maintain some significant differences. With the purpose of contributing to the development of a single metaparadigm for nursing, the following commonly shared themes are identified as forming an appropriate philosophical foundation for the discipline: process, evolution of consciousness, self-transcendence, open systems, harmony, relativity of space-time, pattern, and holism. Views of causality show some divergence between Watson and the other three theorists. Also of particular interest is the finding that Eastern philosophy has provided an important influence, both direct and indirect, on nursing theory. It is recommended that further philosophical exploration of Indian and Chinese world views be conducted and that the above metaparadigmatic themes be more fully developed in future nursing theory development.

As nursing begins to establish its power as a human science, it becomes increasingly important that its philosophical foundation be firmly established. The purpose of this article is to examine the philosophical roots of four contemporary nursing theories and frameworks, to describe their common philosophical themes, and to suggest future lines for theory development on the basis of these themes. The theories and frameworks to be analyzed are Rogers' science of unitary human beings, Newman's theory of expanding consciousness, Watson's theory of human care, and Parse's theory of man-living-health. These theories share many common themes and perspectives, yet also maintain some significant differences, both of which will help to clarify their philosophical stances.

The distinction between philosophy and theory is

About the Author

BARBARA SARTER is currently Associate Professor and Director of the MSN program at the University of Southern California, Los Angeles, where she has been a faculty member since 1984. In addition, she is a Clinical Nurse Specialist at Kenneth Norris Jr. Cancer Hospital, Los Angeles. A certified Clinical Nurse Specialist in medical/surgical nursing, she received certification as a Family Nurse Practitioner from the American Nurses' Association in 1990.

Dr. Sarter is a graduate of the University of Colorado, receiving a B.A. in English (1972) and a B.S.N. in 1974. After practicing as a clinical nurse in New York City for 6 years, she matriculated in the nursing program at New York University, where she received a M.A. (1981) and Ph.D. (1984).

Dr. Sarter describes herself as a practitioner and comments "Sharing the major developmental experiences of life-threatening illness and dying with countless patients has nourished my own under-standing of the meaning of life. The intimacy of caring for the sick as a nurse is a privilege that I cherish. As a teacher, I gain great satisfaction from inspiring and guiding students to be all that they can be." When asked about the future and her role in nursing, she replied, "The goal of my own professional work is to see nursing as an independent health profession with a fully developed philosophical/theoretical base. The current crisis in our health care system presents an important opportunity for nursing to establish itself as a leader in the revolution to reprioritize primary health care as the fundamental right of all persons."

one that has been blurred in the theoretical works of nursing scholars. In fact, some nursing scholars have argued that many of nursing's "theories" are actually "philosophies" (Uys, 1987). It is true that nursing theories are laden with philosophical assumptions which are not always explicitly acknowledged. Hutchison (1977) describes the difference between scientific theory and philosophy as involving the scope of intellectual activity. Whereas scientific theory involves a definite, delineated domain, philosophical thinking deals with unlimited totality, the entire universe. With this distinction in mind, one can argue that nursing's intellectual activity is not only the development of scientific theories, but also the development of a philosophical foundation to place its theories within a larger context.

As part of the structure of a discipline, a philosophical foundation forms the *metaparadigm* of the discipline and ideally should be shared by all its members (Donaldson & Crowley, 1978: Fawcett, 1984). Nursing scholars must develop a metaparadigm that can support a variety of nursing theories, while maintaining a coherent and common philosophical orientation. In the following analysis of the philosophical sources of four major nursing theories, one of the ultimate goals will be to contribute to the development of this metaparadigm for nursing.

Rogers's Science

Rogers's (1970, 1980, 1983, 1986) science of unitary human beings, the oldest and most influential of the four theories to be examined, is an appropriate starting point. Perhaps one of the reasons why Rogers's theory has drawn so much attention and stimulated so much debate is because it appears to be nursing's first attempt to philosophize on a grand scale. Rogerian science attempts to describe the entire universe, while focusing in depth on unitary man within that universe.

A review of Rogers's references and bibliographies is an inspiration to proponents of liberal education. A number of philosophers and scientists have provided important influences on her theoretical formulations. Among the most dominant of the philosophical influences are Ludwig von Bertalanffy, Pierre Teilhard de Chardin, Bertrand Russell, and Michael Polanyi. Scientific theorists have also had a significant influence on Rogers' work. Although they will not be included in this discussion, the ideas of Kurt Lewin, Theodosius

Dobzhansky, and Albert Einstein should be acknowledged in this regard.

Ludwig von Bertalanffy's (1968) rejection of reductionism in favor of a systems view of the world provides an important foundation for Rogerian science. The holistic approach espoused by von Bertalanffy was one of the earliest to receive wide recognition. von Bertalanffy maintains that macroscopic organizational laws occur and need explanation. He also proposes an evolutionary view of living systems, arguing that there is a negentropic trend in nature, due to the fact that nature consists of open systems. This trend implies that there are innate principles of self-organization in the evolutionary process.

The Rogerian view of open systems in a process of negentropic unfolding is virtually identical with von Bertalanffy's. Although the language of negentropy has decreased in her later writings, the concept still holds a pivotal place in the theory, since openness remains one of the foundational concepts of the theory. Open systems, by definition, are negentropic (Sarter, 1987). Von Bertalanffy is not the only theorist to have proposed the concept of open systems and in fact is relatively cautious in his use of the term, limiting it to living organisms, whereas Rogers maintains that there are only open systems and that the universe itself is an open system.

Bertrand Russell, one of the great modern empiricists, appears to also have had a significant influence on Rogers, specifically in the development of her view of noncausality. Russell points out that modern science does not support a law of causality; it merely makes an assumption regarding the uniformity of nature. "The principle 'same cause, same effect,' which philosophers imagine to be vital to science, is therefore utterly otiose" (Russell, 1964, p. 182). Russell identifies a number of philosophical fallacies about causation:

1. Cause and effect must more or less resemble each other.
2. Cause is analogous to volition.
3. The cause compels the effect (but not vice versa).
4. A cause cannot operate when it has ceased to exist.
5. A cause cannot operate except where it is. (Russell, 1964, p. 183).

He also explains that the traditional view of cause and effect is based on a simplified version of an isolated system, not on naturally occurring systems. Russell's careful analysis of causality is not duplicated in Rogers's work, but she accepts his conclusion that traditional views of causation are invalid, maintaining that change is continuously innovative.

Pierre Teilhard de Chardin's view of evolution supports a number of central themes in Rogerian theory. This philosopher is cited by Rogers repeatedly (Rogers, 1970). Teilhard de Chardin views human beings, as well as other evolutes, as centers of conscious energy that are organized into ever more complex and integrated wholes. Energy being inherently conscious at all levels of existence, the evolutionary process consists of an increasing personalization that is ultimately self-transcending into a mystical unity with all. Human self-awareness is a critical point in evolution, when complexity and consciousness become so centered that an entirely new order of experience and understanding emerges (Teilhard de Chardin, 1965, 1969, 1970).

Clearly, Rogers's early theme of an evolutionary trend toward increasing complexity, differentiation, and heterogeneity must have been influenced by Teilhard de Chardin's philosophy. Although she has dropped her characterization of evolution as moving toward increasing complexity and heterogeneity, this trend is implicit in the concept of an open system, as discussed above. Teilhard de Chardin's holism is another important aspect of his work that may have had an influence on Rogers' early theoretical formulations. Teilhard de Chardin's holism is epistemological as well as metaphysical, as is Rogers's. All forms of experience, from sensory to mystical, objective and subjective, are accepted as legitimate sources of knowledge. This is what is meant by epistemological holism. Metaphysically, the primary units of existence are irreducible wholes; consciousness is not a separate aspect but innate in the very substance of the universe, and each evolving unit is coextensive with the entire universe, all knit into one grand unity. Such a view is virtually identical to that presented by Rogers, although she avoids use of the word *consciousness* in favor of *sentience*.

Michael Polanyi's discussion of personal knowledge was also a significant force in the development of Rogers's framework. Polanyi explores the "tacit coefficient" of scientific knowledge, which involves the elements of personal judgment, decision making, intuition, and discerning the Gestalt of a phenomenon or theory. In emphasizing the role of the tacit coefficient or personal knowledge in the development of scientific theory, Polanyi comments that "apart from meaningless sense-impressions there is no experience that abides as a 'fact' without an element of valid interpretation of events. . ." (Polyani, 1946, p. 89). In turn, the interpretation of objective experience involves a weighing of alternative theories that is dependent on the mental satisfaction of the theorist. Verification of theory, then, involves intuition.

Rogers quotes Polanyi when commenting on the relationship between theory and practice: "Almost every major systematic error which has deluded men for thousands of years relied on practical experience" (Polyani, 1958, p. 183). Her discussion of an epistemology for nursing science emphasizes the synthesis of objective and subjective data. One can also speculate that Polanyi's influence may have been operating in the development of Rogers's view of four-dimensionality, in which the importance of subjective awareness is held paramount. In summarizing the influence of Russell and Polanyi on Rogerian science, it may be said that they appear to have been important resources for the development of Rogers's epistemological views. In contrast, Teilhard de Chardin and von Bertalanffy contributed more directly to the actual content of the framework in relation to concepts, propositions, and world view.

Although a complete synopsis of each of the theories under consideration is beyond the scope of this article, it will be appropriate to summarize the key philosophical themes of each theory and the philosophers who influenced these themes. Holism, process, four-dimensionality, evolution, energy fields, openness, noncausality, and pattern are the major philosophical threads of Rogers' theory, and the above discussion has pointed to their probable sources. von Bertalanffy

has discussed extensively the concept of openness. Teilhard de Chardin's work shows links to Rogers's conceptions of evolution, holism, process, and energy fields. Polanyi appears to have directly contributed to the concept of four-dimensionality, and Russell played an important and acknowledged role in the perspective on non-causality.

The key concept of pattern has received increasing emphasis in Rogers's later writings. There does not appear to be a single philosopher who had a particular influence on the development of this concept, although, at the same time that Rogers's thinking was focusing on pattern, there were a number of scientist-philosophers who were developing similar perspectives, such as Capra, Bohm, Pribram, Prigogine, and Bateson (Malinski, 1986). Rogers is familiar with all of these thinkers, and undoubtedly their influence has been important.

Newman's Theory

Newman's (1986) theory of expanding consciousness has strong connections with Rogers's science of unitary human beings. Newman was a graduate student at New York University and acknowledges openly the strong influence of Rogerian science on the development of her own theory of health. Rather than describing the individual as a human energy field, Newman defines a person as a unique pattern of consciousness within a field of absolute consciousness. The critical change from Rogerian science to Newman's theory is the attribution of consciousness to all matter/energy. This is an implied assumption in Rogers's theory (Sarter, 1987), but Newman has made it the foundation of her work. Evolution, then, becomes a process of expanding consciousness.

Newman explicitly acknowledges the direct influence of Teilhard de Chardin, Bentov, Bohm, Young, and Moss on the development of her theory. Of these, the contributions of philosophers Teilhard de Chardin, Bohm, and Young will be examined here. In Newman's theory, Teilhard de Chardin's view of an evolution of complexity/consciousness remains intact, as well as

Teilhard de Chardin's belief that the higher stages of evolution involve an expansion of consciousness toward unity with the entire universe. Newman sounds remarkably like Teilhard de Chardin when she explains that evolution is toward higher levels of consciousness and that persons are centers of energy within an overall pattern of expanding consciousness. The continuation of consciousness after death as part of a universal consciousness is explicitly identified as an idea from the work of Teilhard de Chardin, which confirmed Newman's own personal belief and became incorporated into her theory.

Physicist-philosopher Bohm's theory of the implicate order has contributed to the development of Newman's conception of pattern in the universe as a whole. According to Bohm (1980), the metaphysical ground of being is a multidimensional pattern, unseen, yet generating the explicate, or seen, world. Bohm also rejects mind/matter dualism, viewing them as different aspects of a higher dimensional, implicate order. From this theory is derived Newman's view of health as the visible manifestation of the unseen pattern of person-environment. Bohm's philosophy also supports Newman's holism. The implicate order is a total undivided pattern. Pattern recognition, the basis of nursing intervention, is "moving from looking at parts to looking at patterns. The pattern is information that depicts the whole, understanding of the meaning of all the relationships at once" (Newman, 1986, p. 13). Newman speaks of a holism similar to Rogers's in which not only the individual is an irreducible whole, but ultimately, the entire universe is an indivisible unity. Newman also attributes her view of movement as a manifestation of consciousness to Bohm's description of movement as the immediate experience of the implicate order.

Arthur Young (1976a, 1976b) has had perhaps the most significant influence on the development of Newman's theory, in the sense that Newman's specific delineation of the process of evolution is derived from Young's complex and creative synthesis of science and philosophy. Young's work has the stated purpose of developing a theory of the evolution of the universe that can accommodate and explain the numerous examples of higher consciousness documented in human history. Young maintains that the universe is a process that is put in motion by purpose, developing in seven stages, each of which manifests a new power. A diagram of the arc of process illustrates that the emergence of life marks a turning point. The early stages of evolution are characterized by increasing constraint as light becomes substance. From the emergence of life onward, the process is marked by the conquest of constraint and the development of controlled freedom, as opposed to the random freedom of atomic particles. Einstein's theory of relativity, Bertrand Russell mythic cosmology, Plato, Pythagoras, and Eastern mystical philosophy are Young's acknowledged sources.

Newman applies the principles of Young's arc of process to develop her theory of expanding consciousness. This is an attempt to synthesize her insights regarding movement as an integrating force and the transcendence of space and time through the expansion of consciousness. Young's seven substages of human evolution are incorporated into Newman's theory of expanding consciousness. Her summary statement of this theory is as follows: "We come into being from a state of potential consciousness, are bound in time, find our identity in space, and through movement learn the 'law' of the way things work and make choices that ultimately take us beyond space and time to a state of absolute consciousness" (Newman, 1986, p. 46). Newman equates absolute consciousness with love.

Moss (1981) is also credited by Newman as having been influential in the development of her theory. Moss is a physician, not a philosopher, but his work can be placed within the same tradition as Young and Teilhard de Chardin, process philosophy and mysticism. Moss's focus as a physician is on the personal transformation of consciousness that can occur during illness.

To summarize, the key themes of Newman's theory are pattern, expanding consciousness, movement, process, evolution, space, and time. The concept of pattern was influenced primarily by Bohm. Teilhard de Chardin was influential in the conceptualizations of expanding consciousness, process, and evolution.

Young was an especially strong force in the integration of the concepts of space, time, and movement into a theory of the evolution of consciousness. The roots of these philosophers, in turn, are in relatively and quantum theory, mysticism, and early Greek and Eastern philosophy.

Watson's Theory

Watson (1985) presents perhaps the most philosophically complex of current nursing theories. She is the only nursing theorist to explicitly support the concept of soul and to emphasize the spiritual dimension of human existence. Watson states that her philosophical orientation is existential-phenomenological, spiritual, and based in part upon Eastern philosophy. Watson also draws substantially from the schools of humanistic, existential, and transpersonal psychology. Specific philosophers acknowledged as sources by Watson are Hegel, Marcel, Whitehead, Kierkegaard, and Teilhard de Chardin.

At several points, Watson lists her assumptions, basic beliefs, and value. She assigns special importance in human existence to the soul. Synonyms such as spirit, inner self, and essence are also used for soul. The characteristics of the soul that she identifies are self-awareness, higher and greater degrees of consciousness, inner strength, power, intuitive and mystical experience, and continuation beyond physical death. This conception of soul is characteristic of certain Eastern philosophies, although to generically name the East as a source is meaningless, as Eastern philosophy encompasses the entire range of human thought from materialism to spiritualism. The only specific reference to Eastern philosophy is a book on the *Abhidhamma,* one of the three original Canons of Buddhist thought, which does not uphold the soul or the self as a "real" entity (Robinson & Johnson, 1977). Watson's view of soul is actually more similar to Hindu philosophy, in which the inner self (atman), or soul, endures through thousands of incarnations and merges into the Divine when liberation is attained. Teilhard de Chardin may also have been an influence on these ideas, although his view is less dualistic than Watson's appears to be.

The issue of Watson's dualism is an important one, for it sets her apart philosophically from the other three theorists under consideration. Body, mind, and soul are clearly distinguished from each other and assigned different functions and qualities. Soul is held to be the most powerful force in human existence, being the source of each individual's innate striving toward self-transcendence, or actualization of one's spiritual essence. This separation of soul and mind from body seems to create a dualistic stance. However, Watson would undoubtedly describe herself as holistic in the sense that harmony among the three spheres of body, mind, and soul is held to be the highest form of health and the goal of nursing care.

Another form of dualistic expression occurs in Watson's distinction between subjective and objective experience. In fact, whenever Watson speaks of harmony among various aspects of human life, there is an implicit dualism. The harmony that is identified as desirable includes person/world, perceived self/actual experience of self, actual self/ideal self, person/other, and person/nature. Another particularly significant dichotomy is that between health and illness. Health is harmony; illness is turmoil, or disharmony. Illness may lead to disease in the traditional sense of the word.

Watson's view of time differs from that of Rogers. Rather than rejecting the reality of past, present, and future, that is, rejecting the concept of time altogether, Watson describes them as different modes of being that merge and fuse in human subjective experience. Watson acknowledges the reality of time when describing how each person's causal past and presentational immediacy has the potential to influence the future. Time, however, is transcended in subjective experience. Causality is implicitly accepted as a relational mode in Watson's theory, as can be seen in the expression causal past and in the proposition that a troubled inner soul can lead to illness, which can produced disease.

A strong theme in Watson's theory is that of spiritual evolution, at both the individual and societal levels. Self-transcendence and transcendence of space and time in higher consciousness and mystical experience are held to be indicators of spiritual evolution. The basic inner striving of each person is to fulfill one's evolutionary potential "and in the highest sense, to become more Godlike" (Watson, 1985, p. 57). The evolution of civilizations is not characterized, but is referred to in statements describing the East as more spiritually evolved than the West. Of the philosophical sources acknowledged by Watson, Teilhard de Chardin appears to be the closest to Watson's view of evolution. Hegel as well as Whitehead also deal with the evolution of consciousness, but Hegel views self-consciousness and reason as the highest manifestations of consciousness. Again, it appears that Vedic and Hindu philosophy are indirect sources of Watson's view of evolution, through their influence on popular holistic views.

From the writings of Whitehead (1960), Watson has made an interesting adaptation of the concept of an actual occasion. An actual occasion is the fundamental ontological unit of Whitehead's metaphysics. An individual person or object is a succession of actual occasions, which are characterized by emotion, purpose, valuation, and causation. Every actual occasion is a process of becoming, which perishes once its subjective aim is accomplished. When it perishes, it becomes a datum of consciousness for successive actual occasions. Watson defines her concept of an actual caring occasion (or "event") as "two persons together with their unique life histories and phenomenal field in a human care transaction" (Watson, 1985, p. 58). Although Watson does not further develop this concept along Whitehead's metaphysical lines, her use of the term appears to be an attempt to capture the immediacy and subjectivity of a caring interaction.

Additional key concepts in Watson's theory are person, self, and phenomenal field. Here the influence of Buddhist psychology can be seen. Although there are several distinctive schools of Buddhist thought, some common beliefs are the doctrine of momentariness and the illusion of a permanent self (Hiriyanna, 1949). The person is a being-in-the-world, the experiencing and perceiving organism consisting of three spheres, body, mind, and soul. The self is a process, a perceptual/conceptual Gestalt. The phenomenal field is the subjective reality or individual frame of reference of the person. Implicit in all of these concepts is the idea of process, change, and impermanence. Watson does support the idea of a (more or less) permanent soul. In this her views come closest to those expressed in the *Bhagavadgita,* the most eloquent expression of Upanishadic and early Hindu thought and the most widely read spiritual treatise in the world. The influence of existentialist philosophers can be seen in connection with the ideas of being-in-the-world and phenomenal field.

To summarize, the key philosophical elements of the theory are soul, dualism, harmony, causality and time, spiritual evolution and self-transcendence, actual caring occasion, and self. Watson's conception of soul appears to be most similar to Teilhard de Chardin's and even more similar to that of Hindu philosophy (Sankhya-Yoga) as expressed in the *Bhagavadgita.* Her dualism of soul and body as well as mind and body, again, is most similar to that expressed in the *Bhagavadgita* and texts of the Sankhya-Yoga system of Indian philosophy (Hiriyanna, 1949). The concept of harmony among body, mind, and soul is not attributable to any of the philosophies that serve as sources for Watson; however, it is a commonly used term in popular holistic health views and may be indirectly derived from some Eastern source such as Taoism. Watson's view of causality and time is not traceable to a particular source but appears to be consistent with her stated influence from existentialist philosophy. The perspective on spiritual evolution and self-transcendence, as stated above, appears to be derived from Teilhard de Chardin and Hindu philosophy, which in turn have influenced the transpersonal psychology movement in the West. And, again as indicated above, the concepts of actual caring occasion and self are derived from Whitehead and Buddhist philosophy, respectively.

Parse's Theory

Parse (1981) has constructed a theory of nursing that is probably most explicit in acknowledging its philosophical sources. Parse shows how she has derived her work from her sources. Her creative synthesis of concepts justifies the characterization of her theory for nursing as unique. Parse's acknowledged sources are Rogers and existentialist philosophers Martin Heidegger, Jean-Paul Sartre, and Maurice Merleau-Ponty. From Rogers,

Parse has drawn from the principles of helicy, integrality, and resonancy and the four concepts of energy field, openness, pattern, and four-dimensionality. All nine of Parse's listed assumptions incorporate at least one of the elements from Rogerian theory in a synthesis with at least one of the existential tenets or concepts. It is assumed that the reader is familiar enough with the elements of Rogers's theory that the focus here may turn to existentialism.

The primary concern of the existentialist philosophers is human existence. The human situation is the source of their basic metaphysical categories, the rationale being that this is the aspect of reality that can be understood most fully. The basic question to be answered by the existentialist is "Who am I?" Kierkegaard and Nietzsche were the most influential sources of existentialist thought, which in turn become a fully developed philosophy through the works of Heidegger, Karl Jaspers, Sartre, Albert Camus, Martin Buber, and Paul Tillich. Edmund Husserl has been closely associated with existentialist philosophy through his development of phenomenological philosophy. Husserl focused on the nature of human consciousness, which he characterized as exhibiting intentionality, or objective reference; in other words, the mind is always actively encountering the world. Parse explicitly refers to Husserl's contribution to her work (Parse, 1981, p. 5).

Hutchison (1977) identifies the common themes that are expressed by existentialist writers. The distinction between essence and existence is the defining feature of this philosophy. In man, existence precedes essence; in other words, he knows *that* he is, but not *what* he is. In exploring the nature of man, the qualities of freedom, self-awareness, and self-transcendence are emphasized. Freedom means here man's self-determination, which is realized through the selection of and commitment to values. Closely related to human freedom is anxiety, another theme of existentialist writing. Alienation and nothingness are the result of anxiety in its pathological form. Authentic existence, living fully in the awareness of freedom and its accompanying responsibility, is the cure for alienation. A concern with ethics and human values is another dominant theme of existentialism. Finally, time and history are important foci of concern, for to be human means to have a history.

The tenets that Parse has drawn from existentialism-phenomenology are intentionality, human subjectivity, coconstitution, coexistence, and situated freedom. Although Parse's terminology and definitions are not exact renditions of those to be found in her citations, a careful reading will show her to be true to the meanings of the original sources. The tenets from existentialism and from Rogers are synthesized in the following summary statement of her assumptions: "Man is postulated as a unitary being simultaneously and mutually cocreating with environment rhythmical patterns of relating. As an open being, man freely chooses meaning in situation and bears responsibility for the choices. Man transcends with possibles in negentropically unfolding health" (Parse, 1981, p. 39). The phenomenon of human consciousness dominates this theory, in keeping with its existentialist roots. This becomes even more evident in the three principles of Parse's theory: structuring meaning multidimensionally, cocreating rhythmical patterns of relating, and cotranscending with the possibles. Utilizing a tripartite analysis of consciousness, the three aspects of knowing, feeling, and willing are respectively represented by each of these principles.

Parse's view of health and illness is nondichotomous. As in Newman's theory, health is a process, one of ongoing participation with the world, a synthesis of values, a way of living. Disease is a pattern of man's interrelationship with the world. There is no clear distinction made between health and illness or disease and nondisease. Certain parameters of health are implied by the theory, however. For example, it is maintained that the individual grows more diverse and more complex, chooses values, and molds his or her own ways of living. These behaviors may be viewed as aspects of health. Parse's multiple meanings of health may be grasped by viewing the three principles stated above as principles of health or, more accurately, principles of "man-living-health."

Assumption number four of the theory deals with

Parse's philosophy of *space-time*. Absolute space and time are rejected, replace by the view that these form a unified and multi-dimensional web within which probabilistic patterns of interrelationships unfold. Possibilities and potentialities are active forces in the present; thus, past, present, and future merge, as in Watson's theory.

To summarize, Parse has explicitly derived her assumptions and principles from Rogerian theory and existentialism, producing a creative synthesis that is logically constructed and organized. The rhythmical patterns of human-environment (or person-world) interaction and man's negentropic unfolding are concepts taken from Rogers but interpreted in a new way. The free choosing of meaning and values in life, its attendant self-responsibility and self-transcendence through fulfillment of the potentialities of one's being are aspects of human health that Parse has developed through an application of existentialist thought to the domain of nursing.

Common Philosophical Themes

In reviewing the specific philosophical themes of these four theories and frameworks, a pattern of its own emerges to describe the overall Gestalt. Process is one of the most striking overall themes. There is a view of constant change, but not of random change. The change is evolutionary in a predictable (though never certain) direction. The evolutionary process described by these theorists is not one of physical evolution, but of the evolution of human consciousness. The ways in which this evolution is characterized vary, but one consistent term that appears is self-transcendence. The implications of the view of human evolution as an evolution of consciousness are seen in the definitions of health. Health is this evolution. Human beings as open systems is another dominant view. The interaction between the person and the world is dynamic, continuous, and essential for the evolution described above. Harmony is a related theme that is seen in the writings of the theorists, either harmony within the person or between person and world. Views of space and time are non-linear, fluid, and relative. Space-time forms a matrix in which past and future merge into present. Another key theme is that of pattern. This is one expression of the holism, both epistemological and metaphysical, of the theories.

Keeping in mind the opening comments in this article about the need for a common metaparadigm or world view for the discipline of nursing, it is now clear that in these four theories and frameworks there are consistent philosophical themes that address nursing's metaparadigmatic domain. The themes together form a potentially powerful and coherent metaphysical and epistemological foundation for the further development of a variety of nursing theories. Of particular significance is the impact, both direct and indirect, that Eastern philosophy has had upon the development of nursing theory. Virtually all of the philosophical themes shared in common by these theories have been fully explored by several systems of Indian and Chinese philosophy. It is time that serious attention be paid to the formal systems of thought of the East, both ancient and modern, so that accurate interpretation and application, rather than vague references, can be made. A significant philosophical foundation has been laid for the development of a distinctive and commonly shared disciplinary world view. Nurse scholars should feel proud of the work done to date and commit themselves to further development of this world view. What is needed is nurse philosophers who can deal with philosophically complex issues, drawing upon past tradition as well as their own insights to develop a unique philosophy of and for nursing.

References

Bohm, D. (1980). *Wholeness and the implicate order*. London: Routledge & Kegan Paul.

Donaldson, S., & Crowley, D. (1978). The discipline of nursing. *Nursing Outlook, 26*, 113–120.

Fawcett, J. (1984). *Analysis and evaluation of conceptual models of Nursing*. Philadelphia: F.A. Davis.

Hiriyanna, M. (1949). *Essentials of Indian philosophy*. London: George Allen & Unwin.

Hutchison, J. (1977). *Living options in world philosophy*. Honolulu: University Press of Hawaii.

Malinski, V. (1986). Contemporary science and nursing: Parallels with Rogers. In V. Malinski (Ed.). *Explorations on Martha Rogers's science of unitary human beings* (pp. 15–23). Norwalk, CT: Appleton-Century-Crofts.

Moss, R. (1981). *The I that is we.* Berkeley, CA: Celestial Arts.

Newman, M. (1986). *Health as expanding consciousness,* St. Louis: C.V. Mosby.

Parse, R.R. (1981). *Man-living-health: A theory of nursing.* New York: John Wiley & Sons.

Polanyi, M. (1946). *Science, faith and society.* Chicago: University of Chicago Press.

Polanyi, M. (1958). *Personal knowledge.* Chicago: University of Chicago Press.

Robinson, R., & Johnson, W. (1977). *The Buddhist religion* (2nd ed.). Encino, CA: Dickenson.

Rogers, M. (1970). *An introduction to the theoretical basis of nursing.* Philadelphia: F.A. Davis.

Rogers, M. (1980). Nursing: A science of unitary man. In J. Riehl & C. Roy (Eds.). *Conceptual models for nursing practice* (2nd ed.) (pp. 329–337). Norwalk, CT: Appleton-Century-Crofts.

Rogers, M. (1983). Science of unitary human beings: A paradigm for nursing. In I. Clements & F. Roberts (Eds.). *Family health: A theoretical approach to nursing care.* New York: John Wiley & Sons.

Rogers, M. (1986). Science of unitary human beings. In V. Malinski (Ed.). *Explorations on Martha Rogers's science of unitary human beings.* Norwalk, CT: Appleton-Century-Crofts.

Russell, B. (1964). *Mysticism and logic,* Garden City, NY: Doubleday Anchor (Original work published 1917).

Sarter, B. (1987). *The stream of becoming: Metaphysical foundations of nursing science.* New York: National League for Nursing.

Teilhard de Chardin, P. (1965). *The phenomenon of man* (B. Wall, Trans). New York: Harper.

Teilhard de Chardin, P. (1969). *Human energy* (R. Hague, Trans.). New York: Harcourt Brace Jovanovich.

Teilhard de Chardin, P. (1970). *Activation of energy.* (R. Hague, Trans.). London: Collins.

Uys, L. (1987). Foundational studies in nursing. *Journal of Advanced Nursing, 12,* 275–280.

Von Bertalanffy, L. (1968). *General system theory: Foundations, development, applications.* New York: Braziller.

Watson, J. (1985). *Nursing: Human science and human care: A theory of nursing.* Norwalk, CT: Appleton-Century-Crofts.

Whitehead, A (1960). *Process and reality,* New York: Harper (Original work published 1929).

Young, A. (1976a). *The geometry of meaning.* San Francisco: Robert Briggs.

Young, A. (1976b). *The reflexive universe: Evolution of consciousness.* San Francisco: Robert Briggs.

The Author Comments

In 1986, Rosemary Parse telephoned me to ask me to become a member of the review panel for a new journal she was founding—*Nursing Science Quarterly.* Rosemary also asked me to write an article on nursing theory, from a philosophical perspective. She had enjoyed my first published article in this area and wanted a new perspective for her journal.

Her request came at a perfect time for me. I had been exploring four nursing theorists who particularly excited me—Rogers, Newman, Parse and Watson—and was intrigued by their philosophical richness. Rosemary's request provided the impetus and justification for pursuing this line of inquiry to my full intellectual satisfaction. So, I suggested that I explore the philosophical sources of these New Age theorists. Rosemary was delightfully enthusiastic and supportive.

My exploration of this topic was fascinating and enriching. As much as possible, I went to the original sources of the philosophers who were acknowledged influences on the theorists. The breadth and depth of these philosophical sources deeply impressed me, and has inspired my own further intellectual development. While coming to grasp the philosophical influences on these theorists, I also was struck by the creative leaps they took to develop truly unique theories for our discipline. The discovery of the metaparadigmatic themes common to all these theorists was a serendipitous fruit of this work, one which I hope may stimulate further work on the philosophical foundations of nursing.

I have been gratified to learn that this article has been used as required reading in some graduate level nursing theory courses. I hope it provides its readers with an appreciation of our discipline's intellectual heritage and the prospect of further creativity in nursing scholarship.

—BARBARA J. SARTER

Chapter 13

Theoretical Thinking in Nursing: Problems and Prospects

Hesook Suzie Kim

The development of nursing's knowledge-base for its practice has exercised the minds of nursing scholars in recent years as evidenced in the literature. Many of the nursing theories and conceptual frameworks initially proposed in the 1970s have gone through several revisions and testing by nursing scientists. There are some evidences that nursing's theoretical frameworks are producing an array of explanatory knowledge and some predictive or prescriptive notions about human phenomena and nursing practice. Many doctoral programs in nursing which have been implemented during the past 5 years to a total of more than 40 in the United States have also been instrumental in forcing nursing scientists to seek theoretical bases of their own research and of their students within the nursing perspective.

However, such culmination has received very little systematic scrutiny in the literature as to how far and to what extent the nursing's theoretical development has progressed. Nursing scientists in general are either in-terested in or pressured into 'testing' theories empirically rather than 'evaluating' or 'reflecting' on what theories are being produced or how they are being produced. Of course this is not to say that there have not been any critical analyses of nursing theories. Summaries and critiques of nursing theories and conceptual framewords have been published in recent years as evidenced in such books as Chinn and Jacobs (1983), Fitzpatrick and Wall (1983), Fawcett (1984), and Meleis (1985). However, much of these analyses were limited to evaluation of the contents of theories and conceptual frameworks which I consider to be only one level of analysis.

Inherent in this state of affairs is a lack of systematic framework upon which various levels of questions related to knowledge generation can be posed for the discipline of nursing. In general, questions related to how theories should be developed and what theories should be like are left to scholars in the philosophy of science to grapple with while very little systematic attention is paid to such questions by nursing scholars. In nursing, the products of theoretical work are evaluated only with respect to their contents and forms. My view is that this approach is limiting. A comprehensive system of theory evaluation that poses questions beyond those related to theory's content and form is needed to assess the broader questions of epistemological orientations as well as content adequacy.

This paper attempts to integrate several levels of analysis to examine the nature of theoretical thinking in nursing, beginning with the questions at the level of the philosophy of science and moving to the examination of the contents of theories being developed in nursing. The major assumption underlying this form of analysis is in the belief that the nature of scientific products is influenced by the scientists' views regarding the methods of knowledge generation, the definitions of knowledge structure, and the aims of disciplines as well as the focus of scientific attention.

A Framework for Examining the Nature of Theoretical Thinking

Whether or not a scientist is aware of the connections among his/her theory or research piece and the beliefs about what a theory should be like or what the content of a theory should be and the contributions of the work on the discipline is irrelevant. This is because the articulation between what Popper (1972) calls World 2, a 'subjective' world, and World 3, 'an objective' world occurs in scientific activities regardless of such awareness. What cannot be ignored is the idea that a scientist who is working within the frame of his/her own World 2 (a personal data system) is engaged in creating and adding to a World 3, the objective world of ideas, knowledge, and understanding which becomes interwoven with that particular scientist's perspectives about the world and science.

While it is apparent that most scientists go about with their work, i.e. their scientific activities, without paying very little attention to fundamental questions related to the nature of science and scientific methodol-

ogies, cumulatively their work results in forming prevailing patterns and forms in the discipline's scientific development. Hence the nature of theoretical thinking or theorizing in nursing has to be examined by looking not only into the contents of theories being developed or the products of theory testing but more importantly into the various levels of philosophical and perspective based orientations from which the scientist's work is being developed. From this assumption, I propose a five-level analysis framework for reviewing and evaluating theoretical work in nursing, articulating the following questions. These questions are similar to the ones discussed by Turner (1986) for sociological theorizing.

- What is the kind of knowledge possible for nursing? And, what kinds of theories are possible for nursing?
- What procedures are appropriate for developing this knowledge for nursing? And, what are the appropriate ways to develop nursing theories?
- What is it that nursing should try to develop knowledge about?
- What should nursing theories be concerned with? And, how can we decide what are important questions for nursing science?
- What are the ultimate goals of nursing knowledge being generated?
- What qualifies a given nursing theory to be scientifically sound?

These questions within the five-level framework are shown within the Figure 13-1, indicating the increasing specificity with which descending level influences theorizing and theoretical products in nursing. The five levels are thus specified as (1) the philosophy of science level, (2) the metaparadigm level, (3) the nursing philosophy level, (4) the paradigm level, and (5) the theory level.

The philosophy of science level is concerned with questions related to a scientist's positions regarding the nature of nursing as a science and the nature of scientific theory and theorizing. Analyses at this level will reveal the foundations upon which theories take their form and theorizing progresses. The second level focuses on a scientist's definitions regarding the essential phenomena of nursing requiring scientific attention and the selection of subject matters with which a given

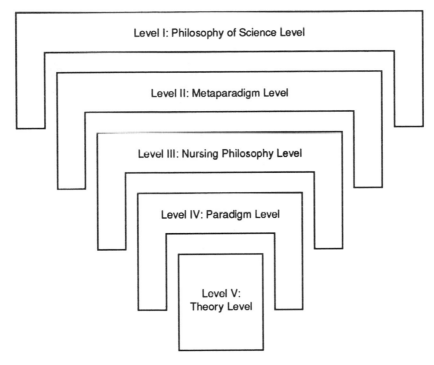

Figure 13-1 *Framework for analysis of theoretical thinking in nursing.*

nursing theory is concerned. This level of analysis can be examined within a metaparadigmatic structure for nursing science as developed by Kim (1983, 1987). What the analysis at this level can reveal is the boundary within which nursing theories are being developed and how such a boundary changes over time within the discipline's revisions regarding the 'critical problems' for scientific attention. While the first level (the philosophy of science level) is concerned with the fundamental positions regarding scientific methodologies for theory development and theory testing, the second level (the metaparadigm level) allows examinations of the 'content' choices which are made for the science.

The third level concerned with nursing philosophy is essential to the extent that a given nursing philosophy directs the development of nursing theories in their orientations for understanding, explanation, prediction, and prescription. Therefore, this level articulates closely with the philosophy of science level by directing the nature of nursing theory being developed in a methodological sense.

The fourth level is concerned with paradigmatic orientations and perspectives from which the actual theorizing is carried out. The term paradigms is used to mean general scientific perspectives and traditions in this discussion, not used in the strict sense with which Kuhn (1962, 1970) described paradigms for the natural sciences. The concept of paradigm for this level is appropriate for our analysis because nursing science is being developed from various scientific traditions, maybe because it is paradigmatic as Kuhn might argue, and furthermore because the critical scientific problems of the discipline seem to require various perspectives for understanding.

The fifth level is concerned with theories themselves. Analyses at this level will reveal the content of a theory with respect to its scope, logic and preciseness (i.e. form) of theoretical statements, testability and use.

While there been many nursing theoreticians who proposed different criteria for theory analysis and evaluation, for example, Stevens (1984), Hardy (1974) and Meleis (1985) among many. These four criteria have been adopted to be critical for the analysis of the contents of theory for nursing within this proposed framework. These four criteria have linkages to the preceding four levels of analysis, in that the questions of scope and use have direct relevance to the metaparadigm and nursing philosophy levels while the questions of form and testability are related to the philosophy of science and paradigm levels.

For the present exposition, this framework is used to scan the status of nursing's theoretical development and point up the areas in which gaps and deficiencies are apparent with respect to our efforts in nursing science. However, many fundamental questions related to the nature of nursing knowledge and scientising of nursing vis à vis nursing practice are lurking unresolved behind the scene of fervour with which scientific knowledge is being produced within nursing. Such questions are most troublesome, for example, as we encounter a nurse at a patient's bedside who is grappling with a decision to apply or not to apply a bed restraint.

Theoretical Development in Nursing: Status, Problems and Prospects

Level 1: Philosophy of Science Questions

Nursing within the last three decades in its attempt to be treated as a legitimate knowledge discipline has embraced the belief that its knowledge has to be scientific and that scientific theories are the foundations upon which knowledge about nursing phenomena may be accumulated. There are three basic questions which have constantly been circumvented by nursing scientists in their quests for nursing knowledge:

1. Is the primary goal of nursing science in understanding or in control?
2. What kinds of knowledge are appropriate for nursing discipline and nursing science?
3. What is (are) the appropriate form(s) of theorizing in nursing?

While it appears that modern nursing is comfortable with the notion that the best way to accumulate knowledge relevant to nursing and nursing practice is through scientific methods, we continue to argue regarding the extent to which the science of nursing should control nursing practice. In addition, dichotomising the science and art of nursing as separate entities requiring some form of integration has been one of the major struggles articulated by many nursing scholars including Florence Nightingale, Henderson, and more recently Carper (1978) and Watson (1981). On the one hand is the belief that nursing practice encompassing the art of nursing goes beyond the scope of nursing science, while the counter argument goes with the belief that nursing practice has to be based on scientific knowledge and the science of nursing. This argument, in a sense, is more fundamentally embedded in the question regarding the nature of nursing science rather than the seeming dichotomy of the science and art. The fundamental question therefore is whether the nursing science is concerned with 'what is' or 'what should be'.

Since all prescriptive theories must be based on the notion of what is the right thing to do, they are based on value premises. The proposal for situation-producing theories as the ultimate goal of nursing in the early years of nursing theory development (Dickoff, James & Wiedenbach, 1968a) had set the stage for nursing science to be normative science for many nursing theorists. Donaldson and Crowley (1978) also argue for the development of prescriptive theories which can govern the clinical practice of nursing. They view 'the syntax of nursing as value systems (both of science and professional ethics). . .' (p 119), and suggest that this syntax influences theory generation in nursing by providing a context from which judgments regarding the appropriateness, reliability and validity of knowledge being developed are made.

Suppe and Jacox (1985) also argue that since situation-producing theories presume goal states as the starting points, they are normative although satisfying as a species of teleological theory within the semantic concept of theories, and indicate that goal selection or the justification of selection are based on nonscientific normative or ethical assumptions requiring extra scientific procedures for analysis.

To the extent that prescriptive theories presume to differentiate what should be desired or preferred from what should not be, they are ideological and normative in nature. However, the procedures followed by developing prescriptive theories in nursing have not incorporated the procedures which are necessary in developing ideological knowledge. One form of argument has been advanced by Beckstrand (1978a, 1978b, 1980) in arguing against practice theories and by proposing that 'the goal of modern 'scientific' practice is to bring about changes in entities through scientific and moral means so that a good is acknowledged and defined within the ethical theory of value is realized or becomes increasingly capable of being realized' (Beckstrand 1978a, p 136). Beckstrand thus believes that scientific theory as value-forming knowledge may be developed separately, requiring juxtapositioning of two bodies of knowledge at the instances of practice.

It appears then that there are at least two schools of thought regarding the nursing science as value-free or value laden. Nursing scientists who believe in the notion that science is 'value-free' will have to be interested in understanding the nature of nursing phenomena as the basic goal of nursing's scientific enterprise, while prescriptive theorists goal of nursing science is in controlling nursing phenomena in selected contexts of goal attainment. This differentiation certainly will result in different types of nursing theories advanced and different methodologies use to develop such theories. Whether or not nursing scientists in general are aware of this differentiation in orientation is highly questionable in the light of the paucity of literature available on the subject.

Somewhat related to the above problem but related to the maturing of nursing as a scientific discipline is the current awareness among the nursing scholars of the role that various philosophies of science have played in influencing the kinds of nursing knowledge being developed. It appears that the debates in the philosophy of science have finally filtered onto nursing scientists, raising sensitivities and questions about the nursing's scientific enterprise as well as their own work in terms of methodologies and contents. This awareness may have been stimulated in recent years by the necessity to delve into the developments in philosophy of science by faculty members in the many newly created doctoral programs in nursing. Hence, we are recently engaged in debating about the nature of nursing science in terms of form and procedures of development (Watson, 1981; Webster, Jacox, & Baldwin, 1981; Hardy, 1983; Gortner, 1983; Uys, 1987) even suggests that many of the so-called nursing theories are pretheoretical and may be considered as foundational studies that try to answer such questions as foundationalism, development of language system, and philosophical analysis regarding the discipline of nursing science.

Nevertheless, the literature indicates that during the past 30 years many nursing scientists who had been trained in the tradition of the received view of science, with or without realizing their commitment to it, led the development of nursing science to the path that emphasized essentialism (Silva, 1977; Jacox, 1974), deductive theory building and formalization (Hardy, 1974; Chinn & Jacobs, 1983; Walker & Avant 1983), operationalization and empirical testing (Fawcett & Downs, 1986) and the rules of confirmation and verification (Silva, 1977; Gortner, 1980).

However, sensitising to the new developments in the philosophy of science with the exposures to and assimilation of the works by Hanson (1958), Popper (1968), Kuhn (1962, 1970), Lakatos and Musgrave (1970), Suppe (1977), Laudan (1978), and Feyrabend (1978) has created a great deal of confusion and uncertainties among nursing scientists in recent years (see Silva & Rothbart, 1984; Suppe & Jacox, 1985). Thus, many theoretical writings by metatheorists and theorists in nursing (e.g., Fawcett, 1980; Stevens, 1984; Meleis, 1985; Rogers, 1983; King, 1981) seem to have embraced selected views regarding the nature and form of nursing science. Some are holdovers from the Received View tradition, while others are encompassing of the new ideas suggestive of the perspective view of Hanson, the semantic conception of theories espoused by Suppe, and the historicism of Kuhn, Laudan, and Shapere, henceforth creating muddiness in the position taken by them regarding the nature and form of nursing theories and theory development. Whether or not this is only transitional and should eventually fall into distinct positions and schools of thought regarding the nature of nursing science has to be borne out by the history, it seems.

Attempts deviating from the earlier efforts in nursing theory development and methodologies for theory testing have become more varied and aggressive in recent years. Phenomenological theories (Parse, 1981; Paterson & Zderad, 1976), inductive theorizing (Benoliel, 1977, 1983; Norris, 1982), use of qualitative methodologies (Munhall, 1982; Watson, 1985), and hermeneutics (Benner, 1983) have been proposed as appropriate or better ways of developing nursing knowledge.

Level II: Metaparadigm Questions

A metaparadigm refers to a boundary structure which consists of items or phenomena for investigation for a given disciplinary perspective. Thus a nursing metaparadigm provides a structure from which the subject matters for nursing may be described and/or selected for scientific attention. Fawcett (1980) uses four essential concepts: person, environment, health, and nursing (Yura & Torres, 1975) as those encompassing the phenomena of interest to nursing science, and suggests these concepts as the components of a metaparadigm for nursing. Meleis (1985) expands this list in what she terms 'domain concepts' for a metaparadigm of nursing theories, and includes nursing client, transitions, interaction, nursing process, environment, nursing therapeutics, and health. Both authors use these metaparadigm concepts to indicate the extensiveness of a given nursing theory in its scope, and suggest that theories describing or dealing with any one of the major concepts are nursing theories—although Fawcett (1984) considers that the most sophisticated nursing theory would encompass all four of the essential concepts.

With a view that these metaparadigms are limited in the specification for the purposes of subject matter selection and of considering what would constitute critical scientific problems, a more comprehensive metaparadigm was proposed for consideration (Kim, 1983, 1987).

A metaparadigm topology of four subdomains for structuring nursing knowledge proposed in my earlier work (Kim, 1987) provides a freedom with which nursing theorists and scientists can select out phenomena of concern for theoretical or empirical attention within the nursing perspective at various levels of scope. This metaparadigm containing four subdomains (the client domain, the client-nurse domain, the practice domain, and the environmental domain) is based on the assumption that the goal of nursing science is to gain knowledge about the nature of human phenomena in the context of nursing practice. With such knowledge, it is possible to understand, explain, or predict human phenomena requiring nursing attention with respect to other human phenomena, environment, client-nurse interaction, or practice. Further, it is also possible to understand the nature of nursing therapeutics and interpret or predict outcomes of nursing practice. Table 13-1 shows a matrix based on this metaparadigm useful in examining the concept selections within nursing theories. It can be used to analyze theories in terms of in what domain the concepts requiring explanation reside and from what domain or domains the concepts providing explanation are selected.

Obviously, the domain of environment does not qualify to be the major domain of interest for explanation in the nursing perspective and is only appropriate in providing the focus of explanation. The matrix therefore can point up within-domain theories and across-domain theories at various degree of scope.

What has been found in our analyses of nursing theories so far is that the general theoretical frameworks, such as Rogers's unitary man model, Orem's self-care model, Roy's adaptation model, and Parse's man-health-living model deal with the client domain concepts in either nonselective or holistic manners, in the form of what Turner (1986) calls 'analytical schemes' rather than as theories containing a network of well developed propositions. Hence, these models may be considered theoretical to the extent that they try to order human phenomena in specific schemata with given orientations for the client domain.

In contrast, many middle range theories being developed and tested in nursing are more specific in the selection of metaparadigm concepts. For example, Johnson's theoretical and empirical work on a theory of self-regulation (1983) is concerned with the concept of identity development, both of them with the metaparadigm orientation in the client domain.

Interests in concepts of the client-nurse domain among nursing scholars are long-standing. Peplau (1962), Orlando (1961), Wiedenbach (1963), and King (1981) have taken concepts from the client-nurse domain for explanation of client phenomena or nursing practice. As it is true of the client domain theories, nursing theories dealing with the client-nurse domain tend to focus on global concepts of interaction and communication rather than on delineated aspects of client-nurse phenomena such as conflict, collaboration, competition, frequency, or quality of interaction.

What is important at this level of analysis is the identification of metaparadigmatic focus with the ultimate purpose of assessing whether or not nursing's theoretical work is adequately and sufficiently dealing with critical problems of the discipline. As one fills the matrix with nursing theories in the process of analysis, it is possible to identify the gaps in theoretical development in nursing. We have thus far limited theoretical

advances in making specific connections between concepts from the client domain and the environment domain and between those from the client domain and the practice domain. Hence, the metaparadigm level questions permit us to examine to what extent a given theory or a collection of theoretical work handle the critical problems or subject matters of interest to the discipline of nursing.

Level III: Nursing Philosophy Questions

As debated by Walker (1971), the term "philosophy of nursing" has been used in several senses in the literature. The specific sense it is adopted for this level of analysis refers to one's beliefs about the nature of humanity and what nursing "should" do about this humanity. These are preparadigmatic choices one has to be committed to in order to streamline one's theoretical thinking, and are closely related to the kinds of philosophic choices one makes in terms of the nature of science and scientific theories. This notion of choice in philosophies of nursing is not universally accepted. Munhall (1982) treats as given that there is an adherence to "a basic philosophy" of individuality and advocacy in nursing. Sarter (1988) points out common philosophical views as well as some divergent ones in her analysis of four nursing theorists' work, and suggests dangerously that the commonly shared philosophical views among the four theories may form "an appropriate philosophical foundation for the discipline." Sarter's conclusion thus is derived with the assumption that nursing science requires a single metaparadigm

Table 13-1
Nursing Domain in Matrix for Identification of Metaparadigm Focus of Theories

Domain of Focus Providing Explanation	Domain of Focus for Theory		
	Client Domain	**Client-Nurse Domain**	**Practice Domain**
Client domain	*		
Client-nurse domain		*	
Practice domain			*
Environment domain			

* Within domain theories.

based on an appropriate philosophical foundation. Sarter therefore equates a common metaparadigm of nursing with a world view, a philosophical foundation for the discipline of nursing. This notion is contrary to the position expressed in this paper, calling for multiple philosophies of nursing as appropriate.

While it is possible that there can be a prevailing philosophy of nursing at a given time, it does not mean that multiplicity in philosophies of nursing is impossible or inappropriate insisting on a unified philosophy of nursing is pigeon-holing the development of theoretical thinking in nursing to only one direction and one paradigm. Certainly for an essentialist who believes in one and only one truth, this view would be appropriate. However, philosophy is an intellectual choice and commitment one makes regarding metaphysics which becomes integrated into the lower level theoretical thinking.

My review, contrary to Sarter's analysis, indicates divergent nursing philosophies with orientations in such positions as rationalism, existentialism, causal determinism, instrumentalism, humanism, and pragmatism. As stated by Bernstein (1986), intellectual currents of a given period may have common philosophical concerns, but philosophical positions culminate into diverse idea systems according to the way the problems of humanity are analyzed. For nursing, this diversity in philosophical orientations will eventually influence the types of praxiology (theories of practice) that get developed.

What is usually portrayed in the nursing literature is a separate treatment of nursing philosophy without integrating it into theoretical positions. Hence, it is often that we encounter a theorist who advocates free will and individualism but whose theory is based on the assumption of normative determinism or behaviouristic holism. It appears that nursing scholars in general take the position that there is a unified nursing philosophy upheld by the nursing community, national or international, and that its significance to theory development is rudimentary at best. My view is contrary to this in that nursing philosophy having a close linkage to the philosophy of science has to be articulated into

theory so that the whole network of theoretical thinking that goes into theory building maintains internal consistency and is based on a compatible thread of idea-system.

Level IV: Paradigm Choices

Paradigm choices in theory development refer to choices related to theoretical tradition and perspective as discussed earlier. A given theoretical tradition for nursing holds specific assumptions about the nature of human phenomena or nursing. A theoretical perspective also advocates specific ideas about theory building and theory testing, thus guides theoretical activities in dealing with selected metaparadigm concepts. The most prevailing paradigm choices which seem to have guided and continue to guide the theoretical work in nursing are:

1. General systems perspective in the tradition of von Bertanlanffy's work
2. Behavioral perspective inclusive of all varieties of stimulus-response and adaptation/coping frameworks
3. Phenomenological perspective
4. Functional perspective
5. Sensory/cognitive perspective
6. Interaction perspective.

Although these seem to be the major paradigms, theories are more often based not on a single perspective but on two or more perspective combined to guide the work.

At the same time, nursing scholars are beginning to pay attention to nontraditional theoretical perspectives such as Habermas' critical theory (Holter, 1988) and hermeneutics and interpretive perspective. (Benner, 1984). It appears that as we become increasingly sophisticated and diversified in asking questions about the nature of critical nursing problems, we seek out alternative explanations based on different theoretical perspectives rather than holding onto those which have offered unsatisfactory answers in the past. This diverse approach to theory building in nursing may eventually fall into major paradigms for the three domains of nursing, as theorists and researchers working independently with concepts from different domains but from similar theoretical perspective begin to realize integration into major theoretical themes.

Level V: Aspects of Theory

This level of analysis is concerned with the content of a theory in terms of key concepts and propositions. Questions of "form" and "testability" refer to the internal structure of a theory, while the questions of "scope" and "use" refer to the degree with which a theory contributes to the development of nursing science. These four are considered to be the elementary, fundamental criteria to evaluate the content of a theory partly in line with Reynolds (1971), Hardy (1978), Stevens (1984), and Meleis (1985).

Form as the criterion of evaluation deals with:

1. The clarity, abstractness and consistency with which key concepts in a theory are specified and derived, and
2. Identification of the types, network and internal structure of propositions and theoretical statements contained within a theory.

An evaluation of a theory with respect to form will reveal the degree of completeness in the development of conceptual system in terms of logic, clarity, and abstractness. On the other hand, testability as the criterion of evaluation deals with the degree with which a theory can be translated for empirical testing. Hence, the more abstract a theory is the more deductive or interpretive steps it would require for empirical testing.

The questions of scope and use have been well articulated by Stevens (1984), and refer to degrees with which a given theory provides explanations for various subject matters in nursing and suggests usefulness in providing the types of knowledge for application. While middle range theories tend to be narrower in scope but are more useful in providing both explanatory and predictive knowledge, grand theories of nursing tend to be broader in scope but very troublesome in terms of utility.

Summary

The foregoing exposition suggests a global approach to evaluate theoretical thinking in nursing. Several issues have come to light in examining the current status of nursing's theoretical work within the proposed framework.

In most of the theoretical pieces of work in nursing, major threads of theoretical thinking are difficult to identify. It seems that even if it were to be an afterthought, any major theoretical work should be committed to certain positions at the four higher levels so that it becomes obvious for the kind of theory that gets developed.

As has been stated by many nursing scholars, the so-called grand nursing theories or conceptual frameworks require further specification to be called theories. There seems to be two ways these frameworks could be developed further:

1. They may be developed into paradigms of nursing by specifying advocated assumptions about the nature of human beings and nursing, theory-building strategy or strategies assumed to appropriate for the perspective, an image of nursing practice the perspective holds, and types of theoretical statements that are possible within the perspective; or
2. They may be developed as bona-fide theories by rigorously following the criteria at the fifth level.

It seems that the time is ripe for nursing scholars working within similar theoretical perspective to come together in order to formulate integrative nursing theories covering concepts from different domains of nursing.

For example, much work in nursing within the symbolic interactionist tradition may be ready to be assimilated into a nursing theory of "self-identity."

Similarly, much of the theoretical and empirical work dealing with how people develop competence in living with chronic illness (for example, cancer) can also be integrated into one nursing theory for further testing.

The community of nursing scholars at large has not dealt with the meaning of prescriptive theories for nursing science and nursing practice. There should be more rigorous debates regarding the normative nature of prescriptive theories and their effects on the development of nursing science and application to nursing practice in the context of scientific philosophy, nursing philosophy, and praxiology. The beliefs that praxiology follows naturally from prescriptive theories and that prescriptive theories are naturally the goal of nursing science are both naive and dangerous.

Certainly, we are becoming increasingly sensitive and competent to carve out those requiring scientific explanation in the nursing perspective. And in doing so, we have created world views of nursing that seem both socially and epistemologically relevant to pursue. However, theoretical thinking in nursing will require a greater degree of specificity in terms of process and products if we are to move away from the intellectual infancy on which we have been comfortably resting. This attempt will require not only a greater degree of specificity, but also a more rigorous self-criticism.

References

Beckstrand, J. (1978a). The notion of a practice theory and the relationship of scientific and ethical knowledge to practice. *Research in Nursing and Health, 1*, 131–136.

Beckstrand, J. (1978b). The need for a practice theory as indicated by the knowledge used in the conduct of practice. *Research in Nursing and Health, 1*, 175–179.

Beckstrand, J. (1980). A critique of several conceptions of practice theory in nursing. *Research in Nursing and Health, 3*, 69–79.

Benner, P. (1983). Uncovering the knowledge embedded in clinical practice. *Image, 15*, 41.

Benner, P. (1984). *From novice to expert: Excellence and power in clinical nursing practice.* Menlo Park, CA: Addison-Wesley.

Benoliel, J. (1977). The role of the family in managing the young diabetic. *The Diabetic Educator, 3*, 5–8.

Benoliel, J. (1983). Grounded theory and qualitative data: The socializing influences of life threatening disease on identity development. In P.J. Wooldridge, M.H. Schmitt, J.K. Skipper Jr., & R.C. Leonard (Eds.). *Behavioral science and nursing theory* (pp. 141–187). St Louis: C.V. Mosby.

Bernstein, R.J. (1986). *Philosophical profiles: Essays in a pragmatic mode.* Cambridge: Polity Press.

Carper, B.A. (1978). Fundamental patterns of knowing in nursing. *Advances in Nursing Science, 1*, 12–23.

Dickoff, J., James, P., & Wiedenbach, E. (1968a). Theory in a practice discipline: Part I, Practice-oriented theory. *Nursing Research, 17*, 415–435.

Dickoff, J., James, P., & Wiedenbach, E. (1968b). Theory in a practice discipline: Part II, Practice-oriented theory. *Nursing Research, 17*, 545–554.

Donaldson, S.K., & Crowley, D.M. (1978). The discipline of nursing. *Nursing Outlook, 26*, 113–120.

Fawcett, J. (1980). A framework for analysis and evaluation of conceptual models of nursing. *Nurse Educator, 5*, 10–14.

Fawcett, J. (1984). *Analysis and evaluation of conceptual models in nursing.* Philadelphia: F.A. Davis.

Fawcett, J., & Downs, F.S. (1986). *The relationship of theory and research.* Norwalk, CT: Appleton-Century-Crofts.

Feyerabend, P. (1978). *Against method.* London: Verso.

Fitzpatrick, J.J., & Whall, A.L. (1983). *Conceptual models of nursing: Analysis and application.* Bowie, MD: Brady.

Gortner, S.R. (1980). Nursing science in transition. *Nursing Research, 29*, 180–183.

Gortner, S.R. (1983). The history and philosophy of nursing science and research. *Advances in Nursing Science, 5*, 1–8.

Hanson, N.R. (1958). *Patterns of discovery.* Cambridge, England: Cambridge University Press.

Hardy, M.E. (1974). Theories: Components, development, evaluation. *Nursing Research, 23*, 100-107.

Hardy, M.E. (1978). Perspectives on nursing theory. *Advances in Nursing Science, 1*, 27–48.

Hardy, M.E. (1983). Metaparadigms and theory development. In N.L. Chaska (Ed.). *The nursing profession: A time to speak* (pp.427–437). New York: McGraw-Hill.

Holter, I.M. (1988). Critical theory: A foundation for the development of nursing theories. *Scholarly Inquiry for Nursing Practice, 2*, 223–232.

Jacox, A. (1974). Theory construction in nursing: An overview. *Nursing Research, 23*, 4–13.

Kim, H.S. (1983). *The nature of theoretical thinking in nursing.* Norwalk, CT: Appleton-Century-Crofts.

Kim, H.S. (1987). Structuring the nursing knowledge system: A topology of four domains. *Scholarly Inquiry for Nursing Practice, 1*, 99–110.

King, I.M. (1981). *A theory for nursing: Systems, concepts, process.* New York: John Wiley & Sons.

Kuhn, T.S. (1962). *The structure of scientific revolutions.* Chicago: University of Chicago Press.

Kuhn, T.S. (1970). *The structure of scientific revolutions* (2nd ed.). Chicago: University of Chicago Press.

Lakatos, I., & Musgrave, A. (Eds.) (1970). *Criticism and the growth of scientific knowledge.* Cambridge, England: Cambridge University Press.

Laudan, L. (1978). *Progress and its problems: Toward a theory of scientific growth.* Berkeley, CA: University of California Press.

Leventhal, H., & Johnson, J.E. (1983). Laboratory and field experimentation: Development of a theory of self-regulation. In P.J. Wooldridge, M.H. Schmitt, J.K. Skipper Jr., & R.C. Leonard (Eds.). *Behavioral science and nursing theory* (p. 262). St. Louis: C.V. Mosby.

Meleis, A.I. (1985). *Theoretical nursing: Development and progress.* Philadelphia: J.B. Lippincott.

Munhall, P.L. (1982). Nursing philosophy and nursing research: In apposition or opposition? *Nursing Research*, *31*, 176–181.

Norris, C.M. (1982). *Concept clarification in nursing.* Rockville, MD: Aspen.

Orlando, I. (1961). *The dynamic nurse-patient relationship.* New York: J.P. Putnam's Sons.

Parse, R.R. (1981). *Man-living-health: A theory of nursing.* New York: John Wiley & Sons.

Paterson, J.G., & Zderad, L.T. (1976). *Humanistic nursing.* New York: John Wiley & Sons.

Peplau, H. (1962). Interpersonal techniques: The crux of psychiatric nursing. *The American Journal of Nursing, 62,* 50–54.

Popper, K.R. (1972). *Objective knowledge.* Oxford, England: Claredon Press.

Reynolds, P.D. (1971). *A primer in theory construction.* Indianapolis, IN: Bobbs-Merrill.

Rogers, M.E. (1983). Science of unitary human being: A paradigm for nursing. In I.W. Clements & F.B. Roberts (Eds.). *Family health: A theoretical approach to nursing.* New York: John Wiley & Sons.

Sarter, B. (1988). Philosophical sources of nursing theory. *Nursing Science Quarterly,1*, 52–59.

Silva, M.C. (1977). Philosophy, science, theory: Interrelationships and implications for nursing research. *Image, 9,* 59–63.

Silva, M., & Rothbart, D. (1984). An analysis of changing trends in philosophy of science on nursing theory development and testing. *Advances in Nursing Science, 6,* 1–13.

Stevens, B.J. (1984). *Nursing theory: Analysis, application, evaluation* (2nd ed.) Boston: Little, Brown.

Suppe, F. (Ed.) (1977). *The structure of scientific theories* (2nd ed.). Urbana, IL: University of Illinois Press.

Suppe, F., & Jacox, A.K. (1985). Philosophy of science and the development of nursing theory. In H.H. Werley & J.J. Fitzpatrick (Eds.). *Annual review of nursing research: Vol. 3* (p. 267). New York: Springer.

Turner, J.H. (1986). *The structure of sociological theory* (4th ed.). Chicago: Dorsey Press.

Uys, L.R. (1987). Foundational studies in nursing. *Journal of Advanced Nursing, 12,* 275–280.

Walker, L.O. (1971). Toward a clearer understanding of the concept of nursing theory. *Nursing Research, 20,* 428–435.

Walker, L.O., & Avant, K.C. (1983). *Strategies for theory construction in nursing.* Norwalk, CT: Appleton-Century-Crofts.

Watson, J. (1981). Nursing's scientific quest. *Nursing Outlook, 29,* 413–416.

Watson, J. (1985). *Nursing: Human science and human care.* Norwalk, CT: Appleton-Century-Crofts.

Webster, G., Jacox, A., & Baldwin, B. (1981). Nursing theory and the ghost of the received view. In J.C. McCloskey & H.K. Grace (Eds.). *Current issues in nursing* (pp. 26–35). Boston: Blackwell.

Wiedenbach, E. (1963). The helping art of nursing. *American Journal of Nursing, 63,* 54–57.

Yura, H., & Torres, G. (1975). Today's conceptual frameworks within baccalaureate nursing programs. In National League for Nursing. *Faculty, curriculum development. Part 3: Conceptual framework: its meaning and function* (pp. 17–25). New York: Author.

The Author Comments

When Dr. Justus Akinsanya asked me to contribute to the volume in *Recent Advances in Nursing* dealing with theories in nursing, I was happy to oblige. For some time, I had been concerned with the lack of systematic linkages among philosophy, theory, and method expressed in much of the theoretical work published in nursing. Initially, many of the ideas for this paper came from discussions I had with my doctoral students and colleagues at the University of Rhode Island, such as Dr. Margaret Hardy and Dr. Donna Schwartz-Barcott. However, the finalization of the paper was stimulated by my exposure to "European thinking" about knowledge generation as I was on my sabbatical leave at the Institute of Nursing Science at the University of Oslo, Norway, during the academic year of 1988–89. For such circumstantial influence on the shaping of this article, I am fondly appreciative of Solzenitzen's notion about how a person's evolution of ideas is shaped by the nature of contexts and experiences.

—HESOOK SUZIE KIM

Chapter 14

Nursing Theorizing
as an Ethical Endeavor

Pamela G. Reed

This article addresses the ethical dimensions of nursing theorizing. Nursing theorizing, whether it occurs primarily at the outset or emerges during the process of inquiry, is inescapably linked to the theorist's value choices and beliefs about human beings, the environment, and health. These choices are reflected in the conceptual frame of one's research. The normative commitment of the conceptual frame is explored using examples from nursing and nonnursing research. Elements of critical ethical reflection are outlined. It is suggested that the discipline's understanding of what constitutes health and how best to promote health, as well as solutions to ethical dilemmas posed by research, may be enhanced by purposeful ethical inquiry that occurs as an integral component of theorizing activities.

Nurses and other scientists who are embracing the postpositivist tradition in science recognize the historical evolution of knowledge: that knowledge is not absolute but changes in interaction with the culture as a whole and with the scientists, theologians, practitioners, philosophers, and others who contribute to perceptions of truth. There is no one truth about the pathway to health that allows theorists, once it is discovered and described, to sit back, content in knowing that they have laid out the facts and cannot be held accountable for the consequences of their theories. No one dominant paradigm exists as a guide for nursing inquiry in the selection of the right worldview, the right perspective on human health and nursing, the right questions and goals, the right method, or the right answers. Instead, development of nursing knowledge seems to be flourishing in what Laudan (1984) described as a "dissensus" rather than consensus among nursing paradigms. Philosophical aims of nursing are changing toward a focus on "continuing a conversation rather than discovering truth"(Rorty, 1979, p. 373).

The nature of the discipline of nursing is such that

About the Author

PAMELA G. REED was born, raised, and educated in Detroit, but now considers Tucson, Arizona (where she has lived since 1983) to be home. Dr. Reed is a three-time graduate of Wayne State University, receiving a B.S.N. (1974), M.S.N. (1976), and Ph.D. (1982). Recently, she has completed postdoctoral coursework in higher education administration at the University of Arizona. Dr. Reed is an Associate Professor at the University of Arizona School of Nursing. Her area of clinical interest is psychiatric-mental health nursing.

Dr. Reed enjoys classical music, traveling, hiking, swimming, and raising her two daughters. She comments that these activities "provide diversity that influences my nursing perspective." When asked about satisfactions that she has experienced in nursing, Dr. Reed replied "I find great satisfaction in being a part of the increased consciousness in nursing of metatheoretical issues as they are relevant to our practice and research."

An active speaker, writer and researcher, Dr. Reed's research interests include spirituality and developmental patterns and mental health in the elderly. When asked about her research and the future, she responded, "One issue concerns my substantive research interest in the area of spirituality and how our philosophical and methodological developments of the discipline will facilitate the study of this human phenomenon in a nonreductionistic yet scientific manner."

the ethical implications of nursing science in general and the ethical implications of the selected conceptual perspective of the individual's research in particular are enormous. This is so not only because the consequences of nursing conceptualizations are intimately linked to promotion of a good of society—health—but also because of the shifting axiology of the discipline. Criteria for what characterizes essential knowledge and for making value choices and judgments in conceptualizing the phenomena of nursing vary across extant nursing paradigms. The indeterminate nature of nursing phenomena is such that these criteria may never, and perhaps should never, be definitively described. Nevertheless, the "assumptions, value choices, and judgments"(Chinn & Jacobs, 1987, p. 80) on which theory is based are ultimately translated into nursing knowledge for actions that directly affect human health. According to Bellah, "what [our theories] say human beings [and health] fundamentally are has inevitable implications about what they ought to be"(Bellah, 1981, p. 15).

Nursing theorizing, then, is an ethical endeavor. Theorizing refers here to the reasoning processes involved in constructing what Kaplan (1964) has termed the "conceptual frame," or the framework or theory in

scientific inquiry. Choices made in theory have ethical consequences in practice. In addition, the act of theorizing alone constitutes a "moral situation"(Dewey, 1948) in that it entails reflective choice and deliberate consideration of what may be better or worse. Thus, both the purpose of nursing inquiry and the nature of the phenomena studied render nursing theorizing its ethical dimension.

Nursing theorizing, whether it occurs at the outset or emerges during the process of inquiry, is inescapably linked to the theorist's value choices and beliefs about human beings, the environment, and health. The message in Nietzsche's "dogma of immaculate perception"(Nietzsche, 1966) extends to qualitative and quantitative methodologies alike. No observation is free from conceptual contamination; observation is already cognition, valuing, and believing (Kaplan, 1965). More precisely, there is no such thing as immaculate conceptualization in theorizing. Regardless of the methodology by which theories are advanced, theorizing likely entails value choices made by the nursing theorist or researcher that ultimately influence the good of society. Kaplan's thesis "that not all value concerns are unscientific, that indeed some of them are called for by the scientific enterprise itself" (Kaplan, 1965, p. 373) is an understatement for nursing science where value-laden terms such as health are the prime focus of inquiry.

The Normative Commitment of the Conceptual Frame

All phases of scientific inquiry in nursing are embedded in "normative commitments"(Bellah, 1981). Deontological judgments of moral value and obligation occur in nursing theorizing, evidenced for example in the theorist's speculations about what may be good for health or well-being, why it may be good, and what ought to be done to promote that good. The distinction between cognitive and normative knowledge is hazy at best and, because of this, ethical inquiry must accompany inquiry into human processes (Bellah, 1981).

Critical ethical reflection is important not only in the testing and application of knowledge, but also in the conceptualization of knowledge. Ethical knowing has been put forth as an essential component of nursing knowledge (Carper, 1978) and fundamental to the development of theory (Chinn & Jacobs, 1987). However, the ethical dimension of selecting or developing a conceptual frame for research has been addressed in the literature by only a few, such as Archbold (1987) or mentioned only in passing (White, 1983).

Ethical issues continues to be addressed in nursing research most characteristically in reference to methodology (Connors, 1988; Moccia, 1988; Munhall, 1988), but also in reference to health care policy (Hinshaw, 1988) and allocation of resources for research (Fowler, 1987). Conspicuous references to the ethical aspects of research methodology and overall purpose of research are found in the American Nurses' Association's *Code of Ethics* (Kansas City: ANA, 1985) and *Human Rights Guidelines* (Kansas City: ANA, 1984). However, selection of a research strategy, generally recognized as a value-laden decision, is often so because the conceptual frame out of which this decision flows is value laden. Careful attention to the values and assumptions operant in the conceptual perspective of a study could facilitate solutions to ethical dilemmas encountered at other points in the research process. Ethical inquiry into the components of an individual's conceptual frame, as prerequisite to the ethical inquiry into the methodology suggested by Munhall (1988) and others, could further enhance the likelihood that the means and ends of research will be morally justified.

The ethical responsibilities associated with scientific knowledge cannot be relegated entirely to the implementors of the research design nor to those who translate the findings in clinical practice. Normative commitments are made in the earliest efforts in theorizing. Dewey (1928) rejected the positivist, continental European image of the scientist as one whose dedication to reason and truth sets him or her apart from the ethical concerns related to the products of science. Dewey denied any dualism between scientific and moral thinking and proclaimed that scientific activity is inherently moralistic in its concern with understanding natural processes and their relationship to the welfare of humankind.

Laudan's (1977, 1981) historicist view on scientific progress reinforces the normative commitment of the conceptual frame in research. Scientific progress is evaluated, according to Laudan, in terms of the problem-solving effectiveness of the discipline's theories. A major problem of interest in nursing is the facilitation of health as a good of society. The nature of nursing is such that, if nurses are to contribute to the scientific progress of their discipline, their theorizing must incorporate a moral dimension that includes logical reasoning and creative reflection on what may be considered good or best vis-à-vis the health of individuals and groups. If nursing theories are to have problem-solving effectiveness, clarification of an individual's ontology, values, and goals must occur not only in reference to implementing the research design as pointed out by Moccia (1988), but also in reference to the act of conceptualizing.

Value-based choices about the sorts of conceptualizations or theories invoked in research influence decisions regarding the problems deemed worthy of study, the perceived societal benefits, definition and measurement of concepts, the types of participant risks worth

taking, acceptable threats to internal and external validity, the interpretation and significance of the findings,
and most importantly the knowledge offered for use in
effecting health in human beings. It is not inconceivable that the conceptual nets (Popper, 1968) cast out by
scientists could be used for catching fish only for their
liking and not necessarily for the good of society.

So powerful is the conceptual frame of a study that
Kaplan (1964) noted one could more easily dispense
with the physical operations of a study than with the
framework that gives meaning to all of the research
activities. The same methodology can constitute a different study and result in different outcomes if the conceptual framework changes. Secondary analysis is an
example of this. Moreover, Laudan (1981) explained
that changes in scientific knowledge occur more often
due to conceptual issues rather than questions of empirical support.

Ethical Implications of Selected Conceptual Frameworks

The ethical implications of theorizing can be illustrated
in examples from nursing and nonnursing literature. In
the nonnursing literature, examples of the ethical significance of conceptual frameworks can be found in classic studies of human development. Human development, like health, is a value-laden concept and not easily
defined. Personal biases have entered into conceptualizations of development with moral consequences.

Developmental Psychology Literature

The late 17th-century conceptualization of the tabula
rasa view of people held moral implications related to
the potential for human development and well-being.
Neither the environment nor the person was perceived
as having an active role in development. The infant, in
particular, was viewed as insignificant in terms of his or
her value in effecting change in the environment; infants were perceived as ineffectual, empty vessels waiting to be filled with information. Research hypotheses
derived from this conceptual stance were directed toward the study of maturity in terms of the acquisition

of a quantity of information using the adult white male
as the standard. This framework limited the scope of
study about sources of human potential and ways in
which development could be enhanced from early life
onward. Primary intervention for the emotional development of infants, for example, was unheard of, since
the infant was not conceptualized as a unique and dynamic being.

The nature vs. nurture controversy was brought to
public scrutiny with Jensen's (1973) well-known conclusions about genetically based racial differences in
intelligence. Jensen was proclaimed as having hood-
winked large segments of government and society into
believing that IQ was genetically based, and as having
an oppressive effect on disadvantaged, primarily black
individuals (Jensen, 1973; Kamin, 1974). The ethical
implications of Jensen's work relate to provision of educational opportunities, hiring practices, and to the self-
concept and self-expectations of certain ethnic groups.
The debate about the heritability of intelligence continues to be fueled by contrasting views about the development of intelligence, particularly by conceptual frameworks such as Jensen's, which dichotomize the
contributions of heredity and environment in development and do not account for the possibility of interaction between the two factors.

The decrement model of human aging provides an
example of the influences that a conceptual frame may
have on human welfare. This model was most popular
15 years ago, although its influences can still be felt
today. The decrement model emphasized quantitative
biological changes that occur with age, such as cardiovascular and perceptual losses (Botwinick, 1973; Horn,
1976). These losses were generalized to the overall process of aging; regression of capabilities was regarded as
a normal process. Young adulthood marked the time of
maximal level of development, after which linear and
irreversible decrement occurred.

Aging was conceptualized as a first in, last out
process, whereby the most recent and complex abilities
are lost first and the earliest and simplest are retained
(Labouvie–Vief & Schell, 1983). The older adult was
conceived of as becoming more childlike with develop-

ment. In addition, the environmental context was not valued as significant in the process of aging. Research based on this model focused solely on ontogenetic rather than contextual factors in development (Labouvie–Vief, 1977). Thus, for example, plasticity, the ability to learn from the environment (now recognized as a characteristic ability of the elderly), was not identified as an issue of aging worthy of study.

The decrement model, in which developmental changes were conceptualized primarily as losses rather than as adaptive or progressive, did little to facilitate means to improve health care, educational programs, and career opportunities of the elderly, not to mention promotion of self-esteem among older adults and a basic societal value for the elderly persons. Research efforts guided by this conceptual frame and directed toward its support could be regarded as unethical, particularly in view of the theorizing and scientific evidence to the contrary that were emerging at the time (Baltes & Baltes, 1977; Labouvie–Vief, 1980; Schaie, 1973).

Nursing Literature

Examples of ethical issues in theorizing exist in current nursing literature, although perhaps they are not yet viewed as being as dramatic as the historical accounts from the developmental psychology literature. A research report on social support by Ellison (1985) increases awareness of the potential dangers in conceptualizing social support as a purely positive phenomenon. Her findings suggest that social support is most health promotive only during certain phases of the lifespan and that social support in other developmental phases may be detrimental to individuals. Personal biases about the desirability of social support that enter the research framework unchecked can have costly effects on well-being when applied in clinical practice.

Boyd's (1985) analysis of the concept of "identification" demonstrates the different meanings the term acquires within various theoretical frameworks. A key point presented was that identification in the parent-child relationship typically has been conceptualized as a one-way, time-limited process in which the child is influenced by the parent. This view contrasts sharply with the mutually interactive and dynamic view of interpersonal relationships depicted in some nursing conceptual frameworks. Research and intervention approaches stemming from a one-sided framework have neglected the potential influence of the child on the parent, including influences on fulfillment of the parental role and the parent's well-being as parent and as a human being.

Narayan and Joslin's (1980) critique of the medical conceptual model of human crisis and their proposal of a nursing model of crisis illustrate the striking difference that a conceptual perspective could make in terms of clinical intervention. In one model, pathogenic risks of crisis are emphasized and a return to the precrisis level of functioning is the treatment goal; in the other model, opportunities for growth enhancement are emphasized and treatment goals acknowledge the human potential for change and further development. Because the definitions of health and goals for intervention differ markedly between the medical and nursing models, it is likely that different outcomes in the client's health and well-being would occur as well. Explicating a conceptual framework of crisis is an ethical endeavor, requiring reflection on one's beliefs about human potential, the level of functioning of which the client is perceived capable, and the ideals the clinician may envision for the client.

There are many nursing phenomena that, when conceptualized for research, stimulate if not demand ethical reflection by the theorist. Personal biases and assumptions about emotional illness, adolescent development, and female sexuality, for example, which typically elicit presumptive notions about the value of time, independence, and other assumed goods, can have moral influences on the types of conceptualizations constructed in the study of these phenomena as they relate to health.

Ethical Reflection— Response to a Calling

In the spirit of Nightingale's ideas, Kaplan stated that science is a "calling" and "cannot flourish if it is always an occupation only" (Kaplan, 1964, p. 379). He explains further that, while one chooses an occupation, a calling chooses the individual and commits him or her to the professional ethic of science—values that guide the conduct of inquiry. The professional ethic of scientific inquiry extends beyond basic moral principles such as beneficence, nonmaleficence, and justice. This ethic is also evident in theorizing about nursing phenomena in a manner unwavered by "habit, by tradition, by the Academy, or by the powers that be"(Kaplan, 1964, p. 380). Normative commitments made in theorizing must not be limited by traditions that exist, either in practice or theory, in hospitals or schools of nursing. The potential for human health is not static, but is ever expanding. Ideas put forth in the conceptual frame must not compromise or constrain this human potential.

Theorists are morally obligated to deliberately examine their motives and values as reflected in their conceptualizations about health and health-related issues. Propositions implicit and explicit to the conceptual frame should be judged not only in reference to what they state but also in reference to what they make more likely (Kaplan, 1964).

Ethical inquiry into one's conceptual frame requires examination of both intrapersonal factors (e.g., worldview, personal and professional experiences) and extrapersonal factors (e.g., historical context, influential others) (DeGroot, 1988) as they influence the motives and purposes underlying one's conceptual frame. Ethical reflection also entails:

- assessment of the moral ideals underlying the concepts of health, human being, environment, and nursing practice that may be represented in the framework;
- creative imagining of the consequences of one's framework;
- depth of personal knowledge;
- moral vision, described by McInerny (1987) as awareness of the deepest beliefs about such things as the value of life and death, and the nature and worth of the environment; and
- an openness to undergo a "transformation of values" (Chinn, 1985) when it is determined that concepts need redefining or theories need reformulating.

An ethical framework in nursing reflects not only a basic concern for human welfare, but also a moral commitment to the discipline. The theorizer must refrain from being lured into conceptualizations "framed in the unique perspective of other disciplines" (Smith, 1988, p.3) that offer more certainty or specificity for the theorists but make little contribution to the aims of nursing. Smith (1988) admonishes nurses to stay tough during the process of theorizing. Moral timidity creates trivial theory. Bellah was highly critical of those who lacked moral vision in their inquiry, who misrepresented human processes with reductionistic and deterministic conceptualizations, and who hid behind the excuse that "our science is still young" (Bellah, 1981, p. 17).

Toward Boldness in Nursing Theorizing

There is movement underfoot to become more deliberate in exploring the philosophical bases of nursing theorizing. Evidence for this can be found not only in the nursing literature over the past decade, but also among graduate students' requests for more courses and course content on the history and philosophy of science, in lunch-hour seminars in which various philosophical views are debated, and in conference proceedings that address philosophical issues as integral to theory development. Doctoral students are embracing a new philosophy of their science, a philosophy that thrives on the indeterminate nature of nursing phenomena, entertains radically new hypotheses, welcomes diversity among paradigms, and values independent thought. At the same time, it is a philosophy that challenges scientists to examine the ethical questions associated with their value choices, judgments, and patterns of reasoning. As nursing turns toward a greater focus on substance rather than structure in the science (Downs, 1988; Fitzpatrick, 1987), increased attention may be given to the ethical dimensions of conceptual processes in research as has been given to the ethical dimensions of the methodological processes in research.

The discipline's understanding of what constitutes health and how best to promote optimal well-being, quality of life, and other values may be clarified by purposeful ethical reflection as a routine occurrence in theorizing. Carper, in explaining the importance of the ethical pattern of knowing, stated that differences in normative judgments may have more to do with disagreements over conceptualizations of health than with a lack of empirical evidence (Carper, 1978). Ethical knowledge about the underpinnings of the conceptual frame may also facilitate solutions to ethical dilemmas encountered in other stages of the research process and in the eventual clinical applications of knowledge.

Nursing scientists today are being challenged to make choices in their theorizing—choices that touch their own identity as well as affect the good of society. Tensions between theory and practice, the conceptual and the operational, help bring into focus the variety of philosophical views and values inherent among nursing paradigms, and the choices one makes in explicating a framework. Is human health best measured and promoted from a reductionistic or holistic perspective or is there yet another perspective? Is the environment best conceptualized as integral or external to human functioning? Is the human cell or human field, or some other human dimension, the fundamental unit of study in nursing?

In nursing's present phase of development as a science, scientists need to explicate the value choices underlying their frameworks in a bold, self-informed manner. Knowledge can be used as sociopolitical power to enforce a theorized good and to effect human health in unforeseeable ways. Ethical inquiry into one's conceptual frame can provide needed constraints on the human tendency to blur the distinction between a researcher's beliefs and societal needs and can also provide the moral vision needed to effectively and humanely solve nursing problems.

References

American Nurses' Association (1985). *Code of ethics*. Kansas City: Author.

American Nurses' Association (1984). *Human rights guidelines*. Kansas City: Author.

Archbold, P.G. (1981). Ethical issues in the selection of a theoretical framework for gerontological nursing research. *Journal of Gerontologic Nursing, 7*, 408–411.

Baltes, M.M., & Baltes, P.B. (1977). The ecopsychological relativity and plasticity of psychological aging: Convergent perspectives of cohort effects and operant psychology. *Psychology, 24*, 179–197.

Bellah, R.N. (1981). The ethical aims of social inquiry. *Teachers College Record, 83*(1), 1–18.

Botwinick, J. (1973). *Aging and behavior*. New York: Springer.

Boyd, C. (1985). Toward an understanding of mother-daughter identification using concept analysis. *Advances in Nursing Science, 7* (3), 78–86.

Carper, B.A. (1978). Fundamental patterns of knowing in nursing. *Advances in Nursing Science, 1*(1), 13–24.

Chinn, P.L. (1985). Quality of life: A values transformation. *Advances in Nursing Science, 8*(1), vii–ix.

Chinn, P.L., & Jacobs, M.K. (1987). *Theory and nursing* (2nd ed.). St Louis: C.V. Mosby.

Connors, D.D. (1988). A continuum of research-participant relationships: An analysis and critique. *Advances in Nursing Science, 10*(4), 32–42.

DeGroot, H.A. (1988). Scientific inquiry in nursing: A model for a new age. *Advances in Nursing Science, 10*(3), 1–21.

Dewey, J. (1928). In J. Rather (Ed.). *The philosophy of John Dewey*. New York: Holt, Rinehart & Winston.

Dewey, J. (1948). *Reconstruction in philosophy*. Boston: Beacon Press.

Downs, F. (1988). Doctoral education: Our claim to the future. *Nursing Outlook, 36*(1), 18–20.

Ellison, E.S. (1985). Social support and the constructive-developmental model. *Western Journal of Nursing Research, 9*, 19–28.

Fitzpatrick, J.J. (1987). Philosophical approach: Empiricism. In C. Bridges & N. Wells (Eds.). *Proceedings of the Fourth Nursing Science Colloquium: Strategies for Nursing Theory Development*. Boston: Boston University School of Nursing.

Fowler, M.D. (1987). Ethical issues in nursing research. *Western Journal of Nursing Research, 9*, 269–271.

Hinshaw, A.S. (1988). Using research to shape health policy. *Nursing Outlook, 36*(1), 21–24.

Hirsch, J. (1975). Jensenism: The bankruptcy of "science" without scholarship. *Educational Theory, 25*, 3–28.

Horn, J.L. (1976). Human abilities: A review of research and theory in the early 1970s. *Annual Review of Psychology, 27*, 437–485.

Jensen, A.R. (1973). Race, intelligence, and genetics: The differences are real. *Psychology Today, 12*, 80–86.

Kamin, L.J. (1974). *The science and politics of IQ*. New York: Halstead.

Kaplan, A. (1964). *The logic of scientific discovery*. New York: Thomas Y. Crowell.

Labouvie–Vief, G. (1977). Adult cognitive development: In search of alternative interpretations. *Merrill-Palmer Quarterly of Behavior and Development, 23*(4), 227–263.

Labouvie–Vief, G. (1980). Adaptive dimensions of adult cognition. In N. Datan & N. Lohmann (Eds.). *Transitions in aging*. New York: Academic Press.

Labouvie–Vief, G., & Schell, D.A. (1983). Learning and memory in later life: A developmental view. In B. Wolman & G. Striker (Eds.). *Handbook of developmental psychology*. Englewood Cliffs, NJ: Prentice-Hall.

Laudan, L. (1977). *Progress and its problems: Toward a theory of scientific growth*. Berkeley, CA: University of California Press.

Laudan, L. (1981). A problem-solving approach to scientific progress. In I. Hacking (Ed.). *Scientific revolutions*. New York: Oxford University Press.

Laudan, L. (1984). *Science and values*. Berkeley, CA: University of California Press.

McInerny, W.F. (1987). Understanding moral issues in health care: Seven essential ideas. *Journal of Professional Nursing, 3*, 268–277.

Moccia, P. (1988). A critique of compromise: Beyond the methods debate. *Advances in Nursing Science, 10*(4), 1–9.

Munhall, P.L. (1988). Ethical considerations in qualitative research. *Western Journal of Nursing Research, 10*, 150–162.

Narayan, S.M., & Joslin, D.J. (1980). Crisis theory and intervention: A critique of the medical model and proposal of a holistic nursing model. *Advances in Nursing Science, 2*(4), 27 40.

Nietzsche, F. (1966). *Beyond good and evil* (W. Kaufmann, trans). New York: Vintage.

Popper, K.R. (1968). *The logic of scientific discovery*. New York: Harper & Row.

Rorty, R. (1979). *Philosophy and the mirror of nature*. Princeton, NJ: Princeton University Press.

Schaie, K.W. (1973). Methodological problems in research on adulthood and aging. In J.R. Nesselroade & H.W. Reese (Eds.). *Life-span developmental psychology: Methodological issues*. New York: Academic Press.

Smith, M.J. (1988). Wallowing while waiting, *Nursing Science Quarterly, 1*(1), 3.

White, G.B. (1983). Philosophical ethics and nursing—a word of caution. In P.L. Chinn (Ed.). *Advances in nursing theory development*. Rockville, MD: Aspen.

The Author Comments

This article has a history; it wasn't developed over a week or even a year. Several factors came together in formulating this paper. An early precursor of the paper occurred while I was a student at Wayne State University in doctoral level nursing seminars in which philosophical and methodological issues of theory development were explored. These discussions stimulated ideas about the ethical dimensions of conceptual and theoretical frameworks used in nursing. Carper's (1978) article (Ed. note: See Chapter 19) on patterns of knowing also supported my thoughts on ethics and its role in not only using but also building knowledge in nursing.

After graduating and while beginning a new teaching position, I became intrigued with the fact that literature and course outlines depicted ethics as an important component of practice and research activities but were silent on this in reference to theory activities— this despite the links acknowledged between theory, practice and research. There seemed to be a "missing link" in terms of the ethical implications of the content of our theories for research and practice. This observation, coupled with the plea from Fitzpatrick, Downs, Meleis and others to better attend to the substance of our theories as we had attended to the syntax of the discipline, further reinforced my ideas. Ethical reflection on the content and process of our theorizing was another way of acknowledging the critical link between theory and practice. It was my view that no matter how "deconstructed" we are, theories at some level influence the way we structure reality and our practice.

The inquisitiveness and progressive thinking of the doctoral nursing students I encountered in teaching a course in metatheory was another critical element in inspiring this article. The relevance of ethical considerations became even clearer as the students critically examined the philosophical underpinnings of nursing theories and theorizing.

Last, I have an ongoing interest about the ethical implications of the theories we choose to develop and ultimately use for practice in this "postpositivist" era—particularly in view of the current thrust toward practical and policy-relevant, mission-oriented research. This focus can serve nursing and nursing's clients well. I hope that the processes required to obtain funding for our research will enhance rather than discourage the endeavor to consider the ethical implications of our theories, the variables we choose to study, and the way in which we conceptualize these variables.

—PAMELA G. REED

Chapter 15

Nursing Values and Science: Toward a Science Philosophy

Susan R. Gortner

Several premises are proposed for nursing science philosophy in contrast to nursing practice philosophy. These include human understanding, a critical tradition that views science as public knowledge, and use of observation, rationality, explanation, and prediction as a guide to therapy. No argument is made for or against a particular philosophy of science (e.g., positivist, historicist, critical theorist). The debates on the fit of philosophic paradigms with research strategies may soon run their course on the North American continent, as they appear to have done in Scandinavia.

The search for meaning in the universe is the subject matter of philosophy. It is not surprising, therefore, that philosophical discussions now characterize those disciplinary fields examining their purpose, significance, and identity. Nursing in the United States, Canada, Great Britain and elsewhere has publicized formally its purpose and obligation to society through statements on standards for practice (American Nurses' Association [ANA], 1973; Canadian Nurses Association [CNA], 1980; Royal College of Nursing [RCN], 1987), codes for practice (ANA, 1976; International Council of Nurses, 1987; RCN, 1987) and social policy statements (ANA, 1980; RCN, 1987). Common themes that might be said to represent nursing philosophy and values commitment are reflected in these statements.

The purpose of this paper is to illustrate how nursing values and philosophy influence thinking about nursing science and research in the United States, Great Britain, and parts of Scandinavia. The position is taken that nursing philosophy represents the belief system of the profession and that it provides perspectives for practice, for scholarship, and for research. This paper will contrast statements of nursing philosophy in the United States and elsewhere and will attempt to show that nursing philosophy can be differentiated from science philosophy. Further, science philosophy

About the Author

SUSAN R. GORTNER grew up in San Francisco and attended Katherine Delmar Burke School for Girls and Stanford University, where she obtained an A.B. degree in social sciences (anthropology, history, and psychology) in 1953. She enrolled in the Frances Payne Bolton (FPB) School of Nursing (at that time at Western Reserve University, now Case Western Reserve) in 1954. She earned a generic master of nursing degree in 1957, graduating with honors and receiving the Cushing Robb Prize for scholarship. While at FPB, she was among the last to go through the tuberculosis and psychiatric rotations.

After graduation, she worked briefly as a clinic nurse for the Maui Pineapple Company, Maui, Hawaii, and then joined the surgical nursing service of Johns Hopkins Hospital, Baltimore. While there, Dr. Gortner worked in the surgical intensive care unit, caring for some of the first patients undergoing cardiopulmonary bypass surgery. She also worked as a clinical instructor and nursing supervisor in surgery. A move to Hawaii and experience as instructor and assistant professor in medical surgical nursing at the University of Hawaii, prompted her decision to go on for a doctoral degree. In 1964, she received a Ph.D. from the University of California, Berkeley. The support of her biochemist husband, an active scientist, was instrumental to her seeking research funds in 1960 and in combining research and academic careers with parenting.

In 1966, Dr. Gortner became special consultant to the Division of Nursing, U.S. Public Health Services, helping evaluate the 1964 Nurse Training Act. In 1967, she became the first nurse scientist to serve as Executive Secretary of the Nursing Research and Patient Care Review Committee, the peer review group for nursing research. This experience, along with later responsibilities as Branch Chief for Research and Research Training, gave her an opportunity to call on a longstanding love of history in documenting the federal efforts on behalf of nursing research development. In 1978, Dr. Gortner accepted the appointment of Professor of Nursing and Associate Dean for research at the University of California, San Francisco. She retired as Associate Dean for Research in 1986.

Dr. Gortner comments "To my longstanding interest in history of nursing and its science now came a companion interest in values and in philosophy of science. Major satisfactions in nursing have included involvement in teaching, in cardiac surgery patient care, and in research. I cannot think but auspiciously for nursing in the future, if it keeps its intellect and accountability in both practice and research."

The author acknowledges numerous persons who have contributed to the literature on nursing science and aided the maturation of her thinking: Marjorie Batey, Jeanne Benoliel, Virginia Cleland, Dorothy Crowley and Sue Donaldson, Florence Downs, Rosemary Ellis, Ada Jacox, Jean Johnson, Rozella Schlotfeldt, former colleagues Doris Bloch and Marie Bourgeois, and recent colleagues Afaf Meleis and Laura Reif. For their efforts in putting the manuscript in final form, the author thanks Cecile Wopat and Cheyney Johansen. She is indebted to Professor Meleis, who provided an opportunity for discussion of this paper in her Doctoral Research Seminar, April 25, 1979, and to doctoral students Mary Ann Curry and Maria O'Rourke, who contributed the points on information transfer and productivity.

can be reframed according to the needs of a discipline for relevant knowledge, empirically and conceptually derived, using a variety of systematic techniques. A philosophic framework for nursing science will be proposed.

Nursing Values

Nursing values portray the concepts of equity, respect for persons and caring (RCN, 1987), health promotion and illness prevention (ANA, 1980; National Center for Nursing Research, 1988), professional competence, and ethical conduct. Fry, who examined the American standards and codes for practice and research, concluded that:

> . . . the concept of nursing embodies the scientific (competence) values of technological skills, scientific inquiry, and knowledge gained by scientific study, as well as humanistic (moral) values of caring and promotion of individual welfare and rights (Fry, 1981, p. 5).

Fry suggests that assumptions underlying American statements emphasize (a) the systematic approach to nursing practice (the nursing process) as the means to provide high quality care, (b) the promotion, maintenance and restoration of health as desirable outcomes of nursing action based on the nursing process (i.e., desired goals or ends), and (c) client participation in the health care plan designed to achieve these outcomes.

The British standards have as their underlying assumptions (a) accountability for practice of a high quality, safety, and effectiveness; (b) client participation in the contractual caring relationship; and (c) personalized, warm, understanding *caring* as the core of service. According to the RCN:

> The nursing system must acknowledge the centrality of care in the overall delivery of its service. . . .it is the skill and art of caring for another person that transforms the action from a technique to a nursing intervention (RCN, 1987, pp. 11–12.)

Other statements in this most recent British document emphasize the commitment to a humanistic philosophy and a patient or client advocacy model. Further, there is virtually no mention of obligation to extend knowledge of practice through research as there is in the American statements or of the "phenomena of concern" as in the American social policy statement (ANA, 1980). Stated differently, this most recent British document does not address scientific accountability in practice (Gortner, 1974), nor does it reflect the consensus reached by American nurses in the 1970s that scientific inquiry was the means by which outcomes of nursing action could be identified.

Although the Scandinavian countries are in the process of developing their standards, the publication by the Nordic Nurses Federation (NNF) of ethical guidelines for nursing research in the Nordic countries acknowledges the nurses' responsibility to "promote health, to prevent illness, to restore health, to prevent death, and to assist to a comfortable death." Further, there is a clear expectation for renewing personal knowledge and skills: "Such an obligation to improve nursing theory and skills implies research in nursing and health care services" (NNF, 1987, p. 7).

The ICN recently revised its position statement on nursing research. The statement reflects interest in the phenomena of concern stated in the ANA's 1980 social policy statement: individual, family, and group responses to actual and potential health problems: "The future of nursing practice and ultimately the future of health care depends on nursing research designed to constantly generate an up-to-date organized body of nursing knowledge" (ICN, 1987, p. 1).

It appears that the term "nursing research" in the NNF and ICN statements is used to describe what in America has come to be called "nursing science" (Gortner, 1980). The United States' usage of nursing science has grown out of a period in our history in which the nature of nursing science was discussed by academic leaders concerned with the preparation of the nurse scientist. In this respect, science, the body of knowledge about the universe, and its manifestations, was distinguished from research, the tool of science (Batey, 1972; Gortner, 1980). This differential terminology now is prevailing in the nursing science institutes at the Universities of Oslo and Bergen as well as at several Finnish universities (Gortner & Lorensen, 1989).

The United States has had an advantage as yet not realized elsewhere in the world of having had government support in the way of grants for nurse scientist training in major universities during the years 1962 to 1972 (Gortner & Nahm, 1977). The periodic forums that brought together the program directors and faculty members from these grantee institutions produced some of the most thoughtful among early statements on nursing science and the nurse's becoming scientist. Of these was Ellis's essay on values and vicissitudes of the scientist nurse, in which scientific research was viewed as the effective tool of the humanist nurse (Ellis, 1970). Batey's (1972) reflections on values relative to research and to science in nursing, as a result of her own nurse scientist training in sociology, recognized (as did Ellis) the tension between science and humanism but argued for the scientific values of organized skepticism, disinterest, and communality. Fry (1981) gives a foundational place to humanistic values in her analysis, arguing that it is the humanistic value scheme, not the scientific one, that guides humane therapy. A further argument is based on the claim made by Fry that scientific values have no moral content in themselves.

The author, 15 years ago, urged greater scientific accountability for nursing based on self-reflection and thoughtful analysis of practice but cautioned against a loss of humanistic values while taking on the scientific (Gortner, 1974). That both science and humanism could be accommodated in nursing without loss of purpose and meaning was noted then and is believed to be possible today. What well may be foundational in humanistic philosophy (concern for person and meaning) can remain as philosophy; it need not be translated into scientific strategies (i.e., interpretive designs) and used to the exclusion of other options. Further, the practice of science and the scientific method, the search for explanations, regularities, and predictions about the human state should not be viewed as being incompatible with professional beliefs about practice and societal and personal worth.

Is Science in Nursing Compatible With Humanism?

For the past two decades, nursing scholars have examined the meaning of nursing through philosophical analysis (Ellis, 1983; Gadow, 1980; Lanara, 1982; Patterson & Zderad, 1976; Vaillot, 1962). Lanara recalled the heritage of classical Greek medicine as a healing art, as part of nursing's caring obligation. Nursing as a profession and as a science of caring has been proposed by several American authors (Benner & Wrubel, 1989; Leininger, 1988; Watson, 1985). These proposals have in common a commitment to personhood, holism, and humanistic attention. Further, there is now considerable literature on the need for scientific approaches that will reflect these commitments (Allen, Benner, & Diekelmann, 1986; Cull-Wilby & Pepin, 1987; Gortner & Schultz, 1988; Schultz, 1987; Silva & Rothbart, 1984; Stevenson & Woods, 1986; Thompson, 1985).

In all but a few of these essays, science is cast against humanism and hermeneutics; the latter is seen as providing true meaning for all human endeavor including scientific work on humans and by humans. Interestingly, European nurses do not support this dialectic; it appears to be peculiarly American, in part because science does not have the certitude, the "gewissenschaft," that it has in the United States. In Norway, "vitenskap" is the term used for science; it has a broader meaning and tradition beyond that of natural science, incorporating many sources of knowledge—not unlike those described by Schultz and Meleis (1988) in a recent account of nursing epistemology. These authors note that valuation of empirical knowledge will require evaluative criteria that are different from either conceptually derived or clinically derived knowledge. Theirs is a refreshing attempt to further understanding values and beliefs about multiple sources of knowledge for a practice field such as nursing.

Changing scientific and philosophical opinions about science in the past two decades have brought about considerable commentary about scientific inquiry and outcome. Science now is viewed as a part of society and not value-free; as such, it is a part of the sociopolitical structure and thus is open to scrutiny. There has been a renewed interest in the history of science, a result of scientists' turning to study their own disciplinary histories as well as philosophy. Kuhn's *Structure of Scientific Revolutions* (Chicago: University of Chicago Press, 1962) was first published in the United States in 1962; Winch's *Idea of a Social Science* (London: Routledge and Kegan Paul, 1958) appeared in Europe about the same time as Kuhn's book, according to Phillips (1987). Also influential around this time was Herbert Marcuse's *One-Dimensional Man* (Boston: Beacon Press, 1964). According to Fjelland (personal communication, July 1989), the writings of Marcuse, who emigrated to the United States, as well as others associated with the Frankfurt school of critical social philosophy, particularly Habermas (1971), fit in well with the student reaction against the American and Northern European "establishment," in which science and objectivity were perceived as being overvalued to the detriment of person and humanity. This reaction also was displayed against positivism, or the received view in philosophy of science. In Scandinavian and northern European universities in the 1970s, Marx as humanitarian rather than as political economist was reexamined along with Hegel and other of the German Idealists (Randi Nord & Eli Haugen Bunch, personal communication, February 4, 1988).

Modern versions of nineteenth century continental philosophy have emerged to influence the science discussions in some disciplinary fields deeply concerned with the human state. Phenomenology, as articulated by Heidegger (1962), Sartre (1963), and Merleau-Ponty (1962), calls for the appreciation of the human being as supreme being and for self-reflection and understanding as the basis of knowing and acting. Cohen (1987) provided an historical account of the phenomenological movement, differentiating these key leaders. Not addressed in her review is the influence of Heidegger on contemporary interpretative philosophy, namely hermeneutics. Leonard (1989) rectified this situation for nursing readers in a recent essay.

According to Bernstein's recent analysis, the issue is less the substitution of hermeneutics for the scientific method as it is acceptance of "the ontological primacy of hermeneutics and its universality" (Bernstein, 1986, p. 96). Hermeneutical understanding can enlighten the human state, a state that has become objectified by scientific advances and technology. Intuition and practical reasoning may well underlie all forms of reasoning including scientific reasoning and the production of scientific knowledge. The foundational nature of hermeneutics for Scandinavian nurse scholars engaged in substantive research programs is a given (Astrid Norberg, personal communication, March 6, 1988). Interestingly, hermeneutics as philosophy has not been transformed there to hermeneutics as method, as it appears to have been transformed in the United States. American scholars might consider this point in reconciling philosophy with modes of inquiry.

The legacy of philosophical positivism continues to guide our beliefs in the scientific method and in careful research strategies and in the conduct of investigations can provide worthwhile and substantial benefits for humankind. The renewed interest in humanism and history has infused us with an appreciation for and sensitivity to the human condition, in the links between objective measures of reality and personal and subjective ones. These links have significant implications for human sciences, among them the health fields.

What seems now to be at stake is whether or not understanding and explanation of the human state can take various forms and whether or not self-understanding and self-theories will be accepted as warranted evidence and thus as measures of "truth." Gergen (1980) suggests that a primary function of such understandings is the capacity to challenge assumptions of the culture, to raise questions about life and to suggest alternative actions: to serve as "generative theory." According to Ziman's (1980) definition, science is public knowledge; if self-defined meanings could be made public and scrutinized, they could be informative, critical, generalizable, and potentially nomothetic. Will such scrutiny distort the faithful interpretation from description that hermeneutical studies aim to present? Probably not, because some excellent public examples now exist in the science literature (Mishel & Murdaugh, 1987). How reproducible and rigorous are the narratives, the data, from such investigations? Herein lies a major debatable question since interpretive studies tend to be idiosyncratic and particularistic, despite cultural and linguistic commonalities. Further, there is no causal requirement for hermeneutical explanation. The explanation is said to lie within the particular history or situation, not in some external human pattern or regularity or "law" that might govern or account for the situation. This lack of causality has serious implications for the human sciences in general and the health sciences in particular. There is loss of generalizability, loss of correspondence with extant theory and diminished power to make "ampliative inferences" that can extend research and therapy. For a practice discipline that needs prescriptive action guides the logic of scientific explanation needs to be coupled with the meaning derived from hermenutical explanation.

Because hermeneutics can make clear practical wisdom, knowledge, and experience, it has great attraction for the clinician and for the art of clinical diagnosis and treatment. It need not be the sole strategy for inquiry, although it may become a key strategy for practice. This leads to the final question: How should research be conducted in the human enterprise called nursing? More specifically, how might a philosophy of nursing science be framed?

Toward a Nursing Science Philosophy

Human understanding is proposed as a premise of nursing science, in keeping with humanistic traditions in ancient and modern philosophy and in nursing philosophy. If accepted as a basic premise, then nursing research would necessarily incorporate means for determining interpretation of the phenomena of concern from the perspective of the client, patient, or care recipient. These interpretations might be subjected to hermeneutic analysis for their meaning, followed by intersubjective consensual validation by participants. To bring the interpretations to intersubjective consensus among scholars requires that they be raised to a level of public information and knowledge, subject to scrutiny, criticism, and further demonstration and empirical testing in other patient-client situations. This strategy might allow for nomothetic explanations as well as idiosyncratic ones.

What is proposed here is what anthropologists would call an emic perspective (Tripp-Reimer, 1984) for most of nursing research. Even if the goal of research is etic, outside the given participant group, one would still argue for consensual validation in the hermeneutic sense (Gortner & Schultz, 1988). But this consensus also has to be brought to the level of public scrutiny, where public this time means other

scholar-scientists in addition to the client or subject or informant.

The public nature of human science knowledge, representing rational, informed opinion about the human state, is proposed as a continued premise of nursing science philosophy, in keeping with traditional and modern views of science (Ziman, 1980). Such knowledge generally is obtained through systematic inquiry, with features of theory/observation compatibility, logic, precision, clarity and reproducibility as is characteristic of "good science" (Gortner, 1987). Such knowledge thrives on criticism and attempts to falsify or substantiate its truth claims. Note here that there is no specification of how this knowledge looks: for purposes of nursing science development, it may represent itself in language or numbers or combinations thereof. What is important is that it is publicized, criticized and tried out. Otherwise it becomes ideology.[1]

Observation as a basic, if not foundational, element of knowledge development in nursing science is proposed as another premise. By this is meant the foundational nature of "observables" of the human state; to be observable means that measurement is possible. What if these are feelings, intuitions, preunderstandings? Can these be "observable"? Indeed yes, and in fact this characteristic or capacity may be a unique feature of nursing science as a form of human science. Nursing's skill in capturing the human situation at a given point of time in the health-illness continuum arises from a tradition of intimate, compassionate, caring, and attentive service. Such intimacy promotes sensitivity to cues in the situation that enlarge understanding and guide action. The means is yet to be developed to reframe these feelings and intuitions in a way that they are "observable" and thus believable by others. The American Academy of Nursing's (1986) scientific

---

[1] A special plea to scholars interested in theory generation and concept discovery is made. Please identify and specify the conditions under which the concept or phenomenon was found. These conditions represent the linkages of the abstraction with reality, increasing the likelihood that the abstraction may be found again. Otherwise who is to know that it is not a fleeting piece of imagination?

sessions recommended the use of triangulation (multi-methods) and pattern-seeking approaches to capture nursing phemonena; these approaches might accommodate investigators of differing interpretive/analytic philosophies. A ''particularistic, pragmatic'' plan for holistic nursing inquiry has been detailed by Schultz (1987). Here the whole (meaning and experiences) is assembled with parts (physiological processes or nursing acts) into a single text, in which the investigator reflectively engages with the data, reasons through dialogue, discovers patterns, and uses these dialectically to construct new understandings and meanings. The conclusion or knowledge claims are then assessed for warrantability using Chisholm's (1982) epistemic principles.

Rationality also is a foundational element in nursing science philosophy. Schultz and Meleis (1988) spoke of conceptual knowledge. Nursing conceptual frameworks and theories can be employed deliberately in investigations to determine their empirical relevance. New theories of the generative sort proposed by Gergen (1980) can be inferred from the data coming from personal histories and clinical ethnographies and from the rationality demanded by critical social theory and feminist scholarship. Rational schemes to describe the relationships supposedly seen in the phenomena of interest also might be proposed through the technique now known as causal modeling. Here, data are examined with regard to previously specified models, through multivariate analytic techniques, and attempts are made to test or generate theories. Here, the ''observables,'' the data, would need transformation from language form to integer form.

Rational philosophies of particular interest to nursing are those employing both critical theory and feminist perspectives. Both are special cases of rationality that apply to situations of social interaction involving authority and power, and both challenge major claims to science based on empirical evidence alone. The arguments for the critical and feminist perspectives have been empirically displayed in research endeavors as well as rationally and ideologically argued by Allen (1985) and Chinn and Wheeler (1985). McLain's (1985) doctoral dissertation and Holter's (1987) theoret-

ical critique are examples of critical theory applications in nursing. An important feminist illustration is Keller's (1985) account of Barbara McClintock's Nobel winning discovery of hybrid corn. The same claims of knowing through intimate attending are made here as have been made by nursing authors in studies of expert caring (Benner and Wrubel, 1989). These claims challenge our contention that scientific knowledge is public knowledge.

Explanatory power is proposed as another premise of philosophy of science in nursing. Human science activities cannot rest only with increased understanding; nor can that understanding be taken as the sole criterion for explanation, as Benner (1985) has proposed. Human patterns and regularities and perhaps even ''laws'' characterize the human state and undergird the whole enterprise of society and human life. Perhaps concern with the mechanistic philosophy of science has prompted the reaction against explication of patterns. But it is argued here that explication is a necessary requirement of nursing science as a clinical and human science, and that eventually such explanations will guide nursing action as therapy. Even if not brought to the prescriptive level, such explanation enhances knowledge about fundamental processes and thus may inform other disciplinary fields.

To understand aids explanation; certainly understanding informs explanation, but explanation in the sense that is being proposed here must suggest what might occur the next time the event or phenomenon occurs. Thus temporality and predictability are assumed in scientific explanations that are within the definition of explanatory power. Whether control of human phenomena is possible or even desirable are both an ethical and scientific question.

To explain means that some causal process or interaction is involved. Here lies one of the greatest areas of disagreement among nurse scholars including our major theorists. It probably will not be resolved in our lifetimes, just as it has not been resolved through the centuries. Explanation in nursing science philosophy can take a variety of forms, some of which have been illustrated in other essays (Gortner, 1983, 1984). Increasingly, statistical inference and the results of cohort studies and clinical trials can enhance the probability of prediction. To sort out pseudoexplanations, these forms of explanation remain logical rather than intuitive, employing the notion of a contrast class, a causal process, a set of clinically and statistically relevant factors (Salmon, 1978). Although forms of explanation may differ, causal inference must remain a key ingredient.

A final premise of science philosophy is that the knowledge generated must also allow for prescriptions that will guide practice. Whether these are clinically or empirically derived, there is the obligation to act or intervene, in keeping with other helping professions. Basic science has no such mandate for application or therapy.

References

Allen, D. (1985). Nursing research and social control: Alternative modes of science that emphasize understanding and emancipation. *Image: Journal of Nursing Scholarship, 17*(2), 58–64.

Allen, D., Benner, P., & Diekelmann, N. (1986). Three paradigms for nursing research: Methodological considerations. In P.L. Chinn (Ed.), *Nursing research methodology: Issues and explanation* (pp. 23–38). Rockville, MD: Aspen Publications.

American Academy of Nursing. (1986). *Setting the agenda for the year 2000: Knowledge development in nursing.* Kansas City: Author.

American Nurses' Association. (1973). *Standards of nursing practice.* Kansas City: Author.

American Nurses' Association (1976). *Code for nurses with interpretive statements.* Kansas City: Author.

American Nurses' Association. (1980). *A social policy statement.* Kansas City: Author.

Batey, M. (1972). Values relative to research and to science as influenced by a sociological perspective. *Nursing Research, 21,* 504–508.

Benner, P. (1985). Quality of life: A phenomenological perspective on explanation, prediction, and understanding in nursing science. *Advances in Nursing Science, 8*(1), 1–16.

Benner, P., & Wrubel, J. (1989). *The primacy of caring: Stress and coping in health and illness.* Menlo Park: Addison-Wesley.

Bernstein, R.J. (1986). *Philosophical profiles.* Philadelphia: University of Pennsylvania Press.

Canadian Nurses Association. (1980). *Definition of nursing practice and standards of practice.* Ottawa: Author.

Chinn, P.L., & Wheeler, C.E. (1985). Feminism and nursing. *Nursing Outlook, 33*(2), 74–77.

Chisholm, R.M. (1982). *The foundations of knowing.* Minneapolis: University of Minnesota Press.

Cohen, M.Z. (1987). A historical overview of the phenomenological movement. *IMAGE: Journal of Nursing Scholarship, 19*(1), 31–34.

Cull-Wilby, B., & Pepin, J. (1987). Towards a coexistence of paradigms in nursing knowledge development. *Journal of Advanced Nursing, 12*(4), 515–521.

Ellis, R. (1970). Values and vicissitudes of the scientist nurse. *Nursing Research, 19,* 440–445.

Ellis. R. (1983). Philosophic inquiry. In H. Werley & J. Fitzpatrick (Eds.), *Annual review of nursing research* (Vol. 1, pp. 211–228). New York: Springer.

Fry, S. (1981). Accountability in research: The relationship of scientific and humanistic values. *Advances in Nursing Science, 4,* 1–13.

Gadow, S. (1980). Existential advocacy: Philosophical foundations of nursing. In E. Stuart & S. Gadow (Eds.), *Nursing: Images and ideals* (pp. 79–101). New York: Springer.

Gergen, K.J. (1980). The emerging crisis in life-span developmental theory. In P. Baltes & O. Brien (Eds.), *Life span development and behavior* (Vol. 3, pp. 31–63). Orlando, FL: Academic Press.

Gortner, S.R. (1974). Scientific accountability in nursing. *Nursing Outlook, 22,* 764–768.

Gortner, S.R. (1980). Nursing science in transition. *Nursing Research, 29*(3), 180–183.

Gortner, S.R. (1983). *Explanation in nursing science: The importance of "why" questions.* Paper presented at the Fifth Annual Graduate Conference: Nursing Knowledge Development, Implementation, and Validation in Practice, University of Portland, Portland, OR.

Gortner, S.R. (1984). Knowledge in a practice discipline: Philosophy and pragmatics. In *Nursing research and policy formation: The case of prospective payment.* Papers of the 1983 Scientific Session of the American Academy of Nursing (pp. 5–17). Kansas City: AAN.

Gortner, S.R. (1987). To build the science. In S.R. Gortner (Ed.), *Nursing science methods: A reader* (pp. 5–15). San Francisco: University of California Press.

Gortner, S.R. & Lorensen, M. (1989). Development of nursing science in Scandinavia. *Nursing Outlook, 37*(3), 123–126.

Gortner, S.R., & Nahm, H. (1977). Overview of nursing research. *Nursing Research, 26,* 10–23.

Gortner, S.R., & Schultz, P.R. (1988). Approaches to nursing science methods. *Image: Journal of Nursing Scholarship, 20*(1), 22–24.

Habermas, J.T. (1971). *Knowledge and human interests* (J. Shapiro, Trans.). Boston: Beacon Press.

Heidegger, M. (1962). *Being and time.* (J. Macquarrie & E. Robinson, Trans.). New York: Harper & Row.

Holter, I.M. (1987). Critical theory. In *Critical theory: An introduction and an exploration of its usefulness as a philosophical foundation for developing nursing theories and for guiding nursing practice and administration* (pp. 8–28). Oslo, Norway: Institutt for Sykepleievitenskap, University of Oslo.

International Council of Nurses. (1987). *Definition: Nursing research.* Geneva: Author.

Keller, E.F. (1985, October). Contending with a masculine bias in the ideals and values of science. Point of view in the *Chronicle of Higher Education.*

Kuhn, T. (1970). Introduction; II, The route to normal science; III, The nature of normal science. In T. Kuhn (Ed.), *Structure of scientific revolutions* (2nd ed., pp. 1–34). Chicago: University of Chicago Press.

Lanara, V. (1982). Development of a scientific foundation for the nursing profession. In K. Lerheim (Ed.), *Proceedings of the Fourth Conference of the Workgroup of European Nurse Researchers* (pp. 98–103). Oslo, Norway: Norwegian Nurses Association.

Leininger, M. (1988). *Care: The essence of nursing and health.* Detroit: Wayne State University Press. (Originally published by Charles Slack, Inc. in 1984).

Leonard, V.W. (1989). A Heideggerian phenomenologic perspective on the concept of person. *Advances in Nursing Science, 11,* 40–55.

Marcuse, H. (1964). *One-Dimensional man.* Boston: Beacon Press.

McLain, B.R. (1985). *Patterns of interaction, decision making, and health care delivery by nurse practitioners and physicians in joint practice.* Unpublished doctoral dissertation. University of San Francisco.

Merleau-Ponty, M. (1962). *Phenomenology of perception.* C. Smith (trans.). London: Routledge and KeganPaul.

Mishel, M.H., & Murdaugh, C.L. (1987). Family adjustment to heart transplantation: Redesigning the dream. *Nursing Research, 36,* 332–338.

National Center for Nursing Research (1988). Nursing science: Serving health through research (Program Announcement). Bethesda, MD: National Institutes of Health.

Nordic Nurses Federation. (1987). *Ethical guidelines for nursing research in the Nordic countries.* Aurskog, Norway: Printing Data Center.

Paterson, J.G., & Zderad, L.T. (Eds.), (1976). *Humanistic nursing.* New York: John Wiley & Sons.

Phillips, D. (1987). The new dynamics of the sciences. In *Philosophy, science, and social inquiry* (pp. 20–36). New York: Pergamon Press.

Royal College of Nursing. (1987). *In pursuit of excellence: A position statement on nursing.* London: Author.

Salmon, W. (1978). Why ask "Why?" An inquiry concerning scientific explanation. *Proceedings and Addresses of the American Philosophical Association, 51,* 683–705.

Sartre, J.P. (1963). *Search for method.* New York: Vintage Books.

Schultz, P.R. (1987). Toward holistic inquiry in nursing: A proposal for synthesis of patterns and methods. *Scholarly Inquiry for Nursing Practice, 1*(2), 135–146.

Schulz, P.R., & Meleis, A.I. (1988). Nursing epistemology: Traditions, insights, questions. *Image: Journal of Nursing Scholarship, 20*(4), 217–221.

Silva, M., & Rothbart, D. (1984). Analysis of changing trends in philosophies of science on nursing theory development and testing. *Advances in Nursing Science, 6*(2) 1–12.

Stevenson, J., & Woods, N.F. (1986). Nursing science and contemporary science: Emerging paradigms. In G.E. Sorensen (Ed.), *Setting the agenda for the year 2000: Knowledge development in nursing* (pp. 6–20). Kansas City: AAN.

Thompson, J.L. (1985). Practical discourse in nursing: Going beyond empiricism and historicism. *Advances in Nursing Science, 7*(4), 59–71.

Tripp-Reimer, T. (1984). Reconceptualizing the construct of health: Integrating emic and etic perspectives. *Research in Nursing and Health, 7,* 101–109.

Vaillot, M.C. (1962). *Commitment to nursing: A philosophical investigation.* Philadelphia: J.B. Lippincott.

Watson, J. (1985). *Nursing: Human science and human caring.* Boulder, CO: Colorado Associated University Press.

Winch, P. (1958). *The idea of a social science and its relation to philosopy.* London: Routledge and Kegan Paul.

Ziman, J. (1980). What is science? In E.D. Klemke, R. Hollinger, & A.D. Kline (Eds.), *Introductory readings in the philosophy of science* (pp. 35–54). Buffalo, NY: Prometheus Books.

The Author Comments

"Nursing Values and Philosophy: Toward a Philosophy of Nursing Science" was conceptualized over a period of several years, as a reaction to the influence phenomenology in general, and hermeneutics in particular, was exerting on American nursing literature. That these philosophies of person might be part of our belief systems without the necessity of having them direct our research programs and strategies was an insight gained abroad during the Fulbright. Readers may not agree that consensus is needed on a philosophy of science for nursing, but may agree that diverse world views can be accommodated in nursing's scientific repertoire.

—SUSAN R. GORTNER

Unit Three

Nursing, Science, and Nursing Science

The term science can be elusive. Although commonly used and familiar, for many it is difficult to define. It is not unusual for definitions of science to be made in conjunction with companion disciplines, for example, the study of living organisms and processes is biological science.

What then is nursing science? For the person with an inadequate definition of science, defining it in terms of nursing may be extremely difficult. Questions are immediately apparent: Is nursing a science, or is it something else? If science is defined by a discipline, then is nursing legitimately a discipline that can define its science?

Unit Three, Nursing Science, and Nursing Science contains fourteen chapters that address these questions and posit some answers. However, the consideration of the meanings of science in nursing is not confined to this unit; these same discussions appear again in future chapters of the book. But, these fourteen articles do provide a comprehensive and specific discussion of the role and meanings of science in the discipline of nursing.

Chapter 16, "The Nature of a Science of Nursing," discusses the need for a specifically identified and explicated body of substantive knowledge that is the "science of nursing." Dorothy E. Johnson defines nursing knowledge and nursing science, and discusses some mechanisms for the development of a body of substantive knowledge in nursing.

Chapter 17, "Values and Vicissitudes of the Scientist Nurse" by Rosemary Ellis, describes some of the difficulties that may be encountered as one becomes a scientist, especially for the nurse who chooses to study in a discipline other than nursing. Although Ellis notes that the problem is not as prevalent today, due to the demise of the Nurse Scientist grants and the increasing availability of doctoral programs in nursing, her comments relating to the difficulty inherent in "becoming a Ph.D." are still pertinent.

Chapter 18, "The Discipline of Nursing" by Sue K. Donaldson and Dorothy Crowley, defines the nature of the nursing discipline in terms of its syntactical and conceptual structures. This article was first presented as the keynote address at the 10th WCHEN Research Conference in April, 1977.

Chapter 19, "Fundamental Patterns of Knowing in Nursing" by Barbara A. Carper, analyzes the kinds of knowledge that exemplify nursing. To do the research that led to this paper, Carper systematically analyzed selected nursing literature to identify the structure of knowledge and patterns of knowing in nursing. Purposes for the study included focusing attention on the question of what it means to know and identifying the kinds of knowledge believed to be most valuable to the discipline.

Chapter 20, "Holistic Man and the Science and Practice of Nursing" by Sarah S. Fuller, presents several definitions of nursing derived from an analysis of recent events. Fuller asks if it might not be best to define nursing and nursing science in terms of the clients that are the focus of nursing. This important question for nurses appears in the literature as a persistent theme.

In Chapter 21, "Nursing Science in Transition," Susan R. Gortner distinguishes science from its inquiry, research. She describes research as "the tool of science" and discusses requirements for increased science: communality, colleagueship, competition, and confirmation.

Two visions of science are presented in Chapters 22 and 23: Harriet R. Feldman elaborates on what she considers science to be and what it might become in "A Science of Nursing—To Be or Not To Be?" and Jean Watson, in "Nursing's Scientific Quest," describes her concern with the relationship between traditional science and the needs of nursing as a human science.

The next two chapters in this unit present historic overviews of the development of nursing science. Gortner, in Chapter 24, and Silva and Rothbart, in Chapter 25, discuss the historic progress of science and present some questions for the future and continuing development of nursing science and knowledge. It is interesting to note the author's individual viewpoints: even though the subject matter of each article is similar, the discussions presented are unique.

The closing four chapters of the unit, by Conway (Chapter 26), Ramos (Chapter 27), Jacobs-Kramer and Chinn (Chapter 28) and Hinshaw (Chapter 29) all speak to the role that science has in developing nursing knowledge. It is interesting to assess the transition of these chapters from the earlier writings about science—the shift to a more conceptual plane is evident.

Understanding nursing science is a difficult task. Often it seems that when one question is answered and there is a consensus of opinion, five new questions are generated. Keeping pace with the changes in nursing science and in the development of nursing knowledge is a challenge. But, if there is a need for a specifically defined body of knowledge in nursing, and if nursing scholars are going to contribute to that knowledge, then keeping pace is not an option, but a requirement.

Chapter 16

The Nature of a Science of Nursing

Dorothy E. Johnson

The question of the existence of a body of substantive knowledge which can be called the science of nursing is a troublesome one for nurses and for members of allied professional groups alike. Yet it is a question of considerable significance for nursing's continued development as a recognized professional discipline. Certainly no profession can long exist without making explicit its theoretical bases for practice so that this knowledge can be communicated, tested, and expanded.

Nursing today faces an important developmental task in the explication of its science. The scope and complexity of the knowledge which can be drawn from the basic and applied sciences makes it difficult to perceive and connect what is pertinent to nursing. The lack of a clearly defined, widely accepted specific goal for professional nursing further complicates the situation. This paper presents some exploratory thoughts on the nature of a science of nursing which may illuminate the problem and provide some direction for research.

It is difficult to find a clear, concise, adequate definition of science. The *Oxford Universal Dictionary* defines science as "a branch of study concerned either with a connected body of demonstrated truths or with observed facts systematically classified and more or less colligated by being brought under general laws, and which includes trustworthy methods for the discovery of new truths within its own domain." While this definition suffices for purposes of this paper, you may wish to refer to Herbert Feigl's (1953) more philosophic discussion.

Although in modern usage the term science, or basic science, frequently is held as synonymous with the natural and physical sciences, it is also accepted by many in reference to the social sciences. These sciences are committed to the task of explaining natural phenomena by scientific investigation and to the systematization of knowledge. The applied sciences, on the other hand, are so named because they draw heavily upon the basic sciences to derive their bodies of knowledge and are committed to the application of knowledge toward some well-defined social goal.

It would appear, however, at least to this unsophisticated observer, that apart from the central tasks to which these sciences, basic and applied, are committed, there probably can be no sharp, unequivocal, clearly drawn line between them. Both are concerned with "a connected body of demonstrated truths." Both utilize the scientific method and "include trustworthy methods for the discovery of new truths." Both contribute through their research to the world's knowledge, and both at one time or another may be concerned with fundamental or practically oriented truths. Both have important social values.

Parenthetically, it may be helpful to take a brief look at some of the interrelationships between the sciences to dismiss, as questions of primarily academic interest, any notion that the individual basic sciences are "pure," superior, of greater fundamental importance, or clearly delineated, either one from the other or from the applied sciences. Every science has a quantitative aspect, so all must depend upon mathematics. Both chemistry and physics are of vital importance to the study of biology, hence the evolution of biochemistry and biophysics. Psychology, now considered a basic science by many, is said to have grown out of the disciplines of physiology and philosophy. In turn, in recent years, it has given birth to a rapidly growing professional field—clinical psychology. Physics, one of the oldest and most respected basic sciences, is ultimately involved in the practical problems of fission-fusion bombs and the atomic-powered electric plant. And philosophy, not usually considered a science at all, is the common father of all.

Disciplines as Sciences

The professional disciplines in general represent applied rather than basic sciences. They are committed to the task of utilizing knowledge to achieve some well-defined social goal. They draw heavily upon the basic sciences to derive their bodies of knowledge. They are

sciences, however, and are concerned with the systematization of knowledge and with its expansion. These characteristics have very direct implications for the development of a science of nursing.

The substantive content of any applied science is interdependent with the social goal of the profession which uses that science. The goals of nursing, both specific and shared, must be established in precise terms, therefore, to give direction to our search for a body of knowledge. There is an ultimate goal held by all health workers: the promotion and maintenance of optimum health of individuals and groups. Toward this ultimate goal, nursing shares with other health workers a number of subsidiary goals: the prevention of illness, the provision of comprehensive care, the promotion of recovery, including rehabilitation, the improvement in health practices and health status, and the expansion of the common body of knowledge of health and disease. In addition, nursing contributes to the achievement of the specific goals of other health workers, notably the physician, through delegated responsibilities. Professional nursing's specific and unique goal—and therefore its primary contribution toward the ultimate goal—is less clearly perceived and less widely accepted than that of medicine, for example, but one viewpoint is briefly presented here to illustrate how the development of a science of nursing can be given direction (Johnson, 1959).

Nursing's Professional Goal

Nursing, like other health professions, is a discipline which focuses primarily on direct service to individuals and groups of individuals. Through that service, nursing's specific professional goal is achieved. Through it, the contribution that nursing can make toward the goals shared with, or specific to other health workers, is realized. Nursing care, of all the components of nursing practice, is probably the medium through which professional nursing's specific goal is achieved. Nursing care, which is provided to individuals or groups under stress of a health-illness nature, has as its primary purpose to relieve tension and discomfort to the end of restoring or maintaining internal and interpersonal equilibrium.[1]

Internal and interpersonal equilibrium—which I hold to be the specific goal of professional nursing—does not imply a state of health or well-being. It is rather a state in which opposing forces—biological, psychological, or social—are balanced momentarily. In a sense, it can be conceived as a resting state in which the individual or group can gather resources or replenish energy for further movement. It is a dynamic state, however, for it is fluid and transitional; rest, over prolonged, can be as destructive as lack of rest. Nursing requires therapeutic as well as supportive measures to assist the patient to achieve this state. It is a state which is an integral part of the change process—whether that change is biological, psychological, or social.

This goal is achieved through activities such as bathing, feeding, explaining, reassuring, and the like, which tend to reduce tension and to offer comfort, gratification, and assistance in relation to basic human needs (biological and psychosocial). Tension is defined as a state of being stretched or strained, whether endogenous or exogenous in origin. It arises from stress. It may be constructive in the sense that it stimulates desirable change. It may also be destructive in that it consumes energy and may immobilize the individual. The dissipation or reduction of destructive tension leads to a state of equilibrium which subsequently makes possible more effective utilization of available energy, facilitating recovery from illness or promoting health.

It is also through the medium of nursing care, as well as through other components or nursing practice, that nursing contributes to the goals shared with, or specific to, other health workers. At times these goals may be the crucial ones; in which case, the nursing practitioner must direct her activities accordingly. Nursing contributes to the achievement of these goals through such activities as health teaching, the adminis-

tration of medications and medical treatment, and observing the patient's response to medical therapy.

Nursing Knowledge

Two kinds of knowledge are needed by the professional nursing practitioner to achieve these goals: ultimate and specific. The accompanying chart (Chart 16-1) presents schematically the derivations of knowledge required in nursing care, and illustrates a concept of the science of nursing. First, there is needed a knowledge of people and how they respond (biologically, psychologically, and socially) to stress. This is indicated on the right-hand side of the chart.

This knowledge of people, derived from both the basic and the applied sciences, is knowledge which we share in common, at least in large measure, with all professional health workers. Nursing is contributing to this body of knowledge by studies such as that of Tudor (1952). An important development in this area in recent years has been the many efforts to correlate concepts from these various disciplines to present a more unified picture of human behavior (Grinker, 1956; Selye, 1956; Simmons & Wolff, 1954). These efforts are adding to our expanding knowledge of the specific patterns of behavior, biologically and psychologically, which can be expected in response to certain stress situations under given circumstances. These predictable patterns of response to stress, as they are validated and expanded, provide an ever more satisfactory basis for diagnosis and for developing remedial modes of intervention—in medicine, in social work, and in nursing.

The second kind of knowledge needed is indicated on the left-hand side of the chart. Knowledge of the science of nursing is necessary if nursing care is to be purposeful and effective, for it provides a conceptual basis and a rationale for the methods or approaches chosen to achieve certain specified and appropriate nursing objectives. The major determinant in the selection of knowledge from the basic and applied sciences pertinent to nursing is nursing's specific and unique professional goal. It is proposed here that the body of

---

[1] The development of this viewpoint was given impetus by Johnson and Martin (1958) and represents, in part, an extension of their concept of the nurse's function. See: A sociological analysis of the nurse role. *American Journal of Nursing 58*, 373.

Chart 16-1
A Schematic Presentation of the Derivations of Knowledge in Nursing Care*

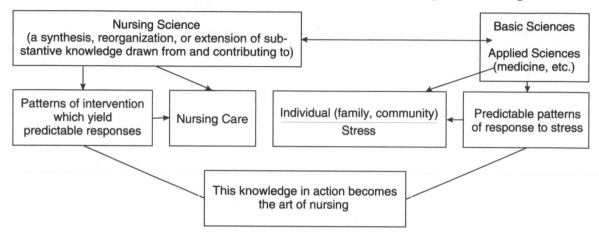

Nursing care is a direct service provided to individuals or groups under stress of a health-illness nature. Stress is broadly interpreted as any situation in which equilibrium is disturbed, producing tension (biological, psychological, social) and discomfort. Our knowledge of people and how they respond to stress (knowledge which we share in common with other professional health workers) provides a basis for a nursing diagnosis. A synthesis, reorganization, or extension of substantive knowledge also drawn from the basic and applied sciences in relation to nursing's specific goal and contribution to patient welfare may lead to concepts and theories of diagnosis and intervention in nursing. Nursing becomes an art when knowledge of nursing and of people is translated into effective action.

* Frances Kreuter, Reva Rubin, Gladys Sorensen, Kathryn Smith, Dorothy Mereness, Pauline Lucas, and Betty Highley are credited for parts of this diagram and for ideas from which it was further developed.

knowledge called the science of nursing consists of a synthesis, reorganization, or extension of concepts drawn from the basic and other applied sciences which in their reformulation tend to become "new" concepts. It is further proposed that these "new" concepts will be concerned largely but not exclusively with the causation, character, and progress of the tensions growing out of stress and disturbing internal or interpersonal equilibrium, or both. They will lead to the development of theories of nursing intervention which will yield predictable (and desirable) responses in patients when implemented in nursing care.

The development and utilization of the science of medicine may offer a helpful analogy at this point. With his knowledge of people and of medical science, the physician makes a diagnosis. The process of diagnosing leads to the identification of the existing medical problem or problems (that is, the nature of the pathological changes which might occur or are occurring) and to selection of appropriate modes of intervention to change the course of events.

By law and by tradition, the physician is charged specifically with the responsibility for preventing and controlling those pathological changes which are manifested in illness or disability. Through the years he has come to recognize and make explicit, at first experientially and later through research, the nature of disease and the therapeutic measures which offer the most reasonable possibility of achieving the desired results. He can describe theoretically, for example, the body's response to invasion by certain infectious agents and knows that certain drugs or treatments, alone or in combination, offer the best possibility of preventing, controlling, or curing in a given situation. He is able to predict, on the basis of verified knowledge, that certain actions on his part will probably result in certain responses on the part of the patient. This predictability, though it may be unreliable for a given individual or situation, is of crucial importance in the development of any science.

Medical science has reached its present status through clear understanding of the specific goals of the profession. This understanding has given direction not only to the activities undertaken in medical practice, but also to the many research efforts which have provided sounder theoretical bases for that practice. There have been many points of departure for these research efforts: keen observation of repetitive actions or reactions, alert analysis of "accidental" events, curiosity about the reason why—to name only a few. In each instance, however, there has been the capacity to tie certain observations or ideas to something already known, establishing a conceptual frame of reference which has led to the asking of more and more precise questions.

Advances in Nursing

Nursing, too, must advance through this slow, tedious process. One might ask: What is the nature of the tensions with which we are dealing? What are their causes? How can we intervene most effectively? We might answer these kinds of questions, descriptively now. Later, answers to more and more precise questions (is it this, or is it that?) will tend to make this knowledge more exact.

Let us look more directly at nursing for a moment and consider our present stage of development. It has long been accepted that nursing's contribution to patient welfare goes beyond effective assistance in the medical care plan. We speak of the identification of nursing problems. And by word of mouth or through experience, we have learned certain ways of handling certain nursing problems. Some nurses know, for example, that appropriate timing may reduce the pain of a daily dressing for the apprehensive patient, that a certain approach together with certain instructions and explanations are most likely to be successful in assisting the postoperative patient to ambulate for the first time, that a back rub and a few words are often effective in inducing sleep when a sedative might otherwise be needed, and that continuous care by the same nurse of the hospitalized infant is sometimes a critical link to favorable progress.

In some instances these modes of intervention have been developed through inference as a result of observations and of knowledge drawn from the basic sciences. In others, trial and error have led to the adoption of certain action patterns because they had been successful in achieving desired results. We have consistently tended to add to our knowledge of people and to rely on scientific investigation as a valid source for that knowledge. Just as consistently, we have tended to depend upon experientially learned action patterns as our source of knowledge of nursing. Only recently we have begun to ask ourselves consciously what the rationale for our actions might be, or whether we might find sound bases in theory for our actions.

It may be helpful to explore a little further one example selected from those given above. It has been observed repeatedly that some hospitalized infants fail to progress as expected under medical therapy. Bakwin (1942) described some years ago the apathy and increasing lethargy shown by some hospitalized infants. The practicing nurse is well aware of the anorexia, failure to gain weight, and even diarrhea which numbers of infants demonstrate, sometimes in increasing severity, after a few days or weeks of hospitalization. Frequently, none of these manifestations can be explained fully, at least as they begin to appear, on the basis of the medical problem or its treatment.

In recent years it has been suggested that this kind of unfavorable progress is related to maternal deprivation or separation anxiety. These are labels used by the behavioral scientists in referring to concepts which define or explain certain mother-child relationships, and they are valid only within the context in which they were developed and tested. Can nursing be satisfied with accepting the immediate inference of these labels for application in a nursing context, that is, to maintain maternal contact or to provide for continuous care of an infant by the same nurse who acts as mother surrogate? Is further investigation essential so that nursing management is really soundly based? Are there tensions generated by this stress-producing situation (hospitalization) about which little is known, and which are properly the business of nursing investigators both alone and in collaboration with other interested scientists? Can certain knowledge drawn from the basic sciences, biological and behavioral, and medicine be tied together with astute nursing observations and ideas to provide a basis for conceptual speculation about the nature of these tensions—their character, cause, or progress—and about remedial intervention?

The Theory of Nursing Diagnoses

The label provided by the behavioral scientist is generally no more satisfactory as a nursing diagnosis than the label provided by the physician. The concepts and research which support these labels are important, however, in the identification of nursing problems, for these contribute to an understanding of people. In their synthesis and with a focus on nursing, these concepts may also provide the substantive knowledge which makes possible a nursing diagnosis, and lead to the development of theories of intervention.

While the accompanying chart was developed in an effort to present graphically the derivations of knowledge used in nursing, it can also be used in presenting the derivations of knowledge in the other health professions. For example, substitute the word "medical" wherever nursing is found in the body of the chart and no further adaptation is needed to make the picture applicable to medicine. As a graphic picture, it is perhaps oversimplified and further analysis might indicate more real differences in the health professions in their sources of knowledge than are now apparent. The major difference between the health professions does not appear to be the sources of their bodies of knowledge, but the selection of concepts from those sources as pertinent to their respective specific social

goals. While the view presented here of professional nursing's specific goal may not be acceptable or valid, it does serve to illustrate that the science of nursing depends primarily upon the acceptance of a specific professional goal, and only secondarily upon nursing's shared goals and delegated responsibilities.

In summary, the science of nursing is conceived as developing through the reformulation of concepts drawn from the basic sciences and certain other applied sciences to yield a body of knowledge fundamental to the development of theories of nursing diagnosis and intervention. It is given direction in its development by recognition of nursing's specific goal and contribution to the ultimate goal of optimum health for all individuals and groups.

There is a foundation on which we can build as we focus on future developments. Present methods and approaches, both technical and supportive, in nursing which have evolved over the years offer a beginning for some research effort since, with few exceptions, their underlying concepts and theories remain to be explored, tested, and made explicit. Content now included in nursing courses can be analyzed with the view to formulating specific nursing concepts which can then be subjected to research. As research in nursing increases in scope and reliability, important contributions will be made to the world's knowledge of people as well as to the science of nursing.

References

Bakwin, H. (1942). Loneliness in infants. *American Journal of Diseases of Children, 63,* 30.

Feigl, H., & Brodbeck, M. (1953). *Readings in the philosophy of science.* New York: Appleton-Century-Crofts.

Grinker, R.R. (Ed.) (1956). *Toward a unified theory of human behavior.* New York: Basic Books.

Johnson, D.E. (1959). A philosophy of nursing. *Nursing Outlook, 7,* 198–200.

Selye, H. (1956). *The stress of life.* New York: McGraw-Hill.

Simmons, L.W., & Wolff, H.G. (1954). *Social science in medicine.* New York: Russell Sage Foundation.

Tudor, G.W. (1952). A socio-psychiatric nursing approach to intervention in a problem of mutual withdrawal on a mental hospital ward. *Psychiatry, 15,* 193–217.

The Author Comments

This was the second of two papers written in tandem. The ideas presented had evolved slowly over a period of more than 10 years as I sought a rational and logical basis for curriculum content and structure in nursing at both the baccalaureate and master's levels. These ideas had been tested and advanced by many discussions with colleagues and students over the years and had been utilized in curriculum development. The papers were written in an effort to make the ideas as explicit as possible so that they might be still further clarified and developed.

Simultaneously, I was involved in a study to determine the feasibility of a doctoral program in nursing. Quite clearly, a doctoral program would require students to study and analyze substantive knowledge in nursing for the purpose of further testing and advancing that knowledge. At that time, there was no widespread agreement on the content to be included in master's-level programs, to say nothing of a doctoral program. It was hoped that the ideas presented in these papers might provide an acceptable as well as a rational basis for the tentative identification of the knowledge to be so utilized. This purpose was not fully achieved for many reasons. Nonetheless, the articles (and the study) provided an important stimulus to my continued thinking about nursing theory and its development.

—DOROTHY E. JOHNSON

Chapter 17

Values and Vicissitudes of the Scientist Nurse

Rosemary Ellis

Nurses have always known that newborns could see. They acted on this belief, in spite of the fact that authorities told them that newborns could not see. Why didn't some nurse study the question of visual development of the infant, and refute the authorities? Why did it wait for the psychologist Robert Fantz (1963) to produce the studies that refute the authorities?

There are probably several answers to this question. Until recently, there have been very few nurses with the skill to investigate the question. Secondly, nurses, in the main, have not valued careful, systematic investigation, especially if it should require subjecting newborns or other dependent people to special testing or strange devices. Probably more importantly, the question of whether babies could see or not was not a problem for the nurse. In spite of the words of the authorities, she could act on her own beliefs; she, and the mother and baby, could ignore the authorities' claims, with no consequences. They did not need to pay

attention to what scientists said about the infant's vision.

The advent of increasing numbers of scientist nurses should make it more likely that something such as the visual development of infants would be studied by nurses. Such scientist nurses, however, will differ from other nurses in the kind, amount, and extent of their formal education. Consequently, they will differ from other nurses in their knowledge, skills, interests, perceptions, and attitudes. Will they differ from the majority of nurses in their values? It seems likely that they will. If scientist nurses are to contribute to the development of nursing, however, there must be some values which scientist nurses and other nurses continue to hold in common. It is to be hoped that one such value would be service to society, expressed as concern and action for health welfare, and the care of the sick.

The route to becoming a scientist nurse, or a career as a scientist nurse, contains experiences and costs which may impede direct expression of this value. Some nurses trained as scientists may even adopt values which supplant the service to society value which underlies nursing. This would not be surprising. A value of knowledge for the sake of knowledge is one that is commonly expressed.

Consider the costs of becoming a nurse scientist through education in some specific discipline. For an appreciable number of years a nurse becoming a scientist usually is removed from daily encounters with a community of nurses, and from living in the environment in which nursing occurs. There is the cost of loss in some nursing skills from disuse, or from the lack of opportunity to keep abreast in a rapidly changing world of nursing practice. There is also the cost in the loss of other learning. While one focuses on learning one discipline, one cannot master others equally important for nursing. The costs affect not only the nurse scientist herself, but may contribute to some estrangement of the nurse scientist from the active nurse practitioner, or to an altered perception of the nurse scientist as a nurse by practicing nurses.

The potential for estrangement is probably related to the motivation underlying a nurse's election of a nurse scientist program or career. Why do nurse scientists choose to bear the costs? The seeking of answers, of knowledge, of status or prestige, of power or influence, of enjoyment, or of special skills are motivation for some. There are probably many more motives, such as avoidance, each with a different potential for producing estrangement from the nurse practitioner.

Whatever the motive for pursuing the career of a nurse scientist, the pursuit is a commitment to a pattern of thought, and of behavior, for years to come. It behooves the nurse scientist to consider how her values relate to those underlying nursing, and to those commonly held by the practitioner in nursing.

The orientation of the nurse scientist to nursing, and to the practice and practitioner in nursing, is essential, if one wants to use the word "nurse" to modify "scientist," or to use the word "nursing" to modify the word "research." Pressures for some discontinuity with nursing can occur in the process of a nurse becoming a scientist.

To truly learn any discipline, one must develop an identity with that discipline. The structures for developing this identity, the spatial or territorial arrangements, and the work relationships, differ somewhat from academic discipline to discipline. Becker and Carper (1956), in an analysis of physiology, engineering, and philosophy, found three significant factors in the development of identity with an occupation. These are the informal peer group, the apprenticeship relationship with professors, and the formal academic structure.

In physiology, the vast world of problems yet to be tackled is the perspective. A careful, building block approach through laboratory studies is the mode. Laboratory groups are the vital work and social orientations. The laboratory is the site for peer group interactions. A major professor as a sponsor, a mentor, and perhaps as a lifetime reference seems the norm. It is not uncommon to find the question "With whom did you study?" to be one of the first questions to be asked of the newcomer physiologist. The answer may influence how the newcomer is perceived or placed. A student typically will select for his investigation some problem specific to the special competence and interest of his mentor. The student will enjoy a close working and social relationship with this mentor which is apt to continue beyond the student's graduation. He spends his time in the same territory as his mentor, and does work with or like that of his mentor. He is physically close to the actual working of his fellow students, has frequent opportunity to observe them in action.

The student in a department of philosophy does not have the specific problem focus, the building block rigor, the laboratory work, the laboratory group, or the same sort of professor-student contacts, characteristic of physiology. The professor does his work secluded in his office. The student may consume the completed work, but he rarely can observe the processes, as his professor works on a philosophical problem. Rarely does the student significantly share in these work processes.

Physiology and philosophy probably represent two extreme models, with other disciplines having models more like one or the other, depending on their "hardness" as science.

The process of acquiring identity with and from an academic discipline cannot help but alter the nurse who lives for a significant number of years, as a graduate student, in that academic environment. There may be some tensions during the period if the expected identity with others in an academic discipline fails to mesh with identity as a nurse. Identity as a nurse may impair the perceptions of significant others as they judge the nurse student against the specifications of the discipline identity. The nurse may find some difficulty in accepting the trappings of the academic acolyte, if these are at odds with the nurse identity. Acquiring full identity with the discipline may make one marginal and suspected in nursing. Failure to acquire the identity makes one marginal and suspected in the discipline. How painful is marginality, and what does one do about it? The answers lie in one's values and primary loyalties, which each one must discover for himself. From the disciplines there is the weight of the problems, the ideologies, the fellows, and the sponsors, from that discipline. There is the burden of loyalty to remain what one has become, so as not to let down the sponsor. For a nonnurse disciple, or the nurse whose primary loyalty is to some discipline, this can have important consequences for career opportunities. It can affect the choice of problems or activities one pursues. For the nurse disciple whose nursing orientation remains a primary loyalty, there is greater freedom to the extent that one may move beyond discipleship more rapidly, because there are few masters in nursing. One may lose some security as one moves somewhat away from a discipline sponsor or colleagues, but one can gain a wide freedom of choice of activities, or problems to pursue. Nursing is not currently characterized by sponsorship, or by loyalty to unique or particular ideologies, as essentials in career development.

To be identified with nursing, the nurses need only exhibit a loyalty to the ethos of nursing. Kolthoff (1968), in writing about the nurse scientist, speaks of old traditions of service in new ways. It is clear that to be identified as a nurse one must retain the nursing tradition of service to man, though one can exhibit allegiance to the tradition in a variety of new ways, based on the knowledge and skills acquired in advanced study. Marginality and suspicion can be overcome, it need not be painful, if the nurse scientist has experienced the satisfaction and enrichment that accrue to the professional in nursing, and finds in these the sources for continued willing adherence to the valuable traditions of nursing. In this is a source for renewal through meaningful work. In this is the source for meaningful relationships with practitioners in nursing.

Such sources would dictate that the problems which scientist nurses choose to study, and their perceptions, attitudes, and values, would be those relevant to nursing. They would be those relevant to a special service to man. The nurse, in contrast to some scientists, would ask "Why?" when she starts a search for knowledge, and the answer to why should contain a relevance or reference to nursing.

One should learn from history or the experiences of others. Medicine is today experiencing some dilemma about the orientation and location of its basic sciences or scientists. Some medical school faculty oriented to clinical practice are deeply concerned about the remoteness from clinical skills or problems of the investigations of their colleagues in biophysics or biochemistry. There is a growing schism between some areas of interest of the medical scientist, and the areas of interest to clinical medicine. Seldin illustrates this as follows:

> Successful and important investigations from a biochemical vantage point may lure the clinical investigator in a direction progressively more remote from clinical medicine. The problems posed by patients no longer elicit curiosity. Deranged physiology becomes too complicated for the powerful but restricted tools of basic biochemistry. The net effect may be research not pertinent to any activity in a clinical department. (Seldin, 1966, pp. 976–979)

It is to be hoped that nursing can avoid this pitfall if nurse scientists are primarily oriented to the values of clinical nursing though they need not themselves be engaged in practice.

Some of the vicissitudes of becoming a nurse scientist have been mentioned or can be inferred from the above discussion of values and orientation. Some of these vicissitudes remain in the career of a nurse scientist, and additional ones develop.

There is always the question of "To whom does the nurse scientist relate for communion?" From whom does she seek exchange, stimulation, and a sense of companionship, in the work world? As a member of a very small minority group, the nurse scientist has a rare-zero distribution in the nursing departments of health or illness agencies, and, with few exceptions, in schools of nursing. Nurses caught up in the exigencies of providing nursing care, or of facilitating the learning of beginners in nursing, are not likely to find appreciable amounts of time to give to the nurse scientist, even if they have the inclination or interest. The pace, the locale, the modus operandi, of the doer and the thinker usually do not coincide. Yet even those who think well alone, or who enjoy the autonomy in research, must, at some point, require the stimulation of response to, validation of, or refutation of, their ideas. For the scientist nurse to achieve this requires that the scientist nurse be willing to become involved to some extent, in the interests, issues, discouragements, and excitements, of the nurse who is not a scientist. Where the values of nursing are evident in the scientist nurse, the gaps between the nonscientist nurse and the scientist nurse are narrowed, to their mutual benefit. The scientist nurse, however, must pick her career arena carefully to ensure that it has the potential for a sense of community in the work world.The choice of where to work, and what to work at, confronts the newly-prepared nurse scientist. Re-entry problems, if one chooses to work in a nursing institution, may plague some nurse scientists. One must become oriented to the institution, to affiliated care agencies, and in some measure, be willing to take on the institution's philosophy and problems. These will be different than those seen as paramount from the graduate student view. There is apt to be a testing by new colleagues of one's identity as a nurse at a time when the new science graduate feels vulnerable or uncertain because of the time-or-distance-from-nursing costs involved in completing a typical doctoral program. Identity challenges recur with any major life transition, and for the nurse scientist, the challenges may come subtly from other nurses.

Then there is the question of "Which language do you speak?" It is amazing to realize how markedly one's language is altered in the process of becoming and being a scientist. Quite unconsciously one begins to use the jargon and special terminology of the world in which one lives. If this is the world of the professional and student in a select discipline, one gradually acquires the language which facilitates communication within the discipline, but does so at the price of impairing communication with those outside the discipline. Even the terms used with some common meaning across sciences, for example the word "variable," if used in communication with the non-scientist, may produce lack of understanding and, possibly, some alienation. Even when one is aware of this hazard, and consciously tries to avoid it, terminology once learned and used creeps into all speech. If one seeks effective communication with nurses, their patients, and their world, one had better use the language of that world, and avoid the terminology of one's scientist training. This requires a continuing conscious attempt to distinguish, and to use appropriately, the languages of two different worlds.

The aforementioned vicissitudes originate from the role of the scientist nurse. What of those in the actual work of the scientist nurse? What of the problems in theoretical study or research relevant to nursing? There are some that arise from the nature of science, and some that arise from the nature of nursing.

First a look at the practice of science. Science is a process for the generation of knowledge. To be useful, the knowledge must be put to some purpose. At times, the scientist's frame of reference may be too narrow for the general good. The development, testing, and introduction of DDT is but one example of some scientist's inadequate frame of reference, a frame of reference inadequate to foresee the important consequences of the use of DDT which are vastly more costly than its benefit. A narrow focus essential to high command of knowledge, techniques, and materials in one sphere, is not the best base from which to consider the universe to which the sphere relates. Analogies to the DDT problem probably could be found in behavioral science practices as well.

Science boundaries are useful for the learner in a scientific community. They limit what he can be expected to master, and give a base for identity of problems. Science boundaries are barriers, rather than benefits, in the *application* of science because of the way they influence the generation and structure of knowledge. Recall the dilemma of medicine. As biochemistry becomes increasingly basic, in the sense of moving to finer and finer particularization, it becomes far less a base for clinical medicine.

A mythical view of science engenders the notion that research finds answers, solves problems, or is an avenue to specific theory. In practice, it is a phase in the vicissitude of theory and research; it is a phase in the alternation of a continuous cycle of theory-research-theory. Far more questions than answers are generated by research. One simply gets another leg up on learning what is yet unknown. In practice, research is more productive for identifying new problems than it is for giving solutions for empirical problems.

Another view of the practice of science that is open to some question is that significant achievement comes *only* from careful, small, rigorous, sequential studies. Serendipity is recognized as occurring, but no statistics are kept to give insight to the frequency with which chance is an important element in the successful practice of science. What is overlooked in serendipity is the priming of the scientist for a sensitivity for relating heretofore unrelated observations or ideas. Such priming can occur in a variety of ways of which rigorously designed methical study is only one. Watson's *The Double Helix* (New York: New American Library, 1969) is a spectacular example of the triumph of the model builder over the "good guy" methical scientist.

Objective scientists run the risk of being blinded by theory. Several years before oceanographers paid serious attention to it, a young woman doing routine tasks in the data analysis laboratory of an oceanographer noted a persistent notch in the tracings of soundings of ridges of the ocean floor. She mentioned it to the oceanographer who dismissed it. It did not fit with his theory. Several years later another bit of information caused the oceanographer to recall the notch. With a new frame of reference, the scientist reviewed the tracings of the notch, and a significant breakthrough in the understanding of ocean floor ridges, and a new theory of continent formation and drift, evolved. Now scientists are saying that the continents of South America and Africa were once joined, something the schoolchild of recent generations intuitively guessed from looking at a map, only to be refuted by the scientist of his time. Theory, inadequate facts and limited focus can be hazards for the unwary scientist.

Now for some problems that arise from the nature of nursing. It is said that one knows nothing about something unless one can quantify it. The present capacity of scientist nurses to quantify important variables for the study of nursing is almost nil. The situation is little better even if one elects to study phenomena or variables which are not those of nursing but of something thought to be relevant for nursing. In this era, if scientist nurses limit their research to that which permits of measurement, they run the risk of limiting themselves to studying trivia or tangents of nursing. One is forced to premature precision by too stringent a requirement of measurability in the present day in nursing.

Nursing is in an acute state of groping. At best, it has some imprecise labels for many thought-to-be important variables, rather than sound and useful tools for measurement. For some time to come, the scientist nurse must balance the requirements of science with the state of nursing. Too rigorous adherence to the ideals of tight design, careful control, and extensively tested methodologies or tools, can be limiting in this day. Very rarely does clinical research permit such adherence. The hazards in less rigid adherence are to be run, if the scientist nurse seeks to explore clinical problems. Koch, in an article on psychology, decries scientist because it produces "ameaningful" thinking. (Ameaningful, as defined by Koch, is the word *meaningful* with the prefix *a* where *a* has the same force as it does in words like *amoral*.) Ameaningful thought or inquiry "assumes that inquiring action is so rigidly and fully regulated by *rule* that in its conception of inquiry if often allows the rules totally to displace their human users" (Koch, 1969, pp. 64–68). The object of inquiry, in such circumstances, appears to become an "ungainly and annoying irrelevance." Scientism and ameaningful inquiry are as possible in nursing as in psychology.

Some of the problems in inquiry of clinical phenomena can be illustrated from the following examples. Some patients give names to their pathology, or to a body part altered by pathology. A patient with a diagnosis of duodenal ulcer disease spoke of "Mr. Peptic," when he spoke of his ulcer site or ulcer disease. A patient with a crippled hand which was being treated by splinting and physiotherapy called the hand "Monkey." A woman with a colostomy called it "Suzie." A patient with ear noise associated with advancing hearing loss called the ear noise "Cricket."

On the assumption that the naming serves some purpose, it would be useful for the nurse to have some understanding of the phenomena. The case of "Monkey" suggested that the use of the name "Monkey" by the patient and her husband served to achieve some distance and objectivity for the crippled hand. It became a special object upon which special attention, tenderness, and love could be lavished. Each evening the husband would carefully rewrap "Monkey" in its splint. The choice of the name "Monkey" suggests some derision, but it also suggests a pet. It could be seen as an effective coping mechanism for a transitional state.

"Mr. Peptic" was used in another way. As the patient discussed his disease, and his regimens for dealing with it, he indicated that "Mr. Peptic" would remind him if he deviated from his regimens very much. "Mr. Peptic" also would not let him do some things. It appears as though "Mr. Peptic" was a way of avoiding activities the patient wanted to avoid. "Mr. Peptic" would not let him go to a party if the patient did not wish to attend it.

The naming phenomenon suggests ego alienation. It also provides a short nickname for ease of communication about a diseased body part or process.

From these fragments one can make a case for further study of the phenomenon of patient or patient relative naming of diseased body parts. But how does one study it? One cannot create the phenomenon; one must wait until it comes along. One cannot think of sampling, but what is the population to be studied? How does one study the phenomenon without altering it by the asking of questions? If one simply observes, what does one observe? Piaget's (1954) study of his three children on which he bases his theory on the development of reality thinking in the young child offers one method. Even this approach offers no easy solution for the inquiry of the naming phenomenon.

Another example can be drawn from interest in patients' use of humor. This is not something which has been studied, yet it may be another coping mechanism. Some patients seem to use humor as means of transcending a painful experience. This use of humor for transcendence has not been systematically explored. How would one proceed?

Another problem which arises in clinical research in nursing is that of retaining data as the patient moves through time. It is not possible in the present state of knowledge of nursing to anticipate all the possibly important variables. What makes a critical difference is not known. One cannot fully anticipate what should be observed and recorded, therefore one has no entry through a rerun of the data for a variable one has not anticipated. The experiment cannot be repeated with identical subjects. In this groping in nursing research, the identification, measurement, collection, and retention of important data, as a patient and nurse move through time, remain problems of great magnitude. Exact repetition of clinical experiments is difficult because of many patient factors beyond the nurses' control, and it is time-consuming.

Further problems in clinical research can be illustrated from an experience with a widely used personality inventory with a patient sample. In the course of studies of eye surgery, stapedectomy, and general surgery patients, in which the writer has been engaged, the Eysenck Personality Inventory was used to measure capacity for introversion (Eysenck, 1963). This variable was thought possibly to be related to having unusual sensory or cognitive experiences under conditions of relative sensory deprivation. One unexpected finding was that the mean scores for various patient groups for the Lie Scale of the Eysenck Personality Inventory exceeded that of the American norms for the instrument. These norms were, however, based on testing of a college population. The difference might be explainable on the mean age differences between the college sample and the patient samples. It might be due to the fact because patients with poor vision or eye patching comprised one of our samples, the test had been administered verbally rather than in the written form. The test manual states that the test may be given verbally or in written form, but the norms are presumably based on written administration. Perhaps a higher Lie Scale score results if one is required to respond verbally to questions like "Would you always declare everything at customs even if you knew you could get away with it?" One might be less willing to say out loud, than with a check-mark, that one has a touch of dishonesty. Could the difference be due to the status of patient? All these elements seemed possible. The point of all this is to illustrate that the very limited use of even common psychological tests with a general hospital population does not provide much base for anticipating the outcomes from such testing. There is little base for interpreting test scores from nonpatient norms. Reliable measurement tools developed and used with nonpatient populations may need re-evaluation for use with patient populations.

A final comment on nursing. Nursing is essentially a special type of human caring. Some perceive human caring and science to be antithetical. Science, for some, conjures up images of test tubes, laboratories and increasing remoteness from the real world. This is not the whole story. Science is also the careful measurement of strain in the pinned hip joint, as a patient goes through various movements attendant to selected nursing activities. Measurement of the strain on a hip union during the movement of the patient by means of a draw sheet, or other nursing maneuvers, is for the ultimate purpose of selection or development of nursing maneuvers that produce the least strain on the healing, reconstructed bone. It is a means of achieving a kind of caring that is not simple sentiment, but a kind of caring that includes deliberate, scientifically selected action. Science can be an effective tool of the humanist. It is not his enemy.

Whitehead (1929) identified three stages in a process of education: the stage of Romance, the stage of Precision, and the stage of Generalization. The stage of Romance is characterized by the freshness of inexperience. Romance gives way to precision as one learns that there are right ways, accepted rules, and ideologies. Over time, one moves to a state of generalization. This last stage is characterized by the production of active wisdom. Knowledge is barren until tested and used. Knowledge alone is insufficient; one also needs wisdom. Whitehead states that wisdom comes from freedom in the presence of knowledge. Science and knowledge are the tools of the scientist nurse. Wisdom is an ultimate goal.

The sequential stages of romance, precision, and generalization characterize the development of the scientist nurse. They also describe a successful nursing career. A young June graduate recently shared the experiences of her first eight months as a staff nurse. She was plunged into responsibilities for which she felt inadequate. Because of the pace and volume of her work, she failed to obtain the satisfactions she had anticipated from nursing. In searching her feelings about nursing, she had come to feel that "nobility is not the thing." Romance had come to an end, as she realized that her romantic view of a Florence Nightingale was not the real world.

Though it is readily understandable why this young nurse feels as she does, one cannot agree with her. From the perspective of more years in nursing, one can see a cycle of romance, to realism, to a return to a sense of nobility that is based on realism. Nobility is the thing in nursing, when "noble" is correctly understood as meaning admirable in dignity of conception, and in manner of expression or execution. There are many ways of expressing or executing nursing. A scientific contribution to the improvement of practice can be a satisfying one for the scientist nurse. It combines the nursing ethos of service to others with great opportunity for self-realization.

References

Becker, H.S., & Carper, J.W. (1956). Development of identification with a profession. *American Journal of Sociology, 61*, 289–298.

Eysenck, S.B.G., & Eysenck, H.J. (1963). *Manual for the Eysenck personality inventory.* San Diego, CA: Educational and Industrial Testing Service.

Fantz, R.L. (1963). Pattern vision in newborn infants. *Science, 140*, 296–297.

Koch, S. (1969, September). Psychology cannot be a coherent science. *Psychology Today, 3*(14), 64–68.

Kolthoff, N. (1968). Evolution of the nurse scientist: Emergence and continued development. *Image, 2*, 11–12.

Piaget, J. (1954). *Construction of reality in the child.* (M. Cook, Trans.). New York: Basic Books.

Seldin, D.W. (1966). Some reflections on the role of basic research and service in clinical departments. *Journal of Clinical Investigation, 45*, 976–979.

Watson, J.D. (1969). *The double helix.* New York: New American Library.

Whitehead, A.N. (1929). *Aims of education and other essays.* New York: Macmillan.

The Author Comments

I prepared this paper for a nurse scientist student conference that was hosted by the University of Colorado School of Nursing. Although I do not recall the conference theme nor what prompted this topic, I had been a member of the Advisory Committee for the Nurse Scientist Grant at Frances Payne Bolton School of Nursing, Case Western Reserve University. I had perceived the strain on some nurses as they tried to study in other disciplines without recognizing the changes required of them in order to become a physiologist, psychologist, sociologist, or other scientist. Too often, students failed to recognize that one does not *earn* a Ph.D., but rather one *becomes* a Ph.D. in some specialized area.

The paper stimulated discussion at the conference and was well received by the audience of nurse scientist students from all the universities with such grants. Since then, my ideas have sharpened but have not changed much. The demise of the Nurse Scientists grants eliminated the prevalence of the problem. I do wish we had used the term *scientist* to modify *nurse* when needed, rather than using *nurse scientist.* Scientist is the key identification. *Nurse* scientist may connote a strange or deviant scientist. Scientist is a general term appropriate for those who are scientists regardless of what they study.

ROSEMARY ELLIS

Chapter 18

The Discipline of Nursing

Sue K. Donaldson

Dorothy M. Crowley

When one considers the gamut of research that nurses are undertaking, all of it is clearly important to the nursing profession, but the knowledge represented by the research problems and methodologies appears to be global. By definition, however, a discipline is not global; it is characterized by a unique perspective, a distinct way of viewing all phenomena, which ultimately defines the limits and nature of its inquiry.

This is the problem that plagues all of us: identification of the essence of nursing research and of the common elements and threads that give coherence to an identifiable body of knowledge. As nurse researchers, we seem to function primarily with tacit rather than explicit knowledge of the broad conceptualizations unique to nursing. We take for granted the nursing perspective as generally accepted and understood, until explanation of the particulars is required. Moreover, nursing authors tend to emphasize speculative formulations and theoretical reflections aimed at deriving the nature of nursing rather than explicating the structure of the body of knowledge that constitutes the discipline of nursing.

Rather than expending a disproportionate amount of effort in the quest for *the* definition of the nature of nursing, it might behoove us—at least at this time—to seek relationships and commonalities in the ideas of writers whose work has influenced (and continues to influence) tacit knowledge of the scope of the field. At least since the time of Nightingale, there has been a remarkable consistency in the recurrent themes that nurse scholars use to explain what they conceive to be the essence or the core of nursing. Three general themes for enquiry emerge:

1. *Concern with principles and laws that govern the life processes, well-being, and optimum functioning of human beings—sick or well.* For example, a concern with the discovery of laws that govern health, knowledge of reparative processes, and prevention was manifest in the late nine-

About the Authors

SUE K. DONALDSON currently holds the Cora Miedl Siehl Chair in Nursing Research at the University of Minnesota School of Nursing, Minneapolis. She also is a Professor in the Department of Physiology, University of Minnesota School of Medicine, where she has been on the faculty since 1984. Previously, she held faculty appointments at Rush University, Chicago, and the University of Washington, Seattle.

Dr. Donaldson studied nursing at Wayne State University in Detroit, earning a B.S.N. (1965) and a M.S.N. (1966). In 1973, she received a Ph.D. in Physiology and Biophysics from the University of Washington, Seattle.

An active researcher, Dr. Donaldson communicates her findings through numerous publications and presentations at professional meetings. She comments "The central focus of my research has been and continues to be the contraction of mammalian striated muscle: excitation-contraction coupling mechanisms, intracellular modulation of tension generation, and muscle pathophysiology. Emphasis is on research at the cellular level. Ongoing studies are related to: (a) effects of acidosis and $MgATP^{2-}$ levels on Ca^{2+}-activated force generation of cardiac and skeletal fibers from adult developing mammalian muscles, and (b) mechanisms governing release of Ca^{2+} from the sarcoplasmic reticulum.

Dr. Donaldson is a member of the ANA, the Biophysical Society, the American Physiological Society, and the American Heart Association. She has served on the editorial boards of *Advances in Nursing Science* and *The American Journal of Physiology: Cell*, the Biophysical Society Council, the American Heart Association National Research Committee and Research Program and Evaluation Committee, the American Heart Association Cardiovascular Nursing Council, and the Physiology Study Section, Division of Research Grants, National Institutes of Health.

DOROTHY M. CROWLEY was born and reared in Mitchell, South Dakota and received a diploma in nursing from the Presentation School of Nursing at McKennan Hospital in Sioux Falls. She continued her education at St. Louis University, receiving a B.S. in Nursing Education (magna cum laude) in 1950. She then earned two graduate degrees at the Catholic University of America: a M.S. in Nursing Education (1953) and a Ph.D. in Sociology (1961). Her master's thesis was on nursing concepts implicit in the Rule of Saint Benedict of Nursia. At the time of her death in 1983, Dr. Crowley was on the faculty of the University of Washington, where she had been teaching since 1965.

Dorothy Crowley was a unique person whose influence long will be felt in the lives of her students, family, and friends. She was interested in the arts and humanities, enjoyed traveling, and got great satisfaction from her work as an educator. A colleague and friend, Elizabeth Worthy, comments "Dorothy was unique in that her scientific background was firmly entrenched as a result of training in the social sciences. Yet her humanity and intense interest in interpersonal interaction was also a major feature of her teaching. Her interest and research in the phenomenon of pain was a good illustration of this dual involvement. For many years, she taught a graduate course on the therapeutic nursing process, which was a revelation to most students and a source of great satisfaction for Dorothy.

Dr. Crowley also was very proud of her accomplishments in the development of nursing science. She was a major energizing force behind the development of a Ph.D. in Nursing Science at the University of Washington School of Nursing in 1977. Dorothy saw the future of nursing as epitomized in the nurse scientist who emerged from the program at the University of Washington; a person who stood tall, was anchored in a scientific discipline with skills in research and teaching, and had a deep commitment to clinical nursing.

teenth or early twentieth century in Nightingale's writings and certainly in Rogers' concern with laws principles governing life processes in the past two decades.

2. *Concern with the patterning of human behavior in interaction with the environment in critical life situations.* As evidence of this theme, Rogers' writings reflect a concern with life rhythms and their relationship to environmental rhythms. Similarly, Johnson's writings in the 1960s focused attention on systems of behavior, pattern-maintenance, and pattern-disruption. The conceptual frames for most nursing curricula today include coping processes, adaptation, and supportive and nonsupportive environments.

3. *Concern with the processes by which positive changes in health status are affected.* Peplau addressed herself to nursing as an interpersonal process, an educative and maturing force; whereas, Kreuter as well as Leininger and others addressed the particular type of process of support system seen as nursing's unique contribution.

These themes suggest boundaries of an area for systematic enquiry and theory development with potential for making the nature of the discipline of nursing more explicit than it is at present.

Integration of nursing research from the level of a conceptual framework for a particular study to the level of more general theories and ultimately to that of a unified body of nursing knowledge has not been pursued to any large extent. Nor have there been widespread efforts on the part of those doing research in nursing to relate individual studies to one another and, thereby, build a larger context for reference. This has contributed to fragmentation of knowledge and confusion about a perspective for nursing research.

As was the case in considering different ideas about the nature and themes of nursing, however, the goal is not to identify a single theory of nursing—rather, we would advocate pluralism. Nevertheless, it would seem desirable to be able to place such theories within the context of a discipline of nursing. More explicit identification of what we are doing in nursing research is imperative if we are to truly function as nurse researchers, rather than as nurses conducting research in other disciplines, and if we are to have nursing theories for the professional practice of nursing. There is also a crucial need for identification of the structure of the discipline of nursing in our educational program. How can we justify doctoral programs in nursing if the discipline of nursing is not defined? Perhaps of even greater importance is the content of these doctoral programs. In fact, the very survival of the profession may be at risk unless the discipline is defined. As Arminger noted "there exists today an unprecedented need for identification of the uniqueness of nursing science and practice, lest overriding forces in contemporary society lead to disintegration of nursing as a distinct profession" (Arminger, 1974, pp. 160–164).

What is needed is the thinking of nurse philosophers and also some philosophizing on the part of the nurse researchers. The problem is not to devise the structure of the discipline of nursing, but to make this structure explicit. Our purpose is to make a beginning along these lines. Throughout this paper, the term "nursing" will refer to the discipline, unless otherwise clarified, and "structure" will refer to the broad conceptualizations and syntax of the discipline, rather than the theories generated within this structure.

Classification of Human Knowledge: Discipline

Traditionally, human knowledge and enquiry have been considered in the context of disciplines. Disciplines reflect true distinctions between bodies of knowledge per se and, as such, become the realm of learning. The Oxford dictionary defines disciplines as "a branch of instruction or education, a department of learning or knowledge." Institutions of higher education are organized around these branches of knowledge into colleges, schools, and departments. Typically, disciplines have evolved as a consequence of a distinct perspective and syntax, which determine what phenomena or abstractions are of interest, in what context such phenomena are to be viewed, what questions are to be raised, what methods of study are to be used, and what canons of evidence and proof are to be required.

As a result of the complex way in which disciplines evolve, disciplines can be and have been identified and organized around a variety of characteristics and combinations of characteristics. Mathematics, for example, has been viewed as distinct from all other disciplines in that its subject matter appears to have no material existence; logic has been set apart because it is concerned with the development of canons of reasoning and evidence, which are utilized in the other disciplines. Thus, it is the unique relationship of logic to the other disciplines that sets it apart, rather than a peculiarity of its subject matter, as was the case for mathematics.

In identifying disciplines and classifying them, we are dealing with the nature and structure of the whole of human knowledge. It should be kept in mind that the number and membership of the disciplines are not agreed and that there is no single accepted organization of even the well accepted disciplines. This is reflected in the diversity of organization of branches of learning in universities and colleges. The broadest classifications of disciplines depend upon a view of the inherent nature of all phenomena. A distinction on the part of the philosophers between the generality of natural phenomena and the particularity of human events leads to a distinction between such sciences as physics and sociology, which seek general laws for repeating behavior, and such disciplines as history, which focuses on unique events, or ethics, which deals with human choices and value orientations (as shown in Figure 18-1). Among the sciences themselves, the biological sciences become distinct from physics and chemistry because they deal with the recognition of the phenomena of life and with living as opposed to nonliving things.

Nursing has both scientific aspects and aspects akin to the arts. For example, human health is considered within nursing in terms of political issues and history as well as in terms of inexorable laws of health. Therefore, nursing as a discipline is broader than nursing science and its uniqueness stems from its perspective rather than its object of enquiry or methodology.

You might well ask: Why bother with pursuing this discussion, especially since there is no agreement as to a single structure of human knowledge? There are at least two reasons: First, the discipline of nursing was not created per se solum, but emerged within the context of the other disciplines. Therefore, we must know its relationship to other disciplines in addition to its structure. Secondly, it must be remembered that the family of disciplines, because each of its members represents knowledge derived within a particular conceptual structure, is subject to revision in the form of fusion, extinction, and multiplication of its members as new conceptualizations emerge. Nursing as a discipline is also subject to change based upon changes in its structural conceptual base; in fact, nurse researchers and scholars have the responsibility of questioning and revising nursing's structure.

According to Shermis (1962), the accepted academic disciplines are all characterized by an impressive body of enduring works, suitable techniques, concerns which are significant and relevant to humans, unifying and inspiring traditions, and considerable scholarly achievements. Although these are not criteria for distinguishing disciplines from nondisciplines, they do provide a basis for acceptance of a branch of learning as a discipline.

But what of emerging disciplines? In the professional field, there typically is an evolutionary process that occurs as the field moves from a vocational level, in which the art and technology are preeminent, to the rationalization of practice and the establishment of a cognitive base for professional practice. It is important to recognize that a discipline emerges as a result of

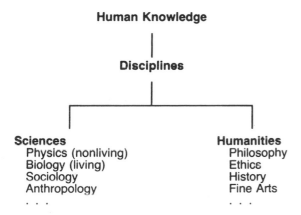

Human Knowledge

Disciplines

Sciences
Physics (nonliving)
Biology (living)
Sociology
Anthropology
. . .

Humanities
Philosophy
Ethics
History
Fine Arts
. . .

Figure 18-1   *Structuring of Human Knowledge*

creative thinking related to significant issues. Because of the vital significance of nursing's perspective, its concern with human health and well-being, and its growth through research and scholarly work, nursing will gain full acceptance in time.

For purposes of this discussion, a distinction between academic disciplines and professional disciplines will be utilized (as illustrated in Figure 18-2). The academic disciplines include sciences such as physics, physiology, and sociology, as well as liberal arts disciplines such as mathematics, history, and philosophy. The aim of academic disciplines is to know, and their theories are descriptive in nature. In contrast, professional disciplines such as law, medicine, and nursing are directed toward practical aims and thus generate prescriptive as well as descriptive theories.

For academic disciplines, the goal is to know, regardless of whether the research is basic or applied. In fact, the distinction between applied and basic research seems appropriate only in relation to descriptive theories, since applied research answers questions related to the applicability of basic theories in practical situations, rather than questions related to *how* basic theories are to be applied. Thus, applied physicists test the practical limits of theories of physics but would not derive information as to the best design for a bridge, for example.

Fields that emphasize applied research would be more correctly termed applied disciplines, or applied branches of academic disciplines, rather than professional disciplines, which have prescriptive theories in addition to descriptive ones. The prescriptive theories characteristic of professional disciplines deal with the actual implementation of knowledge in a practical sense. As Johnson has stated ". . .professional knowledge does not consist of basic science theory which has been validated in practice" (Johnson, 1974, p. 373). In this regard, it is not correct to view professional disciplines simply as applied sciences.

Within the professional discipline there is a need "to know" and to work from descriptive theories in addition to prescriptive ones. As Gortner has pointed out, "some of the work is basic, in that it is applicable to a general understanding of human behavior or responses to illness" (Gortner, 1974, p. 765), and other studies of nursing are applied. Basic and applied research are both needed in a professional discipline because each discipline has a different practical aim which influences the perspective of that field, the way it conceptualizes the relevant world, and the questions it poses for investigation. Therefore, because of the uniqueness of each discipline's perspective and the context in which knowledge from each discipline fits, it is not possible to simply "borrow" theory or knowledge from other disciplines.

Schwab (1964a) has noted that in general the state-

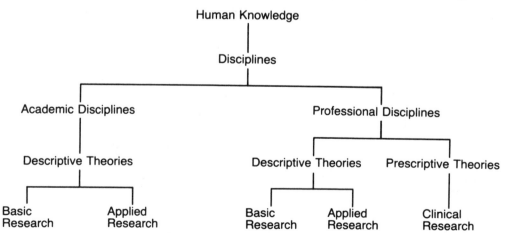

Figure 18-2 *Theories and Research Characteristics of Academic and Professional Disciplines*

ments of a given discipline are like single words of a sentence; their meanings derive more from their context than from their dictionary sense. In other words, statements of disciplines, their conclusions, are properly understood only in the context of the enquiry that produced them. They are true only in that they fit the criteria for truth in the given discipline. From this standpoint, nurse scientists may help in utilization of information from other disciplines, but this will not eliminate the need for undertaking basic research in nursing from nursing's perspective. Viewing phenomena from the perspective of healthy function of individuals in interaction with their environments will generate distinctive research at all levels and a defined, structured body of knowledge.

Even when useful information might be derived from the research of another discipline, the studies are not pursued, either because of lack of interest or because the conditions used invalidate the results for nursing's purpose. For example, a physiologist studying mechanisms underlying a given cellular process may work with intact cells but at a very low temperature, say 0°C, to slow the process down to allow measurement of its kinetic properties. The low temperature does not invalidate the physiologist's conclusions, but may make the data inappropriate in terms of knowing exact rates characteristic of the process at in vivo temperatures. Furthermore, animal and suborganismal, even subcellular, research is valid in its own right in physiology, whereas in nursing the information is ultimately being sought in relation to intact human beings.

Nursing cannot rely upon the academic disciplines to supply its requirement for knowledge of laws and processes. Rather, appropriately prepared nurse researchers must generate and test descriptive theories as necessary and develop their own technology, as has been recommended for other professionals.

Another very important issue is the extent to which each discipline is dependent upon the development of the others. The Comtian view of the sciences, which is a hierarchical one, is noteworthy in this regard, since it has influenced curricula; in turn, these curricula can lead to unwarranted views of the dependence of some disciplines on the others.

Comte held that not only human knowledge in general but also each branch of knowledge passes through states or stages of progress on its way to becoming scientific. He also conceived of the branches of knowledge as evolving in an increasingly complex organizational hierarchy ranging from the physical to the social. As a result of an arbitrary interpretation of Comte's hierarchy in curricula, physics and chemistry have been required, for example, for the mastery of biology, and so on. Although there may be increased efficiency of instruction following this plan, it should be remembered that learners influenced by such curricula may come to view all knowledge as hierarchical. Yet, hierarchical nature of knowledge has not been demonstrated; in fact acceptance of hierarchical structuring of knowledge can be very limiting and should be questioned.

In the first place, there is the danger that one conceive all knowledge of scientific quality as being encompassed by the academic disciplines, with the professions resting on these disciplines for their cognitive base. Secondly, if even the potential for professional disciplines is conceded, it is difficult for proponents of the hierarchical view to envision how professional disciplines could expand their respective bodies of knowledge independently. In contrast, professional disciplines can be viewed as emerging *along with* rather than *from* academic disciplines.

This is not to imply that disciplines are totally independent of each other. Certainly, logical formulations in one discipline cannot ignore the "truths" of the others. The quality of theories and research designs and the validity of conclusions drawn within one discipline are dependent upon their congruence with all of knowledge. Therefore, knowledge in one discipline may set constraints on or enhance the process of enquiry in another. Perhaps the most obvious interrelationship of disciplines is in their associated practice realm.

Every discipline exists in part to provide knowledge which is to be utilized and thus has an associated practice realm has (Figure 18-3). Accordingly, every

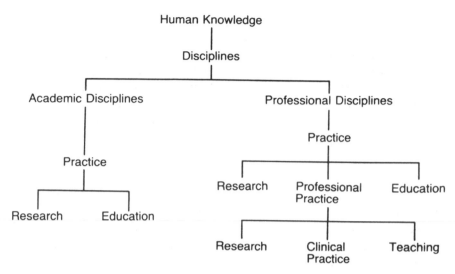

Human Knowledge
|
Disciplines

Academic Disciplines   Professional Disciplines

                                                Practice

                                Research   Professional   Education
                                           Practice

                                    Research   Clinical   Teaching
                                               Practice

                Practice

        Research   Education

Figure 18-3   *Practice Realms of Disciplines*

discipline has educators and researchers who function in this realm to impart the knowledge base to others and expand the knowledge base through research. In addition, professional disciplines have practitioners who deliver a service by engaging in professional practice in the form of clinical service, education, and research.

Sharing of knowledge from many disciplines occurs in the realm of practice associated with each discipline. For example, researchers affiliated with academic disciplines may borrow relevance or reality orientation from observations of professional practitioners and use prescriptive or practice theories from professional disciplines and practice. Similarly, professional disciplines derive knowledge from academic disciplines.

Relationship of the Discipline to Practice

Although the discipline and the profession are inextricably linked and greatly influence each other's substance, they must be distinguished from each other. Failure to recognize the existence of the discipline as a body of knowledge that is separate from the activities of

practitioners has contributed to the fact that nursing has been viewed as a vocation rather than a profession. In turn, this has led to confusion as to whether the discipline of nursing exists.

Part of the problem in viewing a professional discipline as distinct from professional practice stems from the fact that both the discipline and practice evolved interdependently in response to societal needs; as a result, both possess a common practical aim related to these needs (Figure 18-4). Professions evolved because the service they provided was valued. Given the emphasis placed upon science and rationality in the postindustrial age, it is not surprising that there was a strong impetus for establishing a scientific and theoretical base for professional practice. The process of upgrading professional practice also entailed the establishment of closer relations between knowledge serving as the basis of professional practice and knowledge in the academic disciplines. Since the university traditionally has been the locus of development of theoretical knowledge, the professional disciplines were eventually housed there along with the academic disciplines.

The location of professional disciplines such as nursing in institutions such as universities, which are primarily concerned with human knowledge as a prod-

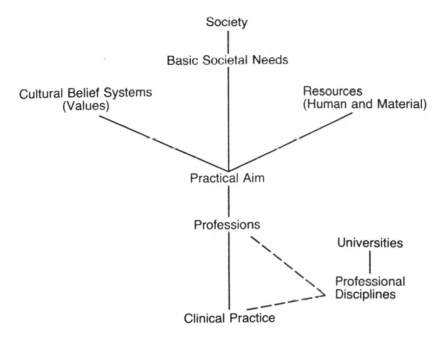

Figure 18-4 *Interdependent Evolution of Discipline and Practice of a Profession*

uct rather than service, does not change the accountability of these disciplines for societal needs and the practical aim of their associated professions. As Johnson has noted, the decisions of what to study and what questions to ask necessarily have stemmed from social decisions about the profession's realm of responsibility in giving services or in clinical practice.

Florence Nightingale (1860) defined the discipline in terms of the responsibility of nursing's practitioners to promote human health based on systematic enquiry into nature's "laws of health." Part of the reason for nursing's struggle in evolving stems from the slow emergence of the recognition of its social relevance. Nurses give service related to the quality of human life; this service is only recently being valued. After all, why should quality of life be considered before biological survival can be assured?

Ethical and moral values inherent in clinical practice have profoundly influenced the perspective and value orientation of the discipline. Thus, nursing has traditionally valued humanitarian service. But in addition, the self-respect and self-determination of clients

are to be preserved. The goal of nursing service is to foster self-caring behavior that leads to individual health and well-being. These values and goals, which are intrinsic to professional practice, have shaped the value orientation of the discipline. As a result of this value orientation, knowledge of the basis of human choices and of methods for fostering individual independence are sought, rather than knowledge of interventions that control and directly manipulate the person per se into a societally determined state of health.

The clinical practice of nursing requires the development of prescriptive theories on the part of the discipline. Much of the early research related to the nursing profession consisted of investigations about nurses, their characteristics and behavior, but these investigations could not actually be considered nursing research. In recent years, the amount of research concerned with theories fundamental to clinical practice has increased.

A key point, however, is that the discipline of nursing should be *governing* clinical practice rather than being defined by it. Of necessity, clinical practice focuses on the individual in the here and now who has a problem requiring relevant and appropriate action. The discipline, in contrast, embodies a knowledge base relevant to all realms of professional practice and which links the past, present and future. Its scope goes far beyond that required for current clinical practice. If the discipline were so narrowly defined, professional nursing could be limited to functioning in the realm of disaster relief rather than serving as a force in the promotion of world health. This is not meant to diminish the importance of problems encountered by nurses in current clinical practice. These problems deserve attention, but they are not the only concern of the discipline.

Part of the problem is that "clinical practice" is too often used synonymously with "professional practice," and clinical practice is narrowly defined. Professional competency goes beyond that required for delivery of health care to individuals, preparation of future practitioners, and conduct of systematic enquiry. For example, McGlothlin (1960) believes that competency includes the need on the part of professionals for social understanding of sufficient breadth to place the practice in the context of society and the need for leadership skills.

Some of the knowledge required for achieving these competencies can only come from the discipline of nursing. Prescriptive theories essential to clinical practice and the appropriate design of nursing research can only be derived from the discipline of nursing. Similarly, although knowledge from political science, history, philosophy, and other disciplines is very important for social understanding, the professional nurse cannot put nursing into a societal context without knowledge derived from the discipline of nursing. This knowledge is obtained in part from nurse philosophers and nurse historians who view nursing as it relates to other disciplines and can articulate how nursing's heritage relates to its perspective. The discipline of nursing must also provide essential components of the knowledge base for preparation of world leaders in the field of health.

The need for philosophical, historical, and similar types of enquiry within the discipline of nursing is crucial not only in terms of providing the knowledge base for professional preparation but also for the development of the discipline. It must be remembered that the discipline is defined by social relevance and value orientations rather than by empirical truths. Thus, the discipline and profession must be continually reevaluated in terms of societal needs and scientific discoveries. Similarly, the entire structure of the discipline may need to be revamped in time, and this should be done by nurse researchers.

For this reason we have been very careful not to equate the discipline of nursing with the science of nursing. As mentioned earlier, only part of nursing employs scientific method. We need doctoral preparation for nurse historians as well as nurse scientists. As Schlotfeldt has pointed out "nursing faculties rarely have among their members scholars who are concerned with establishing the history of nursing science and with identifying the philosophies or conceptualizations of nursing that have influenced the structure of that knowledge at various times in nursing's history" (Schlotfeldt, 1977, p. 8). Once again, the purpose in having nurse philosophers and historians is not to duplicate the efforts of other disciplines, but rather to provide these approaches from the perspective of nursing.

It should be remembered that although nursing requires researchers and scholars who utilize a variety of approaches, all research that is important to the profession of nursing is not derived from the discipline of nursing. Only information and theories stemming from nursing's perspective come from nursing per se. Nursing educators utilize information and theories from education. Even clinical practice should not be viewed as being grounded solely in the discipline of nursing.

In delivering health care, practitioners must in fact draw from many disciplines, such as business administration, medicine, education, and basic sciences. Rarely, if ever, does the skilled clinician rely only on knowledge from one discipline or even rely solely on scientific knowledge. Clinical practice is always to some extent empirical, pragmatic, intuitive, and artistic.

Once we agree that the discipline of nursing does

not have to embody all, the entire whole, of knowledge utilized by the profession of nursing, then we can begin to define the discipline. Nursing is not global in its subject matter and therefore does not subsume part of any other disciplines—for example, education—just because practitioners are educated. Similarly, studies of higher education in nursing that deal with the educational process are not nursing research but educational research. In contrast, a study of the effects of educational techniques on clients' achievement of self-care is within nursing per se. Even though nursing care delivery is greatly affected by attitudes of nurses administration policies, such problems may be studied appropriately in other disciplines.

The purpose in excluding some research from nursing is not to create a ranking of importance or prestige, but rather to make the essence of nursing explicit. Nurses who conduct administrative or educational research may contribute as much to the professional practice of nursing as nurses who conduct nursing research.

In summary, the discipline and clinical practice of nursing share a common social relevance and practical aim. However, the discipline, which is a body of knowl edge, must not be confused with its associated practice realm, which embodies the processes of conducting research, giving service, and educating. Furthermore,

some members of the profession must engage in enquiry that is not immediately applicable to current clinical practice. As a branch of knowledge, the discipline embodies more than the science of nursing and requires researchers who employ a variety of approaches from nursing's perspective. Although the discipline provides crucial and unique content for nurse researchers, clinicians, and educators, these practitioners draw on many disciplines. Appropriately prepared nurses may elect to conduct research within other disciplines because of the critical importance of this non-nursing research to professional practice or the growth of the discipline.

Structure of the Discipline of Nursing

We are now at the point of examining the structure of the discipline. According to Schwab (1964a), disciplines have both substantive and syntactical structures. The substantive structure is composed of conceptualizations which are borrowed or invented, but their inclusion is always based on their fit with the perspective of the discipline. The syntax of a discipline refers to the research methodologies and criteria used to justify the acceptance of statements as true within the discipline (see Figure 18-5).

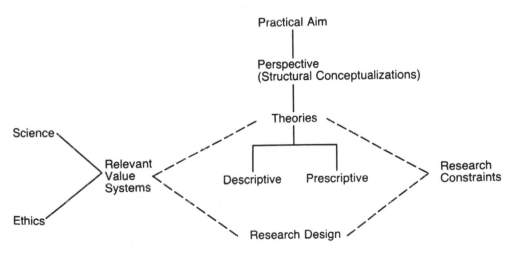

Figure 18-5 *Structure of a Professional Discipline*

We have incorporated the syntax of nursing as value systems (both of science and of professional ethics) and research constraints. Such constraints include consideration of accessibility of controls, congruity with existing knowledge, manifest and latent consequences, and technological feasibility. Both values and constraints influence theory generation and actual research design. In effect, they function to ensure that enquiry will result in conclusions and statements that are appropriate, reliable, and valid for the purpose of the discipline.

Thus, the substantive structure determines primarily the scope and subject of enquiry (what is of interest), and the syntactical structure determines primarily the procedure for conducting research and criteria for acceptability of findings as truth. The findings generated by enquiry are then incorporated into the structure as concepts, theories, and facts—the statements of the discipline. In this paper, we have focused upon the structural conceptualizations, but it should be remembered that the syntax of the discipline is also important, since the syntax determines the extent to which the truth of statements of the discipline is warranted. In contrast, the substantive structure relates to the subject matter of the enquiry. The structural conceptualizations are selected for inclusion in a given discipline with its perspective as a screen.

From its perspective, nursing studies the wholeness or health of humans, recognizing that humans are in continuous interaction with their environments. Nursing's perspective evolves from the practical aim of optimizing of human environments for health. Examples of major conceptualizations in nursing deal with:

1. Distinctions between human and nonhuman beings
2. Distinctions between living and nonliving
3. Nature of environments and humans-environmental interactions from cellular to societal levels
4. Illness versus health and well-being
5. Functioning of the whole human organism versus functioning of the parts
6. Levels of functioning of whole organisms
7. Human characteristics and natural processes, such as consciousness; abstraction; adaptation and healing; growth; change; self-determination; development; aging; dying; reproducing; drive satisfaction; and relating.

The structural conceptions are being utilized, but they are usually not identified or clarified, and rarely questioned. It is important, for example, to know whether health is viewed, in the context of a given theory or design, as a specific state, or as it is defined by each individual.

Depending upon the particular structural conceptualizations utilized, or combinations of them, widely different theories are proposed for testing. Such variation in theories does not lead to different bodies of knowledge, but to different aspects of a single body.

Pluralism of theories promotes productivity; in fact, without testing of a wide variety of theories, progress towards "truth" cannot be made. In physiology, for example, where knowledge of the functions and nature of vital processes of living organisms is sought, a pluralism of theories exists. Many physiologists conceive the functioning of the organism as explainable in terms of the functioning of its parts, whereas others propose an explanation utilizing a conception that the whole is more than the sum of its parts. This dual approach is very useful, regardless of the correctness of the theories, since testable theories are generated that yield empirical evidence related to knowledge of the nature of and mechanisms underlying behavior of living systems. The goal in generating theories is not just to propose an all encompassing theory but to provide testable theories.

Research designed to test hypotheses stemming from theories is very important to the discipline and practitioners when the relationship of nursing theories to the structure of the discipline is explicit. This is the type of research that is easily identified as nursing research. Schwab (1964b) calls this stable enquiry, in that there is no hesitation about what questions to ask or what structural conceptualizations to employ. For example, if the current principles of physiology are organ and function, the researcher engaged in stable enquiry discovers the function of one organ after another.

This type of stable research tends to be the most rewarded, but there is another very important realm of enquiry which must be expanded. We refer to questions relating to the structural conceptualizations and value orientations of the discipline. For example, what is the nature of health? Is health on a continuum with illness? Is health for every person a reasonable goal for society?

At least two major benefits are derived from this second type of research. First the structural conceptual izations are clarified or altered to make them consistent with reality. They should not be accepted as givens. Secondly, the discipline will be continually shaped according to significant themes, those which are of vital significance to man. If nurse researchers are to provide the knowledge base for societal directions in relation to health, they must engage in this type of research.

For the continued growth, significance, and utility of the discipline of nursing, researchers must place their research within the context of the discipline. Theories must also be viewed in terms of the basic structural conceptualizations of the discipline. The responsibility for revising and clarifying the structural conceptions, the very framework, of the discipline of nursing rests with nurse researchers. This means lessening our preoccupation with the process of nursing and pedagogy and placing emphasis on content as substance.

References

Armiger, B. (1974). Scholarship in nursing. *Nursing Outlook, 22,* 160–164.

Gortner, S.R. (1974). Scientific accountability in nursing. *Nursing Outlook, 22,* 764–768.

Johnson, D.E. (1974). Development of theory: A requisite for nursing as a primary health profession. *Nursing Research, 23,* 372–377.

McGlothlin, W.J. (1960). *Patterns of professional education.* New York: G.P. Putnam's Sons.

Nightingale, F. (1860). *Notes on nursing: What it is and what it is not.* London: Harrison.

Schlotfeldt, R.M. (1977). Nursing research: Reflection of values. *Nursing Research, 26,* 4–9.

Schwab, J. (1964a). Structure of the disciplines: Meanings and significances. In G.W. Ford & L. Pugno (Eds.), *The structure of knowledge and the curriculum.* Chicago: Rand McNally.

Schwab, J. (1964b). The structure of the natural sciences. In G. W. Ford & L. Pugno (Eds.), *The structure of knowledge and the curriculum.* Chicago: Rand McNally.

Shermis, S. (1962). On becoming an intellectual discipline. *Phi Delta Kappan, 44,* 84–86.

Bibliography

Argyris, C., & Schon, D.A. (1974). *Theory in practice: Increasing professional effectiveness.* San Francisco: Jossey-Bass.

Davies, J.T. (1965). *The scientific approach.* New York: Academic Press.

Gortner, S.R., & Nahm, H. (1977). An overview of nursing research in the United States. *Nursing Research, 26,* 10–33.

Greenwood, E. (1969). The practice of science and the science of practice. In W.G. Bennis, et al. (Eds.), *The planning of change* (2nd ed.). New York: Holt, Rhinehart and Winston.

Haldane, J.S. (1929). *The sciences and philosophy.* Garden City, N.Y.: Doubleday, Doran.

Henderson, V. (1964). The nature of nursing. *American Journal of Nursing, 64,* 62–68.

Hyde, A. (1975). The phenomenon of caring. *Nursing Research Report, 10,* 2–3ff.

Johnson, D.E. (1961). The significance of nursing care. *American Journal of Nursing, 61,* 63–66.

Kreuter, F.R. (1957). What is good nursing care? *Nursing Outlook, 5,* 302–304.

Leininger, M. (1977). The phenomenon of caring: Part 5. Caring: the essence and central focus of nursing. *Nursing Research Report, 12,* 2.

Merton, R., & Lerner, D. (1969). Social scientists and research policy. In W.G. Bennis, et al. (Eds.), *The planning of change* (2nd ed.). New York: Holt, Rhinehart and Winston.

Parsons, T. & Platt, G.M. (1973). *The American university.* Cambridge, MA: Harvard University Press.

Peplau, H.E. (1952). *Interpersonal relations in nursing: A conceptual frame of reference for psychodynamic nursing.* New York: G.P. Putnam's Sons.

Rogers, M.E. (1970). *Introduction to the theoretical basis of nursing.* Philadelphia: F.A. Davis.

Chapter 19

Fundamental Patterns of Knowing in Nursing

Barbara A. Carper

It is the general conception of any field of inquiry that ultimately determines the kind of knowledge the field aims to develop as well as the manner in which that knowledge is to be organized, tested and applied. The body of knowledge that serves as the rationale for nursing practice has patterns, forms and structure that serve as horizons of expectations and exemplify characteristic ways of thinking about phenomena. Understanding these patterns is essential for the teaching and learning of nursing. Such an understanding does not extend the range of knowledge, but rather involves critical attention to the question of what it means to know and what kinds of knowledge are held to be of most value in the discipline of nursing.

Identifying Patterns of Knowing

Four fundamental patterns of knowing have been identified from an analysis of the conceptual and syntactical structure of nursing knowledge (Carper, 1975). The four patterns are distinguished according to logical type of meaning and designated as: (a) empirics, the science of nursing; (b) aesthetics, the art of nursing; (c) the component of a personal knowledge in nursing; and (d) ethics, the component of moral knowledge in nursing.

Empirics: The Science of Nursing

The term *nursing science* was rarely used in the literature until the late 1950s. However, since that time there has been an increasing emphasis—one might even say a sense of urgency—regarding the development of a body of empirical knowledge specific to nursing. There seems to be general agreement that there is a critical need for knowledge about the empirical world, knowledge that is systematically organized into general laws and theories for the purpose of describing, explaining and predicting phenomena of special concern to the discipline of nursing. Most theory development

From Advances in Nursing Science, *October 1978, 1(1), 13–23. Copyright © 1978 Aspen Systems Corporation. Reprinted with permission from Aspen Systems Corporation.*

About the Author

BARBARA A. CARPER is currently Undergraduate Program Coordinator at the College of Nursing, University of North Carolina at Charlotte. A baccalaureate graduate of Texas Woman's University, Dr. Carper received a M.Ed and an Ed.D. from Columbia University Teacher's College. She also earned a Clinical Certification in Anesthesia from the University of Michigan in 1962.

Dr. Carper has taught nursing on both the graduate and undergraduate levels, with special emphasis on medical-surgical nursing, ethics, and theory development. She spent 1981 through 1982 at Harvard University as a Visiting Scholar in Medical Ethics.

A fellow in the American Academy of Nursing, Dr. Carper is also active in the American Nurses' Association and Sigma Theta Tau and is an elected member of the Nursing Theory Think Tank. Besides her numerous other professional activities, Dr. Carper finds time to review manuscripts as a member of the editorial board of *Advances in Nursing Science*.

and research efforts are primarily engaged in seeking and generating explanations which are systematic and controllable by factual evidence and which can be used in the organization and classification of knowledge.

The pattern of knowing which is generally designated as "nursing science" does not presently exhibit the same degree of highly integrated abstract and systematic explanations characteristic of the more mature sciences, although nursing literature reflects this as an ideal form. Clearly there are a number of coexisting, and in a few instances competing, conceptual structures—none of which has achieved the status of what Kuhn (1962) calls a scientific paradigm. That is, no single conceptual structure is as yet generally accepted as an example of actual scientific practice "which include[s] law, theory, application, and instrumentation together . . . [and] . . . provide[s] models from which spring particular coherent traditions of scientific research" (Kuhn, 1962, p. 10). It could be argued that some of these conceptual structures seem to have greater potential than others for providing explanations that systematically account for observed phenomena and may ultimately permit more accurate prediction and control of them. However, this is a matter to be determined by research designed to test the validity of such explanatory concepts in the context of relevant empirical reality.

New Perspectives

What seems to be a paramount importance, at least at this stage in the development of nursing science, is that these preparadigm conceptual structures and theoretical models present new perspectives for considering the familiar phenomena of health and illness in relation to the human life process; as such they can and should be legitimately counted as discoveries in the discipline. The representation of health as more than the absence of disease is a crucial change; it permits health to be thought of as a dynamic state or process which changes over a given period of time and varies according to circumstances rather than a static either/or entity. The conceptual change in turn makes it possible to raise questions that previously would have been literally unintelligible.

The discovery that one can usefully conceptualize health as something that normally ranges along a continuum has led to attempts to observe, describe and classify variations in health, or levels of wellness, as expressions of a human being's relationship to the internal and external environments. Related research has sought to identify behavioral responses, both physiological and psychological, that may serve as cues by which one can infer the range of normal variations of health. It has also attempted to identify and categorize significant etiological factors which serve to promote or inhibit changes in health status.

Current Stages

The science of nursing at present exhibits aspects of both the "natural history stage of inquiry" and the "stage of deductively formulated theory." The task of the natural history stage is primarily the description and classification of phenomena which are, generally speaking, ascertainable by direct observation and inspection (Northrop, 1959). But current nursing literature clearly reflects a shift from this descriptive and classification form to increasingly theoretical analysis which is directed toward seeking, or inventing, explanations to account for observed and classified empirical facts. This shift is reflected in the change from a largely observational vocabulary to a new, more theoretical vocabulary whose terms have a distinct meaning and definition only in the context of the corresponding explanatory theory.

Explanations in the several open-system conceptual models tend to take the form commonly labeled functional or teleological (Nagel, 1961). For example, the system models explain a person's level of wellness at any particular point in time as a function of current and accumulated effects of interactions with his or her internal and external environments. The concept of adaptation is central to this type of explanation. Adaptation is seen as crucial in the process of responding to environmental demands (usually classified as stressors), and enables an individual to maintain or reestablish the steady state which is designated as the goal of the system. The developmental models often exhibit a more genetic type of explanation in that certain events, the developmental tasks, are believed to be casually relevant or necessary conditions for the normal development of an individual. Thus, the first fundamental pattern of knowing in nursing is empirical, factual, descriptive and ultimately aimed at developing abstract and theoretical explanations. It is exemplary, discursively formulated and publicly verifiable.

Aesthetics: The Art of Nursing

Few, if indeed any, familiar with the professional literature would deny that primary emphasis is placed on the development of the science of nursing. One is almost led to believe that the only valid and reliable knowledge is that which is empirical, factual, objectively descriptive and generalizable. There seems to be a self-conscious reluctance to extend the term knowledge to include those aspects of knowing in nursing that are not the result of empirical investigation. There is, nonetheless, what might be described as a tacit admission that nursing is, at least in part, an art. Not much effort is made to elaborate or to make explicit this aesthetic pattern of knowing in nursing—other than to vaguely associate the "art" with the general category of manual and/or technical skills involved in nursing practice.

Perhaps this reluctance to acknowledge the aesthetic component as a fundamental pattern of knowing in nursing originates in the vigorous efforts made in the not-so-distant past to exorcise the image of the apprentice-type educational system. Within the apprentice system, the art of nursing was closely associated with an imitative learning style and the acquisition of knowledge by accumulation of unrationalized experiences. Another likely source of reluctance is that the definition of the term art has been excessively and inappropriately restricted.

Weitz (1960) suggests that art is too complex and variable to be reduced to a single definition. To conceive the task of aesthetic theory as definition, he says, is logically doomed to failure in that what is called art has not common properties—only recognizable similarities. This fluid and open approach to the understanding and application of the concept of art and aesthetic meaning makes possible a wider consideration of conditions, situations and experiences in nursing that may properly be called aesthetic, including the creative process of discovery in the empirical pattern of knowing.

Aesthetics Versus Scientific Meaning

Despite this open texture of the concept of art, aesthetic meanings can be distinguished from those in science in several important aspects. The recognition "that art is expressive rather than merely formal or descriptive," according to Rader, "is about as well established as any fact in the whole field of aesthetics" (Rader, 1960, p. xvi). An aesthetic experience involves the creation and/or appreciation of a singular, particular, subjective expression of imagined possibilities or equivalent realities which "resists projection into the discursive form of language" (Langer, 1957). Knowledge gained by empirical description is discursively formulated and publicly verifiable. The knowledge gained by subjective acquaintance, the direct feeling of experience, defines discursive formulation. Although an aesthetic expression requires abstraction, it remains specific and unique rather than exemplary and leads us to acknowledge that "knowledge—genuine knowledge, understanding—is considerably wider than our discourse" (Langer, 1957, p. 23).

For Wiedenbach (1964), the art of nursing is made visible through the action taken to provide whatever the patient requires to restore or extend his ability to cope with the demands of his situation. But the action taken, to have an aesthetic quality, requires the active transformation of the immediate object—the patient's behavior—into a direct, nonmediated perception of what is significant in it—that is, what need is actually being expressed by the behavior. This perception of the need expressed is not only responsible for the action taken by the nurse but reflected in it.

The aesthetic process described by Wiedenbach resembles what Dewey (1958) refers to as the difference between recognition and perception. According to Dewey, recognition serves the purpose of identification and is satisfied when a name tag or label is attached according to some stereotype or previously formed scheme of classification. Perception, however, goes beyond recognition in that it includes an active gathering together of details and scattered particulars into an experienced whole for the purpose of seeing what is there. It is perception rather than mere recognition that results in a unity of ends and means which gives the action taken an aesthetic quality.

Orem speaks of the art of nursing as being "ex-

pressed by the individual nurse through her creativity and style in designing and providing nursing that is effective and satisfying" (Orem, 1971, p. 155). The art of nursing is creative in that it requires development of the ability to "envision valid modes of helping in relation to 'results' which are appropriate" (Orem, 1971, p. 69). This again invokes Dewey's (1958) sense of a perceived unity between an action taken and its result—a perception of the means and the end as an organic whole. The experience of helping must be perceived and designed as an integral component of its desired result rather than conceived separately as an independent action imposed on an independent subject. Perhaps this is what is meant by the concept of nursing the whole patient or total patient care. If so, what are the qualities that enable the creation of a design for nursing care that eliminate or would minimize the fragmentation of means and ends?

Aesthetic Pattern of Knowing

Empathy—that is, the capacity for participating in or vicariously experiencing another's feelings—is an important mode in the aesthetic pattern of knowing. One gains knowledge of another person's singular, particular, felt experience through empathic acquaintance (Lee, 1960; Lippo, 1960). Empathy is controlled or moderated by psychic distance or detachment in order to apprehend and abstract what we are attending to, and in this sense is objective. The more skilled the nurse becomes in perceiving and empathizing with the lives of others, the more knowledge or understanding will be gained of alternate modes of perceiving reality. The nurse will thereby have available a larger repertoire of choices in designing and providing nursing care that is effective and satisfying. At the same time, increased awareness of the variety of subjective experiences will heighten the complexity and difficulty of the decision making involved.

The design of nursing care must be accompanied by what Langer refers to as sense of form, the sense of "structure, articulation, a whole resulting from the relation of mutually dependent factors, or more precisely, the way the whole is put together" (Langer, 1957, p.

16). The design, if it is to be aesthetic, must be controlled by the perception of the balance, rhythm, proportion and unity of what is done in relation to the dynamic integration and articulation of the whole. "The doing may be energetic, and the undergoing may be acute and intense," Dewey (1958) says, but "unless they are related to each other to form a whole," what is done becomes merely a matter of mechanical routine or of caprice.

The aesthetic pattern of knowing in nursing involves the perception of abstracted particulars as distinguished from the recognition of abstracted universals. It is the knowing of a unique particular rather than an exemplary class.

The Component of Personal Knowledge

Personal knowledge as a fundamental pattern of knowing in nursing is the most problematic, the most difficult to master and to teach. At the same time, it is perhaps the pattern most essential to understanding the meaning of health in terms of individual well-being. Nursing considered as an interpersonal process involves interactions, relationships and transactions between the nurse and the patient-client. Mitchell points out that "there is growing evidence that the quality of interpersonal contacts has an influence on a person's becoming ill, coping with illness and becoming well" (Mitchell, 1973, p. 49–50). Certainly the phrase "therapeutic use of self" which has become increasingly prominent in the literature implies that the way in which nurses view their own selves and the client is of primary concern in any therapeutic relationship.

Personal knowledge is concerned with the knowing, encountering and actualizing of the concrete, individual self. One does not know *about* the self; one strives simply to *know* the self. This knowing is a standing in relation to another human being and confronting that human being as a person. This "I-Thou" encounter is unmediated by conceptual categories or particulars abstracted from complex organic wholes (Buber, 1970). The relation is one of reciprocity, a state of being that cannot be described or even experienced—it can only

be actualized. Such personal knowing extends not only to other selves but also to relations with one's own self.

It requires what Buber (1970) refers to as the sacrifice of form—i.e., categories or classifications—for a knowing of infinite possibilities, as well as the risk of total commitment.

> Even as a melody is not composed of tones, nor a verse of words, nor a statue of lines—one must pull and tear to turn a unity into a multiplicity—so it is with the human being to whom I say You. . . . I have to do this again and again; but immediately he is no longer You. (Buber, 1970, p. 59)

Maslow (1956) refers to this sacrifice of form as embodying a more efficient perception of reality in that reality is not generalized nor predetermined by a complex of concepts, expectations, beliefs and stereotypes. This results in a greater willingness to accept ambiguity, vagueness and discrepancy of oneself and others. The risk of commitment involved in personal knowledge is what Polanyi calls the "passionate participation in the act of knowing" (Polyani, 1964, p. 17).

The nurse in the therapeutic use of self rejects approaching the patient-client as an object and strives instead to actualize an authentic personal relationship between two persons. The individual is considered as an integrated, open system incorporating movement toward growth and fulfillment of human potential. An authentic personal relation requires the acceptance of others in their freedom to create themselves and the recognition that each person is not a fixed entity, but constantly engaged in the process of becoming. How then should the nurse reconcile this with the social and/or professional responsibility to control and manipulate the environmental variables and even the behavior of the person who is a patient in order to maintain or restore a steady state? If a human being is assumed to be free to choose and chooses behavior outside of accepted norms, how will this affect the action taken in the therapeutic use of self by the nurse? What choices must the nurse make in order to know another self in an authentic relation apart from the category of patient, even when categorizing for the purpose of treatment is essential to the process of nursing?

Assumptions regarding human nature, McKay observes, "range from the existentialist to the cybernetic, from the idea of an information processing machine to one of a many splendored being" (McKay, 1969, p. 399). Many of these assumptions incorporate in one form or another the notion that there is, for all individuals, a characteristic state which they, by virtue of membership in the species, must strive to assume or achieve. Empirical descriptions and classifications reflect the assumption that being human allows for prediction of basic biological, psychological and social behaviors that will be encountered in any given individual.

Certainly empirical knowledge is essential to the purposes of nursing. But nursing also requires that we be alert to the fact that models of human nature and their abstract and generalized categories refer to and describe behaviors and traits that groups have in common. However, none of these categories can ever encompass or express the uniqueness of the individual encountered as a person, as a "self." These and many other similar considerations are involved in the realm of personal knowledge, which can be broadly characterized as subjective, concrete and existential. It is concerned with the kind of knowing that promotes wholeness and integrity in the personal encounter, the achievement of engagement rather than detachment; and it denies the manipulative, impersonal orientation.

Ethics: The Moral Component

Teachers and individual practitioners are becoming increasingly sensitive to the difficult personal choices that must be made within the complex context of modern health care. These choices raise fundamental questions about morally right and wrong action in connection with the care and treatment of illness and the promotion of health. Moral dilemmas arise in situations of ambiguity and uncertainty, when the consequences of one's actions are difficult to predict and traditional principles and ethical codes offer no help or seem to result in contradiction. The moral code which guides the ethical conduct of nurses is based on the primary principle of obligation embodied in the concepts of service to

people and respect for human life. The discipline of nursing is held to be a valuable and essential social service responsible for conserving life, alleviating suffering and promoting health. But appeal to the ethical "rule book" fails to provide answers in terms of difficult individual moral choices which must be made in the teaching and practice of nursing.

The fundamental pattern of knowing identified here as the ethical component of nursing is focused on matters of obligation or what ought to be done. Knowledge of morality goes beyond simply knowing the norms or ethical codes of the discipline. It includes all voluntary actions that are deliberate and subject to the judgment of right and wrong—including judgments of moral value in relation to motives, intentions and traits of character. Nursing is deliberate action, or a series of actions, planned and implemented to accomplish defined goals. Both goals and actions involve choices made, in part, on the basis of normative judgments, both particular and general. On occasion, the principles and norms by which such choices are made may be in conflict.

According to Berthold, "goals are, of course, value judgments not amenable to scientific inquiry and validation" (Berthold, 1968, p. 196). Dickoff, James and Wiedenbach also call attention to the need to be aware that the specification of goals serves as "a norm or standard by which to evaluate activity . . . [and] . . . entails taking them as values—that is, signifies conceiving these goal contents as situations worthy to be brought about" (James & Weidenbach, 1968, p. 422).

For example, a common goal of nursing care in relation to the maintenance or restoration of health is to assist patients to achieve a state in which they are independent. Much of the current practice reflects an attitude of value attached to the goal of independence, and indicates nursing actions to assist patients in assuming full responsibility for themselves at the earliest possible moment or to enable them to retain responsibility to the last possible moment. However, valuing independence and attempting to maintain it may be at the expense of the patient's learning how to live with physical or social dependence when necessary; e.g., in instances when prognosis indicates that independence cannot be regained.

Differences in normative judgments may have more to do with disagreements as to what constitutes a "healthy" state of being than lack of empirical evidence or ambiguity in the application of the term. Slote suggests that the persistence of disputes, or lack of uniformity in the application of cluster terms, such as health, is due to "the difficulty of decisively resolving certain sorts of value questions about what is and is not important." This leads him to conclude "that value judgment is far more involved in the making of what are commonly thought to be factual statements than has been imagined" (Slote, 1966, p. 220).

The ethical pattern of knowing in nursing requires an understanding of different philosophical positions regarding what is good, what ought to be desired, what is right; of different ethical frameworks devised for dealing with the complexities of moral judgments; and of various orientations to the notion of obligation. Moral choices to be made must then be considered in terms of specific action to be taken in specific, concrete situations. The examination of the standards, codes and values by which we decide what is morally right should result in a greater awareness of what is involved in making moral choices and being responsible for the choices made. The knowledge of ethical codes will not provide answers to the moral questions involved in nursing, nor will it eliminate the necessity for having to make moral choices. But it can be hoped that:

The more sensitive teachers and practitioners are to the demands of the process of justification, the more explicit they are about the norms that govern their actions, the more personally engaged they are in assessing surrounding circumstances and potential consequences, the more "ethical" they will be; and we cannot ask much more. (Greene, 1973, p. 221)

Using Patterns of Knowing

A philosophical discussion of patterns of knowing may appear to some as a somewhat idle, if not arbitrary and artificial, undertaking having little or no connection with the practical concerns and difficulties encountered in the day-to-day doing and teaching of nursing. But it represents a personal conviction that there is a need to examine the kinds of knowing that provide the discipline with its particular perspectives and significance. Understanding four fundamental patterns of knowing makes possible an increased awareness of the complexity and diversity of nursing knowledge.

Each pattern may be conceived as necessary for achieving mastery in the discipline, but none of them alone should be considered sufficient. Neither are they mutually exclusive. The teaching and learning of one pattern do not require the rejection or neglect of any of the others. Caring for another requires the achievements of nursing science, that is, the knowledge of empirical facts systematically organized into theoretical explanations regarding the phenomena of health and illness. But creative imagination also plays its part in the syntax of discovery in science, as well as in developing the ability to imagine the consequences of alternate moral choices.

Personal knowledge is essential for ethical choices in that moral action presupposes personal maturity and freedom. If the goals of nursing are to be more than conformance to unexamined norms, if the "ought" is not to be determined simply on the basis of what is possible, then the obligation to care for another human being involves becoming a certain kind of person—and not merely doing certain kinds of things. If the design of nursing care is to be more than habitual or mechanical, the capacity to perceive and interpret the subjective experiences of others and to imaginatively project the effects of nursing actions on their lives becomes a necessary skill.

Nursing thus depends on the specific knowledge of human behavior in health and in illness, the aesthetic perception of significant human experiences, a personal understanding of the unique individuality of the self and the capacity to make choices within concrete situations involving particular moral judgments. Each of these separate but interrelated and interdependent fundamental patterns of knowing should be taught and understood according to its distinctive logic, the restricted circumstances in which it is valid, the kinds of data it subsumes and the methods by which each particular kind of truth is distinguished and warranted.

The major significances to the discipline of nursing in distinguishing patterns of knowing are summarized as: (a) the conclusions of the discipline conceived as subject matter cannot be taught or learned without reference to the structure of the discipline—the representative concepts and methods of inquiry that determine the kind of knowledge gained and limit its meaning, scope and validity; (b) each of the fundamental patterns of knowing represents a necessary but not complete approach to the problems and questions in the discipline; and (c) all knowledge is subject to change and revision. Every solution of an existing problem raises new and unsolved questions. These new and as yet unsolved problems require, at times, new methods of inquiry and different conceptual structures; they change the shape and patterns of knowing. With each change in the shape of knowledge, teaching and learning require looking for different points of contact and connection among ideas and things. This clarifies the effect of each new thing known on other things known and the discovery of new patterns by which each connection modifies the whole.

References

Berthold, J.S. (1968). Symposium on theory development in nursing: Prologue. *Nursing Research, 17,* 196–197.

Buber, M. (1970). *I and thou.* (W. Kaufman, Trans.). New York: Scribner.

Carper, B.A. (1975). Fundamental patterns of knowing in nursing. (Doctoral dissertation, Columbia University Teachers College). *Dissertation Abstracts International, 36,* 4941B. (University Microfilms No. 76-7772).

Dewey, J. (1958). *Art as experience.* New York: Capricorn.

Dickoff, J., James, P., & Wiedenbach, E. (1968). Theory in a practice discipline: Part I, Practice-oriented theory. *Nursing Research, 17,* 415–435.

Greene, M. (1973). *Teacher as stronger.* Belmont, CA: Wadsworth.

Kuhn, T. (1962). *The structure of scientific revolutions.* Chicago: University of Chicago Press.

Langer, S.K. (1957). *Problems of art.* New York: Scribner.

Lee, V. (1960). Empathy. In M. Rader (Ed.), *A modern book of esthetics* (3rd ed.). New York: Holt, Rinehart and Winston.

Lippo, T. (1960). Empathy, inner imitation and sense-feeling. In M. Rader (Ed.), *A modern book of esthetics* (3rd ed.). New York: Holt, Rinehart and Winston.

Maslow, A.H. (1956). Self-actualizing people: A study of psychological health. In C.E. Moustakas (Ed.), *The self.* New York: Harper and Row.

McKay, R. (1969). Theories, models and systems for nursing. *Nursing Research, 18,* 393–399.

Mitchell, P.H. (1973). *Concepts basic to nursing.* New York: McGraw-Hill.

Nagel, E. (1961). *The structure of science.* New York: Harcourt, Brace and World.

Northrop, F.S.C. (1959). *The logic of the sciences and the humanities.* New York: World.

Orem, D.E. (1971). *Nursing: Concepts of practice.* New York: McGraw-Hill.

Polanyi, M. (1964). *Personal knowledge.* New York: Harper and Row.

Rader, M. (1960). Introduction: The meaning of art. In M. Rader (Ed.), *A modern book of esthetics* (3rd ed.). New York: Holt, Rinehart and Winston.

Slote, M.A. (1966). The theory of important criteria. *Journal of Philosophy, 63,* 211–224.

Weitz, M. (1960). The role of theory in aesthetics. In M. Rader (Ed.), *A modern book of esthetics* (3rd ed.). New York: Holt, Rinehart and Winston.

Wiedenbach, E. (1964). *Clinical nursing: A helping art.* New York: Springer.

Reactions

"Personal Knowledge" versus "Self Knowledge." *Advances in Nursing Science,* July 1979, 1(4), viii-ix.

To the Editor:

In reading Dr. Carper's article, "Fundamental Patterns of Knowing in Nursing," in the first issue of *ANS,* we noted a potential confounding of the term "personal knowledge." Carper uses the term to refer to the knowing of the self. In her explication of this pattern of knowing she quotes Polanyi. The use of this quote leads one to think that Polanyi's book is the primary source for the definition of the term.

However, Polanyi uses the term as a technical term related to the nature of man's comprehension and development of scientific knowledge. While he indicates that personal knowledge is a "pattern of knowing," he does not use the term to refer to knowing the self. Polanyi discusses personal knowledge as follows: "We shall find Personal knowledge manifested in the appreciation of probability and of order in the exact sciences, and see it at work even more extensively in the way the descriptive sciences rely on skills and connoisseurship. At all these points the act of knowing includes an appraisal; and this personal coefficient, which shapes all factual knowledge, bridges in doing so the disjunction between subjectivity and objectivity. It implies the claim that man can transcend his own subjectivity by striving passionately to fulfill his personal obligations to universal standards."

Hence there is a discrepancy between Polanyi and Carper's use of the term "personal knowledge," which could confuse the reader. To avoid this result, we would suggest that some other term be used to refer to the pattern of knowing described by Carper. This term might be "knowledge of the self" or just "self-knowledge."

Aside from the previous comments, we found Dr. Carper's article to be informative and thought provoking.

ELLEN C. EGAN, Ph.D.
Associate Professor
JAN BECKSTRAND, Ph.D., R.N.
Assistant Professor
School of Nursing
University of Minnesota
Minneapolis, Minnesota

The Author Comments

The genesis for this article, which is a part of my doctoral dissertation, was my perplexity and confusion as an inexperienced teacher regarding what should be included and excluded from the nursing curriculum. With the rapid accumulation of knowledge, there was an almost irresistible urge to add subject after subject to the already crowded curriculum. Both student and teacher alike became disoriented in a maze of seemingly separate, disarticulated facts.

My search for some meaningful guide to a "sense of the whole" to counteract the feeling of fragmentation led me to attempt to qualitatively analyze the kinds of knowledge that seemed to exemplify nursing. The identification of the fundamental patterns of knowing in nursing was guided by the following questions:

A. What is the conceptual structure of knowledge in nursing?
  1. What are the representative concepts that specify, describe, define and/or classify the phenomena of the field of nursing?
  2. What dominant themes indicate how these concepts are related to each other in a systematic way?
  3. What concepts and/or conceptual models are characteristic in that they direct or control inquiry in the discipline?
B. What is the syntactical structure of knowledge in nursing?
  1. What are the methods of inquiry?
  2. What methods are used to validate/test claims to knowledge?
  3. What methods of inquiry exhibit the patterns of explanation and/or prediction?

—BARBARA A. CARPER

Chapter 20

Holistic Man and the Science and Practice of Nursing

Sarah S. Fuller

It is often said that in the early years following doctoral study the young scientist should be primarily concerned with conducting research. Once established as a competent or seasoned investigator, that same scientist, older now, may be qualified to review and critique the work of other scientists. Then, having been duly recognized as a scholar, the same scientist, much older now, may dare to take a broader view and raise the philosophical issues which may provide direction for future young scientists. If my concern were only for the science of nursing, I would patiently await the passing years so that my views might be clearly derived from my own research and scholarship. But a more immediate concern for the practice of nursing dissuades my patience and prompts me to urge, now, that we consider again the direction of the science and practice of nursing.

In past years there have been many discussions which sought to identify the nature of nursing—what it is and what it is not. We have said that it was both an art and a science. Some said that it was more art than science, since we had no identified body of knowledge on which to base our practice; others said it was a science whose knowledge base had only to be identified. But, as nurses began to become more sophisticated in the ways of science, what had been viewed as the art of nursing came to be relegated to a position of lesser importance. Today, in the practice of nursing, emphasis is on the nursing process with its components of assessment, planning, implementation, and evaluation. Whether any or all of these components are carried out systematically and with any regularity in nursing practice may remain a question, but the method of providing nursing care in a holistic fashion is clearly outlined in the basic steps of the process—a process remarkably akin to the method of generating scientific knowledge. Certainly the methods of the nursing process have refocused our attention on the intellectual and interper-

About the Author

SARAH S. FULLER began her career in nursing in 1964, when she graduated from St. Joseph Hospital School of Nursing in Ottumwa, Iowa. In 1966, she received a B.S.N. from Marycrest College; in 1969, a M.A. in medical-surgical nursing from the University of Iowa. From 1971 to 1975, she studied at the University of Colorado, receiving an M.A. and a Ph.D. in social-personality psychology.

While a student, Dr. Fuller worked in a variety of positions, including staff nurse, clinical specialist, and research associate. In 1977, she joined the faculty at Northern Illinois University, DeKalb. At the time of her death in 1980, Dr. Fuller was a Robert Wood Johnson Faculty Fellow at the University of Colorado Health Sciences Center.

During her professional career, Dr. Fuller published 13 articles and presented at numerous conferences. Her special research interests included stress, anxiety, coping, personal control, and problem solving. Teaching interests focused on psychology in health, adaptation and change, and psychology of aging.

sonal skills that are necessary to the practice of nursing. But adopting the method of science does not necessarily ensure that those particular skills will be used any more scientifically than were nursing arts of bygone days. Assessment tools, standards, and documented plans are now treated with the reverence that once was accorded to well-written procedure manuals. These process methods may, it is true, move nursing toward a more conceptual or knowledge-based form of practice, as some have suggested (Andreoli & Thompson, 1977). But is it not possible that the students of today will show the same unquestioning and undeviating loyalty to these methods as past students have shown for particular methods of making a bed or giving an injection?

As the nursing process has risen to prominence in the past decade, so too have arisen an increasing number of nursing roles. We have the clinical nursing specialist, the practitioner, the primary nurse, the patient care coordinator, the educator, the researcher, the patient advocate; fortunately, we also still have with us the not so prestigious but ever faithful generalist. Although one might debate the wisdom of such role proliferation, it does exist and may be evidence of some unfulfilled needs in nursing practice or in the more general domain of health care. The expansion or narrowing, as the case may be, of roles assumed by nurses seems yet another way of trying to define nursing. Yet again it is definition by function, much as was

attempted nearly 20 years ago (Hughes, Hughes, & Deutscher, 1958). While expanded roles for nurses may result in better health care or greater satisfaction for nurses, there is no assurance that nursing practice so defined will foster a knowledge base for practice or a practice guided by scientific inquiry.

Yet another model of defining nursing has appeared on the horizon in more recent years. As nurses strive to attain the status and ideals of a profession, the phrases that nurses are "autonomous," nurses are "assertive," and nurses "have power" pervade the nursing literature and resound in meeting halls. But does saying a thing make it so? Will autonomy or power gained by political action or proclamation become an enduring characteristic to sustain the practice of nursing? When the political climate changes or the enthusiasm for the slogan wanes, will the practice of nursing be different from what it has been in the past? Or, if it is different, will that difference be for the benefit of human beings in need of nursing care? I doubt it. The autonomy of a profession rests more firmly on the uniqueness of its knowledge—knowledge gathered ever so slowly through the questioning of scientific inquiry. Nursing defined by power does not necessarily beget knowledge. But knowledge most often results in the ascription of power and is accompanied by autonomy.

Nursing has also been implicitly defined by its focus or areas of practice. Thus we have medical-surgical, community health, mental health, maternal-child, and gerontological nursing, as well as many others. The names change from time to time, as do the curricula, which are designed and redesigned with the intention of preparing knowledgeable nurses for practice. But what of the content of these areas of practice? Does one who practices medical-surgical nursing require a different body of knowledge or set of concepts than one who practices gerontological or community health nursing? The proponents of integrated curricula apparently perceive the commonalities, but once again the means appear to have become the end. Though much has been done "in the name of integration," has the practice of nursing been greatly changed or has health care improved (Styles, 1976)?

Even more recently, nursing diagnosis has been heralded as the means of clarifying the nature and extent of nursing problems, and diagnostic taxonomies have been proposed to bring consistency to the research and practice of nursing (Abdellah, 1969; Gebbie & Lavin, 1975). While nursing diagnosis is an appealing idea and represents a greater abstraction than the "21 problems" of past years, does not the approach run the risk of defining nursing practice by consensus rather than by inquiry (Abdellah, Beland, Martin, & Matheney, 1960)? And will the diagnoses derived reflect human problems found *only* in nursing, or will they merely be new names for concepts already identified and studied by our colleagues in the biological, psychological, and sociological sciences?

Research is the method of inquiry characteristic of a science. If unity and order are to be identified in the practice of nursing, the identification will surely come from the quiet pursuit of knowledge using this scientific method. As the 25th anniversary issue of *Nursing Research* (1977) so aptly illustrates, research is being undertaken by nurses and the volume of such study is no longer small.

That the quality of research should have increased to the extent that it has in little more than a quarter of a century gives credence to the ability of nurses to adopt the methods of science. It would nevertheless appear that the identification of a knowledge base for the practice of nursing remains far in the future. It might be said, as Schlotfeldt has noted, that the "conceptualization of a research problem must partly reveal the investigator's conceptualization of the discipline under study" (Schlotfeldt, 1975, pp. 6–7). A review of the research in nursing reveals a fragmented array of studies defying the identification of unity and order in their results as well as in their conceptualizations.

Ellis (1977) found that tasks, technology, and teaching have been the predominant focus of research in medical-surgical nursing. In community health, Highriter (1977) identified great variety in the concerns of research, but the majority of studies represented evaluations of service programs, the performance of techniques, and the performance of specified nursing roles. Barnard and Neal seem to have concluded from their review of research in the area of maternal-child nursing that the elements of nursing remain unknown and that "the basis for nursing actions today is primarily the traditions and dogma that have been handed down as practice beliefs" (Barnard & Neil, 1977, p. 198). The need for a clearer conceptual stance has also been identified for the fields of mental health and gerontological nursing (Gunter & Miller, 1977; Sills, 1977). Perhaps what is most instructive from these several recent reviews is best expressed by Gunter and Miller in their consideration of gerontological nursing: "Gerontological nursing research at this time reflects minimal attention to the integration of knowledge from biology, psychology, and sociology" (Gunter & Miller, 1977, p. 211). The same statement could well be made for most other areas of nursing practice.

Our experiences in research are very much our experiences in nursing practice. And I would suggest that in both domains our course has been ill charted, for whatever reason. We quest for a knowledge base that may already exist, and we confuse methods and roles with our general goal, which surely must be the betterment of the human condition.

Others have said that the science of nursing will consist of a synthesis of knowledge from other disciplines and that nursing's specific and unique professional goal is to determine the appropriate and necessary knowledge (Hadley, 1969; Johnson, 1959). I do not know if there will be or should be a unique professional goal for nursing, but there is definite need for direction. The continued pursuit of what is popular or professionally self-serving will not contribute to the development of nursing science nor is it likely to meet the social necessity for competent nursing care.

Donaldson and Crowley (1978) have recently presented a masterful explication of the discipline of nursing, in which they were quite careful not to equate the discipline with the science of nursing. Nevertheless, their intent seems to have been to provide some coherent direction for the science or nursing by making explicit the perspective of the discipline and placing emphasis on its substantive structure or content. In view of our current plight, to see an emphasis on content rekindles the hope for what might be in nursing. But I believe the direction of the science of nursing must be even more sharply focused, for the substantive structure of the discipline is not strong.

The general focus of nursing seems to be the health of whole human beings in interaction with their environments. This focus is reflected in attempts to develop broad theories and concepts intended to encompass and maintain the integrity of the human being. I would hope that we never lose this humanistic vision. At the same time, to approach the building of science from such a perspective is an impossible task. To mandate that a curriculum be based or organized upon a single conceptual stance is to obscure the dynamic nature of the science and ultimately of the practice of nursing. Similarly, to expect nurses in practice to function well from such a global base is probably unrealistic and may unintentionally render them incompetent.

It may seem an oversimplistic interpretation of a very complex situation, but I believe the heart of the matter is that the organization of our profession lacks logical relationship. This lack of coherence pervades every aspect of nursing; it dissipates our energy and it divides us. The most vocal among us lead us in divergent directions, and because hope springs eternal, we follow each new idea with the fervor of true disciples;

those who do not follow become lost in the abyss of confusion and ultimately lost from nursing. Lest my appraisal seems too harsh, let me say that I do not decry pluralism; certainly we need diverse views and many ideas. In this critical period of our development, however, I believe the most urgent need is for order and stability. I would further submit that the necessary order has been before us for a very long time.

It is neither eccentric nor revolutionary to state that the human being has biological, psychological, and sociological dimensions. These same dimensions exist whether we are speaking of children, adolescents, middle-aged, or elderly adults; they encompass the life span of human beings. Similarly, the same dimensions exist in illness and health, without regard to medical diagnosis; they exist in community as well as in institutional settings. I would suggest, therefore, that we cease to define nursing by functions or role, methods or process, and areas or focus of practice, and consider instead that the knowledge and concepts essential to nursing are already defined by the nature of the human being. The biological, psychological, and sociological dimensions of the human being transcend the traditional boundaries of nursing practice and could, if we would let them, give order to the science of nursing, to the education of nurses at all levels, and to the practice of nursing.

While the whole may be greater than the sum of its parts, as reflected in the general focus of nursing, following this Gestaltian or organismic view to its ultimate conclusion precludes scientific study and thus precludes the discovery of relationships. Without such study the practice of nursing will undoubtedly remain a process of common sense, intuition, or trial and error, none of which is likely to be efficient, economical, or, in the long run, intellectually and emotionally satisfying to nurses in practice.

The greatest tragedy of all, however, is that the ultimate loser is the human being whose needs for nursing care will more often than not go undetected and unresolved unless those needs are systematically studied. Our ultimate aim of service to the whole human being notwithstanding, systematic study requires that research problems be conceptualized within manageable limits or boundaries. The biological, psychological, and sociological dimensions of the human being provide natural, although overlapping, boundaries for the conceptualization of research problems and thus for the ordering of a science of nursing.

In view of our enduring recognition of the contribution of the biological, psychological, and sociological sciences to the discipline of nursing, it is surprising that we have not generally made use of them in our efforts to build a science of nursing. The reluctance to take full advantage of relevant theories and concepts which have been formulated and studied in these sciences may be due to a belief that their adoption would be incompatible with a distinct science of nursing. This kind of defensiveness, however, retards our progress and is difficult to justify when the subject of our study in nursing—i.e., the human being—is the same as in many other sciences.

This is not to say that the essence of nursing is that of an applied science. On the contrary, the uniqueness of nursing may be found in its unusual and simultaneous concern with the relationship of these several dimensions to a condition of health. Nonetheless, the development of nursing science might proceed in a more orderly fashion if health-related research problems were placed within the context of biological, psychological, or sociological conceptualizations. Investigations would not, then, have tasks, technology, teaching, and segregated categories of patients (or clients, if you prefer) as their primary focus. Rather, such entities, when of interest, would be subordinated to the substantive structure of biological, psychological, or sociological concepts related to the health of human beings.

Such an approach would make possible the identification of commonalities across investigations and would stimulate new ideas and further research. The progression of conceptually based research could be expected to result in the reformulation of theories or concepts and in the specification of new ones. Thus, theories in nursing would not be negated but rather given the opportunity to flourish. Their focus, however,

would be on the dimensions of the human being—the subject of nursing—and not on the profession of nursing itself. The question of what is nursing would then become irrelevant and be replaced by the question: What are the needs of human beings which might be met by nursing?

When research in nursing begins to reflect the substantive characteristics of a science whose ultimate concern is the health of human beings, nursing curricula can and surely will assume a similar form and content. That is, the common practice of designing curricula around areas or focus of practice—for example, medical-surgical or community health nursing—will give way to a more logical organization of biological, psychological, and sociological nursing. Within this form, roles, functions, methods, or process can be subordinated to substantive concepts or content. Curricula so organized will have much less of the overlapping and omission of content which currently exists. Faculty members can begin to teach content which is congruent with their research interests and advanced study. The quality of education should improve and bring with it the attendant effects of greater productivity, efficiency, and economy.

At the same time, emphasis would be placed on the human being for whom the profession of nursing exists. Some few schools of nursing around the country have already attempted such organization, although they have generally combined the psychological and sociological dimensions into a single psychosocial category. The organization of these schools, I believe, will eventually become the rule in nursing rather than the exception. If the wealth of content in either the psychological or sociological dimensions is not to become obscured, however, the distinction between them must be maintained for the purposes of research and education.

Curricular transitions, if they are to be substantive and effective, must not be precipitous; they must be as carefully planned as a good research design. Indeed, at this point in our history, it may be wiser to delay major changes in undergraduate curricula until the substantive content of nursing is more fully developed through research. The immediate point of departure needs to be at the level of graduate education—particularly the doctoral level where many new programs are struggling because of the lack of orderly direction. The nurse scientist program provided a natural model for such curricula, but its potential usefulness has yet to be realized. As new doctoral programs are being considered, faculty might be well advised to consider carefully the merits of such a model.

As the form and content of nursing become orderly and consonant with the dimensions of the human being, one can expect greater standardization of curricula at all levels of nursing education. Standardization is badly needed and may ultimately provide the only lasting solution to such critical issues as the articulation of the various levels of nursing education and levels of entry into practice. In other words, an ordered and substantive content in nursing curricula would allow defensible distinctions to be made among the several levels of education and practice.

If education is viewed as the mediating link, the relationship between the science and practice of nursing need not be a capricious one. Nurses in practice require the concepts or knowledge of all three major dimensions of the human being. The exclusion or diminution of any one of them will leave the practicing nurse ill prepared to meet the needs of human beings for nursing care. It is in practice that the whole is greater than the sum of its parts. Nevertheless, the nurse who is not well prepared in each of the component dimensions will not be able to judge when the needs in one dimension must supersede those in another or when the needs are interactive and must be viewed as such for the welfare of the human being.

It is doubtful that nurses beginning in clinical practice experience frustration and disillusionment only because they lack practical experience or because their special capabilities are not valued within the working environment. Rapprochement between nursing education and nursing practice will not be accomplished by placing blame; it may be accomplished by more objectively appraising ourselves. Our common goal is service to human beings in need of nursing care, and we have traditionally opted to meet this goal, both in education and in practice, through various methods, processes, and roles. We have rarely asked ourselves what knowledge or content is necessary to enable nurses to provide competent care.

To achieve our common goal, those nurses who provide direct human services must be knowledgeable of the relationships between and among the several dimensions of the human being and a condition of health. There are times when the biological needs are more imperative for survival than are the psychological or sociological. Because many of our nursing curricula are not strong in the biological content areas (perhaps in overcompensation for past neglect of the psychological and sociological), it should not be surprising that young nurses suddenly faced with the acute and complex biological needs of human beings find themselves overwhelmed by a sense of inadequacy. Nor should we be surprised when we hear of such examples as that of a nurse attempting to relieve a patient's apparent anxiety while ignoring or failing to recognize that his immediate problem was acute hemorrhage.

On the other hand, there are times when the psychological or sociological needs are more salient, as when a patient suffers malnutrition because of loneliness and social isolation. All of the instruction in proper nutritional practices possible will not alleviate such a problem. And, if a nurse fails to recognize or is insufficiently prepared to respond to interactive needs of patients, we need not be surprised when previously competent elderly adults deteriorate before our eyes for the lack of sensory and social stimulation.

The human being is a complex organism, and his needs for nursing care are equally complex. It matters little whether those needs be served by a nurse practitioner, a clinical nursing specialist, or a primary care nurse; the service will be only as competent as the nurse is knowledgeable. But knowledge is more than a compilation of facts; knowledge is understanding and the ability to perceive relationships. Science is the avenue to such knowledge. Thus, we have come full circle in this discourse.

When we have a science of nursing which reorganizes its responsibility for the discovery of relationships among the dimensions of the human being and a condition of health, we may have curricula that will be characterized by their substantive content rather than by their illogical form. Only then will we have a practice of nursing which is guided by the spirit of scientific inquiry and which exists to give service. The results of our efforts should be manifested in the people we serve. If they do not benefit, if health care is not changed, we will have failed.

References

Abdellah, F.G. (1969). The nature of nursing science. *Nursing Research, 18*, 391.

Abdellah, F.G., Beland, I.L., Martin, A., & Matheney, R.V. (1960). *Patient-centered approaches to nursing.* New York: Macmillan.

Andreoli, K.G., & Thompson, C.E. (1977). The nature of science in nursing. *Image, 9*, 32–37.

Barnard, K.E., & Neal, M.V. (1977). Maternal-child nursing research: Review of the past and strategies for the future. *Nursing Research, 26*, 198–200.

Donaldson, S.K., & Crowley, D.M. (1978). The discipline of nursing. *Nursing Outlook, 26*, 113–120.

Ellis, R. (1977). Fallibilities, fragments, and frames: Contemplation on 25 years of research in medical-surgical nursing. *Nursing Research, 26*, 177–182.

Gebbie, K.M., & Lavin, M.A. (Eds.). (1975). *Classification of nursing diagnoses.* St. Louis: C.V. Mosby.

Gunter, L.M., & Miller, J.C. (1977). Toward a nursing gerontology. *Nursing Research, 26*, 208–221.

Hadley, B.J. (1969). Evolution of a conception of nursing. *Nursing Research, 18*, 400–404.

Highriter, M.E. (1977). The status of community health nursing research. *Nursing Research, 26*, 183–192.

Hughes, E.C., Hughes, H.M., & Deutscher, I. (1958). *Twenty thousand nurses tell their story.* Philadelphia: J.B. Lippincott.

Johnson, D.E. (1959). The nature of a science of nursing. *Nursing Outlook, 7*, 291–294.

Schlotfeldt, R.M. (1975). The need for a conceptual framework. In P.J. Verhonick (Ed.), *Nursing Research I.* Boston: Little, Brown.

Sills, G.M. (1977). Research in the field of psychiatric nursing, 1952–1977. *Nursing Research, 26*, 201–207.

Styles, M.M. (1976). In the name of integration. *Nursing Outlook, 24*, 738–744.

Twenty-Fifth Anniversary Issue. (1977). *Nursing Research, 26*, 163–236.

A Colleague Comments

Dr. Sarah S. Fuller was an exceptionally talented nurse scholar. Despite her death early in her professional career, her writings have had a marked impact on theoretical thinking within the nursing profession. The development of nursing knowledge and the conduct of rigorous nursing research were her consuming professional passions. Dr. Fuller's investigative work concerning factors affecting quality of life among the elderly placed her at the forefront of the generation of nursing knowledge critical to humane and holistic care.

Dr. Fuller and I spent many hours discussing approaches to the development of nursing theory and the nature of the substantive structure of nursing knowledge. To converse with Dr. Fuller was to embark on an adventure in thinking. Students were awed by her clarity of thought and articulate manner. She was a highly productive scholar, yet never too busy to spend time in conversation with students who needed support and encouragement in their scholarly pursuits. The memory of Dr. Fuller lives on through her writings. This article is an excellent example of the fine analytical thought that characterized all of her work.

NOLA J. PENDER

Chapter 21

Nursing Science in Transition

Susan R. Gortner

Nursing science, the base of knowledge underlying human behavior and social interaction, under normal and stressful conditions, across the life span, is distinguished from its inquiry (research). Inquiry and, especially, methodology have been afforded greater attention than science. The requirements for increased science are noted: communality, colleagueship, and competition among scientists and continuity and confirmation of scientific activity and evidence.

The credibility of nursing science depends on the rigor and quality of scientific work, the generality of findings, and the reputation and productivity of scholars, both individual and communal. Peer review and acclaim, successful completion of initial and replicated studies, strong investigators, and national and international citation also help to establish credibility. These are the usual means for scientific excellence in any field.

If credibility is based on acknowledged competence and productivity, what is the stage of nursing science, and what are the indicators of quality and output? First, nursing research—the systematic inquiry into problems associated with illness, health, and care—should be contrasted with nursing science—the base of knowledge underlying human behavior and social interaction under normal and stressful conditions—across the life span. Nursing science is a subset of the discipline of nursing (Donaldson & Crowley, 1978). Disciplines are larger entities than their associated sciences and arts. Evolving branches of learning such as nursing may be cast against Shermis' (1962) intellectual criteria for academic disciplines: impressive bodies of enduring works, suitable techniques, concerns significant and relevant to humans, unifying and inspiring traditions, and considerable scholarly achievements. While nursing is not at this level of development, Donaldson and Crowley are optimistic, as am I, about the potential significance of nursing because of its concern with human health and well-being, and the growth of its research and scholarship. The changing nature of that research and the necessary scholarship serves as focus of this article.

Science and Its Inquiry, Research

Science is defined as the body of codified understanding of the natural universe and of human social and individual behavior (Brooks, 1973; Downs, 1979b). Thus, nursing science represents our currently limited understanding of human biology and behavior in health and illness, including the processes by which changes in health status are brought about, the patterns of behavior associated with normal and critical life events, and the principles and laws governing life states and processes (Donaldson & Crowley, 1978; Gortner, Bloch, & Phillips, 1976). Nursing research represents the discrete and aggregated investigations that constitute the profession's major modes and foci of inquiry. What some have mistaken for science is research, the tool of science. Already well begun is the documentation through research, of phenomena in the real world. This empirical orientation has guided us heavily to date because few theoretical explanations or prescriptions were available to provide alternative deductive arguments for the specific situation. Propositions relevant to specific phenomena—for example, maternal-child interaction, self-care, dying—are emerging. While still formative and imprecise, these constructs and hypotheses provide a group of conceptual frameworks capable of guiding the direction of our injury and perhaps aligning such inquiry more closely with the (health/illness) perspective of nursing (Williams, 1979). The transition from data to theory and theory to data requires creative imagination and persistent trials by the scientist. Few have been able to devote the years of life work to accomplish such matters, but those who have, notably Benoliel, Hansen, Jacox, and J. Johnson, contribute greatly to our understanding.

Fundamental Science

For reasons not yet clear, our attention is being directed to inquiry in the sciences that explain human biology and behavior and social interaction. Rather than fascination with the methodological contributions of these sciences, the interest is in which basic laws and relationships explain the phenomena under study. This science base includes both undifferentiated research that is nonspecific to a disease orientation and clinically oriented research that focuses on specific disease processes (U.S. National Institutes of Health [NIH], 1978a). Mere fundamental science holds no immediate hope of clinical application or utility, but contributes to general understanding of events across a wide range of disciplines. As science (not theory), it affords propositions capable of explanation and further proof. On what fundamental science(s), then, does our work lie? I was asked this question on a site visit to a clinical research facility by the director of research, a physician who had listened attentively to a number of clinical nursing studies described in detail. My response, of course, was that the base lies, in the main, in the behavioral and social sciences and, to a lesser extent, in the biological and physical sciences. The questioner observed the similarity between the character of nursing investigations as exemplified by the studies he had heard and the state of clinical medicine 30 years ago that was, predominantly empirical, located within the domain of practice and concerned with treatment.

Indeed, the perspective of nursing inquiry is greatly influenced and defined by clinical practice and not the other way around, as yet. It will be some time before practice is influenced by inquiry and defined by the knowledge store that Donaldson and Crowley call the discipline of nursing. But the question of basic and relevant scientific theory was raised then and is being raised now by increasing numbers of investigators and not exclusively by theorists in isolation from research (Downs, 1979a; Johnson, 1979; Williams, 1979). Such a development augurs well for nursing science, for its disciplines, and for other fields and disciplines as well, especially since the sciences are now competing for resources along with clinical application, technology transfer, and training. The newly identified field of behavioral medicine is a case in point; perusal of its content and parameters as defined by the Yale Conference reveals a striking similarity to nursing research, but there is as yet no formal recognition of one by the other (U.S. NIH, 1978b)—an interesting turn on the issue of credibility.

Ethical and Philosophical Aspects of Science

As though in direct response to Donaldson and Crowley's statement that "what is needed is the thinking of nurse philosophers and also some philosophizing on the part of the nurse researchers" (Donaldson & Crowley, 1978, p. 114), Beckstrand's (1978a, 1978b) two-part article on practice theory and the relation of scientific and ethical knowledge to practice appeared. Drawing heavily on Hempel's (1965) models of scientific logic, Beckstrand made a compelling case against promulgation of practice theory by arguing that the knowledge required for practice is the knowledge of science and ethics. Because practice uses scientific knowledge in attempting to control phenomena (but cannot promise control or assure certainty of outcome), the form of that knowledge is the defense for its use as a major theoretical paradigm. A similar argument is made for ethical theory. A risk/benefit calculus with regard to treatment options is based on the most convincing evidence at the time and the particular needs of the patient. In practice, the clinical evidence may represent insufficient scientific proof but sufficient clinical proof of a desired course of action. The value motivation is beneficence, the obligation to do good and avoid harm. The use of misuse of new knowledge generated through research is not within the domain of nursing science to control. Awareness that practice should be based on knowledge and that knowledge should have veracity is a development of recent years.

The Nature of the Disciplinary-Perspective

Significant themes should be examined with regard to their content and meaning for the discipline of nursing, for the science and the art, and for other fields and disciplines. A useful commentary on nursing's perspective may be obtained from other fields. Is nursing's perspective recognized by other disciplines or by our own? To what extent does our health and human behavior orientation preclude attention to illness states and specifically to disease states?

On another side visit, the institution's faculty and graduate student investigators were asked, "Do you study diseases any more?" Have we gone so far in our rejection of the medical model that we fail to acknowledge not only the biological and psychological dysfunctioning that brings most, if not all, patients to our attention, but also the body of knowledge that explains and describes the pathology? On the other hand, nursing's deliberate concern with the whole human, with life styles, and with health behavior is attractive to those who find the disease orientation limiting and insufficient to explain response to therapy, spontaneous improvement in health status, and high level wellness. "Impressive! I have not heard nursing so described before," remarked one colleague in medicine following a brief presentation of the scope and nature of nursing science and research. Similarly, faculty investigators are called on to participate in forums for the public and to provide data on legislative and policy issues in nursing. Do these movements suggest recognition, beginning belief, or valuation of the perspective? Perhaps so.

The Nature of Scientific Designs

The nature of the scientific designs used in nursing research tends now to be multivariate and multidimensional in recognition that the problems under investigation require such handling and that techniques are now available in statistics to accommodate complex relationships. The classical single variable/treatment investigation applied to an experimental and a control group is not as frequent as it was a decade ago when we began to move away from description as the major scientific approach. Additionally, a combination of quantitative and qualitative strategies can be found in a number of studies, suggesting increased versatility in the methods of science. Investigators are employing designs that allow greater control or manipulation of variables, and they are approaching the naturalistic world with greater sophistication. In the name of increased methodological rigor, will be subject to infatuation with the rituals of science rather than with its substance? Will we make the mistake of equating esoteric research language with quality?

Shaver (1979) castigated educational researchers as being methodologically impeccable, producing a generation of Campbell and Stanley (1966) enthusiasts concerned with questions of sample size, controls, instrumentation, and statistical procedures, but incapable of comprehending the philosophical underpinnings of creative work or the basic orientations of science. In his response to Kerlinger's (1977) presidential address before the American Educational Research Association, Shaver stated that the distinctions between basic and applied research are less important than the incubation of science values during the graduate training period. In keeping with the philosophical view that science is self-testing and self-correcting, studies of differential teaching methods can be examined for implications beyond the original phenomenon and the efficacy of methods. Nursing's analogue to teaching strategies is clinical intervention; many of us would be disquieted if we prematurely put aside appropriate questions of design and procedures. For example, the design and conduct of clinical trials is a fascinating area, one that needs further exploration by nurse scientists concerned with the antecedents and correlates of therapy. In these trials fundamental questions are asked consistently of the data and subsequent trials designed to extend the base. Thus, a remedy proposed by Shaver, and one that has been repeatedly raised in our literature, is the strategy of replication, to demonstrate reliability and generaliz

ability of findings. In her Bicentennial review of nursing research, de Tornyay (1977) commented on the lack of evidence in the literature of replicated studies, attributing such voids to devaluation of replications as non-original endeavors—an unfortunate situation for the state of our science, which rests precariously on single investigations and unconfirmed study findings for the most part.

Principles of Scientific Work
Confirmation

The principle of confirmation is well known in science. If the credibility of nursing research is to be extended beyond our small group of disciples to nonbelievers, the principle of confirmation must be recognized as often as the principles of explanation and description. Similarly, greater attention to substance than to process or, more properly, a more equitable balance between scientific substance (theories and propositions) and scientific methods (tools and techniques) will be important to develop the potential of our research.

Communality

The principle of communality also is well known in science. By this is meant communication: dialogue and exchange of one's work with others, the opportunity for competent opinion of that work, and the promise, if not fulfillment, or colleagueship and collaboration. Batey (1978) and Benoliel (1973) elaborated on this principle as a major norm of science, one that guides scholars with like interests toward one another, that encourages if not requires peer review and acclaim or criticism, and that allows for self-testing and self-correction of knowledge and approaches. Nurse scientists as yet do not fully appreciate the importance of communality for scientific efforts, and as a result these efforts suffer. Few of us have publication records that reflect a consistent and progressive pattern of reporting in the referred scientific literature. Credibility in science rests heavily on the reputation and competence of the individual scientist. How many of us are known to one another by the subject matter of our research, and to what extent is that research competitive beyond the local arena? That is, how would it be viewed nationally? Benoliel commented:

> It is important, it seems to me, to be aware that competition is a part of the reality of academic life and scientific activity. Science and scholarship are essentially a man's form of work, and governed by the rules of the game created by men. Active engagement in the discovery of knowledge requires an aggressive involvement with the substance and the tools of scientific inquiry. It means a willingness to put ideas on the table for debate and discussion. It means developing the capacity to accept critical comments about these ideas without intense feelings of personal attack. (Benoliel, 1973, p.9)

More frequently than infrequently, there is insufficient evidence of competition on local, regional, and national levels for research funds, for scientific meetings, and for publication. The dearth—hurtful individually and collectively—suggests a greater interest on our part in other professional and personal matters than in science. Insufficient productivity among individual scientists leads to lack of recognition within and outside the community. For example, there is virtually no transfer of information from nursing to medicine in the medical literature. Evidence of productivity should not be limited to our own literature, but to citations and presentations of our studies in other fields. We should solicit these opportunities initially on the basis of merit until there is sufficient credibility to prompt spontaneous solicitation. An additional problem is that productivity in nursing is not generally associated with knowledge development.

Also evident throughout nursing research is the phenomenon of single cases and solo investigations and investigators. For reasons still unclear, most investigators attempt to launch research in an individualistic manner much on the order of the doctoral dissertation, but without the benefit of the committee. How important was the access as student to faculty resources that could extend the conceptualization of the problem, suggest and explain the appropriate choice of design,

assist in the selection of instruments, and provide a critical but sympathetic screen for progress!

Competition and Colleagueship

Thus, the initial socialization into science begun in graduate school is rarely maintained, and the expected norms of communality, objectivity, and generalizability are not reinforced. The career patterns of our new doctorates rarely reflect a period of even a year of postdoctoral research under an experienced set of mentors. During this period (i.e., immediately following the doctorate), new scholars move into existing or established programs of research and are assisted to obtain resources for their own research. In the University of California, competition for Academic Senate research funds is by junior untenured faculty or by new appointees in the more senior rank. From my brief tenure on the committee it is clear other disciplines expect young professors will compete for research funds, in modest amounts, to obtain resources for their research. Not infrequently, the new investigator is sponsored by one or more seniors well-established in the programmatic research area who vouch for the applicant, much as the sponsor vouches for the student. This ethic or tradition of continued postdoctorate scholarship is facilitated by additional normative patterns in disciplines other than nursing, namely the assignment of the lightest (rather than the heaviest) teaching loads to new appointees, provision for travel to scientific meetings, initial research space and resources, and firm pressure to become productive as a scientist. Until it is possible for nursing to make the administrative changes to encourage and protect scholarship, no amount of dialogue or extramural funds will correct the situation. Stevenson (1979) called for support of the emerging social institution of science, and Fawcett (1979) addressed these concerns in "Integrating Research into the Faculty Workload," the title of which reflects how nursing views its activities in management and staffing terminology. Sympathetic observers elsewhere on campus are quick to pick up the service patterns of work load, assignments, workday (8 hours/day), workweek (40 hours), and process. Such orientation is antithetical to the concept and practice of scholarship. But the service press is a dominant tradition and one that will resist change. It is essential that it be changed, and it is within our capability to make that change.

Continuity

To the principles of confirmation and communality (including competition and colleagueship) should be added the principle of continuity. By this is meant successive and successful improvements over time in the base of knowledge in a given area. The principle of continuity is fundamental to excellent research programs, to the refinement and modification of ideas over generations of scholars, and to the stability of research resources. Cases in point are the general research support grant programs and the categorical program projects which represent long-standing commitments on the part of the National Institutes of Health. Intellectual ties and methodological talents that are aggregated in deliberate conjugations of investigators have high levels of productivity.

Just as the reputation of the individual scholar should be established, so should the programmatic activities of the scholar group be recognized as valid, creative, and rigorous. I am not convinced that targeted research will extend our productivity and Credibility any further than additional essays, such as this, on the nature of nursing science. Rather, energies should be directed to the science we say we value in order to examine its emerging properties and capacity for proof (confirmation) and explanation. I know of no other way to accomplish this than to be humble in the questions we ask, courageous about the intellectual initiatives we take, skeptical of the answers we obtain (displaying them for others to review), and devoted to and in love with our work (Gortner, 1977; Neusner, 1977).

References

Batey, M.V. (1978). Research communication: Its functions, audiences, and media. *Communicating Nursing Research, 11,* 101–109.

Beckstrand, J. (1978a). The notion of a practice theory and the relationship of scientific and ethical knowledge to practice. *Research in Nursing and Health, 1,* 131–136.

Beckstrand, J. (1978b). The need for a practice theory as indicated by the knowledge used in conduct of practice. *Research in Nursing and Health, 1,* 175–179.

Benoliel, J.Q. (1973). Collaboration and competition in nursing research. *Communicating in Nursing Research, 6,* 1–11.

Brooks, H. (1973). Knowledge and action: The dilemma of science policy in the 70's. *Daedalus, 102,* 125–143.

Campbell, D.T., & Stanley, J.C. (1966). *Experimental and quasi-experimental designs for research.* Chicago: Rand McNally.

De Tornyay, R. (1977). Nursing research in the bicentennial year. *Communicating Nursing Research, 9,* 1–21.

Donaldson, S.K., & Crowley, D.M. (1978). The discipline of nursing. *Nursing Outlook, 26,* 113–120.

Downs, F. (1979a). Clinical and theoretical research. In F.S. Downs & J.W. Fleming (Eds.), *Issues in Nursing Research* (pp. 67–89). New York: Appleton-Century-Crofts.

Downs, F. (1979b). Creativity in science: What it's all about. [Editorial] *Nursing Research, 28,* 324.

Fawcett, J. (1979). Integrating research into the faculty workload. *Nursing Outlook, 27,* 259–262.

Gortner, S.R. (1977). *Nursing research as a university responsibility.* Paper presented at the Intercollegiate Center for Nursing Education, Spokane, WA, and also December 12, 1977, at the University of California, San Francisco School of Nursing.

Gortner, S.R., Bloch, D., & Phillips, T. (1976). Contributions of nursing research to patient care. *Journal of Nursing Administration, 6,* 22–28.

Hempel, C.G. (1965). *Aspects of scientific explanation.* New York: Free Press.

Johnson, J. (1979). Translating research into practice. In *Power: Nursing's challenge for change* (pp. 125–133). Paper presented at the 51st Convention, Honolulu, Hawaii, June 9–14, 1978. Kansas City: American Nurses' Association.

Kerlinger, F.N. (1977). The influence of research on education practice. *Educational Researcher, 6,* 5–12.

Neusner, J. (1977). The scholar's apprentice. *Chronicle of Higher Education, 16,* 40.

Shaver, J.P. (1979). The productivity of educational research and the applied-basic research distinction. *Educational Researcher, 8,* 3–9.

Shermis, S. (1962). On becoming an intellectual discipline. *Phi Delta Kappan, 44,* 84–86.

Stevenson, J.S. (1979). Support for an emerging social institution. In F.S. Downs & J.W. Fleming (Eds.), *Issues in nursing research* (pp. 39–66). New York: Appleton-Century-Crofts.

U.S. National Institutes of Health (1978a). *National Conference on Health Research Principles; October 3 and 4, 1978, Conference Report,* Bethesda, MD: Author.

U.S. National Institutes of Health (1978b). G.E. Schwartz & S.M. Weiss (Eds.), *Yale Conference on Behavioral Medicine* (pp. 8–9). (DHEW Publ. No. (NIH) 78–1424) Bethesda, MD: Author.

Williams, C. (1979). The nature and development of conceptual frameworks. In F.S. Downs & J.W. Fleming (Eds.), *Issues in nursing research* (pp. 89–106). New York: Appleton-Century-Crofts.

The Author Comments

"Nursing Science in Transition" was the keynote address at the 1979 annual meeting for the Western Society for Nursing Research. It was one of my most difficult essays because it attempted to address the movement of nursing into more theoretically based work, including that which had no immediate utility or applicability in science. In this paper I attempted a definition of nursing science, in contrast to the definition of nursing research in the 1975 paper.* "Nursing Science in Transition" makes a distinction, which I believe is valid, between science and its tool, research. Batey has used this distinction in her writings before, and I find it useful. This paper also points out that the contributions of nursing research will fall within the interface of biological and behavioral science, and that the future will see more fundamental work in keeping with discoveries in other fields.

—SUSAN R. GORTNER

---

*Ed. note: Chapter 56, "Research for a Practice Profession."

Chapter 22

A Science of Nursing—
To Be or Not to Be?

Harriet R. Feldman

Science is the attempt to make the chaotic diversity of our sense-experience correspond to a logically uniform system of thought. —ALBERT EINSTEIN

The advancement of knowledge in any area requires examination, integration, synthesis, and evaluation of circumscribed phenomena. The purpose of this paper is to advance knowledge of phenomenon described as "nursing science." Questions will be posed and answered in an attempt to: examine "nursing science," its characteristics and purposes; communicate a position with regard to a methodology of knowledge development; and identify a research problem and how it might articulate with a science of nursing.

What Is Science?

Basic to refining a view of "nursing science" is an investigation of science from several perspectives. Science has been described as both product and process (Greene, 1979; Jacobs & Huether, 1978; Jacox, 1974), the former meaning a body of theoretical knowledge (Andreoli & Thompson, 1977; Einstein, 1950; Johnson, 1974) and the latter referring to a method of inquiry (Beckwith & Miller, 1976; Eccles. 1973) or process of knowing (Heisenberg, 1971; Newman, 1979). In relating this to nursing, one might ask if nursing science is a discrete body of knowledge or a system of investigation. Abdellah defines nursing science as "a body of cumulative scientific knowledge, drawn from the physical, biological, and behavioral sciences, that is uniquely nursing" (Abdellah, 1969, p. 8). Greene combines process and product, claiming her definition "provides a standard to determine whether or not a designated body of knowledge constitutes a science" (Greene, 1979, p. 5). Gortner clearly separates the two, noting that "what some have mistaken for science is research, the tool of science" (Gortner, 1980, p. 180).

About the Author

HARRIET R. FELDMAN is currently Professor and Chairperson of the Department of Nursing at Fairleigh Dickinson University. A native New Yorker, Dr. Feldman received her basic nursing education from Long Island College Hospital School of Nursing. She earned a B.S. in Nursing (1968) and a M.S. with a clinical specialty in medical-surgical nursing (1971) from Adelphi University. In 1984, she received a Ph.D. in Nursing from New York University.

Dr. Feldman has worked in various clinical positions in medical-surgical nursing, including experience as a Clinical Nurse Specialist at Long Island Jewish—Hillside Medical Center. From 1975 to 1987, she held a faculty appointment at Adelphi University.

Dr. Feldman is active in a number of professional organizations, including the New York State Nurses' Association (member, Cabinet on Nursing Research, 1990-92), Southern New York League for Nursing, and Sigma Theta Tau, serving as president of the Alpha Omega Chapter. She has presented at more than 12 conferences and has published scholarly papers in *Advances in Nursing Science, Journal of Advanced Nursing, Nursing Research*, and *Image*. She is cofounder and coeditor of *Scholarly Inquiry for Nursing Practice: An International Journal*. Her research interests focus on pain and pain management.

About her career, Dr. Feldman comments "Although I have truly enjoyed the diversity and multitude of roles experienced in nursing, one of my major satisfactions centers around my involvement in research, whether it is my own, collaborative research with colleagues, or the supervision of my students' research. Another major satisfaction is that of sharing ideas with colleagues, whether in the role of classmate or workmate. To this end I meet regularly with a small group of colleagues, and have done so for about 20 years, to discuss the art and science of nursing and plan strategies for change."

How Have Scientific Disciplines Evolved?

The structuring of knowledge resulted from a need to distinguish between different kinds of knowledge (Silva, 1977). Each of the natural and social sciences emerged because different phenomena were "studied or a different perspective (or frame of reference) was used as a basis for the observations and interpretations made . . . a new body of theoretical knowledge was developed and a new science was born" (Johnson, 1974, p. 372–373). Innate curiosity and concern about man and his environment guided this evolution. Although the path of developing the professional disciplines has been parallel, the force guiding its growth has not; that is, logic and social responsibility have prevailed (Johnson, 1974; Benoliel, 1977).

What Is the Purpose of Science?

The aim or purpose of science is "a comprehension, as *complete* as possible, of the connection between the sense experiences in their totality . . . *by the use of a minimum of primary concepts and relations*" (Einstein, 1950 p. 63). More precisely, it is "the discovery of new knowledge, the expansion of existing knowledge, and/or the reaffirming of previously held knowledge" (Andreoli & Thompson, 1977 p. 33). Kerlinger (1973) describes the purpose of science as theory, and further states the aims to explain, understand, predict and control natural events.

An aim of nursing science is to "define common goals and guide the practice of nursing" (Jacobs & Huether, 1978, p. 64). Edgerton (1973) cites the aims of establishing legitimacy and autonomy as a basis for developing a science of nursing, and sees these as "barriers to improved preparation for problem solving." It is difficult to separate the aim of legitimacy from that of comprehending a discrete body of knowledge in a discipline lacking consensus in many basic areas of definition and development; however, arriving at a distinction will probably expedite the advancement of nursing science.

What Are the Characteristics of Science?

Silva lists the following characteristics of science as a system:

1. Science must show a certain coherence.
2. Science is concerned with definite fields of knowledge.
3. Science is preferably expressed in universal statements.
4. The statements of science must be true or probably true.
5. The statements of science must be logically ordered.
6. Science must explain its investigations and arguments (Silva, 1977, p. 60).

These characteristics combine product and process and may be useful in exploring whether or not, and to what extent a science of nursing exists. Prior to such an investigation, it is necessary for the writer to affirm a position with respect to the earlier questions posed in this paper.

Position Statements

After reviewing a number of articles (Donaldson & Crowley, 1978; Jacobs & Huether, 1978; Johnson, 1978; Murphy, 1978; Sleicher, 1981) it seems reasonable to conclude that at this time there is no science of nursing; that is, there is no identified empirical body of knowledge specific to nursing (the position of science as product, not process, is taken). "Such terms as *embryo, infant, emerging, pre-paradigm,* and *pre-science* are used to describe nursing in its quest to identify and develop a theoretical body of knowledge that gives clear direction to education, research, and practice" (Feldman, 1980, p. 87). Carper (1978) emphasizes the critical need for the sense of urgency about deriving such knowledge. Jacox (1974), in the historical context of science development, takes the position that theory construction is less developed and tested in the "relatively new" science of nursing. While a discrete body of knowledge is not to be found, there seem to be some humble beginnings, particularly with respect to conceptual models. This writer supports such efforts.

As already stated, new sciences evolve because different phenomena or a different perspective on the same phenomena are experienced. The man-environment dyad guides this development. In nursing, specific "building blocks" or subsets have been identified in several conceptual frameworks, namely, man, environment, care providers (nurses), and the end-state of health (Walker, 1971). These subsets, along with definitions and models/frameworks are prerequisite to theory construction, which is, in turn, prerequisite to science. Ultimately, in a practice discipline, science should direct, not be defined by, practice. There should be movement from primarily lower level theory to prescriptive theory construction.

To summarize the writer's position: there is currently no discrete body of knowledge exclusive to nursing; a science of nursing is essential and early beginnings are identifiable; and, the purposes of nursing science are to explain, understand, and predict phenomena relating to man and his environment in order to guide nursing practice.

What Is Envisioned?

Perhaps initial statements of what is *not* envisioned are useful to this discussion. A "grand theory," for example, is neither envisioned nor advocated. Testing basic science theories is *not* supported as a basis for theory development in nursing. Exclusive use of the traditional scientific method of inquiry for deriving nursing knowledge is *not* recommended.

While a "grand theory" does not seem feasible or desirable, the existence of a myriad of conceptual frameworks to build theory is also unrealistic. Johnson (1978) writes about concentrating efforts on the development of a smaller number of conceptual schemata, and this seems most worthwhile. Frameworks used in other disciplines are not specific to nursing's purpose; they are drawn "largely from the work of basic scientists. . . and present only a partial understanding of man . . ." (Johnson, 1978, p. 7). Borrowing is advocated only if concepts, models and theories can be supported or synthesized from a nursing frame of reference (Ellis, 1968; Phillips, 1977) and "worked into a new conceptual set" (Walker, 1971, p. 430). The use of a variety of approaches to the expansion of knowledge is proposed. Creativity, flexibility and openness are envisioned.

Admittedly, the above stance is general, perhaps even vague in the context of communicating an "ideal" or "vision" of nursing science itself. No visible theory unique to nursing has been uncovered by this writer. This makes it very difficult to have an ideal; that is, ideal in relation to what? In envisioning an "ideal," one usually thinks of a "real" that exists or comes close to existence in an ideal state; e.g., my ideal house. In nursing there is little in the way of science to which to relate an ideal. Perhaps the vision cannot be so circumscribed. Perhaps it is simply that "nursing as a professional discipline does not develop independently the knowledge necessary for the practice of nursing. Rather, it draws, as does any applied or professional science, on materials from a wide range of basic disciplines and sciences, translating and adapting them into a form applicable to the achievement of the goals of the profession" (Deloughery, 1972–1973, p. 99).

Examining the Characteristics

A closer examination of the characteristics of nursing science will serve to identify the manifestations of its existence, give evidence of what is needed to meet the stated "visions," and describe how its development should progress.

1. *"Science must constitute a coherent whole of interrelated facts, principles, laws, and theories which are appropriately ordered"* (Silva, 1977, p. 60). Such coherence is far from a reality, although tacit knowledge of recurring themes used by nursing scholars is consistent, suggesting "boundaries of an area for systematic enquiry and theory development . . ." (Donaldson & Crowley, 1978, p. 113). Also, phenomena of interest defined by the various conceptual frameworks are consistent. A concentrated effort toward establishing and interrelating facts, principles, laws, and theories is greatly needed in nursing.

2. Man *"must specialize so that he might know one field, or an aspect of it, well"* (Silva, 1977 p. 60). To this point, knowledge of the nursing field is diffuse. This above quote implies two things for nursing: the need for an acceptable (to the profession) definition of nursing's uniqueness and sub-specialization in the conduct of research. Regarding the former, the "field" of nursing, in order to be "known well," should be developed from a common view of what it is. The latter implication supports a concerted effort of distinct groups of researchers investigating different phenomena so that all "aspects" of the "field" be "known well."

3. *". . . science seeks to discover the universal characteristics of phenomena under investigation"* (Silva, 1977, p. 60).

We are far from expressing universal statements about phenomena; however, present conceptual models are attempting to define and operationalize characteristics of man, environment, health, and nursing process.

4. *"The statements of science must be true or probably true"* (Silva, 1977, p. 60).

What is truth? What is the true nature of things? Does truth change? Perhaps the issue is not that of truth, but of what is accepted by the scientific community at a given time. Kuhn (1970) describes paradigms or belief systems accepted by others. Sufficient anomalies challenge the belief system, giving rise to new paradigms. This replacement theory of science development is characterized by change. Nursing science, in its pre-paradigm state, does not have "truths" or a belief set accepted by its constituents, so it falls short of this characteristic of science. However, while "in the early stages of the development of any science different men confronting the same range of phenomena, but not usually all the same particular phenomena, describe and interpret them in different ways. What is surprising . . . is that such initial divergences should ever largely disappear . . . [but] they do disappear . . ." (Kuhn, 1970, p. 17).

5. *"Science is usually best served through careful observance of scientific methods such as the deductive-inductive or the analytic-synthetic method"* (Silva, 1977, p. 60).

Two points are at issue here: how can we facilitate quality research? and what methods or internal processes of building a body of knowledge are advocated? Feldman (1980) identifies several areas that will build the research enterprise in a quality way: collaborative efforts of nurse researchers involving "think tanks" and networks for sharing information; quality education, including the use of mentors or role models in doctoral programs; and, communication of research findings to clinical practitioners, educators and administrators.

The second question relates to the process and to levels of theory development. The inductive approach to building a science of nursing has been demonstrated to be a useful method of inquiry (Quint, 1967). It probably will be most useful in establishing basic propositions that can be systematically related to one another, thereby facilitating the development of conceptual frameworks. Deductive reasoning involves "taking statements assumed to be true and deriving other statements" (Jacox, 1974, p. 8). Both deduction and induction are needed in theory development. A third method is hypotheticodeductive, which combines inductive and deductive processes and employs hypothesis testing of inferences. Any and all of these processes are encouraged, as long as methodological "rules" are adhered to.

Dickoff and James (1968) have identified four levels of theory: factor-isolating, factor-relating (situation depicting), situation-relating, and situation-producing (prescriptive), the fourth presupposing the existence of the other three. They contend that all theory in a practice discipline is for the sake of practice, and situation-producing theory is for the sake of shaping reality. "To develop useable practice theory, the concepts chosen and the related formulations must be seen in what may be called the mid-range" (Jacobs & Huether, 1978, p. 70). Middle-range theory, according to Merton, guides empirical inquiry. It involves abstractions, (but close enough to observed data to permit testing), deals with delimited aspects of phenomena, and "suggests specific hypotheses which are tested by seeing whether the inferences from them are empirically confirmed" (Merton, 1967, p. 40). Theory development at all levels is desirable. The more research activity toward the systematic, logical ordering of knowledge, the more likely it is that nursing science will advance.

6. *"Scientists have a responsibility not only to report their research findings, but as importantly, to explain the arguments and demonstrations which led them to their conclusions"* (Silva, 1977, p. 60). This relates to accountability and commitment as well as responsibility. The writer strongly encourages the reporting of research methods and findings, and notes the increasing number of research publications in nursing. Other methods of reporting are also supported; e.g., colloquia, peer review panels, informal and formal presentations to nurses at all levels and in all types of practice. A commitment to communicating research will help to insure quality investigations and hypothesis-testing in practice settings.

In summary, the advancement of a science of nursing can be facilitated by defining nursing's uniqueness, promoting scholarliness (Meleis, Wilson & Chater, 1980) and commitment (Sleicher, 1981), collaborating with others (Bishop, 1981), explicating and honing in on definite fields of knowledge, testing models in practice (Johnson, 1978), and communicating research findings. "The science of nursing will grow as nurses who possess the knowledge and tools gained in doctoral study endeavor to state explicitly the unifying characteristics, hypothetical generaliza-

tions, and theories of this emerging science. Only as such nurses establish connections between different phenomena and identify the predictive principles can there be technological application" (Rogers, 1963, p. 95).

Establishing Connections: An Example

A question of interest to this writer is: What is the relationship between perceived pain tolerance and articulation of body concept?

The first step, that is, establishing a connection between the phenomena of pain and body concept, is prerequisite to identifying predictive principles that will guide pain management. Neither of these terms or concepts can be directly observed, but they can be interpreted through their relationships to certain constructs. Fawcett (1978a, 1978b), referring to Dubin's work, describes five types of "units" useful to the construction of theories. These are enumerative, associative, relational, statistical, and summative, and they are the basic building blocks of theories. She further states that the essential units of nursing—i.e., person, environment, health, and nursing—are summative (global, ill-defined), and that less complex, well-defined units are more useful to theory development. While body image is a summative unit, articulation of body concept is enumerative or "a property that will always be present, regardless of the condition of the thing that is observed or imagined" (Fawcett, 1978b, p. 21). Likewise, pain is summative, but pain tolerance would seem to be enumerative.

If a relationship between these two units is established, it would provide a basis for investigating a variety of pain management techniques hypothesized to be effective with individuals of differing body concepts. Once these connections are established, predictive principles can be identified; e.g., an individual with a highly articulated body concept will respond best to "relaxation" as a method of pain management. Certainly, this is most relevant to building nursing knowledge, and particularly to explicating relationships between and among four essential units or building blocks of nursing.

Summary

This paper has presented: views of nursing science, based on readings in the basic and social sciences and nursing; an assessment of the present state of a science of nursing, using specific characteristics of science as a system; methods for facilitating the advancement of nursing knowledge; and, a research question that connects two phenomena of concern to nursing as prerequisite to prediction and prescription. A great deal of thinking and soul searching occurred in formulating and articulating views on nursing science; it is expected that this process will continue for many years.

References

Abdellah, F. (1969). The nature of nursing science. *Nursing Research, 18*, 390–393.

Andreoli, K., & Thompson, C. (1977). The nature of science in nursing. *Image, 9*, 32–37.

Beckwith, J., & Miller, L. (1976). Behind the mask of objective science. *The Sciences, 16*, 16–19.

Benoliel, J.Q. (1977). The interaction between theory and research. *Nursing Outlook, 25*, 108–113.

Bishop, B. (1981). A case for collaboration. *Nursing Outlook, 29*, 110–111.

Carper, B. (1978). Fundamental patterns of knowing in nursing. *Advances in Nursing Science, 1*(1), 13–23.

Deloughery, G. (1972–1973). Some problems in using basic science theory in professional research and study. *Educational Horizons, 51*, 97–99.

Dickoff, J., & James, P. (1968). A theory of theories: a position paper. *Nursing Research, 17*, 197–203.

Donaldson, S., & Crowley, D. (1978). The discipline of nursing. *Nursing Outlook, 26*, 113–120.

Eccles, J. (1973). The disciplines of science with special reference to the neuro-sciences. *Daedalus, 102*, 85–99.

Edgerton, S. (1973). The technological imagination: A philosopher looks at nursing. *Journal of Thought, 1*, 57–65.

Einstein, A. (1950). *Out of my later years.* New York: Philosophical Library.

Ellis, R. (1968). Characteristics of significant theories. *Nursing Research, 17*, 217–222.

Fawcett, J. (1978a). The relationship between theory and research: A double helix. *Advances in Nursing Science, 1*(4), 49–61.

Fawcett, J. (1978b). The 'what' of theory development. In *Theory development: What, why, how?* New York: National League for Nursing.

Feldman, H. (1980). Nursing research in the 1980s: Issues and implications. *Advances in Nursing Science, 3*(4), 85–92.

Flaskerud, J., & Halloran, E. (1980). Areas of agreement in nursing theory development. *Advances in Nursing Science, 3*(1), 1–7.

Gortner, S. (1980). Nursing science in transition. *Nursing Research, 29*, 180–183.

Greene, J. (1979). Science, nursing, and nursing science: A conceptual analysis. *Advances in Nursing Science, 2*(4), 57–64.

Heisenberg, W. (1971). *Physics and beyond: Encounters and conversations.* New York: Harper and Row.

Jacobs, M., & Huether, S. (1978). Nursing science: The theory-practice linkage. *Advances in Nursing Science, 1*(1), 63–73.

Jacox, A. (1974). Theory construction in nursing: An overview. *Nursing Research, 23*, 4–13.

Johnson, D.E. (1968). Theory in nursing: Borrowed and unique. *Nursing Research, 17*, 206–209.

Johnson, D.E. (1974). Development of theory: A requisite for nursing as a primary health profession. *Nursing Research, 23*, 372–377.

Johnson, D.E. (1978). State of the art of theory development in nursing. In *Theory development: What, why, how?* New York: National League for Nursing.

Kerlinger, F. (1973). *Foundations of behavioral research.* New York: Holt, Rinehart, and Winston.

Kuhn, T. (1970). *The structure of scientific revolutions* (2nd ed.). Chicago: The University of Chicago Press.

Meleis, A., Wilson, H., & Chater, S. (1980). Toward scholarliness in doctoral dissertations: An analytical model. *Research in Nursing and Health, 3*, 115–124.

Merton, R. (1967). *On theoretical sociology: Five essays, old and new.* New York: The Free Press.

Murphy, J. (1978). Toward a philosophy of nursing. In N.L. Chaska (Ed.), *The nursing profession: A time to speak.* New York: McGraw-Hill.

Newman, M. (1972). Nursing's theoretical evolution. *Nursing Outlook, 20*, 449–453.

Newman, M. (1979). *Theory development in nursing.* Philadelphia: F.A. Davis.

Parsons, T. (1968). *The structure of social action* (Vol. 1). New York: Free Press.

Phillips, J. (1977). Nursing systems and nursing models. *Image, 9*, 4–7.

Quint, J. (1967). The case for theories generated from empirical data. *Nursing Research, 16*, 109–114.

Rogers, M.E. (1963). Building a strong educational foundation. *American Journal of Nursing, 63*, 94–95.

Silva, M. (1977). Philosophy, science, theory: Interrelationships and implications for nursing research. *Image, 9,* 59–63.

Sleicher, M. (1981). Nursing is not a profession. *Nursing and Health Care, 2,* 186–191.

Turabian, K.L. (1973). *A manual for writers of term papers,* *theses, and dissertations* (4th ed.). Chicago: The University of Chicago Press.

Walker, L. (1971). Toward a clearer understanding of the concept of nursing theory. *Nursing Research, 20,* 428–435.

The Author Comments

In the Fall of 1980, when I was about halfway through the doctoral program at New York University, I enrolled in Divisional Seminar I. This course focused on theory building in nursing and the development of nursing science. Course objectives were (a) to identify the relationship of theory to the development of nursing science, (b) to identify similarities and differences in several approaches to theory development, (c) to develop or refine one's own criteria for the evaluation of nursing theory, and (d) to elaborate a position regarding the kind of theory development that will facilitate the progress of nursing science.

One of the requirements of the course was to write a paper discussing, both philosophically and analytically, a range of views of science and of theory. Students were asked to take a position on what nursing science is today and what it could become, and to discuss the processes by which their vision of nursing science could be actualized. Also included was a discussion of how an actual or intended research effort might articulate with nursing science at large.

The paper I wrote, "A Science of Nursing—To Be or Not To Be?" was so well received by the course professor that I decided to submit it for publication. *Image* was selected because so much of the content of the article connected with the central themes of Sigma Theta Tau's newly proposed 10-year plan. The rest is history.

As an epilogue, the publication was very positively received by many faculty and students at New York University. In fact, the professor who taught Divisional Seminar I used it as an exemplar for students in subsequent course offerings.

—HARRIET R. FELDMAN

Chapter 23

Nursing's Scientific Quest

Jean Watson

Nursing seems to be suffering in its quest for a scientific foundation for its practice. Like the mythological Danaids who kept filling their jars with water only to have it leak through holes, nursing finds its search for scientific underpinnings as elusive as the liquid. Its quest has been influenced by a traditional philosophy of science that is outdated and inappropriate for nursing as are newer concepts from the behavioral sciences. The result has been confusion with nursing and concern about its scientific progress.

In spite of Florence Nightingale's foresight and progressive views on nursing and nursing research, the profession has perpetuated a practice-oriented "doing" culture, almost to the exclusion of its intellectual and scientific development. The term nursing science was rarely used in the nursing literature until the 1950s. Abdellah cites an incident in 1949, whereby a researcher sent a report of a study to a leading nursing journal only to have it returned because "nurses do not do research; they are not interested in research and that furthermore, research has no place in nursing" (Abdellah, 1969, p. 390). However, as nursing education became more associated with higher education in general, nursing norms and expectations began to change. Educators realized that baccalaureate, graduate nursing, and nurse scientist programs required a theoretical-research orientation to prepare students, improve practice, and further nursing's scientific base. Charges were then made that nursing was becoming too removed from practice, too theoretical: Knowing was separated from doing. As recently as the 1960s, there was debate as to whether it was appropriate for nurses to do research, and nursing theory development was questioned or had to be justified (Norris, 1969).

Nursing has indeed received contradictory messages regarding its legitimacy in pursuing research, theory, and scientific advancement both within and outside the profession. Even now nurses have to justify

About the Author

JEAN (HARMAN) WATSON writes "I was born and grew up in West Virginia. However, I have lived, studied, and worked in Colorado for the past 27 years. After completing a nursing diploma program at Lewis Gale School of Nursing, Roanoke, Virginia, I felt deprived of the liberal and broader education I believed necessary to practice and value nursing as a distinct profession. My husband and I moved to Colorado, where he completed law school at the University of Colorado and I returned to school, earning a B.S.N. and a M.S. degree with a specialty in psychiatric nursing. During the same time, I had my daughter Jennifer. After completing my master's, I taught at the University of Wyoming for 3 years while my husband was in the Air Force. During this time, I had my second daughter, Julie. I then returned to Colorado, where my husband resumed law practice and I resumed my doctoral studies in social and clinical psychology, educational psychology, and counseling, receiving a Ph.D. in educational psychology in 1973.

I joined the University of Colorado faculty in the Fall of 1973 and have taught in all programs and levels in the school. I was actively involved in developing the doctoral program in psychosocial nursing and was Director of the doctoral program in 1980 to 1981. When I left for a sabbatical in 1981 through 1982, I was a visiting Kellogg Fellow in Western Australia, and did work in New Zealand, Thailand, Taiwan, and India. I also spent a semester at the University of Virginia as a visiting professor working with their nursing doctoral program. I have been a student of transcendental phenomenology after conducting research in Australia and have studied phenomenology as a methodology for nursing science. Most recently, I have been lecturing and researching on a Fulbright Award in Sweden.

After returning from my sabbatical in 1982, I held the position of Associate Dean for Graduate Programs. I was selected and appointed Dean of the School of Nursing at the University of Colorado Health Science Center in 1984; I served as Dean until 1990.

My personal interests involve my family, international travel, humanities, nursing, and personal mental and spiritual growth. I continue to evolve my philosophy and views about human care in nursing. My work is now studied as a theory and used by several nursing programs in the United States and several foreign countries. I currently am working on a book that builds on all my efforts to date.

Most recently, I have established the Center for Human Caring at the University of Colorado and serve as its Director. Center efforts range from specific curricular activities to piloting and researching new educational-professional practice models of excellence in human caring. The Colorado Center and my efforts are now directed toward offering public and professional forums and institutes, hosting resident scholars from diverse backgrounds, sponsoring interdisciplinary, international programs and projects, and disseminating information through formal and informal educational-research programs and official publications."

and rationalize a theory-research goal far more often than those in other professional or academic disciplines. The reasons are many. In some important ways nursing has been subjected to different social, political, and scientific forces than those in other disciplines.

Historically, medical and male norms influenced nursing's earlier professional practice and educational development and more recently norms from the fields of science and behavioral science have influenced nursing's scientific development. Nursing's established ties and control by doctors and hospitals and society's male-

female role expectations played an important part in nursing's emphasis on "doing," its status, problems with authority, self-denial, and lack of esteem. Its recent attempts in scientific development have often been guided by other fields that are inappropriate models for nursing and have resulted in nurses becoming sociologists, biologists, and psychologists, without their directly addressing nursing problems and issues.

Somewhere in the midst of these strong opposing external forces nursing lost sight of its nursing leaders' call for research aimed fundamentally at the solution of human health problems. Such leaders as Nightingale (1860), Henderson (1964), Krueter (1957), and Hall (1964) were advocates of an integrated approach to scientific study that would capitalize on nursing's richness and complexity and not separate practice from research, the art from the science, the "doing" of nursing from the "knowing," the psychological from the physical, and theory from clinical care.

Nursing needs to take a fresh look at its scientific progress, particularly in light of the insights of these earlier leaders. Perhaps then we can untravel and explain some of the obstacles and find direction in which nursing can move forward as a science in its own right, without apologies or excuses, and with confidence and zeal.

Changes in the Philosophy of Science

During the past three or four decades, the philosophy of science influencing nursing has undergone review and change. Theory concerning the nature of science has largely been the product of philosophers who were either Vienna Circle Logical Positivists, the dominant group in the early 1930s, or others who shared similar views (Webster, Jacox, & Baldwin, 1981). Their orientation to science and its progress consisted of a set of assumptions that became dogma. These assumptions had to do with standards of logic, formalization, objectivity, falsity, truth, observational and operational terms, laws, predictions, and reductionism. Their research was based on a single scientific methodology that was neutral with respect to human values. This set of assumptions has been called the "Received View" of the nature of science, scientific theory, and scientific methodology (Laudan, 1977; Suppe, 1977).

The assumptions of the Received View concerning the nature of science have since been overthrown by those scientists and philosophers who were original proponents of Logical Positivism. During the years that these scientific assumptions were being revised and rejected within the science community, other developing disciplines such as psychology, sociology, education,

and later nursing were trying to adhere to some of the Received View principles. Many of these disciplines still adhere to these principles even though these views have long since been abandoned by others in the science community and are clearly incompatible with the scientific problems and aims of the disciplines in question, especially nursing.

The changing, and at the same time unchanging, views of the history and philosophy of science have contributed to the confusion and ambivalence surrounding nursing's scientific development. The results are that once nursing began its scientific quest, it seemingly accepted uncritically the Received View as the truth about science. Consequently, when scientific advancement became a legitimate pursuit for nursing, nursing theorists and researchers began to translate their understanding of the nature of nursing into Received View notions and attempted to promote nursing research according to its scientific methodology—such as reductionism, quantifiability, objectivity, and operationalization. In the meantime, some of the rich, nonquantifiable, qualitative, subjective, emotional "wholes of nursing" that have long been proposed by nursing's leaders became submerged. Why? Because they weren't scientific or researchable or testable. Some of the components of nursing may never be scientific by the criteria of the Received View, but does that make nursing phenomena bad science?

Dichotomies Within Nursing

Many physicists, philosophers, and mathematicians have been aware of the fundamental problems associated with the Received View of science. Bronowski emphasized that no scientific theory is a collection of facts, that no theory is true or false. He reports, "Science is nothing else than the search to discover unity in the wild variety of nature or . . . in the variety of our experiences. Poetry, painting, the arts are the same search. . ." (Bronowski, 1965, p. 16). He pointed out that the discoveries of science are the act of creation—the same act in original science as well as in original art. Unfortunately, only now are some of the "younger" disciplines—education, psychology, nursing, sociology—seeing the light. As a result, nursing has created a host of false dichotomies as to what is nursing and what is credible and legitimate for the development of nursing science. We are all familiar with the confusions and dichotomies evident in such schisms as:

Nursing art vs Nursing sciences
Nursing profession vs Nursing discipline
Doing vs Knowing
Caring vs Curing
Nursing practice vs Nursing Theory
Subjective vs Objective
Mind vs Body
Psychosocial vs Psychobiological

At the same time, nursing is replete with conflicting methodologies for practice, research, and theory development. Nursing possesses a set of rights and wrongs that are still largely guided by outdated Received View notions. Criteria from psychology, education, sociology, physiology, and formal philosophy still influence nursing research development. The scientific method is considered the one and only process for scientific discovery, experimental quantitative research methodology, and design. Philosophy, in particular, has guided nursing theory development with hierarchical notions of prescriptive theory, predictive theory, descriptive theory, factor-isolating theory, factor-relating theory, as well as created some nurse researchers' preoccupation with syntax, correspondence rules, formalization, and axiomatization. But, clearly nursing's history is full of other notions associated with intuitionism, subjectivism, wholism, traditionalism, utilitarianism, and humanism. The results are sets of conflicting research traditions, leading nursing into a double bind.

If nursing's scientific progress is viewed from a Received View perspective, it may be considered out of step with the mainstream of science because it is largely impressionistic, nonscientific and not readily quantifiable, objective, or formalized. However, in the view of recent scientific influences, largely from the social sciences and education, nursing may be considered more in step with that notion of scientific progress because it has tried to conform to Received View standards. On the other hand, if nursing is viewed from a non-Received View perspective, it is still considered out of step because it has been adhering too closely to the reductionist, logical, positivist view of science. A set of false dichotomies has been established that makes many facets of nursing incompatible. But the situation may change; revisions in nursing's views about research are emerging.

Nursing's Changing Research Tradition

Upon reflection, it appears that early nursing leaders were attempting to create a research tradition for nursing. That is, they tried to establish a set of general assumptions about entities and processes in the domain of study and the appropriate methods to be used for investigating problems and constructing theories (Laudan, 1977). For example, Nightingale talked of a "new art and a new science" and presented nursing as an art that required organized and scientific training. She did not create a false dichotomy between science and art. Later leaders—Virginia Henderson, Lydia Hall, Frances Krueter—promoted concepts of nursing that were consistent with Nightingale. For example, Henderson defined the nurse's role as very subjective and qualitative. She believed the nurse should, ". . .get inside the skin of each of [her] patients in order to know what [he] needs" (Henderson, 1964, p. 63). In describing the richness of this role, she said the nurse is "temporarily the consciousness of the unconscious, the love of life for the suicidal, the leg of the amputee, the eyes of the newly blind, a means of locomotion for the infant, knowledge and confidence for the young mother, the mouthpiece for those too weak or withdrawn to speak and so on" (Henderson, 1964, p. 63). At the same time, she emphasized the necessity of clinical nursing research. Hall believed the uniqueness of nursing was its nurturing aspect of care; she emphasized feelings as well as knowledge. Krueter discussed nursing care as "more related to 'pathos' in that the feelings are touched" (Kreuter, 1957, pp. 302, 304).

While these leaders have strongly influenced the development of nursing and more or less succeeded in promoting a nursing research tradition, nursing has still not actualized what these leaders have described as the essence of nursing or that aspect that is self-directed. One reason is the impact of the later competing and compelling research traditions from other fields, along with the Received View prejudices about the nature of science. It may be more than a coincidence that this transaction and break from the early research tradition, including the generation of a new research tradition, roughly corresponds to the development of nurse scientist programs in which nurses were doctorally prepared in a field outside of nursing. However, as nursing has advanced with its own doctoral programs, it has been subjected to the same processes of scientific development as other sciences—that is, first adopting Received Views ideas and then undergoing its own processes of rejection. For example, consider the following quotes from nurse scientists in the late 1960s and even late 1970s, most of whom were doctorally prepared outside of nursing:

Definitions . . . are operationally defined . . . whenever possible, they should be expressed in observable and quantifiable terms.

The testing of hypotheses either serves to confirm the validity of the theory or leads to a modification of the postulate upon which the theory was based.

All concepts must be subjected to rigorous testing. . .

The art of nursing must not be confused with the science of nursing.

The former concerns itself with intuitive and technical skills and also the more important supportive aspects of nursing; the latter concerns itself with scientific truths. . . (Abdellah, 1969, pp. 391–392)

Our contention is that any practice-minded nursing theory must be a theory of the situation-producing level. (Dickoff & James, 1968, p. 201)

What is significant for nursing . . . is that which pertains to practice. Generation of knowledge for the sake of knowledge is not the raison d'être for the profession. (Ellis, 1968, p. 222)

Theories must be rigorously tested by empirical studies before they can be accepted and then utilized in the real world of nursing practice, clinical research, and education. (Fawcett, 1978, p. 27)

In science, the term theory refers to a set of verified interrelated concepts and theoretical statements. (Hardy, 1978, p. 77)

The clinical practice of nursing requires the development of prescriptive theories. (Donaldson & Crowley, 1977, p. 14)

What a dilemma for nursing's scientific advancement. On one hand, nursing has been told, and we all know in a priori Kantian sense, it is rich, sensitive, complex, caring, subjective, artistic, practice-directed, focused on doing, feelings, and so on. On the other hand, it is presented with insistence on being scientific in the traditional objective Received View sense of science—clearly a double bind. However, more recent authors are suggesting alternative views consistent with Laudan's context for understanding the evolution of the nature of science. The following examples illustrate the change in view during the 1970s and early 1980s that perhaps will generate a new research tradition for nursing.

Nurse scientists must . . . tolerate loosely constructed theoretical notions. (Hardy, 1978, p. 77)

Theorizing is a form of dialogue with reality, an attempt to find meaning in the world one lives in. (Zderad, 1978, p. 39)

Like the nurse scientists, the nurse poets, the nurse artists also share an articulated vision of experience. (Zderad, 1978, p. 48)

Nursing is moving from actions based on facts, or limited units of knowledge (such as nursing procedures), to actions based on theories or broad units of knowledge with wide applicability . . . We are a practice discipline, but we must not be exclusively practice-oriented. (Rinehart, 1978, p. 74)

One of the reasons I have been pursuing cross-cultural studies on caring behaviors and processes is that scientific knowledge of care is limited; and yet, I hold it is the central concept and essence of nursing. (Leininger, 1979, p. xii)

The way to understand nursing is to identify, describe, and research those central humanistic-scientific factors that are essential to effecting positive health change. . . The science of caring combines sciences with the humanities. The science of caring cannot be completely neutral with respect to human values. (Leininger, 1979, p. xii)

The current discussion of the role of the observer

in physics (quantum mechanics and relative theory) challenges the traditional view of the scientist as purely objective. . . The observer, therefore, cannot be a neutral point in the study. . . In the future, it will probably be more important to state the observer's position, values and beliefs, or whatever else is pertinent, as part of the research protocol. (Winstead-Fry, 1980, p. 6)

In recent years, nursing has become disenchanted with traditional approaches to health and illness care. This disenchantment has lead to a re-examination of the concept of health and the role of the nurse . . . (Naravan & Joslin, 1980, p. 27)

These views suggest a new research tradition that can provide nursing with the scientific and social freedom and openness to solve both conceptual and empirical problems. It is an alternative to the Received View and permits nursing to return to the richness and complexities inherent in its social and scientific roots and goals. It may not be totally explanatory, predictive, or directly testable. Its success will be judged as to whether it can provide nursing with some adequate solution to an ever increasing range of empirical conceptual problems (Laudan, 1977).

Nursing is subject to all the problems of an emerging discipline that wishes to make itself credible and respectable. It has been burdened not only by the Received View of the nature of science, but by similar, rigid views associated with women in society, and by traditional ties to a male-dominated medical care system. Nursing now has both the scientific and sexual-social freedom to integrate and synthesize the false dichotomies and explore a whole range of scientific and methodological options. These options are consistent with past visions of nursing as well as the changing views of scientific growth. New alternatives found in nursing doctoral programs rather than in other disciplines may free nursing to recover and restore what it rightfully owns.

References

Abdellah, F.G. (1969). The nature of nursing science. *Nursing Research, 18*, 390–393.

Bronowski, J. (1965). *Science and human values* (rev. ed.). New York: Harper & Row.

Dickoff, J., & James, P. (1968). A theory of theories: a position paper. *Nursing Research, 17*, 197–203.

Donaldson, S.K., & Crowley, D.M. (1977). Discipline of nursing: Structure and relationship to practice. In M.V. Batey (Ed.), *Optimizing environments for health: Nursing's unique perspective.* Communicating Nursing Research, Vol. 10 (pp. 1–22). Boulder, CO: WICHE.

Ellis, R. (1968). Characteristics of significant theories. *Nursing Research, 17*, 217–222.

Fawcett, J. (1978). The 'what' of theory development. In *Theory development: What, why, how?* (NLN Pub. 15–1708, pp. 75–86). New York: National League for Nursing.

Hall, L.E. (1964). Nursing—what is it? *Canadian Nurse, 60*, 150–154.

Hardy, M.E. (1978). Evaluating nursing theory. In *Theory development: What, why, how?* (NLN Pub. 15–1708, pp. 75–86). New York: National League for Nursing.

Henderson, V. (1964). The nature of nursing. *American Journal of Nursing, 64*, 62–68.

Kreuter, F.R. (1957). What is good nursing care? *Nursing Outlook, 5*, 302–304.

Laudan, L. (1977). *Progress and its problems: Towards a theory of scientific growth.* Berkeley, CA: University of California Press.

Leininger, M. (1979). Foreword. In J. Watson (Ed.), *Nursing: The philosophy and science of caring* (p. xii). Boston: Little, Brown.

Naravan, S.M., & Joslin, D.J. (1980). Crisis theory and intervention: A critique of the medical model and proposal of a holistic nursing model. *Advances in Nursing Science, 2*(4), 27–39.

Nightingale, F. (1860). *Notes on nursing: What it is and what it is not.* New York: Appleton.

Norris, C.M. (Ed.). (1969). *Proceedings, First Nursing Theory Conference.* Kansas City: Department of Nursing Education, University of Kansas Medical Center.

Rinehart, J.M. (1978). The 'how' of theory development in nursing. In *Theory development: What, why, how?* (NLN Pub. 15–1708, pp. 75–86). New York: National League for Nursing.

Suppe, F. (Ed.). (1977). *The structure of scientific theories* (2nd ed.). Champaign: University of Illinois Press.

Webster, G., Jacox, A., & Baldwin, B. (1981). Nursing theory and the ghost of the received view. In H. Grace & J. McCloskey (Eds.), *Current issues in nursing* (pp. 26–35). Boston: Blackwell Scientific.

Winstead-Fry, P. (1980). The scientific method and its impact on holistic health. *Advances in Nursing Science, 2*(4), 1–8.

Zderad, L.T. (1978). From here-and-now to theory: Reflexations on 'how.' In *Theory development: what, why, how?* (NLN Pub. 15–1708, pp. 75–86). New York: National League for Nursing.

The Author Comments

The ideas for this article evolved from my concern with nursing's human dimensions and the conflict between traditional science and the view of nursing as a human science. Some of the article was written while traveling in Greece (hence, the Greek mythology); other parts were tied to ideas presented in a Sigma Theta Tau research keynote entitled "The Paradox of Nursing Paradigms."

Later, these ideas and concerns were influenced by my experience in teaching the doctoral theory course at the University of Colorado developed by Dr. Ada Jacox in conjunction with philosopher of science Dr. Glenn Webster. As I worked to refine the course, I linked the concepts associated with the changing nature of science with some of my earlier thinking about nursing being both art and science. At the time I wrote the article, I had completed the book *Nursing, The Philosophy and Science of Caring*, in which I tried to solve some of the same issues related to caring.

In order to stimulate doctoral students, I felt it important to take the concepts from the class and integrate them with my previous thinking and writing. The first draft of this article was presented as a paper to the doctoral students in an attempt to synthesize my views of the material they were studying.

—JEAN WATSON

Chapter 24

The History and Philosophy of Nursing Science and Research

Susan R. Gortner

The research tradition is so young in nursing that only in the past few years has there been comment about the philosophical orientations that might guide research, including methods; discovery in contrast to justification or proof; and ethics and politics. These topics of philosophy of science are now beginning to intrigue many who have been involved with developments in nursing science. For example, one can ask if nursing practice should continue to be the major source of research ideas (as historically it has). One can posit, as has Munhall (1982), that experimental or scientific methods are incompatible with a humanistic, holistic philosophy. Munhall's solution is to discard quantifications. For many of these issues that intrigue us and others, a review of the history of science is illuminating.

Practice as the Source of Knowledge

Early Years

Concepts of nursing practice have influenced the subject matter of research since the beginning of our history. The concerns of the times have varied over the past 150 years, with some early concerns remaining prominent even today. From the Nightingale era onward, the poor quality of care for the sick in hospitals and in the home called attention to the need for qualified caregivers and thus prompted the development of formal programs of nursing education. For over 100 years, education was viewed as the means to the improvement of practice.

At the turn of the century, the concern was for improvement of the public's health. Mortality rates were high due to the major communicable diseases of childhood and adulthood. Maternal and infant health had yet to profit from prenatal care and improved obstetrical practices. Most surgery was done in the home. The literature in professional journals addressed problems associated with tuberculosis, meningitis, scarlet fever, and other communicable diseases. By the early 1920s, case studies began to appear in the literature, as did care plans based around specific groups of patients and procedures. A review of the literature for the period 1930–1960 (Gortner & Nahm, 1977), as well as interviews with such leaders as Lucile Petry Leone, suggest that the need for systematic evaluation of nursing techniques had its origins in the post-depression years. In part, this was because the graduate nurse had returned both to the hospital and to the graduate nursing programs that had begun to develop. Case study presentations also occurred in the field of medicine, in which usual symptomatology was presented, followed by a discussion of medical and nursing therapies.

Nationwide Development

World War II prompted the collection of national data on nursing needs and resources, which heightened the concerns of this period toward identification of professional practice. The Division of Nursing Resources of the United States Public Health Service was formed in 1948. Its staff developed and published guides for institutions on techniques for studying nursing activities (U.S. Public Health Service, 1964). As a result of these guides, a number of "activity" studies were carried out (Roberts, 1964). In 1950, The American Nurses' Association announced plans for a 5-year study of nursing functions and activities. This resulted in the enumeration of functions, standards, and qualifications for practice, as well as the publication *Twenty Thousand Nurses Tell Their Story* (Hughes, Hughes, & Deutscher, 1958). Research in the organization and delivery of health services continued into the late 1950s, often attempting to link nursing staff and unit arrangements to improvement in patient care and patient satisfaction.

Twenty-five years ago, studies of nurses outnumbered studies of patient care 10 to 1. The need for research on problems encountered in patient care began to be addressed at this time. By the early 1960s, the literature was reflecting a shift in focus to the patient instead of the nurse as the object of research. Such a shift was forecast in the 1950 statement of the Chief Nurse Officer of the Public Health Service. Leone (1954) recommended generating a research base through new methods to use nursing skills, nursing care most essential to patient recovery, analysis of nursing techniques, conditions reducing turnover and promoting job satisfaction, use of management theories in the health care arena, and therapeutic effectiveness of interpersonal relationships. It was reemphasized in editorials in the fledgling organ, *Nursing Research*. Both the United States Public Health Service and the American Nurses' Association issued statements of priorities directed toward enlargement of the knowledge base and improvement of patient care.

Thus the efforts to generate a knowledge base for nursing through research have been concentrated in the past two decades. The work has been mainly experiential, not emanating from a solid conceptual or theoretical base until recently. Interest in the theoretical or scientific bases of practice and research was stimulated by the development of programs for training nurse scientists in a number of major universities, by research development activities in these settings, by a growing number of those trained in the scientific methods, and by a tremendous federal investment in the improvement of nursing education over a 15-year period.

Research Development

Early research approaches included the development of critical resources, documentation of need through surveys, use of the conference mechanism, studies of procedures (the technology), case analysis (the art and science), and alliance with other disciplines. Critical resources were identified in terms of numbers of personnel, facilities, and finances.

The survey mechanism was a successful technique for documenting need for personnel and has resulted in a number of classics: the Goldmark report of 1923 (Committee on Nursing and Nursing Education in the United States, 1923), the Committee for the Grading of Nursing Schools reports of 1928 and 1934, and Brown's (1948) *Nursing for the Future*, to name a few. The conference mechanism also has been a successful strategy. Many of these studies were commissioned by conference groups, e.g., the Committee on the Grading of Nursing Schools, the National Nursing Council of the War Years, and the Surgeon General's Consultant Group. This mechanism employed expert panels to convene and deliberate on nursing needs and resources. Other early techniques included the study of procedures and the use of case analysis.

Alliance with other disciplines originated with medicine and education and, as the research base enlarged, also with the social sciences. This alliance has had important implications for the disciplinary technology and modes of inquiry in nursing. The profession has rapidly gained a health-oriented perspective with behavioral, social, and cultural components. Reliance on sociological and anthropological research techniques has provided good capability for description, but perhaps less ability to draw associations and causation.

Current Resources for Research

Current research strategies include:

- enlargement of critical resources with increasing numbers of earned doctorates, increasing postdoctoral activities, and improving the quality of doctoral training
- public support
- colleagueship
- communication
- design and methods, including sampling, instrumentation, multivariate analysis, reproducibility, and generalizability.

Critical resources have an impact on education and practice. Today the research doctorate pool stands at its greatest size since count has been kept. There has been a steady growth in nursing as the major disciplinary field for predoctoral training. Postdoctoral opportunities are being sought by young as well as senior doctorate holders. Public support of research is measured by the size of the private gift and the public tax dollar. The latter has averaged $5 million annually since 1976. There are sufficient numbers of nurse scientists prepared now that some colleagueship within and among institutions is possible in areas of mutual interest. Communication is at an all time high, with two new referred research journals started within the past 3 years and the number of research symposia growing rapidly. Such media are important sources of contact and comment on scientific work. They should provide an opportunity for those beginning to enjoy the meaning of communality.

To assume that the choice of research methods used in nursing was influenced by a particular philosophy of science, e.g., logical positivism, is to attribute too much deliberation or rationality to what was the result of social, political, and economic events. By virtue of their doctoral training in fields other than nursing, nurse scientists brought to the study of nursing those problems and techniques that had served them well in their own doctoral disciplines of sociology, anthropology, biology, psychology, and epidemiology. Socialization into these sciences included the expectation of funding for one's research program. Granting agencies prefer controlled studies in which variables are well specified and instrumentation is precise. What had worked for one science was expected to work for another. Advanced techniques from biostatistics, psychometrics, and computer science were incorporated in the resolution of nursing research problems. Attention is now paid to sampling plans so that enough cases are reported on with sufficient controls to attain some credibility. Design elements are sophisticated enough to allow reproduction and confirmation of findings and to provide some comprehensive treatment of multiple variables under study. A growing body of instruments was evidenced by the recent compilations of research tools. Finally, generalizability has become a critical factor in nursing research efforts. The capacity to affect practice depends heavily on this factor.

Conceptualizations of Nursing and Nursing Science

Nursing has been depicted at various times as a series of tasks and technology (a subset of medicine); as a broad, compassionate, and supportive human service; and, most recently, as a science of human health and behavior across the life span. This current conceptualization includes understanding of biological, behavioral, social, and cultural factors in health and illness and the definition of health outcomes and indicators of health status. These features are reflected in Donaldson and Crowley's (1978) well-publicized themes of inquiry: (a) the principles and laws that govern life processes, well-being, and optimum functioning of human beings; (b) the patterning of human behavior in interaction with the environment in critical life situations; and (c) processes by which positive changes in health status are effected.

Nursing science has been defined as the body of codified understanding of human biology and behavior in health and illness, with particular attention to response states (Barnard, 1980; Gortner, 1980b). There appears to be a growing consensus on the nature of the research paradigms as representing human responses in health and illness. Fawcett (1981) has described person, environment, health, and nursing as elements of a metaparadigm. But while consensus grows among theorists on the subject matter of the discipline and its science, the philosophical orientation of the science is mainly empirical and naturalistic. This orientation involves exploration, description, and classification of phenomena by direct observation and inspection.

It now attempts to incorporate theoretical propositions, however tentative, and seeks to discover relationships. Carper (1978) has described the philosophical base (explanatory base) for many of the present conceptualizations of nursing as teleological, or consequential

and functional. The concept of adaptation, an excellent illustration of such an orientation, is represented in the conceptualizations offered by Roy (1970), Neal (1976), and others. With some exceptions, nursing's current theory is rationally or deductively arrived at, with few empirical verifications. Eventually, the interface will come between the two major modes of inquiry, observation and experimentation, and between the observed phenomena and their logical explanations.

The Philosophy of Science Emerges

The movement from empiricism to rationalism (to theory-laden observations) is heartening—a gain in the level of sophistication of nursing research. There appears to be a move in some settings toward greater specificity of theoretical frameworks and of their concepts and propositions for purposes of empirical testing.

How the empirical testing will be carried out is a matter of debate. Scientific approaches to the study of human health and illness need not eliminate the features of design and methods that have served other sciences well. The logic inherent in the scientific method and the discipline of the method can aid in the identification of correlates of healthy behavior and illness (Winston-Fry, 1980). Science (empirics), art (aesthetics), morality (ethics), and intuition (personal or subjective) all represent sources of knowledge, but nursing research activity has largely concerned itself with the empirics (Carper, 1978). It has been hoped that nursing could maintain its humanistic value orientation as it became more involved in scientific work and thus not repeat the loss of humanism evident in medicine's evolution as a scientific discipline (Gortner, 1974). The profession would be unwise to reject scientific techniques now because of fear of dehumanization or concerns about the validity of analytical approaches. The hypothetico-deductive methods of science can be as much a part of the nursing research repertoire as are the descriptive, inductive, and theory-generating forms. The profession surely can accommodate multiple paradigms (analytic, humanistic) and modes of inquiry (naturalistic, experimental, historical).

Formation of Research Questions

Concepts are ideas or abstractions that form part of our rational perspective and guide the formulation of research questions. Examples of concepts that are frequently in the research literature in nursing include social support, attachment, self-image, pain or discomfort, chronicity, and parenting. Examples of recently completed and ongoing research dealing with these topics may be found in the published proceedings of the 1980 and 1981 meetings of the Western Society for Research in Nursing. Symposia on parenting and nursing, papers on parental assessment, family wellness, and family illness, and instrumentation to measure social support illustrate current scientific interests in only one region of the country.

At another level of abstraction are the following concepts or constructs: health, illness, function and dysfunction, affiliation, adaptation, development, prevention, and promotion. It can be expected that inquiry will be directed toward these constructs and concepts and that the work will be of a more fundamental nature in the future than was true of the past (Gortner, 1980a). The profession is clarifying the sources of its knowledge. It is generally agreed that nursing practice should not be the exclusive source. Accordingly, fundamental knowledge derived from related disciplines and from investigations carried out today in nursing and made relevant to existing theory will be the basic scientific foundation for research.

Areas of Inquiry

Such fundamental questions are generally considered to hold no immediate hope for clinical utility or application in their undifferentiated or basic form. Rather, they contribute a general understanding of events across a wide variety of disciplines. Examples of general areas of fundamental inquiry essential to human health, illness, and recovery include genetic endowment, organ system integrity, psychological well-being, life styles, and culture. Examples of phenomena that have particular relevance for nursing include compliance, chronicity, self-care, social support, parenting, family functioning, and stress.

Besides these areas of fundamental inquiry, there is another area that is concerned with clinical therapeutics. This area has been defined by a number of writers as representing that set of studies of interpersonal and physical techniques that assist patients and families in coping with the effects of illness and in promoting health. The focus is on both the characteristics and outcomes of the interventions, the psychobiological circumstances under which they take place, and the effect they have on modifying psychological and pathophysiological processes (Gortner, Bloch, & Phillips, 1976).

A final area of inquiry that represents a domain of scientific work is investigation of environments. These are viewed as complex multidimensional sets of forces and elements affecting the development and maintenance of healthy and unhealthy states in human beings (Barnard, 1980). Nursing research gives attention to the characteristics of internal and external environments that promote, maintain, and support states of health.

Future Contributions

Nursing science will make a major contribution, as science, in the interface of the biological and social sciences concerned with illness and health. Examples of research questions dealing with the phenomena of chronicity, parenting, and family functioning are as follows:

- How does chronic illness modify self-image?
- What coping mechanisms are effective with chronic and acute pain?
- What factors influence maternal role attainment?
- What constitutes health-seeking behavior among adolescents?
- What is the relationship of family functioning to recovery from episodic illness?

These vital questions have the following features in common. The emphasis is on the psychosocial and biological dimensions of health and illness and on the whole organism. The work produces findings that can be verified and thus contribute to the general understanding of human behavior and response. The questions will ultimately have relevance for the practice field.

As is true of other fields, "good" science in nursing is known by the significance of the questions asked, by the presence of one or more reasonable propositions or hypotheses that can be tested in a verifiable manner, and by the characteristics of creativity, responsibility, and discipline. "Good" scientific work has developed in nursing in a short time. It appears to be well established in a number of areas and settings. The modern university has been a mainstay of important scientific activity in many fields. Will it also house and nurture the fledgling science of nursing, recognizing its potential and its contributions to date? The answer to that critical question may well accelerate or impede nursing's progress as an academic discipline in the next decade.

References

Barnard, K. (1980). Knowledge for practice: Directions for the future. *Nursing Research, 29,* 208–212.

Brown, E.L. (1948). *Nursing for the future.* New York: Russell Sage Foundation.

Carper, B.A. (1978). Fundamental patterns of knowing in nursing. *Advances in Nursing Science, 1*(1), 13–23.

Committee on the Grading of Nursing Schools. (1928). *Nurses, patients and pocketbooks: A report of a study of the economics of nursing.* New York: Author.

Committee on the Grading of Nursing Schools. (1934). *Nursing schools today and tomorrow.* New York: Author.

Committee on Nursing and Nursing Education in the United States. (1923). *Nursing and nursing education in the United States: Report of the committee and report of the survey by Josephine Goldmark, secretary.* New York: Macmillan.

Donaldson, S., & Crowley, D. (1978). The discipline of nursing. *Nursing Outlook, 26,* 113–120.

Fawcett, J. (1981, November). Hallmarks of success in nursing theory development. Paper presented at Vanderbilt University, School of Nursing, Nashville, TN.

Gortner, S.R. (1974). Scientific accountability in nursing. *Nursing Outlook, 22,* 764–768.

Gortner, S.R. (1980a). Nursing research: Out of the past and into the future. *Nursing Research, 29,* 204–207.

Gortner, S.R. (1980b). Nursing science in transition. *Nursing Research, 29,* 180–183.

Gortner, S.R., Bloch, D., & Phillips. T. (1976). Contributions of nursing research to patient care. *Journal of Advanced Nursing, 1,* 507–517.

Gortner, S.R., & Nahm, H. (1977). An overview of nursing research in the United States. *Nursing Research, 26,* 10–33.

Hughes, E.C., Hughes, H.M., & Deutscher, I. (1958). *Twenty thousand nurses tell their story.* Philadelphia: J.B. Lippincott.

Leone, L.P. (1954). *Comments of the need for studies and researchers in nursing.* Unpublished staff paper, historical file. U.S. Public Health Service, Division of Nursing, Nursing Research Branch, Bethesda, MD.

Munhall, P.L. (1982). Nursing philosophy and nursing research: In apposition or opposition? *Nursing Research, 31,* 176–177, 181.

Neal, M.V. (Ed.). (1976, March). *A conceptual basis for maternal child health nursing practice.* Proceedings of a perinatal conference. Baltimore: University of Maryland School of Nursing.

Roberts, D.E., & Hudson, H.H. (1964). *How to study patient progress* (Public Health Service publication No. 1169). Washington, DC: U.S. Department of Health, Education, and Welfare.

Roy, S.C. (1970). Adaptation: A conceptual framework. *Nursing Outlook, 18,* 42–45.

U.S. Public Health Service. (1964). *Patients and personnel speak* (Public Health Service publication No. 527). Washington, DC: U.S. Department of Health, Education, and Welfare.

Winston-Fry, P. (1980). The scientific method and its impact on holistic health. *Advances in Nursing Science, 2*(4), 1–7.

The Author Comments

This recent essay is a culmination of several presentations, beginning with a distinguished scholar's presentation at the University of Pennsylvania, and then at Vanderbilt University, where Jacqueline Fawcett's "Hallmarks of Success In Nursing Theory Development" (1983) also was presented. In my essay, I attempted to depict some major conceptualizations in the history of nursing science and research, and to show how the empirical work and the theoretical or rational work (the development of theory) occurred on parallel and nonintersecting planes for some time. Some comment is made about the nature of methods employed in nursing science; I argue against the position that research methods must be compatible with disciplinary philosophy, whatever that is. No other profession has had such a stringent requirement, and I find it unreasonable. Finally, I argue (as I have for nearly two decades) that the university is the home of knowledge generation as well as knowledge dissemination, and thus it must nurture and support the growing discipline of nursing science.

—SUSAN R. GORTNER

REFERENCE

Fawcett, J. (1983). Hallmarks of success in nursing theory development. In P.L. Chinn (Ed.), *Advances in nursing theory development* (pp. 3–17). Rockville, MD: Aspen Systems.

Chapter 25

An Analysis of Changing Trends in Philosophies of Science on Nursing Theory Development and Testing

Mary Cipriano Silva
Daniel Rothbart

The effects of changing trends in philosophies of science on nursing theory development and testing are analyzed. Two philosophies of science—logical empiricism and historicism—are compared for four variables: (a) components of science, (b) conception of science, (c) assessment of scientific progress, and (d) goal of philosophy of science. These factors serve as the basis for assessing trends in the development and testing of nursing theory from 1964 to the present. The analysis shows a beginning philosophic shift within nursing theory from logical empiricism to historicism and addresses implications and recommendations for future nursing theory development and testing.

Both philosophy of science and nursing theory are in a state of transition. At times this transition is characterized by contradictory, divergent, and confusing points of view that lead to probing questions about the nature of science in general and nursing theory and science in particular. What are the goals and compo-

nents of science? How should science be conceptualized and scientific knowledge assessed? Have nursing theory development and testing kept pace with changing trends in philosophies of science?

The goal of this analysis is to show the influences of changing trends in philosophies of science on nursing theory development and testing and to encourage dialogue among nurses about the future directions of nursing theory.

Philosophies of Science

Since the 1940s, two major schools of philosophical thought have influenced philosophy of science: logical empiricism (1940s–1960s) and historicism (1960s to the present). The most influential proponents of logical empiricism (the orthodox view) included Braithwaite (1953), Ayer (1959), Nagel (1961), Scheffler (1963), Hempel (1965, 1966), and Rudner (1966). These propo-

From Advances in Nursing Science, *January 1984, 6(2), 1–13. Copyright © 1984 by Aspens Systems Corporation.*
Reprinted with permission from Aspen Systems Corporation.

About the Authors

MARY CIPRIANO SILVA was born and raised in Ravenna, Ohio, a small town about 35 miles south of Cleveland. She received her basic nursing education at St. Rita's Hospital in Lima, Ohio, and later earned a B.S.N. and a M.S. from Ohio State University and a Ph.D. in Administration, Supervision, and Curriculum from the University of Maryland. Dr. Silva currently is a Professor of Nursing and Coordinator of the Ph.D. program in Nursing Administration at George Mason University, where she has been a faculty member since 1976. Before moving to the Washington, D.C. area in 1971, Dr. Silva taught at Case Western Reserve University in Cleveland, Ohio, worked as a nurse clinician at Alta Bates Hospital in Berkeley, California, and taught at Stanford University in Palo Alto, California, as a member of the nursing faculty. About the latter position, she comments "Although I consider the Washington, D.C. area 'home,' I left my heart in Palo Alto."

An active writer and speaker, Dr. Silva has published widely in journals of nursing and related disciplines, including *Research in Nursing and Health*, *Advances in Nursing Science*, *International Journal of Nursing Studies*, *Scholarly Inquiry for Nursing Practice: An International Journal*, *TRIAL*, *Journal of Professional Nursing*, and *Annual Review of Nursing Research*. From 1983 to 1984, Dr. Silva was a Kennedy Fellow in Medical Ethics for Nursing Faculty at Georgetown University; during May 1987, she was a visiting scholar at the Hastings Center. In addition, she is a fellow in the American Academy of Nursing and a member of the Council of Nurse Researchers.

On a personal note, Dr. Silva enjoys classical music, art, and interior design. She comments "All three interests influence my professional sense of aesthetics, my sensitivity to the world around me, and my search for the foundations of nursing science."

DANIEL ROTHBART currently resides in Alexandria, Virginia, and is an Associate Professor of Philosophy at George Mason University, where he has been a member of the faculty since 1979. He has received three degrees in philosophy: a B.A. in 1972 from Fairleigh Dickinson University, a M.A. in 1975 from the State University of New York at Binghamton, and a Ph.D. in 1978 from Washington University in St. Louis.

Dr. Rothbart has lectured on medical ethics and philosophy of science around the country and throughout Europe. He was recently appointed a visiting research scholar at the University of Cambridge in England. He has published several articles, book reviews, and chapters in books and is currently preparing a book manuscript titled *Metaphor and the Growth of Scientific Knowledge: A Theory of Metaphoric Innovations in Science*.

About his affiliation with Dr. Silva and writing about nursing, Dr. Rothbart comments "As a philosopher of science, I was excited to learn just how influential philosophy is to nursing theory construction and development of conceptual frameworks. I believe that philosophy is essential for any complete understanding of a knowledge discipline and science. But I know that scientists and theoreticians in most disciplines are generally unaware of the importance of philosophy. I believe that this interaction between philosophy of science and nursing theory should continue because of its mutual benefit."

nents understood the nature of scientific knowledge as an application of logical principles of reasoning.

Although the logical empiricist view dominated the study of philosophy of science for more than two decades, a wave of criticism began in the early 1960s. Logical empiricism was subjected to intense philosophical scrutiny, revolving around the general contention that the orthodox view became too purified in its idealistically formal approach to science. In providing logical rigor and formalization to the nature of scientific knowledge, logical empiricism removed itself from the actual practice of working scientists; the orthodox view approached logic more closely than it did science according to critics. These critics began to reexamine the actual practices of scientists, the patterns of reasoning, and the sociological influences during a historical era. The history of science became an essential element of any adequate philosophical analysis, prompting a new philosophy of science known as historicism.

Major historicists include Hanson (1958), Kuhn (1962, 1970), Lakatos (1968), Toulmin (1972), Laudan (1977), and Feyerabend (1978). Although Kuhn is the best known of these historicists, based on the influential work *The Structure of Scientific Revolutions* (Chicago: University of Chicago Press, 1962, 1970), his philosophical proposals have been widely criticized by other historicists, and Kuhn himself (1977) has had second thoughts about certain aspects of this work.

Therefore, to draw the distinctions between logical empiricism and historicism, it is desirable to focus on the work of Laudan rather than Kuhn. The reasons are threefold: (a) Laudan's works represent the forefront of philosophy of science today; (b) his views are largely shared by other historicists; and (c) his works have gone almost unnoticed by nurse theorists and researchers.

To show fundamental differences regarding theory development, testing, and assessment between logical empiricism and Laudan's version of historicism, these two philosophies are compared for four significant variables: (a) the components of science, (b) the conception of science, (c) the assessment of scientific progress, and (d) the goal of philosophy of science. Table 25-1 summarizes the basic differences between logical empiricism and historicism. These comparisons show the Lifting trends within philosophy of science. From this table one can also surmise implications for the emergent development of new nursing theory.

Components of Science

The components of science, as defined by logical empiricists, are well documented in both the philosophical literature and the nursing literature. Logical empiricists attempt to understand science in terms of theories and the relationships among the components of a theory. A scientific theory is intended to systematically unify all the diverse phenomena of a particular discipline. The unification is achieved by encompassing descriptions of phenomena within an abstract set of statements known as a deductive system.

A deductive system is composed of three major components that are arranged in descending order of abstractness. First, the system's most abstract statements are its assumptions, which introduce the theory's basic concepts through the use of theoretical terms. Secondly, from these theoretical assumptions, propositions are deduced as part of the second level of abstraction. Together these assumptions and propositions systematically organize the entities and processes that presumably "lie behind" the observable phenomena. To complete the theory it is necessary to bridge these principles to empirical generalizations. Toward this goal, bridge principles, still within the second level of abstraction, indicate how the theoretical entities and processes relate to empirical phenomena. Without

Table 25-1
A Comparison of Logical Empiricism and Historicism on Four Parameters of Science

Parameters	Logical Empiricism	Historicism
Components of science	Concepts, theoretical assumptions, empirical generalizations	Concepts, scientific theories, research traditions
Conception of science	Science as product	Science as process
Assessment of scientific progress	Accept theories as probably true Reject theories as probably false	Number of solved problems within a discipline
Goal of philosophy of science	Logical explanation of nature of scientific knowledge	Historical explanation of the nature of scientific knowledge

Note: Although this table highlights the major differences between two philosophies of science, there are some shared views. For example, historicists primarily define science as a human process, but they also examine the products of solved scientific problems.

these principles no empirical explanations or prediction would be possible and the system would be immune to empirical testing. Thirdly, these bridge principles in turn produce empirical generalizations within the lowest level of abstraction. In summary, the components of a scientific system, according to logical empiricists, are a set of statements that are systematically unified within a deductive system and that link theoretical concepts to empirically observable properties through the use of bridge principles (Braithwaite, 1953).

In contrast to the logical empiricists who attempt to understand science in terms of theories, historicists like Laudan (1977) attempt to understand science in terms of research traditions, each of which includes many theories. Although theories are seen by logical empiricists to be specific, short-lived, stable in formulation, and testable, historicists believe research traditions to be global, long-lived, and changeable within the boundaries of an acceptable ontological commitment.

By definition, a research tradition is a broadly based foundation of many theories and is an accepted way of viewing the fundamental phenomena within a discipline. It provides a global backdrop from which theories are constructed and evaluated through a set of guidelines for identifying the fundamental objects of a particular research tradition. Laudan does recognize, however, that the domains of science are not always clear; thus, classification of knowledge into a particular research tradition may be ambiguous. Every discipline has several research traditions, as illustrated by the nursing research traditions of holism and particularism. According to Laudan (1977), three specific components make up a research tradition: (a) specific theories, (b) ontological commitments, and (c) methodological commitments. Some of the specific theories within a given research tradition are new and others are modified versions of older theories that "fit" within the tradition. The function of any theory is to solve scientific problems within the discipline, from the perspective of the research tradition's, ontological commitments. If, for example, one ontological commitment of a research tradition is holism, various theories within this research tradition might address the problem of how to view the person as a holistic being without looking at parts.

In addition to specific theories and ontological commitments, the third component, methodological commitments, is also essential for a research tradition, Methodological commitments define the legitimate methods of inquiry and experimental procedures that are inseparably linked to a research tradition's ontology. To follow the logic of the above example, would not the case study method of inquiry better preserve the ontological commitment to holism than the experimental design method of inquiry with its built-in reductionism?

The components of a scientific system, according to historicists like Laudan, are multiple research traditions, each containing theories that produce a set of ontological viewpoints and methods of inquiry that are not only essentially compatible with the research tradition but also capable of solving problems within it.

Conception of Science

Based on this comparison of the components of science for logical empiricism and historicism, it is apparent that the two schools assume very different views about what science means. Logical empiricists do not understand science in terms of the human activities of working scientists (e.g., experimenting and compiling data). Instead, they conceive of science only in terms of the results of these activities. The term *science* refers only to a product; i.e., a set of statements that purportedly constitute the body of scientific knowledge. The product includes scientific terminology and definitions, propositions, hypotheses, theories, and laws. This conception of science as product rests on the philosophical goal of articulating the logical foundations of scientific knowledge (Rudner, 1966). Within this viewpoint, it is important to recognize that logical empiricists are not interested in how scientific hypotheses are conceived but rather in how they can be sufficiently supported by empirical evidence. Their emphasis is one of theory validation, not theory discovery (Rudner, 1966).

In contrast, historicists understand science as a process of human behavior and thought exhibited by practicing scientists. Historicists would be interested in different questions. What reasoning patterns do practicing scientists use to accept or reject a theory? To what extent are scientists influenced by the theory's empirical findings in contrast to the theory's logical elegance in such a decision? How do external factors such as religious convictions influence the scientist's decision-making judgments? To the historicist, every facet of the scientific process is subject to philosophical examination, including the process of explaining how fruitful theories are conceived by practicing scientists. With greater understanding of this process, historicists hope to develop models for future theory construction. Within this scientific viewpoint, valid data for theory construction include:

- the psychological factors of individual scientists
- the social forces on the community of scientists at a particular time
- the overall historical environment, especially the "nonscientific" influences on scientists.

Assessment of Scientific Progress

The assessment of scientific progress within the logical empiricist tradition rests on the ability to justify a scientific theory by examining the requirements for the theory's truth and the conditions of its falsehood. If a scientist can demonstrate the truth of a theory, the scientist has acquired scientific knowledge.

Certain criteria identify theory as false or true. Generally, if a theory's predictions are repeatedly disconfirmed, the logic of testing requires a rejection of the problematic dimensions of the theory, assuming that the observations are correct (Hempel, 1966). But logical empiricists have more difficulty explaining the method of proving that a theory is true. According to the logic of theory testing, no finite number of experiments can conclusively prove that a theory is true. If a theory passes many severe tests, it is only empirically confirmed; that is, the theory's probability of truth has increased. Therefore, to logical empiricists, scientific progress is assessed by the degree of probability that the theory is true, based on the number and severity of empirical tests it passes.

In addition, logical empiricists consider theoretical reduction an important scientific goal. In theoretical reduction, one theory can be absorbed by or reduced to some other inclusive theory. The philosophical advantage of reduction lies not only with the simplicity of fewer theoretical concepts and laws but also with the insight into the ultimate character of reality (Nagel, 1961).

For historicists, the question of whether philosophy of science should try to explain when, if ever, a theory is true or false is the subject of considerable debate. Many agree with Laudan (1977), who argues that philosophy should not search for distinguishing characteristics of true theories, primarily because practicing scientists rarely evaluate theories in terms of truth or falsity. The history of science includes many instances in which a theory was accepted even though it contained scientific anomalies or produced false experimental predictions. Conversely, some theories have been rejected even though they received the most empirical confirmation. Thus, Laudan argues that questions about truth are essentially irrelevant to scientific progress. The relevant element is the theory's problem-solving effectiveness; a theory's progress is defined by the degree to which it solves more scientific problems than its rivals. As stated by Laudan, *"the solved problem—empirical or conceptual—is the basic unit of scientific progress"* (Laudan , 1977, p. 66).

Historicists such as Laudan find reductionism counterproductive to the goal of solving scientific problems. Research traditions should not be seen as competitors trying to mutually undermine each other rather as collaborators toward the goal of solving scientific problems. This process of synthesizing research traditions, thus expanding them, is called the "integration of research traditions," according to Laudan (1977). Two ways in which this integration may occur are described:

1. One research tradition can be grafted onto another without any major modifications in the components of either.
2. Two or more research traditions may each sacrifice funda-

mental elements that have been refuted while combining their remaining elements in a new way.

An important scientific motivation for integrating research traditions is the goal of explaining different dimensions of the same phenomena under study. For example, in nursing, the integration of divergent research traditions from biology, psychology, and sociology can account for the ontological perspective that individuals are bio-psychosocial beings, which is common in nursing. This pattern of conjoining fundamental perspectives from different traditions is common when scientists develop new interdisciplinary fields of study to account for previously unexplained scientific problems. The integration of research traditions and corresponding theories is shown in Figure 25-1.

Laudan's analysis of integration departs significantly from the logical empiricist contention that science progresses through the elimination of theories by reduction. But the process of integration does not involve elimination by reducing one tradition to another, because both traditions retain their identity. Integration aims at extracting the progressive components of each tradition in a way that produces solutions to previously unsolved problems.

Goal of Philosophy of Science

According to logical empiricists, the ultimate goal of philosophy of science is to present a formalized account of the nature of scientific knowledge. This includes an application of logical principles to questions about the nature of science, since logic provides the eternal principles for relationships between scientific statements. By examining these relationships, the foundation of science is intended to systematically reveal the logical requirements for all scientific knowledge.

Historicists share with logical empiricists the belief that the philosopher's task is to construct a general account of the nature of scientific knowledge. But for historicists like Laudan, such a task must conform to the human elements of scientific evolution and growth. To meet this goal, historicists engage in studies of the actual activities, behavior patterns, and reasoning processes of working scientists. The belief is that philosophy of science must show how science, as it is actually practiced, can yield knowledge about the world. Such examination of the actual practice of scientists is used by historicists as evidence against logical empiricism, because the growth of scientific knowledge seems at times to be aided by illogical and nonrational decision making. It is believed that illogical processes can contribute to creative growth of knowledge within a discipline.

Nursing Theory Development and Testing

Since 1964, nurse scholars have become more aware of the influences of philosophy—in particular philosophy of science—on the development of nursing theory. A review of significant and representative nursing theory literature within three time periods shows the status of nursing theory in regard to logical empiricist and historicist trends in philosophy of science.

1964 to 1969

An important influence on nursing theory development during the 1960s was support given by the Division of Nursing of the U.S. Department of Health, Education, and Welfare (now the Department of Health and Human Services) to nursing schools to sponsor pro-

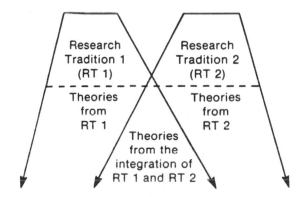

Figure 25-1 *A conceptualization of the integration of research traditions and corresponding theories within historicism.*

grams on the nature and development of nursing science. An analysis of metatheoretical papers from the proceedings of two such conferences—the Symposium on Theory Development in Nursing held at Case Western Reserve University in 1968 and the Conference on the Nature of Science in Nursing held at the University of Colorado in 1969—gives insight into how nurse scholars and others during the late 1960s conceptualized the derivation of nursing knowledge.

In 1968, Dickoff and James presented a version of their position paper on a theory of theories, introducing the idea that significant nursing theory must be situation producing. Although they modified the orthodox view about the purpose of theory—that is, they postulated that theory could be capable of both more than and less than prediction—they, nevertheless, explicitly stated their faithfulness to the logical empiricist tradition. They forthrightly spoke of their work as a broader interpretation of the writings of such philosophers as Nagel (1961) and Hempel (1965, 1966). The language they used to describe theory supports logical empiricism. They spoke of concepts, propositions, set; they assessed scientific progress in terms of truth; and they insisted on a product orientation to science (i.e., production of desired situations).

In 1969, Abdellah discussed the nature of nursing science. Although no mention was made per se of the writings of philosophers who supported logical empiricism, Abdellah's views of what constitutes a scientific theory were nevertheless consistent with their writings; that is, terms must be operationally defined and preferably observable and quantifiable. Postulates are validated by testing deductions, which either helps to confirm the theory or leads to modifications of the postulates. Abdellah concludes that the reward of nurse scientists for their efforts is the discovery and affirmation of truth. Thus, as with Dickoff and James (1968), the criterion for the assessment of scientific progress is an increase in scientific truths.

Other writings (Dickoff, James, & Wiedenbach, 1968a, 1968b) related to nursing theory development and testing during the late 1960s all tended to have a logical empiricist perspective, with the exception of Leininger's (1969) introductory comments to the Conference on the Nature of Science in Nursing, which offered an ethnoscience research methodology to the discovery of scientific knowledge. This approach stresses the viewing of behavior from the subject's perspective rather than the researcher's. This accommodation to subjectivism is more compatible with historicism than with the objectivism of logical empiricism.

1970 to 1975

In the first half of the 1970s, two major trends in nursing theory occurred:

1. Metatheoretical formulations relevant to nursing theory and testing within the logical empiricist tradition were developed to a high degree by such investigators as Jacox (1974) and Hardy (1974).
2. A number of conceptual frameworks for nursing were published; for example, the work of Rogers (1970), King (1971), Orem (1971), and Roy (1974).

According to Jacox (1974), the goal of science is the discovery of truths, and the purpose of scientific theory is description, explanation, and prediction of part of our empirical world. In discussing theory construction, Jacox uses the language of the logical empiricists, including concepts, propositions, axioms, and theorems. Hardy (1974) is even more oriented to the formal logic underlying logical empiricism, discussing nine possible relationships that can exist between concepts and presenting a diagrammatic and matrix presentation of a situation that shows (a) the concepts, (b) the sign of the relationship between concepts, and (c) the nature of the relationships between concepts.

These two articles represented a culmination of the metatheoretical notions about logical empiricism in nursing theory. The irony, of course, is that at the time these and similar reports were making a profound impact on the derivation of theory in nursing, the logical empiricist view-points espoused in them were being strongly repudiated by a growing number of philosophers of science. In other words, nursing's theoretical link to philosophy of science was, from the historicist perspective, about a decade behind the times.

The irony continues in regard to the second trend —the publication of a number of important conceptual frameworks for nursing. Several conceptual frameworks published in the early 1970s were essentially devoid of any explicit linkage to philosophy of science (King, 1971; Orem, 1971). This is no way meant to diminish the quality or significance of these seminal works but only to point out that a situation existed in which the most influential nursing literature on theory construction and testing followed rather than preceded the derivation of the conceptual frameworks, apparently because the metatheoretical movement in nursing was, for the most part, a separate movement from the conceptual framework movement.

1976 to Present

Since 1976, the following trends have occurred:

1. a continued and relatively stable commitment to logical empiricism, although a beginning trend toward historicism is apparent;
2. a revision of several conceptual frameworks for nursing and the introduction of some new frameworks; and
3. a questioning of the adequacy of strictly quantitative research methods to test nursing theory deductions.

The relatively stable commitment to logical empiricism is reflected in the current writings of several nurse authors (Chinn & Jacobs, 1983; Fawcett, 1983; Menke, 1983; Walker & Avant, 1983). However, there are some new trends. For example, in 1979 when Newman introduced a new theory of health, the viewpoint was one of logical empiricism. However, in a recent work (1983), a shift in her thinking is evident. Reflecting the thoughts of Kuhn (a historicist), Newman defines science as "a process of knowing, a process of challenging, and a continuing revolution" (Newman, 1983, p. 387). This emphasis on process (not product) and revolution (not logic) is a noticeable shift in viewpoint from logical empiricism to historicism.

In a recent publication, Hardy (1983) also extensively cited Kuhn in discussing nursing theory. The primary emphasis is on metaparadigms; however, Hardy also seems to agree, at least implicitly, with Kuhn's definition of the development of scientific knowledge as both nonrational and noncumulative. This represents a marked shift in viewpoint from the 1974 Hardy article, which, of all the metatheoretical articles, represented the most rigorous and logically structured formulations in support of logical empiricism. These contradictions in the works of Hardy and other metatheorists are indicative of the pull between orthodox and new ideas in philosophy of science and in nursing theory development and testing.

Although several other nurse authors (Carper, 1978; MacPherson, 1983; Meleis, 1983; Menke, 1983; Munhall, 1982) briefly address Kuhn's *The Structure of Scientific Revolutions*, with the exception of Meleis (1983) they do not discuss Kuhn's more recent writings or mention Laudan's work, which represents the forefront of philosophy of science today. However, Laudan's work is briefly mentioned in an article by Watson (1981) and cited in the bibliographies of books by Parse (1981) and Chinn and Jacobs (1983). Although this attention to the work of Laudan is scant, it is encouraging because it begins to bring the development of nursing theory knowledge in line with current trends in philosophy of science.

The second trend occurring between 1976 and the present is the expansion and revision of the works of those nurse authors who in the early 1970s had developed conceptual frameworks for nursing. For example, first editions of books and other publications were rewritten, expanded, or revised by Orem (1980), King (1981), Roy (1981), Roy and Roberts (1981), and Rogers (1980). Several of these nurse theorists, in an attempt to bring their works more in line with what the nurse metatheorists of the mid-1970s were espousing—logical empiricism—revised their works to explicitly identify such elements as concepts and propositions that are inherent in the orthodox viewpoint.

Thus, an interesting situation has been created: While these nurse theorists have been updating trends in philosophy of science as espoused in the nursing literature of the mid-1970s, those who espoused these views have begun to question them and some no longer espouse them. This is not to say that individuals should not alter their viewpoints but to point out again the seeming separateness of the metatheoretical and conceptual framework movement in nursing and the effect of this separateness on perpetuating traditional or singular viewpoints about philosophy of science.

Two other conceptual frameworks were developed in books published in 1976 by Paterson and Zderad and in 1981 by Parse. Neither book has received much attention in the nursing literature, although there is some evidence that this is changing (Chinn & Jacobs, 1983; King 1981). Could it be that both of these books have a strong existential-phenomenological perspective that, until recently, was out of the mainstream of the thinking of orthodox nurse scientists about philosophy of science? The underlying assumptions these three authors hold about the nature of science are much more in keeping with nontraditional views about philosophy of science than with traditional views. In particular, they see science as process; they envision a strong link between the theory's ontological commitment and its methodological commitment; and they place little emphasis on precise, logical formulations.

The third trend is a shift in emphasis from quantitative to qualitative research methods to test nursing theory deductions. In the late 1970s, nurse scholars (Silva, 1977) began to question the limits of quantitative research methods because they too often sacrificed meaningfulness for rigor. Out of this questioning, articles suggesting alternative approaches to logical empiricism began to appear in the nursing literature (Munhall, 1982; Oiler, 1982; Omery, 1983; Swanson & Chenitz, 1982; Tinkle & Beaton, 1983; Watson, 1981). These approaches were sought because of the inadequacy of logical empiricism to deal with certain phenomena in nursing, in particular, those phenomena dealing with humanism and holism. By exploring alternative philosophies of science and research methodologies that are compatible, it seems possible to study these phenomena in a more meaningful and creative way and, in so doing, to help bridge the gaps among philosophies of science, nursing theory, and nursing research. Historicism is one of the alternative philosophies that holds promise in helping to bridge these gaps.

Implications and Recommendations for the Future

Since every scientific theory is tied to some philosophical framework as the basis for understanding and assessing theory, it is important for the theorists within a given discipline to be aware of the discipline's philosophical orientation. Therefore, nursing theorists should continue to explore the philosophical underpinnings of their discipline in order to integrate the latest advances in nursing theory development and testing with a coherent philosophical foundation.

This review of the trends in nursing theory from 1964 to the present shows not only that nursing theory is presently in a state of transition, but also that many of the changes in nursing theory reflect a reorientation of the underlying philosophy of the discipline. This is evident in the beginning metatheoretical shift away from a strongly empirical and logical orientation to theory construction reminiscent of logical empiricism and toward a more holistic and humanist approach more in line with historicism. There are several implications for nursing theory development and testing;

- Laudan dismisses as counterproductive the logical empirical goal of reducing one theory to another. Rather than trying to restrict the range of possible theories, Laudan encourages theory expansion through a process of integrating components from different research traditions, which results in a multidimensional understanding of the phenomena. Based on this historicist orientation, there should not be a single, conceptual framework for nursing. This orientation suggests, rather, the expansion of nursing theory through the integration of progressive components of the various existing nursing conceptual frameworks, which results in multiple frameworks. This process should be a cooperative endeavor and, if adhered to, should encourage a cooperative rather than a competitive attitude among nurse scholars. In the future some of the conceptual frameworks for nursing may be integrated so that the unimportant elements are sacrificed and the important elements are combined in a new way.

- The historicist's conception of science as a human process, rather than a product of some endeavor, suggests that nursing theory should always be understood as a stage in its evolution and growth. Although nursing theory is experiencing shifts in its evolution, the result of the transition will not be some final and static body of knowledge. Like any scientific discipline, nursing theory construction will never culminate in some static set of eternal truths but will represent one episode in its evolving history.
- Historicism strongly encourages a careful study of the actual practices, belief systems, and external factors influencing a community of scientists within a given discipline. This has a direct bearing on the type of data relevant for any theory construction. Thus, data for nursing theory development and testing will include the common practices of nurse clinicians, the social and psychological factors affecting the profession of nursing, the widely held beliefs of the community of nurses, and the reasoning patterns of individual nurse theorists. A result of integrating these data will be a nursing theory that more explicitly addresses the human dimensions of nursing and the practitioners of nursing.
- Scientific progress for Laudan reduces to the number of solved problems within a discipline. Therefore, the assessment of progress in nursing theory development and testing will be less rigid and more practical than suggested by a logical empiricist orientation. That is, there will be less emphasis on truth and error as the criteria for assessing scientific progress and more emphasis on the actual solution to nursing care problems. This shift should help to bridge the gap between those persons who are primarily nurse scholars and those who are primarily nurse clinicians. The clinician, of course, is in an ideal position to both understand and assess whether, and to what degree, a nursing care problem has been solved. Within this framework, the nurse clinician should be highly valued as an integral part of the process of nursing theory development and testing.

Based on the changing trends in philosophies of science and nursing theory, four recommendations are made:

1. Creation of liaisons between departments of nursing and departments of philosophy to help nurse scholars, theoreticians, researchers, and clinicians stay abreast of changes in philosophy of science;
2. Establishment of closer, cooperative working relationships among nurse metatheorists, theoreticians, researchers, and clinicians with a common goal of solving problems of significance in nursing;
3. Exploration of innovative, qualitative methods for testing

nursing theory that are in keeping with the historicist tradition; and
4. Continued and explicit emphasis in nursing theory courses on the interrelationships among philosophies of science, nursing theory, and nursing research.

If the above recommendations are implemented, they should help to establish and maintain an open dialogue, which portends a healthy and promising future for the advancement of nursing science.

References

Abdellah, F.G. (1969). The nature of nursing science. *Nursing Research, 18*, 390–393.

Ayer, A.J. (1959). Editor's introduction. In A.J. Ayer (Ed.), *Logical positivism* (pp. 3–28). New York: Free Press.

Braithwaite, R.B. (1953). *Scientific explanation: A study of the function of theory, probability and law in science.* London: Cambridge University Press.

Carper, B.A. (1978). Fundamental patterns of knowing in nursing. *Advances in Nursing Science, 1*(1), 13–23.

Chinn, P.L., & Jacobs, M.K. (1983). *Theory and nursing: A systematic approach.* St. Louis: C.V. Mosby.

Conference on the Nature of Science in Nursing (1969). *Nursing Research, 18*, 388–411.

Dickoff, J., & James, P. (1968). A theory of theories: A position paper. *Nursing Research, 17*, 197–203.

Dickoff, J., James, P., & Wiedenbach, E. (1968a). Theory in a practice discipline: Part I. Practice-oriented theory. *Nursing Research, 17*, 415–435.

Dickoff, J., James, P., & Wiedenbach, E. (1968b). Theory in a practice discipline: Part II. Practice-oriented research. *Nursing Research, 17*, 545–554.

Fawcett, J. (1983). Hallmarks of success in nursing theory development. In P.L. Chinn (Ed.), *Advances in nursing theory development* (pp. 3–17). Rockville, MD: Aspen Systems.

Feyerabend, P. (1978). *Against method: Outline of an anarchistic theory of knowledge.* London: Verso.

Fitzpatrick, J.J., & Whall, A.L. (1983). *Conceptual models of nursing: Analysis and application.* Bowie, MD: Brady.

Hanson, N.R. (1958). *Patterns of discovery: An inquiry into the conceptual foundation of science.* London: The Syndics of the Cambridge University Press.

Hardy, M.E. (1974). Theories: Components, development, evaluation. *Nursing Research, 23*, 100–107.

Hardy, M.E. (1983). Metaparadigms and theory development. In N.L. Chaska (Ed.), *The nursing profession: A time to speak* (pp. 427–437). New York: McGraw-Hill.

Hempel, C.G. (1965). *Aspects of scientific explanation and other essays in the philosophy of science.* New York: Free Press.

Hempel, C.G. (1966). *Philosophy of natural science.* Englewood Cliffs, NJ: Prentice Hall.

Jacox, A. (1974). Theory construction in nursing: An overview. *Nursing Research, 23,* 4–13.

King, I.M. (1971). *Toward a theory for nursing: General concepts of human behavior.* New York: John Wiley & Sons.

King, I.M. (1981). *A theory for nursing: Systems, concepts, process.* New York: John Wiley & Sons.

Kuhn, T.S. (1962). *The structure of scientific revolutions.* Chicago: The University of Chicago Press.

Kuhn, T.S. (1970). *The structure of scientific revolutions* (2nd ed.). Chicago: The University of Chicago Press.

Kuhn, T.S. (1977). Second thoughts on paradigms. In F. Suppe (Ed.), *The structure of scientific theory* (pp. 459–482). Urbana, IL: University of Illinois Press.

Lakatos, I. (1968). Changes in the problem of inductive logic. In I. Lakatos (Ed.), *The problem of inductive logic* (pp. 315–417). Amsterdam: North-Holland.

Laudan, L. (1977). *Progress and its problems: Toward a theory of scientific growth.* Berkeley, CA: University of California Press.

Leininger, M.M. (1969). Nature of science in nursing. *Nursing Research, 18,* 388–389.

MacPherson, K.I. (1983). Feminist methods: A new paradigm for nursing research. *Advances in Nursing Science, 5*(2), 17–25.

Meleis, A.I. (1983). A model for theory description, analysis, and critique. In N.L. Chaska (Ed.), *The nursing profession: A time to speak* (pp. 438–452). New York: McGraw-Hill.

Menke, E.M. (1983). Critical analysis of theory development in nursing. In N.L. Chaska (Ed.), *The nursing profession: A time to speak* (pp. 416–426). New York: McGraw-Hill.

Munhall, P.L. (1982). Nursing philosophy and nursing research: In apposition or opposition? *Nursing Research, 31,* 176–177, 181.

Nagel, E. (1961). *The structure of science: Problems in the logic of scientific explanation.* New York: Harcourt Brace & World.

Newman, M.A. (1979). *Theory development in nursing.* Philadelphia: F.A. Davis.

Newman, M.A. (1983). The continuing revolution: A history of nursing science. In N.L. Chaska (Ed.), *The nursing profession: A time to speak* (pp. 385–393). New York: McGraw-Hill.

Oiler, C. (1982). The phenomenological approach in nursing research. *Nursing Research, 31,* 178–181.

Omery, A. (1983). Phenomenology: A method for nursing research. *Advances in Nursing Science, 5*(2), 49–63.

Orem, D.E. (1971). *Nursing: Concepts of practice.* New York: McGraw-Hill.

Orem, D.E. (1980). *Nursing: Concepts of practice* (2nd ed.). New York: McGraw-Hill.

Parse, R.R. (1981). *Man-living-health: A theory of nursing.* New York: John Wiley & Sons.

Paterson, J.G., & Zderad, L.T. (1976). *Humanistic nursing.* New York: John Wiley & Sons.

Rogers, M.E. (1970). *An introduction to the theoretical basis of nursing.* Philadelphia: F.A. Davis.

Rogers, M.E. (1980). Nursing: A science of unitary man. In J.P. Riehl & C. Roy (Eds.), *Conceptual models for nursing practice* (2nd ed.) (pp. 329–337). New York: Appleton-Century-Crofts.

Roy, C. (1974). The Roy adaptation model. In J.P. Riehl & C. Roy (Eds.), *Conceptual models for nursing practice* (pp. 135–144). New York: Appleton-Century-Crofts.

Roy, C. (1981). *Introduction to nursing: An adaptation model.* Englewood Cliffs, NJ: Prentice-Hall.

Roy, C., & Roberts, S.L. (1981). *Theory construction in nursing: An adaptation model.* Englewood Cliffs, NJ: Prentice-Hall.

Rudner, R.S. (1966). *Philosophy of social science.* Englewood Cliffs, NJ: Prentice-Hall.

Scheffler, I. (1963). *The anatomy of inquiry: Philosophical studies in the theory of science.* New York: Knopf.

Silva, M.C. Philosophy, science, theory: Interrelationships and implications for nursing research. *Image, 9,* 59–63.

Swanson, J.M., & Chenitz, W.C. (1982). Why qualitative research in nursing? *Nursing Outlook, 30,* 241–245.

Symposium on Theory Development in Nursing (1968). *Nursing Research, 17,* 196–222.

Tinkle, M.B., & Beaton, J.L. (1983). Toward a new view of science: Implications for nursing research. *Advances in Nursing Science, 5*(2), 27–36.

Toulmin, S. (1972). *Human understanding* (Vol. 1). Princeton, NJ: Princeton University Press.

Walker, L.O., & Avant, K.C. (1983). *Strategies for theory construction in nursing.* Norwalk, CT: Appleton-Century-Crofts.

Watson, J. (1981). Nursing's scientific quest. *Nursing Outlook, 29,* 413–416.

Reaction. . .

Nursing Theory Development: Another Look

To the editor:

In their article, "An Analysis of Changing Trends in Philosophies of Science on Nursing Theory Development and Testing" (*Advances in Nursing Science* 6(2), January 1984), Silva and Rothbart conducted a historical analysis of the development of nursing theories that contrasted with the changing philosophies of science from 1964 to the present. Although their analysis is interesting, it leaves the reader suspended regarding their opinion on why these trends occurred and whether they should be considered aberrant behavior or developmentally expected. The authors are clearly advocating a historical approach to the basis of nursing theory, but their treatment of external factors responsible for the devotion of nurse researchers to logical empiricism is not convincing.

One must first examine the rationale on which theory building was based and ask why it was constructed on the altar of positivism. If one looks at the beginning nursing theorists, it becomes apparent that they felt a theory must have some reality base (Abdellah, 1969; Johnson, 1959). They sought ideas that would be clearly explainable in the everyday observations of nursing care. Taking cues from the biomedical model, they attempted to ground theory in observations, trying to find or discover nursing truths.

That is still a sticking point today. Are there priority nursing principles that data collectors such as Benner (1984) may yet find? This is not to endorse total devotion to empirics, but a large anomaly has developed in that we are devoting much time to theory development without adequate data collection. It must be understood that, in a developing discipline, it was easier to justify spending time and money on classic methods rather than on trying to solve as-yet undefined problems.

One note of caution regarding the historical approach is that it requires a careful study of external factors. A reality is that, as doctoral programs—the profession's breeding ground for young researchers—increase in number, most teaching will continue to be done by faculty steeped in quantitative methodology. Faculty teaching in doctoral programs are people who have little background in qualitative versus quantitative research. The result will be continued emphasis on logical positivism in nursing.

Meleis (1985) has a valid criticism with which I agree. What dictates that nursing must follow the tradition of philosophy of sciences? This question deserves consideration. Nursing theory is not necessarily subject to the laws of the hard sciences. Instead, macrotheorists must examine what nursing is and ask: is it a science, an art, or neither? Observers of nursing progress must also assess how that profession embraces or relinquishes its theories. In a community in which its researchers are separated by a wide gap from its practitioners, the observer must choose carefully when deciding what factors influence its frameworks. Are nursing theorists creating new frameworks or just describing frameworks that fit the observable phenomena?

Studying the development of nursing theory is fascinating but can be hazardous to one who relies on traditional referent points of scientific progress. One must be careful to take into account the distinctiveness of the nursing perspective and the unique approach nursing may use to articulate its place among the disciplines.

JOHN G. TWOMEY, JR., R.N., M.S.
Doctoral Student in Nursing University of Virginia
Charlottesville, Virginia

REFERENCES

Abdellah, F.G. (1969). The nature of nursing science. *Nursing Research, 18,* 390–393.

Benner, P. (1984). *From novice to expert: Excellence and power in clinical nursing.* Reading, MA: Addison-Wesley.

Johnson, D.E. (1959). A philosophy of nursing. *Nursing Outlook, 7,* 198–200.

Meleis, A. (1985). *Theoretical nursing: Development and progress.* Philadelphia: J.B. Lippincott.

The Authors Comment

The ideas for this article arose over a decade ago when, during my doctoral studies, I was introduced to logical empiricism as the accepted mode for scientific inquiry. Although I was able to see strengths in this approach, I also found it limiting. I discussed some of these limitations in "Philosophy, Science, Theory: Interrelationships and Implications for Nursing Research," published in *Image* in 1977.* Since that time, I have continued to question the emphasis on a singular mode of scientific inquiry, but until recently almost all of the metatheoretical literature in nursing gave the impression that logical empiricism was the only acceptable mode.

Because every discipline has more than one point of view, all of which change over time, during 1982 I asked Dan Rothbart of the Department of Philosophy and Religion at George Mason University what major shifts had occurred in philosophy of science over the past decade. Dan, who specializes in philosophy of science, told me about the shift from logical empiricism to historicism. In the spring of 1982, we agreed to write a manuscript on these shifts, as well as on the effect of these shifts on nursing theory development and testing. Over the next year, we reorganized and revised the manuscript several times and then submitted it to *Advances in Nursing Science* in June 1983.

Since our article appeared in *Advances in Nursing Science* in January 1984, we have received many favorable comments on it, as well as some excellent suggestions for further elaboration and clarification. We are pleased with this feedback because, as we said in the introduction, one of our goals was "to encourage dialogue among nurses about the future directions of nursing theory." To the extent that this goal is accomplished, we believe that nursing science has been advanced.

—MARY SILVA

During 1982, Mary Silva, a professor in the School of Nursing at George Mason University, asked me about the influence of philosophy on nursing theory. Subsequently, we each read articles and books within the other's discipline and discovered that the philosophical ideas incorporated in nursing theory since 1964 were somewhat outdated. We found that most of nursing theory literature embraces a logical empiricist philosophy of science, even though the philosophy of science has evolved significantly away from logical empiricism. Thomas Kuhn's work has sparked a rival philosophical school with many prominent advocates, such as Larry Laudan. Based on our reading and discussion, we came to believe that a historicist philosophy would have a profound effect on constructing nursing theory, conceptual frameworks, and research methods.

We wrote the article in the following manner: First, I discussed the evolution of philosophy of science from logical empiricism of the 1940s to historicism of the 1980s. Second, Mary reviewed the significant nursing theory literature to show the status of nursing theory in regard to logical empiricist and historicist philosophies. Finally, we wrote the third section on the implications of these changes and recommendations for the future.

—DANIEL ROTHBART

---

*Ed. note: Chapter 58.

Chapter 26

Toward Greater Specificity in Defining Nursing's Metaparadigm

Mary E. Conway

The thesis presented is that nursing in its disciplinary context cannot appropriately be considered a concept in the metaparadigm of nursing science. Nursing as a discipline is guided by theories and prescriptions that emanate from puzzles solved in the domain of nursing science. Failure to distinguish between the science of nursing and its disciplinary aspects in building conceptual frameworks will retard the growth of science. The merits of three competing paradigms—normal science, historical facts, and social facts—are discussed. None of these paradigms is adequate for discovery in nursing science. Efforts to develop knowledge around the phenomena of central concern to nursing may advance more rapidly if theory building follows a set of rules, as yet undefined, that incorporates the methods of both normal science and historical tradition.

In recent literature, attention has been focused on the present stage of theory development in nursing and the projected direction of its future evolution. The case has been made that nurse theorists have been moving away from an earlier adherence to the logical empiricist tradition and toward the holistic or historicist tradition (Silva & Rothbart, 1984). This movement is understandable, given the concern of nursing with holism and the integrity of individuals, and given the fact that the ho-

listic tradition in the philosophy of science accommodates these concerns. Concomitant with the movement away from logical empiricism, a few scholars have asserted that nursing is at a preparadigm stage in the development of its science (Hardy, 1983). Fawcett (1984) recently claimed that nursing now has an identifiable metaparadigm. This judgment is made on evidence that a majority of nurse theorists, including conceptual model builders, explicitly recognize four

About the Author

MARY E. CONWAY is currently the Dean and Professor Emeritus of the School of Nursing at the Medical College of Georgia in Augusta, Georgia. Dr. Conway began her nursing career in 1947 when she received a B.S. in Nursing from Columbia University. She worked as a staff nurse, head nurse, supervisor, and research assistant for 10 years in New York and Massachusetts. In 1957, she enrolled at the University of Minnesota, from which she received a M.N.A in Nursing Administration in 1958. After another 10 years of varied administrative positions she then began full-time study for her Ph.D. in Sociology at Boston University in 1968. After receiving her doctorate, Dr. Conway joined the BU faculty for 4 years until 1976. She moved to Milwaukee, assuming the position of Dean of the School of Nursing at the University of Wisconsin. She has held her current position since 1980.

Dr. Conway is an active writer, having published more than 20 articles and three books. She is a Fellow in the American Academy of Nursing, having been inducted in 1975. In 1985, she received the Mary Tolle Wright Award for Leadership from Sigma Theta Tau, one of the Honor Society's highest honors.

concepts of central concern to the discipline: man, environment, health, and nursing. These concepts have appeared consistently in the conceptual frameworks developed by nurses.

Whether nursing science has a metaparadigm is debatable, but an even more important issue is whether *nursing* is, or appropriately can be, considered to be a *central concern* of the discipline's science development. Nursing, by at least one definition, is a set of psychomotor and cognitive acts performed by an educated professional on behalf of another individual, toward goals of promoting health or helping the other to cope with illness. By another definition, nursing is the discipline within which scholars "build" science by efforts analogous to those of scientists such as molecular biologists, who theorize, solve puzzles, and experiment to add to knowledge in the subfield of molecular biology. Molecular biology *qua biology* is not a concept of central concern to biologists. Similarly, the acts of professionals who practice within the discipline of nursing are not of prime importance to those concerned with the discipline's science. "Concern with oneself as an actor is concern with something fundamentally different [than instrumental knowledge]" (Eckberg & Hill, 1979). The question posed for this discussion is: Can nursing be properly considered a metaparadigm concept of nursing science?

The Science Versus the Discipline of Nursing

There is a lack of consensus in the literature regarding what may be considered the present stage of development in nursing science. This is understandable because science is evolving, and its theories and principles are always open to the possibility of disconfirmation by the discovery of new evidence (Popper, 1959). Competing views of nursing theory, definitions of its major concepts, and acceptable methods for developing and testing theory abound (Fawcett, 1984; Rogers, 1980; Jacox, 1974; Neuman, 1982). As a science in a given discipline matures, there is a tendency toward more intersubjectivity among its scholars and one or more clearly distinguishable lines of inquiry. In "normal" science, the discoveries or solutions to puzzles made by one generation of researchers are built on by succeeding generations.

A widely accepted world view of a discipline that shapes the direction and methods of its researchers is often referred to as a paradigm (Kuhn, 1970). According to Kuhn, substitution of a new paradigm occurs only when the existing world and what is empirically known of it no longer is understandable in terms of extant scientific theories or when the existing paradigm "has ceased to function adequately in the exploration of an aspect of nature to which that paradigm itself had previously led the way" (Kuhn, 1970, p. 92). Kuhn calls this a scientific revolution. The science of nursing has not yet reached the paradigmatic stage; thus, the various lines of theory development and research pursued by its scholars may be considered to be preparadigmatic efforts.

However, Fawcett (1984) pointed out "some major and persistent themes" in the nursing literature that to some extent are guiding an increasing number of researchers. The serious student or neophyte researcher who reviews the literature explaining these concepts and themes will find as many questions raised as answered. A fundamental epistemological problem is the recurring use of the term *nursing* within a variety of contexts and at varying levels of abstraction.

A small number of nurse scholars have recognized this lack of specificity in the usage of the word nursing and the problem this creates in attempts to arrive at a consensus, or paradigm, in enlarging the body of nursing science, Donaldson and Crowley have made a helpful contribution toward clarification of the term and have distinguished between two major contexts in which they say nursing ought to be viewed:

> Failure to recognize the existence of the discipline as a body of knowledge that is separate from the activities of practitioners has contributed to the fact that nursing has been viewed as a vocation rather than a profession. In turn, this has led to confusion as to whether the *discipline* of nursing exists (Donaldson & Crowley, 1978, p. 117.

They argue that another important reason for keeping a clear distinction between the science and the discipline is that the discipline is defined by its social relevance and, thus, may need to be altered on the basis of societal needs. But this is not necessarily true for nursing *science.* It appears that Hardy also conceives of a science of nursing as distinct from a *practice* of nursing. In explaining her concept of a "community of scientists," she wrote "Such groups [scientists] work under a common cognitive umbrella or metaparadigm whether they be biologists, psychologists or physicists"(Hardy, 1983, p. 430). She also stated that

"Nurse-scientists are not yet at the point of seeing themselves as a community of scientists developing a body of knowledge that is distinct from other groups in the health field"(Hardy, 1983, p. 431). The contextual use of the terms scientist, cognitive umbrella, and body of knowledge leaves little doubt that she was describing a *science* and the endeavors of scientists, not clinicians.

The distinction between a science and the practice of a discipline has been attempted by other scholars. In a discourse tracing the evolution of theory development in nursing from a logical empiricist tradition to that of a holistic or historical tradition, Silva and Rothbart (1984) repeatedly used the phrases "components of science," "phenomena within the discipline," and "metatheoretical formulations relevant to nursing." Because they do not refer to the acts of nurses or the practice of nursing, it can be concluded that their sole focus was the science of nursing.

Paradigm and Metaparadigm

Arguments about whether nursing science is at a stage representative of a preparadigm, metaparadigm, or paradigm are unlikely to promote or impede the actual development of nursing as a body of science. It is relevant, however, to consider the extent to which nursing is evolving toward a paradigm, since a paradigm is generally considered the most highly evolved stage of a science. A paradigm provides a road map for scholars in a discipline and assists in the accumulation of knowledge about selected phenomena of concern to the discipline. It is a concept common to all science, but it does not have a common, universally interpreted definition. For example, Masterman (1970) counted 21 different connotations in usage in Kuhn's original explanation of the concept of the paradigm in science.

After studying Kuhn's work, Masterman concluded that it is simpler to understand the notion of a paradigm by asking what it does rather than what it is. Based on a selection of statements from Kuhn, she wrote:

> If we ask, however, what a paradigm does, it becomes clear at once (assuming always the existence of normal

science) that the construct sense of 'paradigm,' and not the metaphysical sense or metaparadigm, is the fundamental one. For only with an artifact can you solve a puzzle. . . . It remains true that for any puzzle which is really a puzzle to be solved by using a paradigm, this paradigm must be a construct, an artifact, a system, or a tool together with the manual of instructions for doing it successfully and a method of interpretation of what it does (Masterman, 1970, p. 70).

From this description, it can be deduced that the paradigm, according to Kuhn, is a more highly evolved stage of science and that puzzle solving is its essential feature.

The cumulative work of scholars in both the physical and biological sciences has been guided by the type of paradigm described by Kuhn. Some social scientists (Ritzer, 1975; Friedrichs, 1970) have challenged the Kuhnian paradigm as being too narrow to be applicable to the social sciences, especially sociology. Ritzer (1975) asserted that a paradigm for the social sciences represents the broadest consensus of all scientists in the discipline; Friedrichs (1970) contended that the most important dimension of the paradigm in the social sciences is that it encompasses social scientists' image of themselves as scientific agents. The research of some nurse scholars is done within a broad social consensus rather than a true paradigm. As examples of this orientation, Hardy (1983) cited the construct of grounded theory (Glaser & Strauss, 1967) and the concept that a patient with a chronic illness takes on a *social identity* (Quint, 1969).

Because of the variety of definitions of paradigm from which the working scientist may select, there is an additional dilemma. Which definition will nurse scientists accept? Nurses must eventually agree on a definition, since without such a consensual base, it is doubtful that agreement can be reached on the puzzles and phenomena central to nursing. Ritzer's (1975) broader social definition of paradigm has appeal for a large number of scholars because of its apparent absence of fixed boundaries or rigid rules regarding the directions of research within a discipline. The social definition of a paradigm, however, fails to serve one of the important purposes of the paradigm: the demarca-

tion of one discipline's body of knowledge from that of another.

Nursing may never achieve an uncontested body of knowledge it can claim as its own science. However, for both pragmatic and philosophical reasons, theorists and researchers must continue the quest. Without a clearly defined science as the basis for practice, there can be no claim by practitioners in the discipline to a societally protected professional role.

Conceptual Models

A brief consideration of three nurse theorists' conceptual models provides the basis for a conclusion about nursing science's stage of evolution in Kuhnian terms.

Rogers (1970) has explicated a highly abstract conceptualization of mankind/environment. Man is defined as a unitary being in continuous, mutual, simultaneous interaction with the environment. In a later development of theoretical thinking, Rogers (1980) named this definition the principle of complementarity. Three principles are integral to Rogers's conception of unitary man—the principles of homeodynamics: helicy, resonancy, and complementarity. Rogers notes that these principles "have validity only within the context of this conceptual system of unitary man" (Rogers, 1980, p. 333). The principle of complementarity specifically excludes the idea of *causality*; that is, energy exchange across boundaries of the human-environmental field may bring about an alteration in the total system, but the addition of a variable does not *cause* a change in the human field.

This highly abstract conceptualization of man as a unitary being poses problems for nurse researchers because the usual methods of deductive research do not seem appropriate. Acceptable measures for rhythmicity, human field acceleration, and repatterning have yet to be developed.

Orem, like Rogers, views man as a unity—but here the similarity between the two conceptualizations ends. Orem stated than an individual is "a unity that can be viewed as functioning biologically, symbolically, and socially" (Orem, 1980, p. 120). And although Orem defined health as a state of wholeness or integrity, her conception of the individual as functioning in these three spheres suggests the prospect of analyzing the individual as a three-dimensional system rather than as an integrated whole.

Orem's model was constructed for a pragmatic purpose: to highlight the purpose of nursing, which is to provide appropriate assistance to individuals who have a self-care deficit in maintaining personal health. Orem conceptualizes a deficit relationship between the individual's "therapeutic self-care demand" and the self-care that can be marshalled. Three types of nursing systems are presumed to be available to persons with self-care deficits: (a) wholly compensatory, (b) partly compensatory, and (c) supportive-educative. Several concepts are not fully clarified in Orem's model. For example, it is unclear whether illness occurs when a self-care deficit is present; when parameters of the environment are not identified; or how a physical self-care deficit may be related or unrelated to a mental self-care deficit (Fawcett, 1984). Unlike Rogers's model, Orem's conceptual model contains elements of both nursing science and disciplinary practice.

Another model is that of Neuman, who postulated a wellness-illness model based on general systems theory in which an individual is defined as "an interacting open system in his total interface with his environment and is at all times either in a dynamic state of wellness or ill health in varying degrees" (Neumann, 1982, p. 9). A line of defense, buffers, and stressors are key concepts. At first glance, this conceptualization of the person seems almost identical to that of Rogers. A key point of difference, however, is Neuman's acknowledgement that within the environment (client system), "variables *affect* man and man in turn affects the variables found in the environment"(Neumann, 1982, p. 8). The word affect suggests a causal relationship between man and environment, but Rogers (1970) specifically excludes causality in her conceptualization of unitary man. Nursing is also a central concept in Neuman's model, with nursing's concern being the response of the individual to all environmental stressors.

These conceptual models do not provide evidence of Kuhn's interpretation that the paradigm must pro-

vide a puzzle-solving key. However, they do exemplify an additional function of a paradigm: delineation of an important set of beliefs. These examples demonstrate the belief of nurse scientists in the integrity of the individual and the inseparability of the person and the environment for the purpose of nursing. These conceptual models differ one from another in at least three important aspects:

1. They are at differing levels of abstraction.
2. The concepts are differentially defined.
3. The linkages between and among the concepts are not universally specified.

Thus, a preparadigm exists to the extent that these models are representative of nursing science.

Holistic/Humanitarian Approach

Watson's work is representative of the previously noted shift among nursing's theorists toward adoption of a holistic/humanitarian approach in developing theory. Watson contends that there is a *science of caring* and that this science is central to nursing. She has set forth seven basic assumptions and ten *carative factors* as the basis for a science of caring. The notion of a nursing core organized to encompass the carative factors is central to this concept. "The term core refers to those aspects of nursing that are intrinsic to the actual nurse-patient/client process that produces therapeutic results in the person being served. I refer to this basic core of nursing as comprising the philosophy and science of caring"(Watson, 1979, p. xv).

Watson has argued strongly for a humanistic perspective in developing knowledge to support a science of caring; for example, the first carative factor calls for "the formation of a humanistic-altruistic system of values" (Watson, 1979, p. 9). Despite this strong insistence on the humanistic approach to a science of caring, she is ambivalent about whether the scientific (normal science) method or some other method is more appropriate in studying the science of caring. "Just because the existence of something [caring] cannot be validated scientifically does not mean that it does not exist. . . . The scientific problem solving method is necessary for the science of caring to study, guide, direct and research knowledge and practice."(Watson, 1979, p. 56).

Apparently, Watson resolved the conflict by concluding that the scientific method is appropriate for nursing science, "as long as scientists use the basic assumptions and criteria for determining the nature of reality" (Watson, 1979, p. 58). Presumably, the assumptions and criteria are those delineated earlier as carative factors.

How is Watson's conceptualization of a science of caring related to the *persistent themes* previously alluded to in the conceptual frameworks of a large number of theorists? Does the construct of a "science of caring" compete with a science of nursing? Caring, as a construct, is central to the practice of nursing, but conceiving of it as a science promotes the undesirable blurring of the distinction between the science of nursing and its discipline. Caring, as it relates to the more highly abstract conceptual models of nursing, is a derived construct or instrumentality that is the aggregate of the therapeutic acts performed by nurses. In this disciplinary context, it represents a value central to the practice of nursing.

If the examples of nursing science's prevalent themes and concepts considered here are representative of the present status of knowledge development, this evolutionary phase of nursing's science conforms closely to Hardy's (1983) definition of the preparadigm. There are divergent schools of thought, concern for the same range of phenomena, and no single set of rules to direct further theory building.

Linking Nursing's Two Domains

The solving of nursing's puzzles is a joint enterprise of theorists, researchers, and practitioners. However, the way in which this responsibility is carried out must differ, given the primary responsibility inherent in each of the three roles. Practitioners need not take on the burdens that properly belong to theorists and researchers, but the important end is that "the discipline of nursing should be governing clinical practice rather than being defined by it" (Donaldson & Crowley, 1978, p. 118).

In an attempt to clarify the relationship between the domain of theory and the domain of practice, Kim (1983) has asserted that conceptual systems are important to both domains. She holds that ways of acting in the world of nursing action must be determined by scientific explanations or prescriptions.

In other words, our need to understand and explain scientific problems that reside in the domain of client and environment are for this ultimate purpose [prescriptions] as well. More specifically, only those theoretical postulates and empirical questions that have ultimate significance for the contents of nursing action can be considered to be within the nursing frame of reference, and require scientific answers for the nursing angle of vision. The starting point, then, for a scientific study of nursing is in thinking of nursing activities as "purposive" (Kim, 1983, p. 118).

Initially, Kim seems to separate scientific explanation from the "world of nursing action." However, the concluding assertion in this excerpt raises a question as to its exact meaning. If actions are prescribed on the basis of findings from scientific study, how can the *starting point* for a scientific study of nursing logically be in "thinking of nursing actions as purposive?" Kim assumes two loci of action: the client-nurse system and the nurse system. Kim points out that observation cannot be used to infer the nurse's perceptions in regard to the client. She believes that the majority of nursing actions outside the client-nurse system belong *in the nurse system* at the conceptual level. Thus, she states: "I believe that such behaviors can be explained and predicted within the theoretical constructs for the nurse system phenomena" (Kim, 1983, pp. 120-121).

Another conceptualization of the relationship between the domain of theory and that of practice is a system's schema, in which *knowledge* is conceived as the output variable (Conway, 1979). Two antecedent conditions are postulated: the existence of a body of theorists and a body of practitioners. In this model, the word *discipline* encompasses both. Theorists set forth theories and postulates (inputs). Throughputs in the model consist of the testing of hypotheses, their reformulation, and in collaboration with practitioners, the systematically application of findings in the practice domain. Both theorist and practitioner are represented in the practice domain as sharing responsibility for evaluating the outcomes of prescriptions derived from research findings and applied to the care of clients. This model would have appeal only for theorists and researchers who adhere to the logical-empirical tradition, since it does not take into account various "ways of seeing" or unique perceptions of "nursing's reality" (Watson, 1979).

It appears that the realization of a paradigm to guide both theory and research efforts lies in the future. There will have to be some intellectual accommodation between adherents of the logical-deductive method of science and adherents of the philosophy of science, since present evidence indicates that both perspectives offer important insights on nursing's central concerns. To the extent that both perspectives can aid in the discovery of nursing knowledge, both should be used.

Some researchers say nursing has a unique perspective that guides the formulation of its research questions in the absence of specified criteria for judging what a nursing question is (Gorenberg, 1983). This begs the all-important issue of whether the majority of the questions researched in the past represent the *real* puzzles of nursing science. In most instances, nursing research reflects the researcher's view of an important question, which presumably is justified by searching the literature to determine questions that have not been answered by previous research.

Fawcett (1984) has demonstrated substantial evidence for the existence of themes and concepts central to nursing's concerns in the conceptual frameworks of nurse theorists. But there is no consensus or world view regarding directions for the further development of nursing science. To move toward such a consensus, a clarification of nursing preparadigm should be attempted so that a road map leading to the metaparadigm can be drawn. A series of questions designed to distinguish between nursing's central concerns on the basis of whether each is a disciplinary concern or a

science concern might be a useful step in narrowing the preparadigm. If nursing is ultimately to acquire a body of theoretical knowledge having discernible boundaries and the potential for governing practice, it is essential that the appropriate distinction is maintained between the science of nursing and its discipline.

References

Conway, M. (1979). Knowledge generation and transmission: A role for the nurse administrator. *Nursing Administration Quarterly*, *3*(4), 29–41.

Donaldson, S., & Crowley, D. (1978). The discipline of nursing. *Nursing Outlook*, *26*, 113–120.

Eckberg, D.L., & Hill, L. (1979). The paradigm concept and sociology: A critical review. *American Sociology Review*, *44*, 925–937.

Fawcett, J. (1984). The metaparadigm of nursing: Present status and future refinements. *Image*, *16*, 84–87.

Friedrichs, R.W. (1970). *A sociology of sociology*. New York: Free Press.

Glaser, B., & Strauss, A. (1967). *The discovery of grounded theory: Strategies for qualitative research*. Chicago: Aldine.

Gorenberg, B. (1983). The research tradition of nursing: An emerging issue. *Nursing Research*, *32*, 347–349.

Hardy, M. (1983). Metaparadigms and theory development. In N.L. Chaska (Ed.), *The nursing profession: A time to speak* (pp. 427–437). New York: McGraw-Hill.

Jacox, A. (1974). Theory construction in nursing: An overview. *Nursing Research*, *23*, 4–13.

Kim, H.S. (1983). *The nature of theoretical thinking in nursing*. New York: Appleton-Century-Crofts.

Kuhn, T.S. (1970). *The nature of scientific revolutions* (2nd ed.). Chicago: University of Chicago Press.

Masterman, M. (1970). The nature of a paradigm. In I. Lakatos & A. Musgrave (Eds.), *Criticism and the growth of knowledge* (pp. 59–89). Cambridge, England: Cambridge University Press.

Neuman, B. (1982). *The Neuman systems model*. Norwalk, CT: Appleton-Century-Crofts.

Orem, D.E. (1980). *Nursing: Concept of practice* (2nd ed.). New York: McGraw-Hill.

Popper, K. (1959). *The logic of scientific discovery*. New York: Basic Books.

Quint, J. (1969). Becoming a diabetic: A study of emerging identity. Doctoral dissertation, University of California, San Francisco.

Ritzer, G. (1975). *Sociology: A multiple paradigm science*. Boston: Allyn & Bacon.

Rogers, M.E. (1970). *An introduction to the theoretical basis of nursing*. Philadelphia: F.A. Davis.

Rogers, M.E. (1980). A science of unitary man. In J. Riehl &

C. Roy (Eds.), *Conceptual models for nursing practice* (pp. 329–337). New York: Appleton-Century-Crofts.

Silva, M.C., & Rothbart, D. (1984). An analysis of changing trends in philosophies of science on nursing theory development and testing. *Advances in Nursing Science, 6(2), 1–13.*

Watson, J. (1979). *The philosophy and science of caring.* Boston: Little, Brown.

The Author Comments

I was prompted to explore the issue of nursing's so-called metaparadigm as identified by Fawcett and others by the thought that this declaration was premature and intellectually unjustified. I attempted to support this belief in this article, originally published in *Advances in Nursing Science* in 1985.

Admittedly, the question of the appropriateness of the so-called metaparadigm is open to debate. At the heart of the question, I believe, is the discipline's lack of common definitions of paradigm and metaparadigm and the *purpose* to be served by a paradigm for nursing. After much reflection, reading, and discussion with other nurse scholars, I have begun to question just how important it is that nursing declare its own metaparadigm. I think that it is less important than I once believed, and now subscribe to the view that several paradigms may best guide nursing research..

—MARY E. CONWAY

Chapter 27

Adopting an Evolutionary Lens: An Optimistic Approach to Discovering Strength in Nursing

Mary Carol Ramos

Appropriately, the state of the art of nursing is in constant review. Philosophy of science, particularly the work of Thomas Kuhn, has traditionally provided the criteria upon which these introspective evaluative processes are based. More recent developments in philosophy of science have introduced alternative models, such as Toulmin's evolutionary model, which might yield a more cogent, optimistic assessment of theoretical progress within nursing. Specific shortcomings of Kuhn's model and possible advantages of one evolutionary model are explored with comparative outcomes presented. Evidence of emerging evaluative criteria within nursing is also explicated.

Nurse scholars are appropriately conscientious in assessing their discipline's theoretical progress; healthy introspective critique and evaluation have characterized nursing during the past decades (Meleis, 1985). However, proportionately less attention has been given to the choice of criteria used in the process, criteria that have an enormous influence on the outcomes. Through self-examination, nursing ideally can evaluate its progress, trace the growth of its knowledge, and perceive change in its understanding of epistemological issues that pose questions for the discipline. But despite the inherent advantages of constant evaluation, a pessimis-

tic attitude or a tendency to underestimate strength (Hardy, 1978; Wooldridge, 1971) may emerge, partially due to the choice of evaluative criteria. In all likelihood, the present state of the art within nursing is more optimistic and healthy than might be perceived through the habitual use of outmoded, only partially applicable, evaluative tools.

The Revolutionary Model

Historically, nursing has turned to philosophy of science when evaluating disciplinary change in its cog-

About the Author

MARY CAROL RAMOS was born in Grand Rapids, Michigan and began her nursing education at Bronson Methodist Hospital, Kalamazoo, receiving a diploma in nursing in 1969. She then went on to study nursing at several schools and colleges in Michigan and Texas, earning a B.S.N. from the University of Texas Medical Branch, Galveston, in 1975 and a M.S. in Psychology from Lamar University, Beaumont, Texas in 1984. She then moved to Virginia and matriculated at the University of Virginia in 1985, from which she received a M.S.N. in Psychiatric-Mental Health Nursing in 1987 and a Ph.D. in Nursing in 1990. For her doctoral research, Dr. Ramos studied empathy in the nurse-patient relationship. Just as she has experienced a little bit of everything in nursing education, Dr. Ramos also has had wide-ranging employment experiences, including recent research assistantships at the University of Virginia.

When asked about nursing and its impact on her life, Dr. Ramos commented "Nursing history has done a great deal to inform my perspective of our progress and future. Interviewing practitioners for my dissertation research has given me great optimism—there are many well qualified people in nursing giving excellent care. I believe that as a group we can make a difference if we can be satisfied with our progress, strive to coalesce as a power force, and project our patient care goals onto developing health care policy." In a personal vein, she continued "Being a single parent to two adolescents who persist in telling me to "chill out" has helped me to be careful when setting priorities and attempting optimism about personal and professional issues. Having experienced nursing education at *all* levels, I feel well qualified to make observations."

nitive, ethical, and methodological realms. Philosophy of science offers criteria for ascertaining whether progress has occurred within a discipline by explicating models of scientific change. As knowledge within a discipline unfolds, is applied to disciplinary goals, and is disseminated, conceptual change can be examined. In evaluating the state of knowledge in nursing, authors most often cite one of the pioneers in philosophy of science, Thomas Kuhn. In his "revolutionary theory," he asserts that change within science has been characterized by "paradigm shifts," revolutions in accepted thought patterns that occur in a predictable manner after dissension grows between experts in a field (Kuhn, 1962, 1977). Nursing embraced Kuhn heavily in 1978, notably with Hardy's scholarly article applying his model to developing nursing science (Hardy, 1978). She equated the plethora of theoretical notions in nursing to the context of Kuhn's preparadigmatic stage. Her original observations are still valid; since there is widespread disagreement in nursing as to theory use and development and the value of theoretical underpinnings, nurses have not converged, and there is no "normal science" Hardy, 1978). Thus

nurses have become familiar with the word "paradigm" and have grown comfortable with the description of nursing as preparadigmatic. The nursing literature frequently refers to Kuhn's ideas and variously applies them to nursing and its development.

Possible Deficiencies in Kuhn's Model for Nursing

Although Kuhn's revolutionary model is widely accepted in the nursing literature, shortcomings in its application to many disciplines, including the human science of nursing, have become evident with the passage of time. Part of the frustration stems from his vague terminology; especially difficult is the multiple use of the word paradigm (Masterman, 1970). Is a paradigm in nursing a model, conceptual framework, theory, or metatheory? Consequently, criteria for identifying points of conceptual agreement and disagreement within nursing are not clear. Nursing is characterized as existing in a preparadigmatic state, where multiple schools of thought exist in a morass of confusion. Present levels of knowledge and theory cannot be evaluated (Hardy, 1978); progress is nearly impossible to trace.

The waning applicability of Kuhn's ideas partly relates to change within nursing. His model was predicated on historical study of the physical sciences (Kuhn, 1962). Nurse scientists of the 1970s, possibly seeking to emulate the credibility of the physical sciences, and well acquainted with quantitative approaches, described emergent nursing theory in Kuhnian terms. However, as nursing begins to emerge from the positivistic tradition (Webster, Jacox, & Baldwin, 1981; Suppe & Jacox, 1985) with its dependence on correspondence rules and a strict, classically empirical approach, perhaps a more open, encompassing explanation of change within the discipline is needed.

To further complicate the Kuhnian plight, the relationship between practice and theory in nursing is not easily explainable in terms of the revolutionary model. Since the writings of Dickoff, James, and Weidenbach (1968) and others (Conant, 1967; Ellis, 1969), there has been an ongoing effort to explore the interface between the scholarly, intellectual, and practical facets of nursing. Kuhn offers little insight into this relationship. In light of his evaluative criteria, there exists an uneasy truce between practice and theory, with evidence of suspicion in both camps. The credibility of theory is questioned by practitioners, sometimes resulting in a defensive stance by both.

The Metaparadigm: A Realistic Expectation?

In order to defend its utility and existence, scholars sometimes approach emergent nursing theory with strict criteria (Ellis, 1968; Hardy, 1974; Fawcett, 1984) as to its appearance, content, and relationship to practice, presumably in an attempt to formalize theory into a Kuhnian paradigm acceptable to all of nursing. Identification of a Kuhnian metaparadigm has occupied a number of nursing scholars. Presumably, its explication would define nursing as a discipline, where progress could be measured in Kuhnian terms (through the oc-

currence of revolutions in thought). Some would add that theory could develop only under the auspices of a unified metaparadigm (Conway, 1985).

Despite extensive growth within nursing, with scholarly work in progress, it frustrates Kuhnians to note that there may be no clear evidence of impending revolution, growing consensus, or emergence of agreement on an all-inclusive theory (metaparadigm) for nursing, one which demonstrates incommensurability with competing frameworks. The uniqueness of nursing does not emerge. There is no explanation for the cumulative nature of much of nursing's knowledge. Growth in nursing is not evident, and a frustrating lack of tools with which to measure progress persists.

There is no evidence that nursing, as a human science, rather than a compact physical science, is ever going to gain disciplinary status in Kuhnian terms. Kuhn's framework, then, loses explanatory power for nursing, since progress cannot be measured with clarity or ease, nor is choice between paradigms or bodies of suppositions guided by criteria. The wisdom of using Kuhn's model seems to fade in light of emerging alternatives from the realm of philosophy of science.

An Evolutionary Model

In his book, *Human Understanding*, philosopher of science Stephen Toulmin offers one alternative to Kuhn's revolutionary model. Toulmin's framework contrasts with Kuhn's in many dimensions. In reviewing Kuhn's explanation of scientific change, Toulmin asserts that Kuhn had difficulty demonstrating scientific revolutions historically (Toulmin, 1972). Moreover, he notes that Kuhn made no attempt to elucidate the mechanisms or reasons for consensus, on which the emergence of a metaparadigm depends. Another major criticism is Kuhn's lack of consideration for the importance of *conceptual change*. Thus Toulmin casts doubt on the utility of Kuhn's framework and seeks to remedy the deficits of the revolutionary model through the explication of an evolutionary model.

Toulmin's work presents three main themes: (a) a new definition of discipline, one encompassing a clearer role for practice; (b) an evolutionary approach toward change in disciplinary thought; and (c) a new account of human understanding, emphasizing the role of concepts and the relationship between disciplines and their accepted conceptual repertoires. In a Kantian mode, Toulmin attempts to combine the importance of empirical data and modern rationalist thought.

Toulmin's model, then, deals with the role and use of concepts as a model for change within scientific endeavors. He perceives conceptual change as an evolutionary process, with "intellectual innovation balanced against a continuing process of critical selection" (Toulmin, 1972, p. 140) rather than sporadic revolutions signaling the adoption of a novel conceptual system. For Toulmin, concepts unify knowledge. He examines the relationship between empirical and conceptual issues, and the way concepts are integrated into knowledge by the individual disciplinarian. Concepts are used to explain activities, he says, although conceptual systems cannot define or dictate a science. Concepts, rather, are of import in their use, their "explanatory activity" (Toulmin, 1972, p. 173). In Darwinian language, he postulates how disciplines develop and grow, and how the practice element of some disciplines is woven into that development. Concepts within a discipline inform and reflect the disciplinary world view. Conceptual usefulness changes as research and practice foci change. Conceptual boundaries between disciplines are also fluid, as problems change. In a Kantian sense, concepts represent the world. They must not be reified, nor should the metaphors they generate; concepts are merely tools to preserve, articulate, and help generate knowledge.

Conceptual change parallels historical change in disciplines, but the goal of scientific enterprise is not the ideal concept, for there is no ideal form. There is no formal axiomatic system to be rigidly replaced in a revolutionary manner. Conceptual change takes place almost imperceptibly, through progressive transformation of understanding and authority. Toulmin suggests that all motion is forward motion. Therefore, all change is for the better. Disciplines are not pursuing Kantian noumenal Truth, but simply a clearer path to understanding the world and its concepts. This realistic view

of continual growth seems to fit nursing particularly well.

Integration of Practice

Common, shared concepts, rather than a metaparadigm, define a discipline, according to Toulmin. Concepts that are of interest usually pertain to a set of problems encountered in a practice situation. Although his criteria would typify nursing as a "would-be" discipline, he incorporates an integral role for practice. Disciplines, he says, are intellectual endeavors; but the problems with which the disciplinarian struggles arise from the practice arena (Toulmin, 1972). Thus he addresses the age-old dilemma in nursing regarding the role of practice, theory, and research. They are integrally interwoven, the fabric of the endeavor. Because nursing cannot be practiced without conceptualization, concepts reflect the state of knowledge in practice settings. When practice changes, responding to environmental and social change, the discipline changes. For example, problems for Nightingale in the Crimea centered around sanitation issues. Decades later, sanitation problems were still encountered by nurses at the Henry Street Settlement. They probably used some concepts familiar to Nightingale, but they also had new knowledge in sanitation and applied epidemiological techniques. In addition, they would add other conceptual frameworks in striving to deliver nonthreatening health care to needy immigrants. Thus the conceptual body of knowledge changed and grew. It continues to grow, into the hospital setting, and out to the community. As problems grow and change, so do the concepts that explain and inform the discipline. Those concepts that are important at any moment are those pertaining to the problems encountered in practice.

The conceptual problems of the discipline (Laudan, 1972) demand answers, and conceptual growth is stimulated by such problems. Solved problems in practice constitute growth in knowledge development; conceptual definition and growth increase the explanatory power of the disciplinary body of knowledge. Consequently, the evolution of a discipline can be traced through conceptual change. Small increments of change can be appreciated in Toulmin's framework; in Kuhnian terms, such progress is not easily noted.

Dissent and Growth

There are other advantages in looking to Toulmin's model for the evaluation of nursing. It represents a system open to input from all levels of nursing. Growth in practice, academia, and research interact to promote the welfare of the whole of nursing. Rather than seeking total consensus in order to accomplish disciplinary growth, Toulmin sees room for dissent—disciplinarians need not agree on every conceptual definition pertaining to their work and thought. Dissension plays as large a role as consensus, since in Toulmin's framework, there is no search for the "correct" answer. Some discussion in nursing (Thompson, 1985; Chinn, 1986) has recognized the value in discourse and conceptual debate within the discipline. Continuous interchange of thought takes place, with intellectual debate serving to refine the ideas.

When applied to practice, those ideas that advance the discipline are preserved, and those that fail to serve are abandoned, to be resurrected when utility demands. In an evolutionary framework, Toulmin likens this to Darwin's "ecological niche." When environmental circumstances permit, species survive. Otherwise, they perish. Within nursing, the utility of disciplinary knowledge within practice will preserve that knowledge. Otherwise, it will be shelved until (and only when) that knowledge is demanded pragmatically. However, knowledge that is not used does not cease to exist. In nursing, that becomes evident in many situations, such as the emergence of older ideals of environmental management in public health practice, cast in the new image of home health care in the changing delivery system.

Evolution Toward Self-Evaluation

The keystone of any discipline, according to Toulmin, is the concept. The concept is integral to nursing. The foundations of theory and practice and struggles to ex-

plicate the uniqueness of nursing center on conceptualization. Concepts and their application, relative to knowledge, epitomize the growth of nursing as a discipline. Nursing and its progress should be measured in terms of concepts, whether the traditional ideal of man, health, nursing, and environment (Fawcett, 1984; Flaskerud & Halloran, 1980) or the emergent ideals of a new practitioner. Nursing must be open to emergent uses of traditional concepts as well as the advent of new conceptual ideals. Knowledge cannot grow unless scholars understand that nothing is irrelevant in principle. Closure must be avoided.

Concepts change with the empirical needs of the practice. The body of conceptual knowledge is constantly evolving in response to the forces around it. Neophytes are given the body of conceptual knowledge and values as the "transmit" of the discipline, and they are encouraged to modify it in a creative, open manner (Toulmin, 1972, p. 158). In Toulmin's model, there is not only room, but also a demand for creativity, and a need for constructive dissent within the discipline. Both are necessary for the health of the conceptual body (perhaps necessitating an examination of the tendency to suppress creativity). Agreement and disagreement must be articulated, separate from personal identities. Evaluation is continual and is practiced by all those in direct contact with the body of knowledge. Meaning is gained through intellectual debate; communication between disciplinarians is of paramount importance. Through these refining processes, nurses will gain conceptual understanding and develop intradisciplinary criteria with which to evaluate nursing and communicate its progress and value to others.

One outgrowth of the evolutionary process is already strong within nursing, the embracing of new modes of inquiry (Benner, 1985; Benoliel, 1984; Goodwin & Goodwin, 1984; Smith, 1981). Increasing flexibility within the research community toward less empirical methodologies has stimulated an appreciation of certain characteristics and processes within nursing that are not quantifiable. That realization, coupled with nursing's ties with academia, has given rise to an acceptance of creative alternatives to standard, empirical methodology in acquiring and transmitting knowledge.

Toulmin and the Present State of Nursing

Toulmin's framework can help nursing to understand its present state, in terms of concepts, research questions, and the relationship between theory and practice. Disciplinary knowledge evolves through explanations garnered in research. Research problems are generated in practice. Thus, according to Laudan (1972), the "solved problem" becomes part of disciplinary knowledge. Whatever methodology is cogent is utilized. Nursing is given the freedom to enlarge its idea of science and consider itself scientific if that is indeed valuable to its identity.

In view of Toulmin's framework, then, nursing need not strive after a metaparadigm; it is not even advisable at this stage of development. The most meaningful activity centers around definition of an existing "transmit," the body of knowledge, values, and social skills to be passed on to new nurses. Together nurses can calmly and pragmatically evaluate nursing knowledge and how well it solves problems in practice, and how its language and understanding of relevant concepts can be refined to better advance communication between disciplinarians. New modes of practice and research can communicate to the novice the scope of expert knowledge and the behavioral repertoire of the expert (Benner, 1984; Benner & Wrubel, 1982). Problems in practice can be addressed using overt and tacit knowledge, expanding even on Carper's (1978) classic modalities. There is comfort in Toulmin's notion that practitioners and researchers can be "two men," utilizing those with theoretically facile minds (but perhaps limited psychomotor skill) in theorizing, while others do the practice.

The future holds great promise. Articulation of goals, values, and purpose will stimulate the emergence of philosophical criteria for evaluating change, evaluation carried out by and for nursing by the new philosophers of nursing. New insight will result from pragmatic evaluation of concepts and conceptual change. Nursing will grow to accept the differences between nursing and the more "compact" disciplines, appreciate the waxing and waning of theoretical frameworks, and enjoy debate in the intellectual forum. The relative roles of theorizing, evaluating, and practicing will intertwine; different corps of nurses will do each and communicate openly. The future for nursing is bright, if evaluated in light of nursing's relative newness in the academic world and the stunning progress made during this century, conceptually and pragmatically. The state of the art for nursing is one of health, prosperity, and promise, magnified through the use of a suitable framework in viewing its strengths.

References

Beckstrand, J. (1978). The notion of a practice theory and the relationship of scientific and ethical knowledge to practice. *Research in Nursing and Health, 1*, 131–136.

Benner, P. (1984). *From novice to expert*. Menlo Park, CA: Addison-Wesley.

Benner, P. (1985). Quality of life: A phenomenological perspective on explanation, prediction, and understanding in nursing science. *Advances in Nursing Science, 8*(1), 1–14.

Benner, P., & Wrubel, J. (1982). Skilled clinical knowledge: The value of perceptual awareness. *Nurse Educator, 7*, 11–17.

Benoliel, J.Q. (1984). Advancing nursing science: Qualitative approaches. Proceedings of the 1984 conference of the Western Society for Research in Nursing. *Western Journal of Nursing Research, 6*(3), 1–9.

Chinn, P.L. (1986). Getting older, getting wiser? *Advances in Nursing Science, 8*(3), v–vi.

Conant, L.H. (1967). Closing the practice-theory gap. *Nursing Outlook, 15*(11), 37–39.

Dickoff, J., James, P., & Weidenbach, E. (1968). Theory in a practice discipline. Part I: Practice-oriented theory. *Nursing Research, 17*(5), 415–435.

Ellis, R. (1968). Characteristics of significant theories. *Nursing Research, 17*(3), 217–222.

Ellis, R. (1969). The practitioner as theorist. *American Journal of Nursing, 69*, 428–435.

Fawcett, J. (1984). *Analysis and evaluation of conceptual modes of nursing*. Philadelphia: F.A. Davis.

Flaskerud, J.H., & Halloran, E.J. (1980). Areas of agreement in nursing theory development. *Advances in Nursing Science, 3*(1), 1–7.

Goodwin, L.D., & Goodwin, W.L. (1984). Qualitative vs. quantitative research or qualitative and quantitative research? *Nursing Research, 33*(6), 378–380.

Hardy, M.E. (1974). Theories: Components, development evaluation. *Nursing Research, 23*(2), 100–107.

Hardy, M.E. (1978). Perspectives on nursing theory. *Advances in Nursing Science, 1*(1), 27–48.

Kuhn, T.S. (1962). *The structure of scientific revolutions*. Chicago: University of Chicago Press.

Kuhn, T.S. (1977). *The essential tension*. Chicago: University of Chicago Press.

Laudan, L (1972). *Progress and its problems*. Berkeley, CA: University of California Press.

Masterman, M. (1970). The nature of a paradigm, In I. Lakatos & A. Musgrave (Eds.), *Criticism and the growth of knowledge*. Cambridge, England: Cambridge University Press.

Meleis, A.I. (1985). *Theoretical nursing: Development and progress*. Philadelphia: J.B. Lippincott.

Smith, J.A. (1981). The idea of health: A philosophical inquiry. *Advances in Nursing Science*, *3*(3), 43–50.

Suppe, F., & Jacox, A.K. (1985). Philosophy of science and the development of nursing theory. In H.H. Werley & J.J. Fitzpatrick (Eds.), *Annual review of nursing research* (pp. 241–267). New York: Springer.

Toulmin, S. (1972). *Human understanding*. Princeton, NJ: Princeton University Press.

Webster, G., Jacox, A., & Baldwin, B. (1981). Nursing theory and the ghost of the received view. In J. McCloskey & H. Grace (Eds.), *Current issues in nursing* (pp. 26–43). Boston: Blackwell.

Wooldridge, P.J. (1971). Metatheories of nursing: A commentary on Dr. Walker's article. *Nursing Research*, *20*(6), 494–495.

Bibliography

Carper, B.A. (1978). Fundamental patterns of knowing in nursing. *Advances in Nursing Science*, *1*(1), 13–23.

Collins, R.M., & Fielder, J.H. (1981). Beckstrand's concept of practice theory: A critique. *Res Nurs Health*, *4*, 317–321.

Conway, M.E. (1985). Toward greater specificity in defining nursing's metaparadigm. *Advances in Nursing Science*, *7*(4), 73–81.

Hall, B.A. (1981). The change paradigm in nursing: Growth versus persistence. *Advances in Nursing Science*, *3*(4), 1 6.

Jacox, A.K., & Webster, G. (1986). Competing theories of science. In L.H. Nicoll (Ed.), *Perspectives on nursing theory* (pp. 335–341). Boston: Little, Brown.

MacPherson, K.I. (1983). Feminist methods: A new paradigm for nursing research. *Advances in Nursing Science*, *5*(2), 17–25.

Meleis, A.I., & May, K. (1981). Nursing theory and scholarliness in the doctoral program. *Advances in Nursing Science*, *4*(1), 31–41.

Munhall, P.L. (1982). Ethical juxtapositions in nursing research. *Topics in Clinical Nursing*, *4*(1), 66–73.

Munhall, P.L. (1982). Nursing philosophy and nursing research: In apposition or opposition? *Nursing Research*, *31*(3), 176–181.

Munhall, P.L. (1983). Methodological fallacies: A critical self-appraisal. *Advances in Nursing Science*, *5*(4), 41–49.

Silva, M.C., & Rothbart, D. (1984). An analysis of changing trends in philosophies of science on nursing theory development and testing. *Advances in Nursing Science*, *6*(2), 1–13.

Thompson, J.L. (1985). Practical discourse in nursing: Going beyond empiricism and historicism. *Advances in Nursing Science*, *7*(4), 59–71.

Walker, L.O. (1971). Toward a clearer understanding of the concept of nursing theory. *Nursing Research*, *20*(5), 428–435.

Woolridge, P.J. (1986). The author comments . . . In L.H. Nicoll (Ed.), *Perspectives on nursing theory* (pp. 42–43). Boston: Little, Brown.

The Author Comments

Simultaneous immersion in philosophical, theoretical, and historical literature provided the premise for this paper. Historical inquiry provided a new appreciation of the progress of our profession in slightly more than a century. Our modest beginnings as a domestic vocation have given rise to academic standing and a growing cadre of highly educated professionals. Review of the theoretical literature, however, revealed an underappreciation of what I perceived, in an historical sense, to be great strength in nursing knowledge. Metatheoretical analysis in nursing became rather common during the 1970s, but the criteria used to evaluate disciplinary knowledge were drawn from philosophy of science, notably the work of Thomas Kuhn. Given a lack of metatheory specializing in "philosophy of nursing," this was perhaps the best alternative. However, Kuhn's criteria were devised to assess physical, not human, sciences; the fit between the criteria and the subject matter was, perhaps, tenuous. Kuhn's criteria reflected an Aristotelian dichotomy between theoretical and applied knowledge. The notion that applied knowledge is inferior to "pure science" was deeply ingrained in our culture and reflected in Kuhn's work. Nursing, with a strong practice component, was automatically subordinate to bench science in his schema.

As nurse scientists, we want to answer the classic epistemological questions: "Do we know?" "How do we know?" and "How do we know that we know?" We want to perceive forward motion. A model to evaluate such progress should be flexible enough to allow for the richness within nursing, including our complex, practice-bound value system. This notion is not impossible, given a loosening view of science as an activity. It is presently accepted that science is not value-free, that science does not grow in an orderly fashion, that science is not built on a foundation of pure observation, and that science is not totally goal-oriented. Although Toulmin's evolutionary model is also not the ideal for evaluation of nursing as a discipline, it is critical that we test different criteria to trace our progress. If there are no criteria that can be drawn directly from nursing philosophers, let us know that measurement of our advancement must be done carefully. As a philosopher friend suggested, "There is no way to measure the length of a caterpillar with a ruler that says, 'not yet a butterfly'."

—MARY CAROL RAMOS

Chapter 28

Perspectives on Knowing: A Model of Nursing Knowledge

Maeona K. Jacobs-Kramer
Peggy L. Chinn

In the premiere issue of Advances in Nursing Science *(October, 1978), Barbara Carper detailed a typology of nursing knowledge. Carper's ideas have been appreciated and commented upon extensively in the nursing literature, with little extension of her work. This article describes a model of nursing knowledge that builds from Carper's initial formulation. The model begins with an interpretation of Carper's four original knowledge patterns: empirics, ethics, aesthetics, and personal. Each pattern is considered in relation to: (a) developmental processes and product outcomes associated with its creation; (b) expressions of the pattern; and (c) process context for assessing credibility of knowledge associated with the pattern. The position taken is that all knowledge patterns must be integrated to enable deliberate clinical choices. A failure to integrate knowledge patterns impedes choice and produces negative care outcomes.*

In the premiere issue of *Advances in Nursing Science*, Barbara Carper (1978) set forth a typology of knowledge forms utilized in nursing. Since the appearance of this article, Carper's work has been widely cited, appreciated, and commented upon in nursing. Moreover, there is an increasing literature concerning the necessity for nursing knowledge other than traditional empirics (Allen, Benner, & Diekelmann, 1986; Benner, 1984; Benner & Tanner, 1987; Chinn, 1985). The interest in developing and using alternate knowledge forms as well as exploiting the full range of empirics is consistent with the aims and methods of a human science which is recognized as a legitimate orientation for nursing (Meleis, 1987; Watson, 1985). Pursuing the tenets of human science within nursing raises many questions and issues regarding the aims and purposes of nursing knowledge, as well as how it is developed, transmitted, and evaluated. Although Carper's work was significant in that it named knowledge forms in addition to empirics and set them out for debate and discussion, it remains for nurses collectively to consider how knowledge patterns other than empirics are devel-

About the Authors

MAEONA K. KRAMER (formerly Jacobs) is currently a Professor in the Parent-Child and Adult Nursing Programs at the College of Nursing, University of Utah, in Salt Lake City. She grew up in rural Akron, Michigan, a town she describes as "a small farming community in the thumb area," and studied nursing in Michigan, receiving a diploma from St. Joseph Hospital School of Nursing and B.S.N., M.S.N., and Ph.D. degrees from Wayne State University. In early 1972, she accepted a faculty appointment at the University of Utah and now considers the West, particularly the intermountain area, to be home.

Dr. Kramer's specialty is nursing theory, nursing metatheory, and philosophy of nursing knowledge. Besides publishing various journal articles in these areas, she has coauthored (with Peggy L. Chinn) a beginning text in theory titled *Theory and Nursing: A Systematic Approach* (St. Louis: C.V. Mosby, 1983). Her early clinical interest was in cardiovascular nursing, and she has published on various aspects of cardiac functioning in both healthy and ill adults in several journals, including *Research in Nursing and Health* and *Western Journal of Nursing Research*. Her work on the management of dependent pregnancy edema in healthy women has appeared in *Nursing Research*. Dr. Kramer was a founding foresister of Cassandra: Radical Feminist Nurses' Network and is active in the network both locally and nationally. She also holds membership in WICHN (Western Interstate Commission for Higher Education in Nursing), WSRN (Western Society for Research in Nursing), ANA, and Sigma Theta Tau.

When asked about nursing theory and her thoughts about the future, Dr. Kramer comments "I believe we need to begin teaching metatheory in the undergraduate programs. Perhaps 'metaknowledge' would be a better way to phrase it. Our new graduates need to know how theory, practice, and research relate to make a difference. This can be done more effectively if we realistically examine theory within the context of other forms of knowledge and if we begin to examine it sooner in our educational programs."

PEGGY L. CHINN currently lives in Denver, Colorado, but considers Hawaii to be home. She received a B.S. with a major in Nursing from the University of Hawaii in 1964, then continued her education at the University of Utah, receiving an M.S. with honors in Child Nursing in 1970 and a Ph.D. in Educational Psychology in 1971. Currently, Dr. Chinn is a Professor of Nursing at the University of Colorado, Health Sciences Center and the Center for Human Caring, where she teaches graduate courses in theory, research, and nursing as a human science. Before coming to the University of Colorado in 1990, Dr. Chinn held faculty appointments at Wright State University, Texas Women's University, the University of Utah, and the State University of New York at Buffalo.

Besides holding her teaching position, Dr. Chinn serves as editor of *Advances in Nursing Science*. As editor, she has formulated and evaluated the journal's purpose and philosophy and is involved in reviewing manuscripts, planning content and editorials, and guiding ongoing development and evaluation. She believes that another important role of an editor is advising prospective authors during early stages of manuscript development.

Dr. Chinn is an active feminist; her participation in feminist activities on various levels has helped to shape her nursing perspective. She is cofounder and member of Cassandra: Radical Feminist Nurses' Network, and has presented on various aspects of feminism at a number of Cassandra gatherings around the country as well as publishing several articles on similar themes in the newsjournal. Recently she coauthored, with Charlene Eldridge Wheeler, a book on feminist process titled *Peace and Power: A Handbook of Feminist Process* (New York: National League for Nursing, 1989, 2nd ed.). Her current research interest is in developing a methodology for the art of nursing that draws on both feminist and critical theory.

Dr. Chinn has been involved in curriculum revolution work for the National League for Nursing for the past 3 years. In Fall 1990, she spent several months at Deakin University, Geelong, Victoria, Australia, assisting with curriculum development, teaching feminist theory and theory development, and researching concepts in the curriculum.

oped and used, transmitted, evaluated, and integrated into practice.

The purpose of this paper is to develop a model that constructs a perspective on the generation, transmission, and evaluation of knowledge forms other than traditional empirics and to consider the purpose for which nursing knowledge is created. It builds upon and modifies a beginning conceptualization published by us in 1987 (Chinn & Jacobs, 1987), while retaining its essential features. In this article the four knowledge patterns originally named by Carper (1978), empirical, ethical, personal, and aesthetic knowledge, form the basis of the model. Each of the patterns is extended by considering how it is created, expressed, and assessed. Our interpretive overview of the knowledge patterns is followed by a discussion of the creative, expressive, and assessment dimensions of the model.

Overview of Knowledge Patterns

Empirical knowledge—the science of nursing—is the pattern most closely associated with traditional science. Empirical knowledge represents knowledge that accrues from sensory experience. Empirics is classically expressed as principles, laws, and theories that have general applicability. It comprises knowledge acquired and transmitted through understanding the meanings of commonly held language symbols— that which is public, verifiable, and common. Empirics rests upon assumptions of linear time and a degree of temporal stability for phenomena represented by this pattern.

Ethical knowledge relates to matters of duty, rights, obligations, and moral imperatives. Ethical knowledge and reasoning processes are invoked when it is necessary to make a decision about a deliberate, voluntary action that is subject to the judgment "right" or "wrong." Ethical knowledge also directs judgments and actions which, though not moral imperatives, obligations, or duties, may be good, noble, or honorable actions. Although ethical knowledge is communicable through language symbols, it is not public, verifiable, and common in the same sense as empirics. Legitimate disagreements can exist over whether or not the same

course of action is "right" or "wrong," "ethical" or "unethical," "noble, honorable, and good" or not.

Personal knowledge is awareness of self and others in a relationship. It involves encountering and actualizing the self. Personal knowledge transcends objective reality, forms, and stereotypes and is not mediated by the symbols of language. That is, knowledge of self and others can be transmitted independent of written discourse. One comes to know self and others through living and lived immediate experience.

Aesthetic knowledge—the art of nursing—is knowledge gained by subjective acquaintance. Whereas empirical knowledge involves the abstraction of generalities, aesthetic knowledge requires abstracting that which is individual, particular, and unique. This knowledge pattern represents an immediate knowing that is based on comprehending specific and unique situational particulars, integrating those particulars into a balanced and unified whole, and acting in relation to projected outcomes. Our interpretation and modification of Carper's (1978) knowledge patterns form the basis for considering how each knowledge pattern is created, expressed, and assessed.

Empirics: Creative, Expressive, and Assessment Dimensions

The creative dimension expresses the interrelationship between the processes of knowledge creation and the product created. To consider the creative dimension is to consider what the knowledge pattern is useful for, and how—through use of knowledge within the pattern—knowing and knowledge are extended and modified. For empirics, processes within the creative dimension include the familiar research approaches of describing, explaining, and predicting. The product—empirical knowledge—is used to describe, explain, and predict, and as empirics are invoked for describing, explaining, and predicting, the process accrues information that is germane to extending and modifying it. In addition to formal research processes, clinicians in their practice may use empirically derived knowledge or data that describes, explains, or predicts features of clinical experience, such as stress-coping. As clinicians apply empirical knowledge, client responses provide information about its adequacy. These responses, in turn, provide a basis for modification of that knowledge. Appreciation of processes operating within the model's creative dimension is central to understanding how the emerging product and ongoing process are expressed.

The expressive dimension of the model is conceptualized as a means to represent the form of knowledge expression associated with the pattern. That is, knowledge expression considers how patterns of knowing can be exhibited as knowledge. For empirics, descriptive, explanatory, and predictive knowledge can be expressed as facts, theories, models, and descriptions that impart understanding. Empirics tends to take forms that are rather "naturally static," since empirical knowledge is bounded, linear, and symbolically represented. Empirical knowledge related to stress-coping might be expressed as models and theories, interpretive descriptions of the meaning of stress, facts reflecting its incidence, and clinical opinions about how to manage stressful experiences. How knowledge is expressed is significant for considering processes invoked when knowledge is examined for credibility—the assessment dimension.

The third dimension of the model is assessment, which provides for an examination of the separate knowledge forms. Assessment of knowledge involves three aspects: First, a critical question asked of each knowledge pattern to discern the adequacy of the pattern as a pattern; second, the process context that is specific to the ongoing creation; and third, a unique credibility index that is associated with each knowledge pattern. Not only do knowledge patterns differ in how they are created and expressed, but they differ in processes and methods for assessing their value and utility. While assessment addresses the credibility of each pattern as a unique pattern, this does not equate with the evaluation of knowledge that emerges from integration of all knowledge patterns. Each knowledge pattern can be evaluated as credible in and of itself, but its ultimate value is addressed when the knowledge pattern is inte-

grated with other forms of knowing and applied to a specific care situation. For example, it is possible to create a very "good" empirically based theory that many not result in a "good" client outcome when clinically applied.

Empirical knowledge is assessed by invoking the critical questions "What does this represent?" and "How is it representative?" These questions imply an assessment of how some reality is expressed and how that expression functions as a form of human knowledge. The process and context for addressing these empirical questions is replication. In replication, the knowledge must be repeatable across similar contexts. Validity is the index of credibility. The knowledge must be demonstrated to be what it is thought to be.

Assessment of stress-coping theory involves discerning what reality the theory represents and determining the adequacy of the linkages between behavioral expressions and interpretations of stress and theoretical knowledge about stress. As questions of validity and reliability are addressed, the limitations and value of stress/coping theory become more fully known. Engagement in this process of determining credibility is useful for continuing to develop empirical knowledge. Table 28-1 summarizes the features of the creative, expressive, and assessment dimensions for all knowledge patterns. Table 28-2 summarizes the essen-

Table 28-1
Summary of Model's Features: Creative, Expressive, and Assessment Dimensions

Dimensions	Features
Creative	Captures how knowledge is generated and extended through its use. Implies process product interaction; implies motion.
Expressive	Captures how knowledge pattern is exhibited and recognized. Knowledge display with "stasis" of time.
Assessment	Provides for examination of knowledge by: (1) asking critical questions of knowledge form; (2) within a process context; and (3) using a pattern-specific credibility index.

tial elements of each dimension for empirics as discussed, as well as for ethics, personal, and esthetic knowledge, to be considered next.

Ethics: Creative, Expressive and Assessment Dimensions

The creative dimension of ethical knowledge involves valuing, clarifying, and advocating. This pattern is both created by and extended through these processes. Individuals and groups come to hold various positions about what is right and ethical through learning and internalizing values, clarifying the emerging values, and advocacy of these values for self and others. As the process of valuing, clarifying, and advocacy proceed, ethical knowledge continues to emerge.

Ethical knowledge is expressed through codes and standards, and more formally in normative ethical theories. These forms represent common patterns of ethical knowledge expression. Ethical knowledge, however, can also be expressed in descriptions of ethical decision making. Such descriptions elucidate important contextual features that determine how an ethical judg-

ment is finally made. Descriptions can also address the reasoning processes used in reaching a course of action. Ethics also shares some characteristics with empirics in the expressive dimension. That is, ethical knowledge can be expressed as theory and, even if not in theoretical form, it is linear, discursive, and mediated by language symbols.

Even though ethical knowledge is expressed in a form similar to empirics, ethical forms of knowledge are assessed quite differently. It is the justness, rightness, and responsibleness of ethical knowledge that is sought as the standard of judgment when this knowledge pattern is assessed rather than reproduction or replicability. The critical questions asked of ethical knowledge are: "Is this right?" "Is this just?" The process context involved in asking these questions is dialogue, while the credibility index is justness. With ethical knowledge it is not sufficient to logically analyze an ethical decision with reference to a normative ethical theory, professional code, or standard. Rather, dialogue is required to share understanding of contextual meaning and elucidate reasoning processes. Since in examining the credibility of ethical knowledge the reference

Table 28–2
Summary of Essential Elements: Model of Nursing Knowledge

Dimension	Empirics	Ethics	Personal	Esthetics
Creative	Describing	Valuing	Encountering	Engaging
	Explaining	Clarifying	Focusing	Interpreting
	Predicting	Advocating	Realizing	Envisioning
Expressive	Facts	Codes	Self: authentic and	Art-act
	Theories	Standards	disclosed	
	Models	Normative-ethical theories		
	Descriptions to impart understanding	Descriptions of ethical decision making		
Assessment				
Critical question	What does this represent? How is it representative?	Is this right? Is this just?	Do I know what I do? Do I do what I know?	What does this mean?
Process/context	Replication	Dialogue	Response and reflection	Criticism
Credibility index	Validity	Justness	Congruity	Consensual meaning

point is not externally located empirical reality, multiple ethical positions in relation to a single situation may be justified.

To illustrate, nurses can be expected to possess or have at their disposal a storehouse of ethical values, principles, and precepts that are derived, in part, from the codes of the profession, societal norms and values, and individual professional experiences. We express these values in practice by valuing, advocating, and clarifying health care options, and in so doing we contribute to the emergence of ethical patterns of knowing.

For nurses, processes of client advocacy and clarifying the meaning of life and living have potential to alter the prevailing values of the health care system. Having experience with the predominant ethical position that life equates with physical processes, we are coming to view life and living as requiring a dimension of quality that goes beyond physical existence. The emergence of a changed value or conceptualization of life and living can then be reflected in ethical knowledge forms such as descriptive opinions about the nature of quality and life living, or professional codes related to nursing when physical life can no longer be sustained. The newly emerged knowledge forms express both what was done and what ought to be done and can be subsequently assessed through a process of dialogue with others.

Personal Knowledge: Creative, Expressive, and Assessment Dimensions

The personal knowledge pattern expresses knowledge of self—an individual in relationship with others. The creative dimension of personal knowledge involves experiencing the self—encountering and focusing on self while realizing its realities and potentialities. Like other knowledge patterns, personal knowledge is conceptualized as useful for facilitating the processes of experiencing, encountering, and focusing, and these processes evolve ongoing knowledge of self.

The expressive dimension of personal knowledge

is the self as authentic and disclosed. Authenticity implies what the personal self actually is at any moment and is not meant to connote what finally emerges after a lifetime of work. The authentic self is known privately, while the disclosed self can be revealed to others. Unlike empirical and ethical knowledge, this knowledge pattern is not represented in language. Though it is possible to write about self as authentic and disclosed, it is not possible to write about or record "self." Personal knowledge is expressed as our selves, through the self.

The assessment dimension of personal knowledge requires a focus on the self as privately known and expressed to others. Assessment of self is a process carried out by the self through a rich inner life, but not solely in the context of aloneness. Assessment involves examining the expression form — the self - for congruity of the authentic self with the disclosed self. The intent of this conceptualization is closely aligned with Watson's (1985) notion of "I-Me" congruity. Critical questions address the credibility index of congruity. Asking to what extent we "know what we do" and "do what we know" creates awareness of both the authentic and disclosed self. This enables personal movement toward inner strength, genuineness, and authenticity —characteristics associated with congruity. Reflection and response is the process context associated with assessment of self as a pattern of knowing. As the individual examines self, perceptions and insights are reflected and responded to by others. The reflected responses provide insight about the individual self and its congruity.

In caring encounters, nurse and client participate in a sharing of their unique selves. During the encounter, what is disclosed becomes a basis for knowledge about the authenticity of self and other. The unique situation of client and nurse encounter makes possible disclosure of self, one to another. As client and nurse focus on the client's situation, heightened awareness of what each person feels or "knows" and how they act or "do" emerges in the encounter. Personal knowing grows to the extent that actions are in concert with the whole of inner experience.

Aesthetics: Creative, Expressive, and Assessment Dimensions

The pattern of aesthetics is a difficult pattern to comprehend because it can be conceptualized as both a separate knowledge form and a synthesis of all knowledge forms. As a separate pattern, it constitutes knowledge about artful nursing practice—knowledge that is expressed with difficulty because it is fully dependent on and integrates context. For example, expert nurses may be able to provide some insight into the esthetic knowledge they possess and use in caring for clients. Specifics of how they have used and expect to employ such knowledge, however, defy description because they do not "know" what they will do until they are in a situation, and what they "know" changes with the situation. Although the expression of aesthetic knowledge is only partially describable in language, it is fully comprehensible when the whole of experience is considered.

As the synthesis of knowledge patterns, aesthetics can be viewed as the total knowledge spectrum integrated in practice. The creative dimension of aesthetics involves engaging, interpreting, and envisioning. Aesthetics requires engagement in the moment and the "all-at-once" interpretation of a situation to project an outcome and act in relation to what is envisioned. As nurses encounter clients in practice contexts, aesthetic knowledge is integrated with all other forms of knowing to form and continue forming patterns of engagement, interpreting, and envisioning. New knowledge emerges in this process.

Although the creative dimension of aesthetics is associated with engagement, interpreting, and envisioning, its creation depends upon the artful enfoldment of all knowledge patterns. Aesthetics as a separate knowledge pattern enfolds itself with empirical, ethical, and personal knowledge to bring about a harmonious and pleasing whole—an artful nursing act.

Aesthetic knowledge finds expression in the art-act of nursing. Like personal knowledge, the expression of aesthetic knowledge is not in language. We can unfold our art and retrospectively recollect and write about its features, and we can record it using electronic media, but the knowledge form itself is not what we write or record. The knowledge form is the art-act.

The assessment of aesthetic knowledge involves a consideration of meaning in those aspects of the art-act that can be represented. The art-act is responded to by criticism, which is the process context by which the knowledge pattern is assessed. Criticism can be thought of as an explanation of a judgment that finally reduces to the simple statement: "This means that" (Bleich, 1978). Criticism assumes that interpretation of meaning is motivated behavior and that meaning is constructed in relation to some purpose. The critical question asked of the art-act is, "What does this mean?" Criticism requires empathy and an intent to fully appreciate what the actors meant to convey. As the art-act is criticized, credibility is discerned by reaching for consensus—a full and rich understanding of the art-act that brings together the perspectives of a community of co-askers who construct and confer meanings. Seeking consensual meaning as motivated behavior implies a desire and need to create knowledge on one's behalf. It does not imply mere agreement or acquiescence to some meaning but connotes deep understanding of intents, a reconciliation of self with others.

To summarize, as nurses encounter clinical situations, knowledge is brought to those encounters that can be conceived of as having different patterns: empirics, ethics, personal, and esthetic. Nurses possess: (a) objective, empirically based knowledge such as stress-coping theory and statistics about stress phenomena; (b) knowledge of what is ethically right and good; (c) personal knowledge of themselves and how they relate to others; and (d) knowledge about how they might esthetically approach, balance, and integrate this knowledge in differing clinical situations. To some extent, individual nurses and the profession collectively can examine these knowledge patterns separately for credibility to heighten awareness of the state of knowledge within them.

As practice contexts are encountered, processes within the creative dimension of aesthetics are initiated. Through the process of engagement, interpreting, and envisioning, "past" knowledge is enfolded into aesthetics, and clients are uniquely cared for. As caring processes continue, new knowledge emerges. When the nursing context is "exited," the art-act as the experience of nurse and client can be unfolded to reveal the newly emerged separate knowledge patterns. These separate knowledge patterns can be individually examined for their contributions to the total art-act, how they are altered as a result of their enfoldment during the encounter, and where the knowledge base was problematic. The total art-act, as the expression of aesthetics, can also be exhibited and criticized. This exhibition of the total art-act is always imperfect, yet it can be recollected, recreated in language, and observed as it occurs in nursing situations. Both the recreation of nursing's art and its natural observation provide a means of examining practice.

Toward a Credibility Index for Nursing Practice

Processes within the creative dimension of aesthetics enfold the separate knowledge forms that are exhibited as an ongoing art-act. The art-act of nursing, and not separate knowledge forms, provides an avenue for examination of the credibility of nursing practice. Valid empirics, just ethics, and congruent selves are important, and critical questions within each knowledge pattern need to be asked and answered. An examination of the art-act that integrates all knowledge patterns as expressed in practice provides a comprehensive, context-sensitive means for enfolding multiple knowledge patterns. This shift toward integration of all knowledge patterns will move nursing away from a quest for structural truth and toward a search for dynamic meaning (Munhall, 1986).

A focus on the art-act toward the evolution of dynamic consensual meaning is to be valued, because it promotes choice and freedom from the constraints of considering only one knowledge pattern as credible. Choice and freedom are values consistent with promotion of health. As nurses exercise the freedom to examine practice as art and analyze all patterns of knowing expressed through practice, their effectiveness as promoters of health will be enhanced.

References

Allen, D., Benner, P., & Diekelmann, N.L. (1986). Three paradigms for nursing research: Methodological implications. In P.L. Chinn (Ed.), *Nursing research methodology* (pp. 23–38). Rockville, MD: Aspen.

Benner, P. (1984). *From novice to expert: Excellence and power in clinical nursing practice.* Menlo Park, CA: Addison-Wesley.

Benner, P., & Tanner, C. (1987). How expert nurses use intuition. *American Journal of Nursing, 87*(1), 23–31.

Bleich, D. (1978). *Subjective criticism.* Baltimore and London: Johns Hopkins University Press.

Carper, B.A. (1978). Fundamental patterns of knowing in nursing. *Advances in Nursing Science, 1*(1), 13–23.

Chinn, P.L. (1985). Debunking myths in nursing theory and research. *Image, 17*(2), 45–49.

Chinn, P.L., & Jacobs, M.K. (1987). *Theory and nursing: A systematic approach* (2nd ed), St. Louis: C.V. Mosby.

Meleis, A.I. (1987). ReVisions in knowledge development: A passion for substance. *Scholarly Inquiry for Nursing Practice, 1*(1), 5–19.

Munhall, P.L. (1986). Methodological issues in nursing research: Beyond a wax apple. *Advances in Nursing Science, 8*(3), 1–5.

Watson, J. (1985). *Nursing: Human science and human care.* Norwalk, CT: Appleton-Century-Crofts.

Response to "Perspectives on Knowing: A Model of Nursing Knowledge"

Barbara A. Carper

The article by Jacobs-Kramer and Chinn proposes, a model for generating, transmitting, evaluating, and integrating into practice the four fundamental patterns of knowing in nursing originally identified by Carper (1978): empirical, ethical, personal, and esthetic knowledge. Each of the four patterns was conceptualized in relation to three dimensions: (a) the creative dimension of knowledge generation and its extension through use, (b) the expressive dimension of formulating and communicating knowledge produced, and (c) the assessment dimension, which addresses the processes and methods for determining the credibility of each pattern. The model, as presented, extends and modifies a previously published framework for examining science and alternative ways of knowing and understanding patterns of knowledge for nursing practice that are not admissible form the perspective of the empirical scientific tradition (Chinn & Jacobs, 1987).

The elaboration of this model is timely in that generating and disseminating knowledge is a recog-nized priority for the profession (Diers, 1987). It may also be risky, deviant, and necessary, because the positivistic way, although recognized as limited in generating knowledge for practice, is still the prevailing norm (Munhall, 1982; Stevenson & Woods, 1986; Watson, 1985). The current challenges to this prevailing norm of knowledge development, however, are directed primarily toward methodological issues and addressed *only within the scientific pattern of knowing.*

To propose a model for developing, disseminating, and using knowledge forms outside of the scientific realm is inherently risky. Doing so poses a threat to the gain in professional status and prestige associated with developing an academically rigorous, science-based body of knowledge for nursing practice. It is difficult to disregard the fact that the "relative status of the various professions is largely correlated with the extent to which they are able to present themselves as rigorous practitioners of a science-based professional knowledge" (Schon, 1987, p. 9). It is equally difficult to risk exposure to criticism from those who maintain that the only valid, reliable, and legitimate knowledge is quantitative, theoretical, generalizable, and replicable by proposing what appears to be widely divergent and, certainly, logically distinct types of knowledge as necessary for nursing practice.

Schultz (1987) identifies the emerging discourse and debates concerning appropriate methods of inquiry for knowledge development in nursing as originating from questions posed by epistemology and ontology. Although seemingly remote from the everyday realities of practice, these questions are critically important in providing norms for discerning among competing knowledge claims those sufficiently dependable and credible to serve as grounds for practice. Meleis (1985) has identified similar questions related to theory development in nursing. The epistemological perspective of nursing knowledge on which this model is premised raises questions regarding the nature of truth and the criteria for accepting or rejecting knowledge as legitimate and valid. Issues regarding the aims and purposes of nursing knowledge and the relationship of knowledge to practice inherent in the patterns of knowing question some of the epistemological assumptions of contemporary nursing. If nursing knowledge is paradigmatically scientific knowledge, and if nursing practice is the systematic application of empirical knowledge to yield problem solutions, then this model presents a deviant perspective of knowledge necessary for practice.

On reflection, perhaps, this perspective is not as deviant as it may seem to some when considered in light of an emerging concern in other science-based practice or service-oriented professions such as medicine and engineering. Schon presents a convincing argument that there is a growing crisis of confidence in professional knowledge and education for practice based on "a flawed conception of professional competence and its relationship to scientific and scholarly research [which is] rooted in the prevailing epistemology of practice" (Schon, 1987, p. 12). The problems that professional practitioners must solve are rarely straightforward and frequently are complex. Often practice problems do not present themselves as clear, well-defined problems but as messy, indeterminant situations that cannot be solved simply by the application of scientific or technical knowledge:

> These indeterminant zones of practice—uncertainty, uniqueness and value conflict—escape the canons of technical rationality. When the problematic situation is uncertain, technical problem solving depends on the prior construction of a well-formed problem—which is not itself a technical task. When a practitioner recognizes a situation as unique, she cannot handle it solely by applying theories or techniques derived from her store of professional knowledge. And in situations of value conflicts, there are no clear and self-consistent ends to guide the technical selection of means. (Schon, 1987. p. 6)

Limited evidence suggests a growing awareness of the gap between the prevailing scientific knowledge and the preparation of practitioners to deal competently with situations characterized by uncertainty, uniqueness, and conflict. Benoliel observed that Benner's (1984) description of nurses' competencies illustrates "the complexity of nursing practice and the range of knowledge involved in making judgments and decisions in clinical situations" (Benoliel, 1987, p. 150). Furthermore, her study provided evidence that expert nurses used empirics, ethics, and personal knowledge, and "the action they took reflected as esthetic sense of what was significant in the situation and contributed to care that can best be described as holistic" (Benoliel, 1987, p. 151).

In developing their model, Chinn and Jacobs-Kramer recognize and respond to the plurality of ways of knowing. This model reflects the richness and complexity of the phenomena, problems, and aspects of reality with which nursing is legitimately engaged. It may also be a stimulus to others to address a formulation to Schultz's question, "Is there an epistemological position that can be argued to undergird a discipline which integrates or synthesizes knowledge generated from such diverse patterns of knowing (Carper, 1978) as science, aesthetics, personal knowledge, and ethics?" (Schultz, 1987, p. 137). It may be risky. It may be deviant. But it is necessary.

References

Benner, P. (1984). *From novice to expert.* Menlo Park, CA: Addison-Wesley.

Benoliel, J.Q. (1987). Response to "Toward holistic inquiry in nursing: A proposal for synthesis of patterns and methods." *Scholarly Inquiry for Nursing Practice, 1*(2), 147–152.

Carper, B.A. (1978). Fundamental patterns of knowing in nursing. *Advances in Nursing Science, 1*(1), 13–23.

Chinn, P.L., & Jacobs, M.K. (1987). *Theory and nursing: A systematic approach* (2nd ed.). St. Louis: C.V. Mosby.

Diers, D. (1987). Editorial: On research in nursing practice. *Image, 19*(3), 106.

Meleis, A.I. (1985). *Theoretical nursing: Development and progress.* Philadelphia: J.B. Lippincott.

Munhall, P.L. (1982). Nursing philosophy and nursing research: In apposition or opposition? *Nursing Research, 31*(3), 176–177, 181.

Schon, D.A. (1987). *Educating the reflective practitioner.* San Francisco: Jossey-Bass.

Schultz, P.R. (1987). Toward holistic inquiry in nursing: A proposal for synthesis of patterns and methods. *Scholarly Inquiry for Nursing Practice, 1*(2), 135–146.

Stevenson, J.S., & Woods, N.F. (1986). Nursing science and contemporary science: Emerging paradigms. In G.E. Sorensen (Ed.), *Setting the agenda for the year 2000: Knowledge development in nursing* (pp. 6–20). Kansas City: American Academy of Nursing.

Watson, J. (1985). Reflections on different methodologies for the future of nursing. In M.M. Leininger (Ed.), *Qualitative research methods of nursing.* Orlando, FL: Grune and Stratton.

The Authors Comment

We wrote this article shortly after completing the revision for the second edition of *Theory and Nursing* (St. Louis: C.V. Mosby, 1987). During the revision process for the second edition, we had many long discussions around the knowing patterns. We explored and carefully considered how to best conceptualize and express our ideas, particularly as they related to (a) the creative, expressive and assessment dimensions of each pattern, (b) the nature of aesthetics as both an integrating and separate pattern, and (c) the relevance of the knowing patterns for clinical practice. These discussions not only deepened our appreciation and understanding of what we were trying to convey, but also added complexity to our understanding of the knowing patterns. Throughout our discussions, we were acutely aware of the difficulty of expressing such complex and interrelated ideas in writing. This article could be considered both an extension and a parallel version of the knowing patterns as contained in the second edition of *Theory and Nursing.* This article also provided an important intermediary understanding of the knowing patterns that helped us conceptualize the current version of the knowing patterns for the third edition of *Theory and Nursing* (St. Louis: C.V. Mosby, 1991).

—MAEONA K. KRAMER AND PEGGY L. CHINN

Chapter 29

Nursing Science: The Challenge to Develop Knowledge

Ada Sue Hinshaw

The development of knowledge for nursing poses an exciting, scholarly adventure for the profession's scientists. A series of challenges are involved: the challenge to develop the substantive content needed for practice within nursing's disciplinary perspective, the challenge to sustain excellence in the developing science base and in the preparation of nurse researchers, and the challenge of disseminating stable, appropriate research results to the profession's clinicians and to the public. Nursing is entering into a new era, moving from the stage of establishing structures to support nursing research and building the cadre of scientists needed to conduct investigations, to the stage of focusing on the identification and study of the phenomena which comprise the body of knowledge needed for practice. A number of directions or priorities for nursing research are evident for the future. The questions of concern are how to centralize nursing's scientific endeavors and resources as well as prepare researchers who are on the cutting edge or frontiers of science, and what strategies can be used to facilitate excellence in these efforts. The dilemma of transferring research findings into practice in a timely but scientifically appropriate manner requires a partnership between practitioners and researchers. Both are committed to making clinical decisions based on accurate, relevant information. Such research based practice requires a merger of the talents and expertise of those providing practice and those developing the knowledge base for the profession.

Developing nursing science is a scholarly adventure, one guided by purpose and goals and undertaken with a boldness, sense of freedom, and creativity merged with intellectual rigor and integrity. Developing nursing science entails generating knowledge which can be used by any discipline but is specifically focused on providing information to underlie nursing practice and health care. Nursing, as a profession, has a societal mandate to provide health care for clients at different points in the health/illness and developmental continuum in diverse practice settings. In order to responsibly fulfill society's mandate. The profession must generate

About the Author

ADA SUE HINSHAW was born in Kansas and still considers that state to be home. She received a B.S. from the University of Kansas in 1961, a M.S.N. from Yale University in 1963, and a M.A. in Sociology (1973) and a Ph.D. in Sociology (1975) from the University of Arizona.

A well-known nurse researcher and scholar, Dr. Hinshaw currently is the Director of the National Center for Nursing Research, a position she assumed in 1987. Before this appointment, she had been the Director of Research at the University of Arizona College of Nursing. Commenting on her research interests, Dr. Hinshaw stated "To me, nursing research is an adventure. I enjoy conducting research and experiencing the excitement of pursuing the discovery of knowledge coupled with the logical process of scientific inquiry." When asked about other satisfactions in the area of nursing research, she replied, "I see great promise in building and facilitating research programs for nursing with colleagues in the nursing scientific community, as well as with multidisciplinary colleagues. For the future, my goal is to be involved in facilitating the transfer and utilization of knowledge in nursing practice. It is extremely satisfying to generate relevant research studies from critical clinical issues, conduct the investigations and facilitate the use of the findings in practice when appropriate."

a relevant, accurate, and reliable knowledge base to guide nursing practice.

The scholarly adventure of generating nursing science entails a commitment to the process of discovery and systematic inquiry. The idea of discovery is central to nursing as a profession and has been the hallmark of many of its leaders. Fulton (1987) analyzes the contributions of Virginia Henderson to the science of nursing, for example, as embodying the concept of discovery. O'Hear, in characterizing Popper's philosophy, suggests the essence of science entails the "boldness and freest adventure yet of the inquiring human spirit"(O'Hear, 1985, p. 45). Whether the discovery process is focused on more basic, possibly not immediately usable information, or directly applicable problems and data, the ultimate purpose of the process is to provide guidance for nursing care and the promotion or improvement of the health of the public.

The development of knowledge reflects the interface between nursing science and research. The sciences are defined as "bodies of human knowledge based on general principles about a delimited range of phenomena derived from empirical observations" (Hinshaw, in press, p. 3). It involves experiences of the senses, which can be empirically tested. Science does not reflect idiosyncratic individual experiences but rather the "consensus of a scientific community and its repertoire of research" (Gortner & Schultz, 1988, p. 22).

Nursing science as a body of knowledge has been defined in several ways. Basically, it can be characterized as consisting of defined concepts/constructs describing various human responses to health and illness as well as therapeutic nursing actions in systematically specified relationships (adapted from Kerlinger, 1986). Viewing nursing science in relationship to practice, it can be defined as the body of knowledge generated and tested from the nursing perspective in order to ultimately provide relevant substantiated information for the guidance of practice (Hinshaw, 1987). In one of her earlier definitions, Gortner provided an often-cited definition of nursing science as reflecting nursing's understanding:

> of human biology and behavior and health and illness, including the processes by which changes in health status are brought about, the patterns of behavior associated with normal and critical life events, and the principles and laws governing life states and processes (Gortner, 1980, p. 180).

Recently, this definition was placed in perspective with Gortner and Schultz's statement that the goal of nursing science "is to represent nature, in particular human nature, to understand it and explain it for the benefit of mankind"(Gortner & Schultz, 1988, p. 23).

Although science is not the same as the process of systematic inquiry by which it is evolved, science is shaped by the characteristics of the research process and the selection preferences of the scientific community's investigators (DeGroot, 1988). Nursing research can be defined as "the systematic process of inquiry which utilizes a variety of methodological approaches to investigate the questions and concepts of interest in nursing" (Hinshaw, 1987, p. 5). Multiple modes of scientific inquiry can be used for accomplishing the goal of nursing science and for developing the substantive fields of knowledge for the discipline.

This discussion of nursing science and research reflects the assumptions outlined by Meleis and May (1981, p. 32–33). The three assumptions are:

- Nursing science is in an evolving, developing stage.
- Nursing science incorporates the constructs which the profession's theorists agree form the boundaries of the profession's mission: clients, nurses, and environments within a health/illness context.
- There is a pluralistic ethic or tradition in nursing which underlies scientific work and the selection of methodological approaches.

A series of challenges are involved with developing nursing science. First, and of highest priority, is the challenge to develop the substantive content of the knowledge base through systematic inquiry. The second challenge is to sustain the excellence of the developing science base for nursing. The third challenge is the transfer of stable, appropriate research results to nursing and health care because, as a service profession, the ultimate purpose of science is its applicability in nursing practice. Each of these challenges is a major issue in generating a body of knowledge for nursing which is societally relevant and scientifically rigorous.

The Challenge to Develop Knowledge

Nursing is entering into a new era in terms of knowledge development. Stevenson (1988) suggests that the discipline is moving from an initial stage of "knowledge development" to a more advanced stage. The first stage was primarily involved with the research training of a cadre of nurse investigators and the establishment of the environmental structures to facilitate research in academic and clinical settings: for example, offices of research and laboratories for investigators. The current stage, she suggests, will reflect more concentrated work on the actual development of the substantive content needed for the discipline.

Visions and Revisions of Knowledge Development

The phrase "visions and revisions of knowledge development" was coined by one of nursing's foremost theoreticians, Afaf I. Meleis (1987). Meleis suggests the central focus of the new revision in knowledge development will be on the substance and content of the nursing discipline. Agreeing with Stevenson, she cites major debates in the nursing literature which speak to the roles of holism versus particularism in the care of clients and in the development of knowledge, on the more or least congruent methodologies for nursing research, and to philosophical dilemmas as they relate to selective methodologies for building nursing science. Although such debates are important, Meleis concludes that they detract or draw attention away from the major issue in knowledge development, which is the identification of the substance and major phenomena for which the nursing discipline is accountable.

The basic tenet of the arguments emerging in the discipline's literature is that the new era for knowledge development must turn from methodological and philosophical debates to a mutual concentration of investigators with different perspectives on the development of knowledge. Nursing's ability to fulfill its promise both as a science and practice depends on the scholars confronting and accepting the challenge of identifying the major phenomena basic to the discipline's perspective of health care. In this manner, a knowledge base can be built and refined congruent with that perspective to guide the practice of nursing's professionals.

Nursing's Disciplinary Perspective

The development and testing of a strong, accurate body of knowledge does not occur in a vacuum but rather reflects a specific disciplinary perspective (Hinshaw, 1987). In their classic article, "The Discipline of Nursing," Donaldson and Crowley provide an excellent conceptualization of the structuring of human knowledge. According to their framework, human knowledge is structured in terms of unique disciplines. The disciplines have:

> . . . evolved as a consequence of a distinct perspective and syntax which determines what phenomenon or abstraction of interest will be considered, in what context such phenomena are to be viewed, what questions are to be raised scientifically, what methods of study are to be used and what evidence or proof is required (Donaldson & Crowley, 1978, p. 114).

As Donaldson and Crowley note, the definitions of these disciplines are not agreed upon, and there is no single organization for even the well-established disciplines. However, disciplines do reflect differences between developed bodies of knowledge.

Health care disciplines reflect unique perspectives which represent an integration of the sciences and the humanities. The science base of the disciplines focuses on the general biological, physiological, and social/behavioral patterns needed to provide care whereas the humanities bring the moral and ethical as well as individual perspective. According to Davis, the humanities "express and provide experience and orientation that is both aesthetic and ethical and communicate(s) an individual vision of life to others"(Davis, 1985, p. 377).

Certain collective values and ethics which are held in common by the professionals in a discipline guide and provide the perspective for the unique body of knowledge. For example, in nursing, several basic tenets which guide practice as well as the development of the body of knowledge include:

- Individuals respond holistically to health and illness situations.
- Nursing focuses on the care processes of health and illness.
- Nursing focuses on individuals and their families during responses to health and illness not on the illness.

Such basic values and premises guide the professional's decisions in practice, the questions raised for systematic inquiry, and the interpretation of research findings.

Directions for Knowledge Development

Considering the perspective and values of nursing, a number of scholars have risked suggesting which major phenomena may ultimately be the focus of scientific knowledge developed for the nursing discipline. Several authors have suggested the central tenet and process of the nursing discipline is the concept of care and the process of caring (Leininger, 1984; Aamodt, 1978). In a recent editorial, Diers (1988) disagrees with this premise, stating that it is presumptuous of nursing to assume only they "care." This debate emphasizes the need for definition and study of the care concept. Other theorists have suggested a basic commitment to the phenomenon of holism (Stevenson, 1988; Meleis, 1987), health and wellness (Pender, 1982), self care (Orem, 1985), cultural orientation (Leininger, 1978; Tripp-Reimer, 1986), and patterning (Crawford, 1982) as central phenomena for the discipline.

There is relative consensus for major phenomena involved in the broad conceptual paradigm of nursing: person, health, environment, and nursing (Meleis, 1987; Fawcett, 1984). However, even with the commitment to and consensus concerning these four broad phenomena, knowledge to be developed and useful in practice will need to be much more specific in nature.

A number of professional organizations have published statements outlining the substantive priority areas in which they recommend directions for nursing research through the year 2000. These priority position papers provide excellent data on the content areas of nursing science which are most needed for nursing practice, education, and administration. The American Nurses' Association policy statement on nursing research, *Directions for Nursing Research: Toward the Twenty-First Century* (Kansas City: ANA, 1985), outlines 11 research priorities for the 21st century. The first five are related to nursing practice, while one each cites the importance of the delivery of nursing care, nursing education and the historical/professional aspects of nursing. Examples of several priority needs for information are:

- promoting health, well-being, and ability to care for oneself among all age, social, and cultural groups

- minimizing or preventing behaviorally and environmentally induced health problems that compromise the quality of life and reduce productivity
- minimizing the negative effects of new health technologies on the adaptive abilities of individuals and families experiencing acute or chronic health problems (ANA, 1985, pp. 2–3).

In the June 1988 issue of *American Nurse*, Hesook Suzie Kim, chair of the ANA Cabinet on Nursing Research, cited four areas of priority for nurse researchers: "nursing care of preterm infants, nursing care of cancer patients, women's health, and long term care of older people and children" (McCarthy, 1988, p. 1). Lowery, chair of the ANA Council of Nurse Researchers, suggested nurse investigators focus on major issues such as shortened hospital stays and AIDS—issues of paramount concern to society (McCarthy, 1988). For the Association of Critical Care Nurses, the major knowledge priorities consisted of the following types of questions:

- What are the most effective ways of promoting optimum sleep-rest patterns in the critically ill patient and preventing sleep deprivation?
- In light of the nursing shortage, especially in critical care nursing, what measures can be taken to prevent or lessen burnout among critical care nurses?
- What type of orientation program for critical care nurses is most effective in terms of cost, safety, and long-term retention?
- What effects do verbal and environmental stimuli have on increased intracranial pressure in the head injured patient?
- What are the most effective, least anxiety-producing techniques for weaning various types of patients from ventilators? (Lewandowski & Kositsky, 1983)

Three of these five priorities are clinical and patient-centered, whereas one is focused on orientation of the critical care nurse and the stress problems plaguing these specialty practitioners. The American Organization of Nurse Executives' (AONE) statement of research priorities is one of the most recent with four categories for knowledge development. The first one focuses on the influence of delivery systems on patient care, and the others suggest that the development of information on the delivery system is needed. The four categories for research and an example of the questions posed for each area are:

Category 1, Practice and administrative systems: What is the cost/quality impact of differing systems of nursing care delivery (primary, modular, team, functional, standards of practice based, nursing diagnosis-based, and so forth)? What nontraditional systems can provide high quality nursing care at an acceptable cost?

Category 2, Support services: What is the impact of the level of support services on the requirements for the effectiveness of the professional nursing staff?

Category 3, Documentation: What is the most effective and time-conserving nursing documentation system that meets professional, legislative, and reimbursement requirements?

Category 4, Education: What type of personnel are needed in nursing service settings, and what level of educational preparation is required? (AONE, 1986, pp.53–54)

The National League for Nursing (NLN) cites four priorities for nursing research; (a) patient care outcomes related to home care, (b) clinical decision making and its effects on patient care outcomes, (c) maximizing the capacity for self-care in individuals with chronic illness, and (d) patterns of health care delivery for the AIDS patient in the community (NLN, 1988). The American College of Nurse Midwives (ACNM) research concerns place a priority emphasis on the processes and decisions for care as related to client outcomes (ACNM, 1988). In addition, ACNM stresses studying the care environment as it affects patient outcomes. Other areas of suggested priority also dealt with professional and educational issues. Several specialty organizations emphasized rehabilitation problems and questions as well as the testing of preventive interventions (Rehabilitation Nursing Foundation, 1988; American Association of Neuroscience Nurses, 1988; American Association of Spinal Cord Injury Nurses, 1988).

Evolving Clinical Nursing Research Priorities

One attempt to provide a blueprint for the development of knowledge is currently being conducted by the National Center for Nursing Research (NCNR) with the nursing scientific and professional community. The development of a National Nursing Research Agenda (NNRA) for NCNR requires evolving clinical nursing research priorities. Evolving clinical nursing research priorities will provide a systematic plan or blueprint for knowledge development in the discipline. Given the mandate of NCNR, which is the conduct, support, and dissemination of basic and clinical nursing research, or research to guide patient care, in conjunction with the heavy emphasis placed by the profession on clinical nursing research priorities, it is logical to begin the evolution of the NNRA with the identification of clinical nursing research priorities. Whereas a clinical research agenda provides guidance for only part of the information needed for the profession, knowledge development in this area is the central focus of a practice discipline such as nursing.

Essentially, the NNRA will serve as a guide for the use of federal resources in knowledge development for the discipline. A word of caution—only a portion of the resources will be used for these targeted research endeavors. The majority of federal resources will be maintained for allocation to the individual investigator creative project, which may or may not fit within the research priorities as defined by the professional and scientific community.

A number of sources have been used for accumulating information from the professionals and scholars in nursing to guide the development of this research agenda. An analysis was conducted of the published priority statements by the professional organizations. In addition, such organizations were provided the opportunity and encouraged to submit an updated statement of research priorities for the discipline from the perspective of their particular organization. In addition, individuals in the nursing science community have been actively involved in the identification of the clinical nursing research priorities. A steering committee consisting of NCNR Advisory Council members as well as NCNR staff guide the process of the development of the NNRA. Thus, collaborative endeavors between the professionals and scientists in the discipline and the staff of the NCNR were assured from the very onset of the process. The initial broad clinical nursing research priorities were evolved by a conference group of approximately 50 seasoned scientists working with the staff. These scientists represented the various programmatic areas of research in nursing as well as diverse methodological approaches, and diverse philosophical stances on the development of knowledge. From the initial consensus conference, seven broad priorities were evolved by the steering committee from the information provided by participating conference colleagues. These have been organized into three stages; all have been agreed upon and approved by the NCNR Advisory Council. The three stages of clinical nursing research priorities are as follows:

Stage 1

HIV-positive patients, partners, and families. Although the nursing profession and nurse researchers do not generally work within an illness orientation, society demands attention to this epidemic. Biopsychosocial components of care for clients and patients who are HIV positive (both adults and children) and their partners and caregivers need to be examined. Ethical aspects of clinical decision making, as well as health promotion/disease prevention issues will be included. Attention to this problem for minority groups is important.

Low-birth-weight infants and mothers. Included in this priority is nursing care of mothers at risk for having low-birth-weight infants, with a focus on prevention of premature delivery and on the care of low birth weight infants. The study of relevant, innovative nursing care delivery patterns is also included in this priority. Nurses have access to mothers and fathers in early pregnancy. In the study of both prevention and care, special attention is to be given to: (a) minority/disadvantaged populations, because of their high risk for prematurity; (b) the role of the family in support of mother and infant, because decisions regarding care are often made by the family, rather than by the individual; and (c) the adolescent population, because they are at high risk for unwanted pregnancies, compromising maternal behaviors, and emotional and physical abuse.

Stage 2

Long-term care. This will include the study of long-term care of the elderly, with priority given to nursing home care, including the prevention of iatrogenic complications. Important issues to be attended to are self-care, patient and caregiver coping and adaptation, and quality of nursing care, including continuity of care through discharge. Often, caregivers of frail elderly are themselves older people.

System management. Clinical assessment of and intervention for the relief of patient symptoms (singly or interaction), such as pain, sleeplessness, fatigue, and nausea and vomiting, are the focus of this proposed priority. The priority should be developed to blend bio-psycho-social parameters and to be relevant to diverse settings. Strategies for symptom assessment and management need to be generated and tested.

Information systems. Two major areas are to be developed: standardized data sets which document nursing care across settings, and taxonomies to classify nursing phenomena and allow for the common use of terms. Systems need to be compatible and built on what already exists. The specific research issues need to be developed, and may include issues related to the link between resources and patient outcomes.

Stage 3

Health promotion. Of interest in this area is the basic science, which may be biobehavioral, and the testing of interventions. The most critical issue for study is the fundamental psychosocial mechanisms underlying the maintenance of health promotion behaviors, with an emphasis on lifestyle and the need to take responsibility for one's own health. Included in this priority should be basic and intervention research regarding the acquisition of health promoting behaviors among children. Nursing needs to be cognizant of an important concept in this priority, namely the concept of "tailoring," which is the planning of care tailored to a specific population group.

Technology dependency across the lifespan. The priority outlines problems of interest in technology dependency and individual and family responses to technology across the life span, including attention to the needs of children. Much patient care technology is found in critical care settings. In addition, prevention of iatrogenic complications is a critical issue in the use of technology (Hinshaw, Heinrich, & Bloch, 1988).

The definition of these broad clinical nursing research priorities is only a beginning. As Stevenson (1988) notes in a recent presentation, broad nursing research priorities do not give the needed direction required for knowledge development. In concurrence with this basic premise, priority expert panels will be formed around each of the defined areas. These expert panels will have represented both nurse scientist and scientists from other disciplines, and a number of consultants who will refine the ideas which need to be targeted for nursing research. This will entail; (a) assessing the current state of the science in each of the areas, (b) identifying nursing's particular perspective and strongest potential contribution in terms of knowledge and practice, and (c) identifying a set of recommenda-

tions about future research directions within the priority area.

Future Nonsubstantive Trends Central to Developing Nursing Science

A number of trends are central to the development of nursing science regardless of the content focus or direction. First, a value for both basic and clinical practice types of research will underlie the science of nursing. Basic research is defined as studies which provide information needed to guide the conduct of clinical research and allow investigators to explain and understand relationships among and underlying clinical ideas. Practice or clinical practice research can be defined as studies which focus on nursing therapeutics or interventions and their impact on the quality of care and desired patient outcomes (Bloch, 1981). Both types of information are needed to build nursing science. Clinical studies testing the influence of nursing interventions on patient outcomes cannot be conducted until the basic exploratory and descriptive information and mechanisms from which to define effective interventions and the desired outcomes are understood and available.

However, a trend toward an increased use of correlational and experimental designs as well as causal model testing suggests nursing research is building on its heavy descriptive body of knowledge to consider relationships among factors which influence practice outcomes (Brown, Tanner, & Padrick, 1984). Ultimately understanding the relationships in practice is the critical knowledge needed to manipulate nursing interventions and the health care environment to achieve the desired practice outcomes for clients.

However, such emphasis on the explanation and prediction of practice relationships will not mean a decrease in the use of methods which are more qualitative in nature. Because of the numerous practice concepts or questions about which nursing knows little, the qualitative strategies will continue to be a strong part of the nurse scientist's methodologies. In addition, qualitative approaches provide a rich type of information which is highly valued by both the clinician and researcher regardless of the purpose of the project and scientific state of the art. In the future, nursing researchers can be expected to combine the best and most systematically rigorous of the quantitative and qualitative methodologies in their research designs. This will provide a rich diverse data base from which to consider either new concepts or causal relationships.

Nursing science will reflect, to a greater extent, an interface between its physical, physiological nature and the psychological, sociological processes. A strength of the current nursing research base is its emphasis on the client's psychological and sociological concerns; for example, distress responses to surgery, family's coping responses to the care of a loved one, and maternal/paternal responses to parenting. However, recently there has been an increase in attention to the more physical, physiological responses to illness. Examples include the management of pain, enhancement of functional capacity, and the prevention of iatrogenic conditions from life-saving medical treatments. Thus, the emphasis on the physical, physiological nursing practice questions can be expected to increase and be more evenly balanced with the current strength in studying the psychosocial aspects of nursing practice.

The Challenge to Sustain Excellence in Nursing Science

It is important during the evolution of nursing science to systematically assess, maintain, and monitor the growing knowledge base for excellence. Excellence in science has been judged from a number of perspectives.

Gortner and Schultz (1988) provide a recent cataloguing of well-accepted criteria for judging excellence in science: significance, theory-observation congruency, generalizability, science, reproducibility, precision, and intersubjectivity. Significance refers to the contribution of knowledge or research findings to practice as well as to the broader body of knowledge. Theory-observation compatibility involves the empirical testing of theory through observations according to the level of theory development; for example, factor isolating to the goal-oriented predictability of causal relationships (Dickoff, James, & Wiedenbach, 1968). A variety of methodological approaches appropriate to the level of theory could be used to obtain the empirical

observations. Reproducibility is defined as replicating the findings under similar conceptual, clinical, and/or methodological approaches (Connelly, 1986). Testing the theory under multiple clinical conditions and diverse health care setting to determine if the findings remain consistent provides generalizability to the science. Precision is the degree of sensitivity and accuracy with which research findings can be repeated in additional research or when used in practice. Intersubjectivity combines several of the other scientific characteristics and refers to "evidence and knowledge claims which can be corroborated by others" (Gortner & Schultz, 1988, p. 22). This characteristic refers to the high value for scientific consensus across investigations and descriptions.

These criteria are applicable regardless of the methodological or philosophical approach used in developing the knowledge. Both Benner (1985), in considering the phenomenological perspective on theory development and research, and Norbeck, in her article on the "Defense of Empiricism" (Norbeck, 1987), selectively refer to these criteria. However, understanding and using these criteria under diverse philosophical research approaches needs further study.

The norms of science are often used to judge the merit of the inquiry process and resultant knowledge base (Merton, 1979; Barber, 1952; Storer, 1966). These criteria, which are interdisciplinary across the social sciences, include universalism, commonality, disinterestedness, and organized skepticism. Jacobs-Kramer and Chinn (1988, p. 133) suggest three criteria which can be used to assess models and the information base accessed through different ways of knowing: empirical or scientific, ethical, and personal and aesthetic. These criteria include creativity, expressiveness, and assessment. Creativity is defined as how the knowledge is generated, placed in conceptual perspective, and extended. Expressive refers to how the knowledge pattern is exhibited and recognized, while assessment provides for examination of the knowledge under several conditions.

Two other operational criteria need to be used to judge excellence in science: the development or existence of substantiated bodies of knowledge specific to areas of critical concern in the profession, and the evolving information base on the "cutting edge" of the science. Both of these characteristics are crucial to developing a science base which is creditable and usable.

Building Substantiated Areas of Knowledge

Brown, Tanner, and Padrick (1984) noted that a major limitation in their study of reported nursing research studies was the failure to build a cumulative science. In order to amass knowledge which is creditable and usable, a series of studies needs to constitute the information base for any area of study. The historical pattern in nursing research has been a more "shotgun" approach; that is, one or only two studies in any one substantive field. This pattern has been the result of limited resources for research support and training in relation to a field of research which is broad and diverse. There are several notable exceptions to this pattern: Johnson's (1973) program of research relating sensory information to distress responses of patients undergoing traumatic procedures, and Walike et al.'s (1975) studies on reducing diarrhea in tube-fed patients.

However, it is important that the nursing scientific community adopt strategies to systematically develop a cumulative science. A cumulative body of knowledge includes building on colleagues' as well as on one's own research. It involves generating multiple studies in specific content areas in order to have substantiated and replicated findings from which to develop further research questions and for application in practice. Several strategies can be proposed; building individual research programs and facilitating the development of cadres of researchers focused on similar areas of content.

Building individual research programs

One major strategy for developing depth in nursing science is to philosophically adopt a "research program" orientation in nursing as the model for systematic inquiry. By definition, a research program is the series of projects comprising an area of study undertaken by an individual investigator. Characteristically, a researcher may be involved in the area of study for a number of years and move from one phase of the research into another, always building on the results and experiences of the former phase(s). For this stance to be adopted requires that investigators conceptualize their research from the beginning in phases or stages and understand the commitment to continuing the development of knowledge in a specific field.

Funding sources need to be available which allow for the initial use of intramural funds internal to an academic or clinical institution and expanding over time to extramural funding from public and private sources. An example of such a pattern of support would be competing for an American Nurses Foundation or Sigma Theta Tau small grant initially. Later, a First Independent Research Support and Transition (FIRST) application for federal support could be submitted as an early step toward obtaining a research project grant (RO1), which can be viewed as the beginning of a series of competing continuations and supplements, ultimately leading to a Method to Extend Research in Time (MERIT) award.

Developing cadres of nurse researchers in similar areas of content

In generating a cumulative science. nursing researchers need to develop networks for promoting the sharing of results and communication of ideas among investigators with similar interests and research programs. This essentially mandates the existence of a scientific community for researchers. The major characteristics of a scientific community are: (a) commonality or the sharing of ideas and research endeavors; (b) colleagueship, which entails the support of scientific accomplishments and concerns; and (c) constructive competition, of which a major feature is the questioning of ideas and striving to extend each others' endeavors (Hinshaw, 1983; Gortner, 1980). A number of nursing scientific communities are evident at the national level (e.g., Council of Nurse Researchers) and regional level (e.g., Western Society for Researching in Nursing and Midwest Nursing Research Society).

Another strategy for developing cadres of nurse researchers includes coordinating individuals conducting research in like areas of study within an academic or clinical agency or through sponsorship of a professional organization. Such organizational arrangements promote interaction of ideas and the ability to build on each others' scientific endeavors. Many diverse strategies will be developed to accomplish the goal of building cadres of investigators in similar areas of study in order to provide depth in nursing science.

Maintaining nursing research at the "cutting edge"

As the knowledge base for nursing practice grows, it is imperative that the research be maintained at the "cutting edge" of science. This will require that nurse investigators be in the forefront with their knowledge of the substantive area as well as the methods needed for their field of study. Several strategies will enhance the scientist's ability to have a "state of the art" grasp of their research arena: (a) a commitment to ongoing postdoctoral education in their investigative field, and (b) an interdisciplinary understanding of their substantive area of study.

Career trajectory for research education. To remain on the "cutting edge" of any scientific field requires consistent reeducation and study. Developing the philosophical orientation to research which acknowledges the need to return to intense study at periodic intervals allows the investigator to remain updated on the content and methodological issues of the field. Immersion into a scientific program of research begins most intensely with a postdoctoral experience, which allows investigators to become engrossed in their research program before acquiring a number of other responsibilities, such as in university and service positions. Often, due to the demands of academic or clinical positions, it is important to be able to return to full-time study and again become immersed in research during a midcareer stage. In addition, individuals who are mentors and seasoned scientists have multiple demands on their energy and need time to reimmerse themselves in their science for an intensive experience. Thus, a career trajectory for research training is needed to provide the time for continual learning and relearning as an important facet of remaining on the "cutting edge" of science.

Interdisciplinary relationships. A second strategy for staying in the forefront of the developing scientific body of knowledge is maintaining strong relationships with interdisciplinary colleagues in fields of study pertinent to the investigative endeavors of the nurse researcher. The research questions posed, like the clinical issues handled in practice, are complex and often require multiple perspectives. The scientific efforts are often on the interface of knowledge being developed in several disciplines including nursing. If nurse investigators are aware of the advances in knowledge in the social, behavioral, and biological sciences specific to their field of study, then their ability to stay on the "cutting edge" of the field will be facilitated.

Transferring Research Findings

One of the major challenges which continues to confront the profession is the ability to transfer research results into practice in a timely and effective manner. Nursing is not alone in this dilemma; other service professions such as medicine and dentistry grapple with the issue as well.

Several characteristics of the dilemma account for its complexity. One, there are multiple audiences for whom the research findings must be transferred and used. Results must be made available for the use of the nursing professionals as well as for those individuals and groups who are the focus of nursing care. In addition, the research findings must also be apparent to the general public because such results provide a way of legitimizing nursing practice and influencing public policy on health care. Two, the problem of translating research into practice is complex because of the breadth of the nursing research field and the diverse nature of the information that must be disseminated. Three, the issue is complex because of the numbers and types of practitioners in various settings to whom the information must be targeted for utilization.

Two basic principles need to be understood in terms of this author's approach to research utilization. One, the clinician, administrator, educator, and researcher are all responsible for the transfer and utilization of investigative findings; and two, the findings will be transferred and used in the sense of principles and concepts and not in terms of procedures or standardized rules.

In the future, research will be an acknowledged way of life of all nurse professionals. Each will integrate research as a part of professional practice, ranging from the process of utilization or application of information in clinical and administrative decision making to the explicit merger of research into curriculum patterns, both graduate and undergraduate, to the individual whose primary role responsibility is that of conducting and disseminating research information. As such, research will be a part of all job descriptions including clinicians, administrators, educators, and nurse scientists. The degree to which research is the focal point of the professional positions will vary, of course, by the roles and types of education that individuals have chosen in their careers. For the baccalaureate practitioner, the research involvement will entail applying research findings in clinical practice decisions. The masters-prepared clinical specialists can be expected to generate numerous research questions in tandem with the practicing clinician, whereas both can be expected to participate in the research process when new information is being sought and studies are being conducted. The nurse investigator who has chosen to pursue an earned doctorate and acquire the knowledge and skills specific to the conduct, implementation, and dissemination of research will be responsible for the generation and testing of the body of nursing information which is needed to guide practice as well as its application. Because all professionals will be part of the research generation, testing, and interpretation process, the ability to transfer, use and be comfortable with manipulating and understanding research results will be evident.

Lindeman (1984) has suggested the manner in which research results need to be transferred is in terms of principles and concepts—not by standardized procedures. The point is an important one, professionals do not function by rote, *even from their own developed knowledge base*. Each patient's or client's care is individualized. The knowledge base as transferred and used, is weighted and applied as best fits and benefits particular clients and their specific needs.

The process of disseminating and utilizing information which has been generated and tested by nurse researchers is extremely important in a profession such as nursing. Both basic and clinical research programs are pursued for the purpose of being applicable and ultimately useful to improve patient care and to guide practice (Horsley, Crane, Crabtree, & Wood, 1983).

Conclusion

The challenges involved with generating and testing nursing science provide the spice for the scholarly adventure. The nursing scientific and professional community have confronted the challenge to develop knowledge for the discipline with clinical sensitivity, scientific rigor, and integrity. The research programs being developed focus on significant health care issues of society through the appropriate processes of systematic inquiry. The multiple scientific communities available at the institutional, regional, national, and international levels provide support and maintenance for dealing with the challenge of assuring excellence in the evolving knowledge base. The final challenge of transferring the research findings into practice is best handled through a shared partnership between the scientists and the clinicians, educators, or administrators in the profession.

References

Aamodt, A.M. (1978). The care component in a health and healing system. In E.E. Bauwens (Ed.), *The anthropology of health.* St. Louis: C.V. Mosby.

American Association of Neuroscience Nurses. (1988). Correspondence to NCNR regarding organizational research priorities.

American Association of Spinal Cord Injury Nurses. (1988). Correspondence to NCNR regarding organizational research priorities.

American College of Nurse Midwives. (1988). Correspondence to NCNR regarding organizational research priorities.

American Nurses' Association Cabinet on Nursing Research. (1985). *Directions for nursing research: Toward the twenty-first century.* Kansas City: Author.

American Organization of Nurse Executives. (1986). *Final report of the ad hoc committee on nursing administra-*

tion research. Chicago: American Hospital Association Nurse Executive Sourcebook Series Number One.

Barber, B. (1952). *Science and the social order.* New York: Collier Books.

Benner, P. (1985). Quality of life: A phenomenological perspective on explanation, prediction, and understanding in nursing science. *Advances in Nursing Science, 8*(1), 1–14.

Bloch, D. (1981). A conceptualization of nursing research and nursing science. In J.C. McCloskey & H.K. Grace (Eds.), *Current issues in nursing* (pp. 81–93). Boston: Blackwell Publications.

Brown, J S., Tanner, C.A., & Padrick, K.P. (1984). Nursing's search for scientific knowledge. *Nursing Research, 33,* 26–32.

Connelly, C.E. (1986). Replication research in nursing. *International Journal of Nursing Studies, 23,* 71–77.

Crawford, G. (1982). The concept of pattern in nursing: Conceptual development and measurement. *Advances in Nursing Science, 5*(1), 1–6.

Davis, A.J. (1985). Ethical issues in nursing research. *Western Journal of Nursing Research, 7,* 377–379.

DeGroot, H.A. (1988). Scientific inquiry in nursing: A model for a new age. *Advances in Nursing Science, 10*(3), 1–21.

Dickoff, J., James, P., & Wiedenbach, E. (1968). Theory in a practice discipline (Part I): Practice-oriented discipline. *Nursing Research, 17,* 415–435.

Diers, D. (1988). On clinical scholarship (again). *Image, 20,* 2.

Donaldson, S.K., & Crowley, D.M. (1978). The discipline of nursing. *Nursing Outlook,* 114.

Fawcett, J. (1984). The metaparadigm of nursing: Present status and future refinements. *Image, 16,* 84–87.

Fulton, J.S. (1987). Virginia Henderson: Theorist, prophet, poet. *Advances in Nursing Science, 10,* 1–9.

Gortner, S.R. (1980). Nursing science in transition. *Nursing Research, 29,* 180–183.

Gortner, S.R., & Schultz, P.R. (1988). Approaches to nursing science methods. *Image, 20,* 22–27.

Hinshaw, A.S. (1983). The image of nursing research: Issues and strategies. Keynote address: 16th Annual Communicating Nursing Research Conference. Published in *Communicating Nursing Research, 16,* 1–13.

Hinshaw, A.S. (1987, November). Integrating the sciences and humanities in health care. Annual Elizabeth Sterling Soule Lecture, University of Washington, Seattle.

Hinshaw, A.S. (in press). National Center for Nursing Research: A commitment to excellence in science. In J.C. McCloskey & H.K. Grace (Eds.), *Current issues in nursing* (3rd ed.).

Hinshaw, A.S., Heinrich, J., & Bloch, D. (1988). Evolving clinical nursing research priorities. *Journal of Professional Nursing, 4,* 398. 458–459.

Horsley, J., Crane, J., Crabtree, M.K., & Wood, D.J. (1983). *Using research to improve nursing practice: A guide.* Orlando: Grune and Stratton (Conduct and Utilization of Research in Practice Project).

Jacobs-Kramer, M.K., & Chinn, P.L. (1988). Perspectives on knowing: A model of nursing knowledge. *Scholarly Inquiry for Nursing Practice: An International Journal, 2,* 129–144.

Johnson, J.E. (1973). Effects of accurate expectations about sensations on the sensory and distress components of pain. *Journal of Personality and Social Psychology, 27,* 261–275.

Kerlinger, F.N. (1986). *Foundations of behavioral research* (3rd ed.). New York: Holt, Rinehart, and Winston.

Leininger, M.M. (1978). *Transcultural nursing: Concepts, theories, and practices.* New York: John Wiley & Sons.

Leininger, M.M. (1984). *Care: The essence of nursing and health.* Thorofare, NJ: Charles B. Slack.

Lewandowski, L.A., & Kositsky, A.M. (1983). Research priorities for critical-care nursing: A study by the American Association of Critical-Care Nurses. *Heart and Lung, 12,* 35–44.

Lindeman, C.A. (1984). Dissemination of nursing research. *Image, 16,* 57–58.

McCarthy, P. (1988). Researchers take on major nursing issues. *The American Nurse, 20,* 1,12.

Meleis, A.I. (1987). Revisions in knowledge development: A passion for substance. *Scholarly Inquiry for Nursing Practice: An International Journal, 1,* 5–19.

Meleis, A.I., & May, K. (1981). Nursing theory and scholarliness in the doctoral program. *Advances in Nursing Science, 4,* 31–41.

Merton, R.F. (1979). *The sociology of science: An episodic memoir.* Carbondale, IL: Southern Illinois University Press.

National League for Nursing (1988). Correspondence to NCNR regarding organizational research objectives.

Norbeck, J.S. (1987). In defense of empiricism. *Image, 19,* 28–30.

O'Hear, A. (1985). Popper and the philosophy of science. *New Scientist, 7,* 43–44.

Orem, D. (1985). *Nursing: Concepts of practice* (3rd ed). New York: McGraw-Hill.

Pender, N.J. (1982). *Health promotion and nursing practice.* Norwalk, CT: Appleton-Century-Crofts.

Rehabilitation Nursing Foundation (1988). Correspondence to NCNR regarding organizational research objectives.

Stevenson, J.S. (1988). Nursing knowledge development: Into era II. *Journal of Professional Nursing, 4,* 152–162.

Storer, N.W. (1966). *The social system of science,* New York: Holt, Rinehart & Winston.

Tripp-Reimer, T. (1986). Health heritage project: A research proposal submitted to the Division of Nursing. *Western Journal of Nursing Research, 8,* 207–224.

Walike, B.C., Walike, J.W., Hanson, R.L., Grant, M., Kubo, W., Bergstrom, N., Wong, H.L., Padilla, G., & Williams, K. (1975). Nasogastric tube feeding: Clinical complications and current progress of research. *Northwest Health Team Approach, 2,* 33–41.

The Author Comments

"Nursing Science: The Challenge to Develop Knowledge" was generated by the need to organize and formally convey the challenges that, in my judgment, were confronting the discipline in the mid 1980s, as nursing scholars pursued the science required for nursing practice. These challenges—particularly the development of knowledge for nursing practice and the need to sustain excellence in nursing science—provided guidance for the early initiatives undertaken at the National Center for Nursing Research; that is, developing the National Nursing Research Agenda (NNRA), establishing a trajectory for research training and career development, enhancing collaboration among disciplines for scientific endeavors, and developing an intramural research program. A major strategy for sustaining excellence in the developing knowledge base for practice is the promotion of depth in the profession's research programs in relation to important areas of study. The NNRA is the process implemented as one of the first NCNR initiatives to identify priority areas for investigation. The intent is to focus scientific endeavors and federal resources on the areas identified by the nursing community to develop clusters of studies which is expected to promote depth in the evolving body of knowledge.

Facilitating nurse scientists' commitment to a trajectory of research training and career development is a critical strategy for promoting excellence in the profession's knowledge base. Ensuring that investigators maintain the "cutting edge" of their science, both substantively and methodologically, is the goal of adopting a career trajectory toward research training. Periodically devoting time and effort to updating scientific knowledge and skills or learning new techniques as research programs need to take a different direction, is crucial to staying at the forefront of an investigator's field of scholarship. Establishing a full range of federal mechanisms for supporting research training and career development across the research trajectory, from beginning researcher to senior investigator, was accomplished in the NCNR's early years. Training and development awards exist for predoctoral, postdoctoral, mid-career and senior points on the career trajectory. In order to facilitate a well-prepared cadre of nurse scientists, emphasis has been on postdoctoral study and the establishment of institutional training programs in research intensive environments.

Enhancing collaboration among scientists of multiple disciplines is important given the complexity of the clinical and research questions pursued by nurse researchers. the questions require diverse perspectives and areas of expertise. Multidisciplinary collaboration has promoted the merger of the expertise of investigators from different disciplines to evolve the knowledge needed for nursing practice. To promote such collaboration, the NCNR often cosponsors program initiatives with other NIH institutes, centers and divisions and specifically requests that applications for certain types of research awards provide evidence of collaboration with other disciplines; e.g., the Specialized and Exploratory Centers and the Institutional Training Grants.

Developing a knowledge base for nursing practice where there are gaps in the research conducted by the extramural community is the major focus of the intramural research program at NCNR. When major health care crises exist and the opportunity and timing for studies from the extramural community is limited, protocols can be generated and conducted more rapidly in the intramural program. As fruitful areas of research are evident, these can be shared, replicated and extended with scientists in the extramural community.

The challenge of disseminating stable, appropriate research findings to the practicing professional and the public will guide numerous initiatives for the NCNR as findings are available from research programs. While the earlier investments of the NCNR are in research and research training support, priorities will need to shift to dissemination as results that can guide practice become available.

—ADA SUE HINSHAW

Unit Four

Theory Building: Development, Analysis, Evaluation

The fifteen chapters in Unit Four, Theory Building: Development, Analysis, Evaluation, take a different approach to theory than do those in the preceding three units. As is probably evident to the reader, a great deal of the discussion of theory has revolved around the type of theory that is necessary and appropriate for nursing. One relevant point that must not be ignored in this debate is, "Where will theory come from?"

In order to effectively answer that question, it is necessary to stop and look at theory, both in the classical sense and in its more current evolutionary phase. The articles in Unit IV attempt to do that, and subsequently, to address issues relating to theory development.

Chapter 30, "Characteristics of Significant Theories" by Rosemary Ellis was a paper presented at the Case Western Reserve University theory symposium in October, 1967. That conference was one of the first forums where nurse scholars came together to discuss issues related to theory in nursing. Likewise, Chapter 31, "Theories, Models and Systems for Nursing" by Rose McKay, was a presentation at the second nurse scientist conference, "The Nature of Science in Nursing" held at the University of Colorado. Dr. McKay was one of the planners of the conference, along with Dr. Madeleine Leininger, Dr. Betty Jo Hadley, and Dr. Kathryn Smith.

Chapter 32, "Development of Theory: A Requisite for Nursing as a Primary Health Profession" by Dorothy E. Johnson focuses on the methods of building nursing knowledge and identifies some of the difficulties that may be present in the process. Johnson also considers models and suggests a rudimentary framework for analysis and evaluation of conceptualizations in nursing. Also of interest in Chapter 32 is the lengthy response from Zbilut in which he elaborates on many of the points made by Johnson in her essay.

Chapter 33, "Theory Construction in Nursing: An Overview" by Ada K. Jacox, presents a view of classical theory development and suggests ways this might be incorporated into the development of theories in nursing. Jacox states in her comments that she believes this article is outdated. It has been included in this anthology, however, for two very specific reasons. First, when this article was published it was widely read and quoted, and as such is a necessary component of the historical evolution of theory development. Second, Jacox defines many of the terms that are commonly used in the theory literature, such as concept, construct, and proposition. This article is a good reference for clear understanding of other readings about theory.

Chapter 34, "Competing Theories of Science" by Ada Jacox and Glenn Webster, was included as an illustration of Jacox's more recent thinking. Jacox requested the opportunity to include in this anthology something more current and relevant to the ongoing activity in nursing development. Jacox and Webster discuss the rejection of the Received View by philosophers of science and consider the nature of other competing views of science. This article clearly illustrates a juxtaposition of ideas and the development of understanding that has occurred for Jacox since 1974.

Chapter 35, "Theories: Components, Development, Evaluation" by Margaret E. Hardy, is similar to Jacox's discussion of classical theory structure. Both Jacox and Hardy pursued doctoral study in sociology, and their approaches to theory presented in Chapters 33 and 35 clearly reflect this orientation.Chapters 36, 37, 39, and 42 might all have been placed consecutively if the chapters had not been ordered chronologically. This is an example of how many categorical schemata and arbitrary and context dependent. The focus in all four chapters is on models. John R. Phillips, "Nursing Systems and Nursing Models," presents a concise overview of the nature of models and discusses uses of models in nursing. Chinn and Kramer, in "A Model for Theory Development in Nursing," provide an example of how a model might be used to develop theory. They include a graphic representation of the model they developed. "Models for Nursing" by Bush and "Models and Model Building in Nursing" by Lancaster and Lancaster elaborate on the discussion first introduced by Phillips in Chapter 36.

Chapters 38 and 40 could also be perceived as being logically connected. Crawford, Dufault, and Rudy, "Evolving Issues in Theory Development," and Flaskerud and Halloran, "Areas of Agreement in Nursing Theory Development," all encourage the reader to step back and look at what has occurred in theory development. The authors point out what progress has been made and provide some tentative ideas for future development.

Chapter 41, "A Framework for Analysis and Evaluation of Conceptual Models of Nursing" by Jacqueline Fawcett, is a very useful article. Fawcett's focus is pragmatic: she provides a nuts and bolts discussion of how logically to analyze and evaluate conceptualizations in nursing. Fawcett has continued to develop this framework and applies it to several conceptual models in nursing in her recent texts (see Chapter 41 for the reference). While Fawcett's approach may be pragmatic, she is not atheoretical. True understanding can only come after a complete and thorough critique of the nature of conceptualizations that provide structure for nursing knowledge.

In Chapter 43, "Conceptual Issues in Nursing," Rosemary Ellis argues for a need to understand the nature of nursing knowledge in order to transmit it. Always practical and down-to-earth, Ellis recognized confusion among nurses due to multiple uses of words such as theory, model, health, environment, and nursing. Her purpose in writing this article was to try to clarify some of the issues related to theory development. The essay is an appropriate close to Unit IV, forcing the reader to stop and reflect on the many different points that have been presented in the twelve chapters.

Many argue that the whole is greater than the sum of the parts. But sometimes, in the process of learning, it is useful to look at individual components in order to have an understanding of how each contributes to the whole. The articles in Unit Four present different components of theory, and a variety of ways to understand and analyze the components. The caveat for the reader, though, is not to automatically assume that by analyzing parts a clear understanding of the nature of theory can be achieved. Theory development is more than an additive process.

Chapter 30

Characteristics of Significant Theories

Rosemary Ellis

Theory development relevant to the profession of nursing requires attention to the stated or implied preposition used to connect the word *theory,* or the term *theory development,* to the word *nursing.* The preposition serves to give a sense of placement, direction, or other relationship. Think of the different meanings of the phrases *theories of nursing, theories in nursing,* or *theories for nursing.* It is the intent here to discuss characteristics of theories which are significant for nursing.

The need to attend to the expressed or implied preposition has been mentioned because one is exposed, with increasing frequency, to the term *nursing theory.* This term can be ambiguous. It is used to mean a "generalized theory capable of supporting an overall concept of a process of nursing," as Putnam (1965) uses it. In this sense, it means a theory of nursing. The term is also used more loosely to indicate some, or one, of the concepts used as a basis for explaining or understanding certain nursing practices.

For purposes of the present discussion, the word theory should be understood in its meanings of: "a coherent set of hypothetical, conceptual, and pragmatic principles forming a general frame of reference for a field of inquiry (as for deducing principles, formulating hypotheses for testing, undertaking actions)," "a systematic analysis, elucidation, or definition of a concept," or "a hypothetical entity or structure explaining or relating an observed set of facts" (Webster's, 1961). The task of this paper is to set forth a case for theory development *for* nursing, and to discuss characteristics of significant theories where significance is determined with reference to nursing.

The phrase *for nursing* implies that the discussion will be concerned only with theories, or characteristics of theories, that are relevant to that function which has to do with helping individuals to cope with health problems when their own strength, will, or knowledge is insufficient. Improvement in the practice that achieves this function is the appropriate goal of theory development for nursing. It is this goal which defines the need for theory development, and which, for this writer, determines what is significant theory. It determines what theories, or theories of what, are significant.

Nursing does not occur apart from a patient. This is not to say that all nursing is done in the physical presence of a patient, but that which is nursing is something for or with a patient. It is something that has to do with the patient's response to pathology or the therapy for it, not with the treatment of pathology per se. Nursing also cannot be defined apart from the patient; the definition centers on functions for the patient. Nursing is not defined by the activities of the nurse but by what the patient receives from them. It is not even the process itself; it is the effects of the process. A significant theory for nursing, therefore, is one that enlightens us about the patient, and what happens to him. With this orientation, studies of nurses may or may not contribute to the development of significant theories for nursing. They have the potential for such a contribution only if they treat the variable nurse as one unit in an interrelationship of units, with patient as an essential one in the structure. Theories which treat the nurse as a determinant in the patient response would seem to have this potential. Theories about why, or what people enter the profession of nursing are far less apt to have this potential.

Purposes of Theory Development

Before discussion of the characteristics which make a theory significant for nursing, consider some reasons why nurses need to be concerned with theory development. One elementary purpose for developing theories is to attempt to distinguish fact from pseudofact. Fact is defined as the close agreement of many observations of the same phenomena. By making explicit the phenomena observed, the conditions or context for the observations, and any inferred relationships, one is forced to recognize failure to conceptualize, or observe, potentially relevant variables. If close agreement is not obtained over many observations, either conceptualization is inadequate, or significant variables have not been identified or included.

A second purpose for theory development is that nursing requires the attempt to structure converging facts from a number of fields. This convergence is necessary to the understanding of human beings, especially human beings with health problems. There is no science of human beings. Knowledge about them is drawn from many fields, such as anatomy, physiology, sociology, and psychology. Not one of these fields supplies all the knowledge necessary for the undertaking of nursing human beings. The parts supplied by various fields do not always fit together to make a whole. Nurses and others are far from being able to put forth any grand theories which effectively combine the knowledges about humans already generated from many fields. However, nurses attempt to do this, in effect, in order to nurse. The attempt is essential if one seeks the holistic approach to an individual. Holism, if used as the appropriate view for aiding a patient, requires that one be concerned with any factor, be it physiological, social or any other, which affects the patient's health. It requires that the factors be treated in combination, not in isolation. It also means that the combination is not the same as the sum over each factor. Nursing requires the recognition of the inseparability and interdependence of many factors. Very few concepts or theories from other disciplines effectively enlighten us about the dynamics of interdependent biological and behavioral relationships.

There are theories about illnesses defined as psychosomatic. Rarely do these include propositions to describe, or explain, how psychological factors actually effect the observed physiological changes. What are the mechanisms involved in the translation of a psychological state into biological pathology? The answer is likely to require the synthesis of knowledge across several fields. Recognition of the interrelationships of biological and psychological factors is the first step toward explaining them and their consequences. For the most part, present knowledge, or theory, is at the level of recognition only. Nursing cannot be achieved through the application of theory or knowledge from several fields unless there is some synthesis. Until formal synthesis is forthcoming, the struggle toward an holistic approach for nursing is held back. Whether synthesis will be produced from the basic sciences remains to be seen. What source will provide a theory of incontinence that will treat of all the factors that appear to be involved? Such theory would seem essential for the prevention of the problem, or the treatment or rehabilitation, to the extent possible, of the patient who has this problem.

Another reason for nurses to be concerned with theory development and not merely application, is that theory, or theoretical knowledge, is used to give direction to practice. Only use in practice, and careful observations of results, offer the opportunity for the essential criticism of a theory's usefulness. Practice can and should test theory. Theory must not be used uncritically. It often is. One can find some examples from nursing where a concept is accepted generally and used without question, where there is very little support for it. One such concept is that of *stages of development.*

There is evidence for a certain order in the progression of development. There is little evidence to support the concept of *stages* in this progression. Stage implies a step-like progression with at least brief plateaus, instead of a slope or gradual continual increase. What evidence is there that stage is the model for the "shape" of development?

Stage is also the term in a model of the course of illness. Stages of illness are believed to exist, but why staging is the model rather than a smooth line of some shape is not clear. That stage may be an inappropriate model here is suggested by the difficulty in defining a stage of illness that is discrete and delimited. Inadequacies of language no doubt contribute. (What is the word to designate a particular point on a curve or a straight line and its position relative to other such points?) But it may make an important difference if individuals are perceived as being in one stage or another where stages are mutually exclusive and in the nature of plateaus, in contrast to being perceived as in some gradual process which is with constant increment and without plateau.

Nurses may need to decide which model is most appropriate.

Theory is also useful as a framework for the retrieval and use of generated and stored knowledge which lies in libraries. With a framework there is a guide to knowledges already available but not used, which could produce beneficial innovations. A dentist recently commented that theory development was the most critical current need for development in the treatment of dental caries. According to this dentist, treatment is based on a theory developed decades ago. The theory generally is regarded as inadequate and outdated. Treatment has not changed, however, because no one has come up with a better theory. There is no guide for the direction of change in practice. The dentist also speculated that the separate bits of knowledge to construct a new treatment probably exist in materials already in libraries. It cannot be retrieved and pieced together without some theory as a guide.

Characteristics

The above purposes or reasons for nurses' involvement in theory development do not exhaust all possible ones. They are imperative reasons. It is with references to these purposes that characteristics of significant theories for nursing will be discussed.

Scope

Scope is one characteristic important to the significance of a theory. A theory has scope if it covers and relates a number of smaller generalizations or concepts and provides at least a potential framework for ordering observations about a variety of phenomena. The broader the scope, in terms of the number and variety of facts or concepts related, the greater is the significance of the theory. Ideally, theories most important for nursing would be those that encompass both biological and behavioral observations, and have the potential for explaining their relationships. For nursing, the scope should be judged in terms of the generalizations and phenomena pertinent to an individual of the human species in the circumstances which cause him to be labeled by the concept *patient.*

Some of the theories which support current practices lack the scope necessary for nursing. It was long accepted that absolute bed rest was important for proper recovery from major surgery.Less than 30 years ago many surgeons insisted upon three weeks of bed rest for the patient who had had herniorraphy. Now nurses accept, often unquestioned, the benefits of ambulation in the early recovery from surgery and its concomitants. Both the insistence on absolute bed rest and the insistence on early ambulation stem from conceptualizations based on biological knowledge. There is support for the practice of early ambulation, or maintenance of mobility, in the findings on the effects of stasis, and of the organic changes which accompany immobilization at bed rest over long periods of time. The conceptualizations, however, do not all treat all psychological factors which might enter into recovery from surgery. The non-biological effects of insistence upon early ambulation, and of insistence that the individual resume his care of his body as early as physically possible need to be explored. Biological imperatives may need to be reconciled with psychological ones.

If nursing deals with recovery of the person as well as the body, theory which directs practice must have the scope to cover both. There is need to consider the time and the circumstances necessary for the integration of the event of surgery in addition to those which are expeditious for recovery of the body after surgery.

Complexity

Another characteristic of significant theories is that they have complexity; they treat of multiple variables or relationships, or of the complexity of a single variable. Simple postulations are not particularly valuable if they express only ideas which are readily apparent. There is no objection to the postulation; it simply does not, of itself, stimulate many new insights. If a postulation is of something not obvious, it is most likely complex.

What is complex is often not recognized as such. Incomplete conceptualizations, expressed as simple postulations, are apt to carry the hazards of illusory comprehension. For the scholar, this is unfortunate. For the practitioner who uses the postulation, the consequences may be more severe if he prescribes for others.

Testability

Another characteristic of theories to be used for nursing is that their tentativeness be clearly visible. They should be clearly recognizable as hypothetical. Usefulness of a theory depends upon its being understood as a construct. Constructs are amenable to change. They are frequently changed by their authors. Control over a construct may be lost to the author once it is placed in the public domain. It may not be erased or revised by the public when it should be. The appearance of impermanence of theories is essential if no sufficient scientific evidence accompanies their presentation. The presentation is warranted, but it must be accompanied by the caution that it be used with care and scrutiny.

Testability of a theory at a general level, however, is not requisite for use or for significance. It would be desirable. The more useful theories at this time may be those with scope and complexity to the point that they cannot, in toto, be operationalized or scientifically tested in any other way. Testability can be sacrificed in our era in favor of scope, complexity, and clinical usefulness. This is to say that elegance and complexity of structure are to be preferred to precision in the meaning of concepts in the present state of knowledge.

Usefulness

Another prime characteristic, essential for significance of theories for nursing, is that of usefulness for clinical practice. Clinical practice must be the touchstone for determining what theories are significant, and what knowledge nurses must, and should, spend time pursuing.

Theories which may be significant by other criteria are not significant for nursing if they fail in their usefulness for developing or guiding practice. An example of such a theory that may not yet be significant for nursing, but which is deemed significant for other fields, can be found in the construct *dependence.*

Dependence is convenient as a label, but conceptualizations about it are as yet inadequate to the task of guiding nursing practice with adult patients in any important way. Dependence is recognized as a component in illness, it is observed, but what theory guides what the nurse does about it? The global concept dependence includes physical dependence, social dependence, knowledge dependence, or emotional dependence. Theories do not clearly indicate the interrelationships among these. They predominately have to do with a psychological dependence only. Existing theories about dependence expound its genesis. They often contain the implication that independence is the to-be-desired and pursued state. There are many circumstances for which this seems appropriate. The practitioner of nursing, however, deals with dependence as an inevitable accompaniment of whatever calls forth the need for nursing. Theories of the genesis of dependence are not wholly adequate for nursing when an adult suddenly becomes dependent due to illness or accident. Theories with the value of independence are not useful guides for what is to be done about it if it is suddenly or gradually lost forever.

Certainly a goal of nursing is to assist the patient to a state in which he no longer needs the professional. But theory does not give the guidelines for determining the optimum rate to move, or how to treat dependence when prognosis indicates that the patient cannot regain independence.

If our value for independence is prepotent, attempts will be made to have the patient assume full responsibility for himself at the earliest possible moment or to retain responsibility for himself to the last possible moment. Much current practice reflects this. What is often unspecified is responsibility for what. Attempts often are made to move the patient to resumption of independence in management of his physical care without concomitantly allowing him resumption of independence for activities or decisions that have to do with his job, home, or other social responsibilities. One could speculate the resumption of independence, or at least abandonment of imposed dependence, for the adult patient, should progress in a rapidly accelerated miniature of earlier life development. Practice would support such theory.

Valuing independence and attempting to maintain it to the last moment may, however, be at the expense of learning how to live with dependence. This should be considered when circumstances predict that dependence cannot be avoided, as in chronic debilitating or degenerative disease. Reinforcement of independence by the nurse conveys a high value for it. At what point in time, or in the course of disease which produces erosion of physical independence, does reinforcement of independence hamper acceptance of reality-based dependence? If physical dependence is inevitable, do practices that convey high value for independence increase discomfort with dependence? Do they do the patient unnecessary harm or delay adjustment to the inevitable? They might make the patient unable or less able to accept dependence, may make him fear he will be less valued as he becomes dependent. Stress can be heightened unknowingly if at the time the patient is becoming dependent, independence is the value and the expectation the nurse appears to have. The patient's welfare might be better served if in this case of increasing loss of functioning, he could learn that he will be accepted and valued when dependent. This could enable him to retain more easily his sense of worth in the face of deterioration of his body.

This dilemma for the nurse is the choice between reinforcement of independence, or creation of an environment in which the patient is enabled to learn that he can be respected in spite of his physical dependence, can learn to be comfortable with dependence. Perhaps the choices are not mutually exclusive, though they seem so. What is important is that existent theories do not provide help for the practitioner. In this sense they are not yet significant for nursing.

Implicit Values

An implication of the above discussion of dependence is that another characteristic of significant theories is that implicit values are recognized and made explicit.

Theories of behavior usually contain some implication of the normative or desired behaviors which are not made explicit. Independence usually is treated as the desired norm or goal state without reference to the values which cause this to be so, and without consideration of the values with which it might conflict.

Information Generation

Another characteristic of significant theories is that they are capable of generating a great deal of new information. Hypotheses which are highly probable may be so simply because they state what is apparent empirically and can contribute little that is new (Popper, 1954). A theory that generates many hypotheses, even some without high probability, or some that are difficult to test, contribute significantly to understanding. Even theories which do not have other characteristics of significance may be significant if they generate hypotheses of some sort.

Hypotheses logically derived, that fail to be supported by empirical evidence, may serve to call attention to variables that were not thought of previously. Variables essential for an effect, or those that can negate effect, may be illuminated, the special case discovered. Incomplete or imperfect theories are better than no theory at all in generating new ideas and new practices. They may be significant. The imperative is to embark on theorizing even at the simplest level, and to cherish the efforts of those who attempt theorizing and the testing of it.

A student's hypothesis about a relationship between stress and helplessness provoked a recognition of the complexity of the concept helplessness. The initial proposition was that feelings of helplessness would be associated with feelings of stress. The study suggested that there is no simple relationship. Under some conditions an individual may feel himself very helpless. If he perceives that he, or the one for whom he is responsible (as in caring for a spouse at home who is in the terminal stages of cancer), is the recipient of adequate help from others, he is not necessarily under high stress with helplessness. He can feel very helpless, but is not threatened by the feeling because others, such as the visiting

nurse, help him share and carry out his responsibilities of care. They offer back-up security that, in effect, prevents the feeling that the responsibility is unmanageable. Theory is needed to begin to understand and explore feelings of helplessness and their consequences.

Thinking about helplessness generated recognition of a possible clinical dilemma. Under what conditions should one attempt to offer to act for the person who feels helpless? If one can help him avoid stress by doing for him, should one? Or should the task be to help the individual to gain the competence and confidence to deal with the situation and so to help him attempt to deal with his feelings of helplessness? If the situation provoking his helplessness is self-limiting the dilemma may arise. The nature of a nurse's intervention, what she actually does and the outcomes are likely to be different for one choice versus the other. Avoidance of stress, and skill in learning what is necessary to overcome helplessness, may not be simultaneously attainable. What theory guides a decision? The gaps in our knowledge and recognition of the inadequacies of existing theories are one result of a very simple hypothesis which itself was stimulated by reading about crisis theories. It could be a significant hypothesis for nursing.

Meaningful Terminology

A final characteristic of theories significant for nursing would be that they are couched in terminology which can be used meaningfully with, or applied to, phenomena observed in nursing. This might not appear much of a problem, but terminology from one science is used for what appear to be analogous phenomena in another context. The terms, used in this second context, may be expressive, descriptive, and serve as a useful label for the phenomena, but they may have lost their special terminological meaning. The danger is that the loss may not be recognized. An erroneous assumption of analogy is connoted and perpetuated.

Count (1964, p. 95) illustrates the problem in calling attention to the difference between the physical science terms pressure and force, and these concepts as used in social science. The laws which pertain to pressure and force, and these concepts as used in social science. The laws which pertain to pressure and force in physical science cannot be duplicated in meaningful formulas or units of measure in social science.

It is tempting to borrow terminology. An example of one tempting term is "regression in the service of the ego." It appeals as a descriptive label for some of the phenomena observed in illness. An adult defined as ill may be exempted from some responsibilities, is allowed more license for egocentric behavior than when he is well, and for reasons of physical changes, may be fed, bathed, and assisted with toileting. If such a state is functional for recovery, it could readily be called regression in the service of the ego. The phenomenon may not be analogous to those observed by psychologists who use the term to label the conceptualization to "explain" such things as humor, artistic creativity, problem solving, and empathy (Schafer, 1958, p. 121). Until the analogy is established, use of the term for phenomena in nursing should be avoided even though a more useful label is lacking.

Other terms of phrases attractive for nursing may sound so similar as to be confused in use. *Levels of consciousness* as used in conjunction with anesthesiology or coma is not synonymous with the term *altered states of consciousness* as the psychologist uses it. Unless a nurse who uses them knows the terminologic meaning of phrases from specific fields, they can be confused or used indiscriminately when both psychological and physiological states are involved.

Other Relevant Considerations

Several final thoughts are offered not as characteristics of significant theories for nursing but because they seem relevant. The first is that ultimately, for nursing practice, theories or theoretical formulations will be needed that will predict or explain phenomena for individuals, not groups. Simply knowing that when grouping is based on a cultural factor, that groups differ in their behavior with pain, is not very useful for nursing practice. It does not allow the prediction or presumption that any given individual will behave as the majority of his cultural group appear to behave. It may be claimed that at least the group-based finding could alert

the nurse to the probability that a patient from a given cultural group will behave in a certain way. This may or may not be useful. Operating on the prediction is unsafe. It can be biasing and lessen sensitivity to deviations of the individual from specific cultural norms. It may set up expectations which are actually not beneficial for a given patient.

A second thought is that the assumption of the uniqueness of individuals is also not very useful for nursing. When the assumption implies that one knows nothing about an individual until one has encountered and assessed him, it denies the patterning and order in nature. Classification as human begins to tell one something of the structure, basic needs, and of some processes the individual will have. At best, the assumption of uniqueness is useful only as a caveat. It indicates there is risk in prediction and that one must look for individual differences.

Summary

A position has been taken that there is a need for nurses to undertake theory development. Application of theories developed from various sciences cannot be done uncritically. Existing theories, or theories likely to be developed from a single science, are not apt to be complete enough for an holistic view of man. The holistic view seems most suitable for the function of nursing as it is currently defined in the profession of nursing.

Theories that are significant for nursing are those that include the patient as an essential component. They are also those that enlighten us about the patient. Various characteristics of theories, such as scope, complexity, testability, implicit values and others, have been discussed as determinants of significance of theories for nursing. The ultimate test of the significance of a theory for nursing lies in its usefulness for the practice of nursing.

Both methodological development and theory development are essential for the inquiry which can facilitate improvement in nursing practice. The domain of nursing practice should delimit the domain appropriate to theory development for nursing. Theory, whether begged, borrowed, derived, or originated by nurses, is significant for nursing if it can enlighten nursing practice.

The first obligation of the professional in nursing is the responsibility for nursing practice or its improvement. This is not to say that contribution to general or specific knowledge is less desirable. It is to say that such concern is less our responsibility than is that for practice. What is significant for nursing, what theory, what knowledge the professional nurse should spend time pursuing, is that which pertains to practice. Generation of knowledge for the sake of knowledge is not the raison d'etre for the profession of nursing—*nursing is.*

References

Count, E.W. (1964). Dimensions of fact in anthropology. In E.W. Count & G.T. Bowles (Eds.), *Fact and theory in social science.* Syracuse, NY: Syracuse University Press.

Popper, K. (1954). Degree of confirmation. *British Journal of Philosophy and Science, 5,* 146.

Putnam, P. A. (1965). Conceptual approach to nursing theory. *Nursing Science, 3,* 430-442.

Schafer, R. (1958). Repression in the service of the ego: The relevance of a psychoanalytic concept for personality assessment. In G. Lindzey et al. (Eds.), *Assessment of human motives.* New York: Holt, Rinehart and Winston.

Webster's Third New International Dictionary (1961) (Unabridged ed.). Springfield, MA: Merriam.

The Author Comments

I was invited to write this paper to explore what theory was needed for nursing—theory about nurses or theory about patients. I chose to argue that theory that could improve nursing practice was what was needed. I attempted to stress the inadequacies of (then) dependence on theory from other disciplines and the failure to attend to the phenomena and circumstances of nursing as they occur as a source for theory development. The paper still is constantly cited, but my "Characteristics" subheadings often are used *inappropriately* in analyses of schema that I do not consider theory. This paper provided one early argument for paying attention to the phenomena in practice as subject matter for theory development in nursing. Nurse scientists of the day were often selecting concepts or variables for research and theory development from theories or interests acquired in the field in which they did doctoral work. These concepts seemed to me too often removed from involvement and concern with phenomena in clinical practice.

—ROSEMARY ELLIS

Chapter 31

Theories, Models, and Systems for Nursing

Rose McKay

The nurse performs her actions with integrity, understanding, and skill. When she acts with integrity, she acts in accordance with the value system developed by the profession. When she acts with understanding, she has the knowledge necessary to identify a rationale for, and the probable result of her actions. When she acts with skill, she is able to achieve a high degree of correlation between her intentions and the results produced by her actions. Professional practice is a combination of believing, knowing, and doing. The value system has its source in philosophy, ethics, and religion. The knowledge comes from science and the methods of practice, at least in part, from the subtleties of interpersonal interaction. It is evident that nursing is not all science; the ethical and aesthetic elements cannot be disregarded. As a profession grows all three areas change— value assumptions are redefined, knowledge is extended, and skill is perfected—but it is the acquisition of knowledge and the organizing of it into meaningful patterns which enriches professional practice. The qual-

ity of service is related to the individual practitioners' knowledge and understanding improves not only as nurses increase their experience but also as they draw upon and contribute to the development of an expanding body of theory.

Theories

Theories are not mere decorative extensions of facts. They are the capstone of all scientific work since the understanding which is the goal of science is expressed in terms of theoretical formulations. In a complex applied area such as nursing it is unrealistic to demand acceptance of a single proposal which will be satisfactory to all researchers and practitioners. It is to be expected that there will be a variety of suggestions which have as their goal the systematic ordering of ideas about the phenomena of the field of inquiry. Specialized theories will probably deal with the phenomena at particular levels. Until we know which frames of reference are

About the Author

ROSE MCKAY is well known and respected by colleagues and students in nursing for her contribution to the development of nursing theory. Her doctoral dissertation *The Process of Theory Development in Nursing*, written in 1965 at Columbia University, was conceived and written before many of us recognized the value of theory for the development of nursing as a discipline.

Rose was born in New York City in 1926 and grew up there. She was always interested in the source of knowledge—whether it be the origin of words, ideas, or historical thoughts. As a young girl, she spent many hours reading in the stillness and coolness of the neighborhood library. After graduating from a Catholic high school, she studied nursing at the College of Mt. St. Vincent in New York. Following graduation in 1947, she worked as a public health nurse for the New York City Department of Health from 1947 through 1953.

She began graduate study at Teacher's College at Columbia University in 1948 and completed her master's degree in 1952. She then commenced her academic career as a nurse educator in 1953 and taught at various universities until her death in May, 1983. Her expertise grew in the areas of curriculum, methods of instruction, and theory development.

going to be the most useful, it will surely be desirable to retain alternative frameworks and to take considerable pains to develop means for transition from one framework to the other.

A definition of theory is relatively easy in the more sophisticated physical sciences. A definition of this term which might be suitable for all empirical generalizations, conceptual frameworks, working hypotheses, representational models and deductive schemes called theory in other areas, is more difficult. In a vague sense the word means a general conceptual background to some field of practical activity. A more technical interpretation used in highly quantified sciences is a hypothesis that has been verified by observation. More commonly the word theory is used to refer to a logically interconnected set of such confirmed hypotheses. In this sense it is essentially a system of logical statements which are comprehensive, consistent, and parsimonious and which generate testable hypotheses. It is assumed that verification is provisional rather than absolute.

The field of nursing, at present, might use the word theory in a rather modest sense. While we should not remain content with mere factual data, averages, or correlations on which the researcher has imposed little rationale, neither should we aspire to a large scale deductive scheme with theorems rigorously derived from postulates and axioms.

Models

Taxonomies, paradigms, and models can help to explain phenomena, predict results of actions, and serve as influences for improved practice. *Taxonomy* is the process of classification of phenomena, according to some system; *paradigms* are patterns or schemes which attempt to organize or describe a process; and *models* are symbolic representations of perceptual phenomena. Meadows has said that "the formulation of a model consists in conceptually marking off a perceptual complex. It involves, moreover, replacing part or parts of a perceptual complex by some representation or symbol. Every model is a pattern of symbols, rules, and processes regarded as matching, in part or in totality, an existing perceptual complex. Each model stipulates thus some correspondence with reality and some verifiability between model and reality" (Meadows, 1957, p. 4).

Models vary in two ways. They vary first in their level of abstraction. At the lowest point are the iconic or pictorial models which attempt to reproduce the important or relevant features of an event being studied for the purpose of making possible closer scrutiny and manipulation. Relationships can not easily be made pictorial. At a middle point on the continuum are the descriptive models. These may be used to present not so much the features of a situation as the structure of the relationships within the reality setting. These models are more abstract and selective and they permit the development of hypotheses. At a higher level are the more abstract mathematical models. Max Black identifies the advantages of mathematical analysis in any empirical investigation as "precision in formulating relations, ease of inference via mathematical calculations and intuitive grasp of the structure revealed" (Black, 1962, p. 225). This level would probably also include stochastic systems and correlations. In some presentations the term model is synonymous with theory, though it may be reserved for those theories which are either highly speculative or quantified or most likely both (Brodbeck, 1963; Miller, 1951). In these cases, the use of the word "model" emphasizes the tentative and unconfirmed nature of the hypothesis in question.

Models may vary secondly in terms of the metaphor that they utilize. Meadows (1957) has indicated that historically the two dominant metaphors have been the machine and the organism. Depending on the cultural milieu one of them has been dominant.

Until fairly recently the machine has been the dominant metaphor in modern scientific theory. This view regarded man as an inert instrument performing tasks assigned to him. All effects of interaction were ignored. In institutions the use of this model led to operations specified by the system, the level of specialization was kept low and basic decisions were not an individual responsibility. The assembly line approach in manufacturing is the typical example. The heritage of this model can easily be seen in the role of nurses in hospitals today. They are regarded as givens rather than variables in the system and the idea of fixed positions and interchangeable personnel is firmly established. Specialization is deemphasized and a reasonable division of labor is the goal. The idea of nurses as "cogs in the machinery" while not often expressed is still widely utilized.

Currently the open, self-maintaining and self-regulating biological system is the dominant model in many fields—an organismic rather than a mechanical image.

Models at each level of abstraction and patterned after their selected metaphor offer both assistance and difficulties to their users. While development of mathematical models can remain as an inevitable but distant goal, in many areas, including ours, current progress permits representation only in iconic or descriptive terms.

In selecting metaphors the best approach would seem to be to use whichever seems suitable (some include "field" as a third type of metaphor). The human individual can certainly be represented best as an organism. However, certain human processes might best be visualized as a type of feedback mechanism which is essentially a machine model.

While machine metaphors can and should be used to explore certain areas, for both philosophical and practical reasons, we can probably agree that the organismic model is the dominant one for nursing.

For clarification at this point we should mention several other terms which are frequently used in relation to models and model construction. The first is *analogue*. An analogue is that which is assumed to be similar in nature and function to some other thing. It is an observable example of the metaphor on which a particular model is based. For example, Hobbes' analogue of the state as a leviathan suggests we should observe a monster whale if we want to make inferences about the action of the state. In the same way "angel of mercy" might be an analogue for nurse, or a computer an analogue for an individual. One important quality of analogues is that while there are similarities there are also differences. This way of thinking is as ancient as man. In the past it often produced inspiring but scientifically sterile metaphors. With the development of analytic methodology in science it receded as a source for significant hypotheses.

A second term frequently used in describing models is *isomorphy* or *isomorphism*. While a model is described as a formal identity between a conceptual system and a real one, isomorphism is a formal identity between two conceptual systems. Two theories whose laws have the same form are isomorphic or structurally similar to each other. In the case of two theories, one of which is less well developed, the concepts of the better known area are replaced in the laws by the concepts of the new area. This replacement results in a set of laws about the new area. If observation shows these new hypotheses to be verified then the two theories are isomorphic. An example of this is pointed out by Bondi (1955) when he recommends examination of theories of terrestrial physics as a basis for any theory of the internal constitution of the stars. One of the situations to be avoided is the utilization of theories about which little is known as models for areas about which even less is known. A basic requirement for the less well developed area is that it has its concepts or constructs identified and defined.

Scientists wish to predict and models become a device by which assumptions are transformed into postulates—conceptualizations of reality to be tested. Griffiths (1963) points out that some assumptions concerning the use of models are that: (a) the world is knowable in general, (b) order can be imposed on the phenomena under study, (c) models are culture bound (e.g., Darwin's model of survival of the fittest is thought to be related to the free enterprise economic system of his period), and (d) that all models are constructs of systems.

Systems

In the last decade an interesting new connection has developed among scientists from such divergent fields as physics, biology, political science, psychology, and sociology. These scientists have become identified as general systems theorists. They believe that it is possible to represent all forms of inanimate and animate matter as systems which have common properties though present in different forms. They also hold that universal laws can be found which described the structure of these systems and their manner of functioning. Let us briefly review some of the possible reasons for this development.

The unifying principle of the analytical method has been the language of mathematics. Attempts to extend this method to the study of living processes were only partially successful and this formed the basis for arguments between vitalism and reductionism. Concepts of biology such as life, birth, and adaptation seem too complex to be dealt with by analytical method. In regard to human behavior, the field of the social scientists, the problem of producing mathematical formula representing a relationship between variables becomes even more severe. The concept of organism in biology, of individual in psychology, of institution in sociology, of nation in political science, and of culture in anthropology are indispensable to these fields. Each of these wholes presents itself naturally because we perceive it as such. According to Rapoport, "A whole which functions as a whole by virtue of the interdependence of its parts is called a system" (Rapoport, 1968, p. 17). The method which aims at discovering how this "wholeness" functioning is brought about in the widest variety of systems has been called general systems theory. Hall and Fagen have presented a very clear statement which defines system. They describe it as "a set of objects together with relationships between the objects and between their attributes" (Hall & Fagen 1950, p. 18). That is, the essential components of a system are the *objects* which are the parts of the system, the properties of the objects identified as *attributes,* and the *relationship* among the objects and their attributes which holds the system together.

Besides the differences in models which are used for symbolization of systems (in metaphor and level of abstractness) systems may also be differentiated in terms of another characteristic; i.e., whether they are open systems or closed systems. An example of a closed system is a chemical reaction confined in a reaction vessel. An example of an open system is a living organism. The essential difference is that open systems are related to and exchange matter with their environment while closed systems do not. Even living organisms tend at times to act like closed systems—an isolated community or a withdrawn individual might be considered a system tending toward closure.

A significant aspect of this differentiation between closed and open systems is in relation to certain funda mental dynamic processes which govern the operation of each. When isolated from their environments closed systems are subject to the action of the Second Law of Thermodynamics. This law states that the entropy or measure of disorder of a closed system will always increase toward a maximum attained in equilibrium. Closed systems, therefore, move toward a state of homogeneity, a leveling of all differences, of maximum disorganization.

The Second Law applies to all systems but in the case of living systems another force, called negative entropy is also working. This tends toward the achievement of a more complex order and heterogeneity. von Bertalanffy states that "Self-differentiating systems that evolve toward higher complexity (decreasing entropy) are for thermo-dynamic reasons possible only as open systems importing matter containing free energy to an amount over-compensating the increase in entropy due to irreversible processes within the system (import of negative entropy)" (von Bertalanaffy, 1968, p. 16).

Both closed and open systems are capable of attaining stationary states. But the nature of this state is different in each system. In the closed system in accor dance with the Second Law of Thermodynamics a state of equilibrium *must* eventually be reached. In an open system a state in which the system appears to be stationary *may* be achieved provided certain conditions are given. This result is called a *steady state*. The composition of the system remains constant but there is a continuous exchange and flow of component material.

Properties characteristic of systems in general (according to Hearn, 1958) are as follows:

1. Every order of system except the smallest has *subsystems*.
2. All but the largest have *suprasystems* consisting of the system and its environment (Hearn, 1958, pp. 38–51). There are factors in both the system and the environment which affect their respective structure and function. The factors in the system or subsystem are called *variables;* those in the environment are called *parameters.*
3. Every system has a *boundary* which distinguishes it from its environment. It may be determined in various ways but it is in every case an arbitrary distinction. James Miller (1955) has suggested that the boundary is the region where greater energy is required for transmission across it than for transmission immediately outside that region or immediately inside it.
4. The *environment* of a system is everything external to its boundary. Higher order systems, therefore, are always part of the environment of lower order systems. For each system moreover, there may be both a proximal and a distal environment. The *proximal environment* is that of which the system is aware, the *distal environment* affects the behavior of the system but is beyond the awareness of the system.

It is easily recognized that the realities of human existence are more complex than any conceptual system which attempts to describe it. James Miller says "you cannot judge a model in terms of appearances (seeming to have nothing to do with the warm reality of human life) but rather by its effectiveness in explaining and predicting" (Miller, 1955, p. 523). With this in mind, the organismic model at the middle range or descriptive level seems to offer the best overall integrating basis for representing human beings as individuals and in groups.

Characteristics of the Organismic Open System

All the characteristics of systems in general also apply to organismic open systems. They have subsystems, they are part of a suprasystem, each has a boundary. They have system variables and environmental parameters. They have environments both proximal and distal. Open systems in addition have the properties previously mentioned; i.e., they exchange both energy and information with their environment. (Inputs *and* outputs of both energy and information.) Open systems also maintain themselves in steady states.

After any disturbance a system tends to reestablish its steady state. When a component is added, the organism reacts in a way so as to reestablish a steady state similar to the original. If the stimulus is prolonged or if external conditions change in any major way the system can react in such a way as to establish another steady state. Thus another quality of open systems is the process of *self-regulation*. Order, predictability and manipulation of the environment are integral parts of the self-regulating, adaptation overlay of human beings when considered as open systems.

Closely related to the concept of steady state is the concept of *equifinality* first identified by Driesch. In contrast to equilibrium states in closed systems which are determined by initial conditions, the open system may attain, according to Bertalanffy, "a time independent of initial conditions and determined by only the system parameters" (von Bertalanffy, 1968, p. 18). The phenomenon of equifinality can be illustrated in man, as in sea urchins, when a normal individual of each type can develop from a complete ovum or from each half of a divided ovum (identical twins are the product of the splitting of one ovum just as two sea urchins were the result of Driesch's experiment). This means that for every species there is a typical or characteristic state. Indeed there is, for every individual, a characteristic state which he by nature must strive to assume. Perhaps more precisely there are states for each successive stage of development around which the individual strives to maintain the steady state which is characteristic of that stage.

This concept could be very important in nursing since according to this structure illness can be regarded as the life process regulating toward normalcy after disturbance owing to the equifinality of biological systems—and perhaps with our assistance and intervention. Recovery would be an expression of the dynamics of living systems maintaining and reestablishing so far as possible the original steady state. Chronic disease or disability would be an altered steady state between available input-output balance (entropy tendency) and equifinal state.

Equifinality could also explain growth. In childhood organization is greater than disorganization and the organism becomes more and more differentiated; i.e., as it grows. In old age disorganization is greater than organization, and at death entropy has full reign. This may be a too simplistic view of aging. A recent article by Goldman proposed that aging is the "relentless if slow increase in the degree of disorganization of an organism due to the accumulation of uncorrected deviations from its fully organized condition" (Gold-

man, 1968, pp. 14–15). This leads to a loss of choice in the number of things the organism can do and this loss of choice is an indicator of the degree of aging.

The problem of temporal as well as functional organization of organismic open systems is another interesting area in regard to the concept of equifinality. For example, it has been shown that even without environmental cues such as light and temperatures certain circadian rhythms persist. This would argue for the existence of some sort of internal impetus. This type of teleological behavior and others such as fetal movements without external stimuli would support the concept of equifinality.

Two additional phenomena of open systems are yet to be described. First is the dynamic interplay of subsystems operating as functional processes which maintain the steady state. Bertalanffy (1968, p. 16) also offers the idea of "leading part." (In an individual this subsystem would be the brain, in a group the leader).

The open system can be maintained in or near a steady state by feedback processes. Thermoregulation in warm blooded animals is one of the best examples of this process in living organisms, thermostats or other types of servomechanisms in inanimate systems. Weiner defines feedback as "the property of being able to adjust future conduct by past performance. It may be simple, as the common reflex or it may be of a higher order feedback in which past experience is used not only to regulate specific movements but also whole policies of behavior. Such a policy—feedback may, and often does, appear to be what we know under one aspect as a conditioned reflex, and under another as learning" (Weiner, 1954, p. 33). These (thermostat and thermoregulator) are examples of negative feedback. It is important to note that feedback can also be positive; i.e., if a thermostat were to add more fuel as the environment became warmer. *Amplification* is another type of feedback. Chain reactions of any sort are examples of this type. von Bertalanffy comments concerning the relationship between feedback and the dynamic interplay of processes. "At first, systems—biological, neurological, psychological, or social—are governed by dynamic interaction of their components; later on, fixed arrangements and conditions of constraint are established which render the system and its parts more efficient, but also gradually diminish and eventually abolish its equipotentiality" (von Bertalanffy, 1955, p. 79). In addition to the process of *progressive segregation* wherein the system divides into a hierarchical order of subordinate systems which gain a certain independence of each other, the process of *progressive mechanization* wherein certain processes became set as fixed arrangements is also ongoing. The consequences of these two processes are that negative entropy is developed and life is maintained, but restraints are imposed on the free interplay of the functional subsystems which would seem to limit the degree to which the system can achieve its potentiality.

While many of these preceding concepts come from the physical or biological sciences, von Bertalanffy maintains that there is a formal identity or isomorphism between these concepts and the more complex levels of organization beyond individual; i.e., groups, communities, and societies. Systems at whatever level are subject to the same universal laws.

The power of any model to add to organization and understanding depends to a large part on the central integrating idea. System of the organismic type seems to be directly related in so many ways to the underlying processes, values, and actions in the field of nursing. We are involved in our professional role with individuals, groups, and communities. If all can be regarded as systems, and there are properties common to all, it seems that the principles which define their operations form a part, at least, of a concept of nursing.

An open organismic system exchanging information and energy with its environment seems to be a most productive way of conceptualizing individuals, groups, and communities. Nursing is a biopsychosocial process. The predominating emphasis of the physical and biological science might be seen as energy transfer. Social sciences deal with verbal or symbolic behavior. Systems, concepts, and theory deal with both information and energy transfer and with the relationship between them in open systems. Nursing could be conceived of as a dyadic system between the nurse and the

patient and as such could be analyzed according to the inputs and outputs of information and/or energy exchanged. Nursing functions could be interpreted as bringing a source of energy or information from the distal to the proximal environment in order to maintain the steady state, or as serving as a receptor for "spilling" along any dimension when the input was excessive and maintenance of steady state required increased output.

It is obvious that such process interpretations are abstract and general. The concept of equifinality allows for individualization but the profession will have to specify through development of its philosophy and ethic the values and goals for action within this complex.

A possible limitation of the utility of this construct for the analysis of phenomena to be studied is its necessarily high level of abstraction. The proposition that all systems have boundaries and subsystems is universal but it fails to specify the functional interrelationship of these subsystems or the system parameters which increase or decrease the permeability of the boundary. This high level of abstraction need become an impediment only if we made no attempt to relate it to our use by deduction and testing. While nurse-scientists in biology, sociology, psychology, and anthropology are making contributions related to their disciplinary field of study, a level of abstraction which could utilize all these contributions to foster inter disciplinary communication and practical application would seem to be not only desirable but possibly essential. We have already experienced the communication difficulties which arise for example when biologists try to communicate with anthropologists. An interesting question might be—what are the system boundaries for a nurse-scientist? Is communication and interaction more feasible within the disciplinary group or within the nursing group or only within the group which consists of those who are alike on both dimensions? A high level abstraction which can furnish a framework and a language for understanding and which already has adherents in the disciplinary areas would seem to be a definite asset.

At this point it might be well to mention that those

who are interested in the field of general systems usually include conceptual approaches such as cybernetics, information theory, game and network theory, and applied fields such as system engineering and operations research under the systems approach. They are considered to be adaptations of the open systems model or self-regulating feedback systems. System engineering is oriented toward scientific planning design, evaluation and construction man-machine systems, e.g., air travel. We could easily think of applications of this approach in coordinating the entire organization for an intensive care unit where the patient-analogue computer-nurse system could be studied.

Another area of problems might lie in identifying the degree of openness and closedness of systems. At any one time an individual subsystem or a group subsystem might function as a closed system while the rest were functioning as open systems. This question seems to offer a wide open field for questions pertinent to investigation. Is the group member who does not participate an example of a subsystem closure? The patient with severe physiological energy demands whose information processing system is not available for input might also be thought of in this way. Some studies done in coronary care units show that information given to patients during the first few days after an attack is usually not remembered; there is almost complete amnesia. Information given at a later time is remembered. Is questioning by a patient before a new therapeutic experience an example of an internal strain which elicits efforts to achieve inputs of energy and/or information that will reduce strain and tend more toward the steady state? What is the result of illness in terms of reduction of the equipotential level? Is it related to a gradual reduction in the equilibratory range of the equipotential steady state? Would nursing action vary if, in relation to the out-of-phase variable, the reaction was hyper or hypo to the steady state? What inputs and subsystems functions maintain the usual chaotic state of many busy hospital units but prevent the out-of-phase reaction of panic? These and other questions become immediately available—and there is a framework for deducing pertinent hypotheses.

A source of theorems or propositions based on general systems theory has been developed by Miller. While these formulations have been criticized by Buck (1956) some do seem to be particularly appropriate for investigation in our field.

One states "when reduction of several strains is not possible simultaneously the order in which they are reduced in systems which survive is from strongest to weakest if the effort required for their reduction is identical" (Miller, 1955, p. 528). Investigation of the priority for handling of presenting problems might reveal ways in which to equalize effort so that this priority could be established. Important health goals are sometimes neglected because the effort required for this solution is directed toward other higher strain system demands such as maintaining the established life pattern in a steady state.

Another of James Miller's propositions is that "there is always a constant systematic distortion—or better alteration—between input of energy or information into a system and output from that system" (Miller, 1955, p. 524). This is a familiar problem to nurses. How often have we failed to communicate or achieve other desired effects because of this distortion. (In other formulations such as information theory this distortion would be called "noise" and systemic "noise levels" are monitored for feedback which affects input signals.) A second proposition related to this one is "the distortion of a system is the sum of effects of processes which subtract from input to reduce strains in subsystems or add to output to reduce such strains" (Miller, 1955, p. 525). This proposition seems to provide a rational explanation for the cause of the distortion and may even lead to predictions in regard to the form and direction which distortion may take. Miller offers 19 propositions in his article. While they may not all be equally helpful a number of them seem to offer a basis for investigation of the multivariable complexities of the nurse-patient interaction milieu.

In nursing education as well, the use of general systems theory may have some implications. As our practice becomes ever more demanding of knowledge from an increasing variety of disciplines the question of input overload becomes a significant one. How do the students react to this variety of requirements and contents? Can they absorb all of them, do they screen out? What is the amount of stored information and the extent of ignored signals? Up to a maximum the system can absorb a great amount of information and energy but what is the system tolerance level? Does this factor affect recruitment and retention?

The additional problem in nursing education of finding a rationale for a sequence of professional courses which include necessary content from a variety of disciplinary sources as well as their specific application in nursing itself is a challenge most faculties are facing. The answer to this problem is not easily found. General systems theory could offer a possible focus around which to organize the curriculum. The problem of where to begin is not answered, of course. Should the introductory unit be the cell, the individual, the group? The method for utilization of this content is not indicated, either. Applications in the nursing setting could be developed however. A model of nursing action in wellness and illness based on a general system approach is not impossible. It would no doubt include variations of the dyadic system structure and function in relation to the degree of system distortion especially of the subsystem (patient) caused by strain along any one of several variables. It would also have to allow for a suprasystem of nursing team or health team. The degree of control of the nurse of significant system parameters for the maintenance of steady state would also need to be considered. Another question might be what are the equifinal stages of this dyadic system? Is the achievement of entropy a desirable goal in this case?

Summary

Much of what has been said is conjectural. Certainly the task ahead of us is very great before contributions from this theory can become tangible. The first step perhaps is to develop models specifying important system variables for investigation. Three suggested by Kaufman (1958) are time, stress, and perception. These too are at a fairly high level of abstraction but it is a beginning. Others might be as Goldman (1968) projected: aging, noise and choice. Energy (input sources and internal supply) distortion, purpose, progressive mechanization, temporal distortion, comfort, and entropy are other concepts to consider. The important step to be taken next would be to deduce the hypothesis which could lead to a testing and validation in the reality setting. The taxonomic development of the subsystems of the larger systems is another task which must precede study of the functional relationships in groups and communities.

The superiority of programmatic research has been amply demonstrated in every field. The hope that this approach might provide a possible framework for a comprehensive program has influenced the worth of this model for me.

Knowledge is essential to our practice. If it can be codified it can more easily be communicated and extended. If there is not a strong factual base we must work from assumptions. But our assumptions regarding the nature of man range from the existentialist to the cybernetic, from the idea of an information processing machine to one of a many splendored being. Today a model of the open organismic system has been offered for your consideration. Even if I am committed to the concept of an open system, I am an even more dedicated adherent of the open mind. We may still have much to learn from our initial encounters with these ideas. We have even more to learn from an attitude of thoughtful consideration and frank criticism.

References

Black, M. (1962). *Models and metaphors,* Ithaca, NY: Cornell University Press.

Bondi, H. (1955). Astronomy and cosmology. In J.R. Newman (Ed.), *What is science?* New York: Simon and Schuster.

Brodbeck, M. (1963) Logic and scientific method in research on teaching. In N.L. Gage (Ed.), *Handbook of research in teaching* (pp. 44–93). Chicago: Rand McNally.

Buck, R.C. (1956). On the logic of general behavior systems theory. In H. Feigl & M. Scriver (Eds.), *Foundations of science and the concepts of psychology and psychoanaly-*

sis (pp. 223–228). *Minnesota studies in the philosophy of science,* Minneapolis: University of Minnesota Press.

Goldman, S. (1968). Aging, noise and choice. *Perspectives in Biology and Medicine, 12,* 12–30.

Griffiths, D.E. (1963). Some assumptions underlying the use of models in research. In J.A. Culbertson & S.P. Hencley (Eds.), *Educational research; new perspectives* (pp. 121–140). Danville, IL: Interstate.

Hall, A.D., & Fagen, R.E. (1950). General systems. In L. von Bertalanffy and A. Rapoport (Eds.), *Yearbook of the society for the advancement of general systems theory.* Ann Arbor, MI: Braun Brumfield.

Hearn, G. (1958). *Theory building in social work.* Toronto: University of Toronto Press.

Kaufman, M.A. (1958). *Identification of theoretical bases for nursing practice.* Doctoral dissertation, University of California, Los Angeles.

Meadows, P. (1957). Models, systems and science. *American Sociological Review, 22,* 4.

Miller, J. (1955). Toward a general theory for the behavioral sciences. *American Psychologist, 10,* 516–28.

Miller, N.E. (1951). Comments on theoretical models. *Journal of Personality, 20,* 82–100.

Rapoport, A. (1968). Foreword. In W. Buckley (Ed.), *Modern systems research for the behavioral scientist.* Chicago: Aldine.

von Bertalanffy, L.V. (1955). General systems theory. *Main Currents of Modern Thought, 2,* 79.

von Bertalanffy, L.V. (1968). General systems theory; a critical review. In W. Buckley (Ed.), *Modern systems research for the behavioral scientist.* Chicago: Aldine.

Wiener, N. (1954). *Human use of human beings* (2nd ed.). New York: Doubleday Anchor.

A Colleague Comments

I first met Rose McKay in 1975, when she joined a WCHEN-sponsored task force to develop a taxonomy for nursing. It was typical of Rose to devote her energies to the effort to develop a logical scheme that would describe our practice. As I worked with Rose at the University of Colorado in her position as chairperson of the graduate program of Community Health Nursing, I observed firsthand her commitment to identifying the knowledge base of nursing.

Collaborating with her in writing two articles about the identification of curriculum models for community health nursing was a stimulating and challenging experience for me. During the writing of these articles (September, 1982 to May, 1983), Rose's visual acuity was impaired. She was awaiting surgery for a cataract and then recovering from the surgery and waiting until she could be fitted with reading glasses.

During those 7 months, we excitedly discussed our project and wrote the articles. During the writing of the second article, I would read Rose the results of the data analysis. She would listen carefully, then start talking rapidly about the interpretation of the findings. As each article took shape, every line was carefully examined, reworked, and honed to ensure that the thought was clear and communicated the intention of our thinking.

In May 1983, at age 57, Rose died suddenly from a heart attack in Santiago, Chile, where she was conducting a nursing theory workshop with Sister Callista Roy. She died doing for others. Her contribution to nursing is important, and I encourage nurses to read her writings. She was ahead of her time and we can all benefit from her creative thinking.

—MARY E. SEGALL

Chapter 32

Development of Theory: A Requisite for Nursing as a Primary Health Profession

Dorothy E. Johnson

Problems nurse scientists and nurse educators face in influencing the direction and progress of nursing as a profession and a scientific discipline are discussed.

Since its first recorded use in the midfifteenth century, the word "profession" has been defined as a learned vocation (Cogan, 1953). While scholars may differ to some extent on the distinguishing characteristics of a profession, there is universal agreement that a theoretical body of knowledge is an essential attribute (Cogan, 1953; Goode, 1960; New, 1965). A profession's service to society is an intellectual one, and a sound, scientific basis for that service is indispensable. Moreover, a profession is responsible for creating the constantly increasing body of knowledge upon which its service depends (Goode, 1960; New, 1965). If nursing is indeed an emerging profession, nurses must be able to identify clearly and develop continually the theoretical body of knowledge upon which practice must rest.

The Status of Nursing Science

Progress toward this end is not an easy task, however, as many a sincere and industrious nurse scientist has discovered. Investigators in other disciplines forge ahead, building on the work of their founding fathers. But there are no scientific giants in nursing's heritage on whose shoulders present-day investigators can stand. There is no circumscribed body of knowledge. There is not even a particular group of facts or empirical generalizations widely recognized and accepted as offering the rudiments of nursing science that can provide a foundation for further work. Even the focus of scientific concern considered appropriate for this profession varies markedly among investigators and within the profession at large. Given such a situation, the prospective scientist in nursing is left without support and without direction. Small wonder then that our scientists tend to be relatively unproductive and our research reports, though increasing in number and producing a variety of findings, have yet to reflect a cumulative effect to any degree.

The prospective nurse investigator might well search for direction, consciously and rationally, by attempting to answer two relevant and related questions, at least to her own satisfaction, before she sets about her work. The seeker of answers will recognize that in each instance more than one alternative exists and must be examined and that the answers selected will reflect underlying social decisions. The most obvious question is: For what purpose is a theoretical body of knowledge intended? Or, what is the nature of the service nursing offers, for which knowledge is needed? Secondly, given this responsibility, what phenomena must be studied and what kinds of questions must be asked to develop the needed knowledge?

Evolution of Scientific Disciplines

Nurses and nursing probably are rarities in the scientific world in facing such questions so deliberately and self-consciously. Indeed, the necessity for doing so is questioned not only by individuals in other disciplines but also by many nurses. But nursing has not followed the path of evolutionary progress characteristic of other scientific disciplines. Scientific endeavor began thousands of years ago, with observations of the natural world generated by innate curiosity or pragmatic concern. Later, but still centuries ago, the search for truth was strengthened and stimulated by the rise of philosophy. Over the years, as facts were uncovered and relationships established concerning man and his universe, the several natural and social sciences emerged gradually as independent and distinct fields of inquiry. Each of the sciences developed by seeking partial understanding of the world through a focus on selected phenomena from a particular perspective. Each emerged as some investigators addressed the phenomena of concern to a parent discipline from a new perspective or

turned their attention to a different kind of phenomenon with still other questions. Because a different kind of phenomenon was studied or a different perspective (or frame of reference) was used as a basis for the observations and interpretations made, a new body of theoretical knowledge was developed and a new science was born. From a pragmatic interest in metals and in the heavenly bodies gradually emerged the sciences of chemistry and astronomy, while interest in all material phenomena under the rubric of natural philosophy led to the disciplines of physics and biology. And, eventually, the concern for understanding man manifested so early by the Greeks was rounded out by the births of the several social sciences in the seventeenth, eighteenth, and nineteenth centuries.

Sciences, then, become differentiated from one another on the basis of what is studied and the perspective used to raise questions, make observations, and interpret evidence. Since several sciences may, and often do, study the same phenomenon, it is the distinctive perspective of each science which most clearly discriminates it from others. Emergence of the now recognized and accepted basic disciplines is an historical product, brought about by the more or less arbitrary decisions of investigators, as phenomena for study were selected and the particular questions to be asked were identified. The emergence of the professional disciplines is also an historical product, and these disciplines generally have followed the same evolutionary path in that there was a gradual growth of knowledge through the study of selected phenomena from a distinctive perspective. The direction of growth for these disciplines, however, has been governed to an extent by logic—or at least by social responsibility. Professional decisions of what to study and what questions to ask necessarily have gone hand in hand with social decisions about the profession's realm of responsibility.

The Professions as Sciences

The focus of any profession's scientific concern is interdependent with the profession's service, its social function. Given the task of safeguarding some significant social value for the members of society, the members of a profession are obligated to develop the theoretical and technological means by which this responsibility can be met. Ascribed long ago, medicine's social responsibility has been stated aptly and colorfully by the historian, Lynn White: "to free mankind from the ills of the flesh" (White, 1963, p. 52). Given this task, physicians have created over the years a large and continuously growing body of knowledge as a means of understanding and controlling man's bodily ills. They have done so by identifying, describing, and explaining all manner of disorders or disturbances in man's biological being and by developing the rationale necessary to their prevention and management. In essence, this statement of an explicit, ideal goal in patient care for the physician established for the medical investigator then proper object for study— the living human body—and pointed to the socially relevant perspective—the identification and control of biological system disorders.

If nursing's social responsibility had been clearly and precisely formulated as an ideal goal in patient care many years ago, perhaps we, too, would have been building upon previously established theory. But nursing's history is quite different from that of medicine, despite a certain similarity in the ages of the two fields. The significant differences are many; I will mention only two. First, nursing is an occupation whose form of service, until recently, was not considered particularly socially valuable and certainly not very critical in social life. What matter the quality of life if biological survival could not be insured? Furthermore, the service given was practical, not intellectual in nature, requiring in the main strong legs, strong arms, and a certain amount of human compassion. This service with its underlying pragmatic concern—the care of the sick, the injured, and the helpless (Bullough & Bullough, 1964)—did not lead easily to the development of knowledge. Unlike the case with metals or heavenly bodies, or even disease, nursing's service encompasses a wide range of objects and events of a less tangible nature and its purpose has been difficult to identify or describe in symbolic terms. As a concern focused on essentially social objects and events, nursing antedated the social sciences. But the possibility of theoretical knowledge in nursing could scarcely be envisioned when there had been little or no development in a significant component of its basic science foundations. Nursing stands today, as a field of practice without a scientific heritage —an occupation created by society long ago to offer a distinctive service, but one still-ill-defined in practical terms, a profession without the theoretical base it seems to require.

There is a controversial point which should be mentioned here although it is somewhat unrelated to the preceding discussion. The issue concerns the nature of an applied science and the relationship of knowledge in an applied science to that of a basic science. At the most fundamental level, all professions (and that includes the professional outgrowths of the basic sciences) are applied sciences in that theoretical knowledge is developed and used to achieve practical ends. Moreover, theory construction in the professions usually draws upon and builds from the foundation provided by one or more of the basic sciences. In general, however, a theoretical body of professional knowledge cannot be developed simply by the testing of basic science theories; or, to put it another way, professional knowledge does not consist of basic science theory which has been validated in practice.

The professional fields also are in the business of describing and explaining selected aspects of reality, a reality that with few exceptions differs from that considered by any one of the basic sciences.[1] Furthermore, as Dickoff and James (1968) pointed out, professional disciplines are obligated to go a step further than explanation and prediction in theory construction, to the development of prescriptive theory. Specifically, the phenomenon of interest and the perspective utilized in the several professions differs from those of the several basic sciences, and so different and unique bodies of theoretical knowledge are developed. Each of the biological sciences, for example, focuses on the biological

---

[1] Those professional fields that are applied branches of only one basic science, e.g., applied physics, or the counseling-psychotherapy branch of psychology, are exceptions to this generalization.

organism, and each has added partial understanding of the structure and function of that organism. Only medicine, however, has focused on disturbances in the system as a whole and on their management.

This issue would be no trouble at all, were it not for the fact that many prospective nurse scientists have had advanced education and research training in one or another of the basic sciences rather than in nursing. In this process, they have necessarily acquired the scientific orientation of that discipline; that is, they have learned to direct their attention toward those aspects of the world of interest to that discipline and to use the discipline's frame of reference in raising questions about the world. Moreover, it is a reasonable observation that more than a few basic scientists tend to be somewhat prejudicial in their judgments and somewhat limited in their understanding of the professions and their research tasks. Consequently, a not uncommon view among them is that the professions, as applied sciences, convert basic science laws into principles of practice through the testing of these laws (Greenwood, 1961). This point of view has been transmitted to many nurses who then limit their research efforts to those seen as appropriate in the discipline of orientation. While this may be productive for the basic discipline, it will not necessarily further the cause of nursing. And to the extent that it clouds the thinking, it creates a potentially serious problem for nursing.

Alternative Routes to Theory Development

The would-be nurse scientist as well as a faculty contemplating curriculum development at the highest level face problems for which several choices are possible. There is the laissez-faire alternative; that is, either intentionally or unwittingly letting the future course of events evolve as it will. Each nurse scientist would continue to follow her own scientific orientation, whatever its origin; and educational programs would continue to emerge and expand within a more or less rational, explicit, and cohesive framework. It is conceivable, of course, that our unconscious ties and strong commit-

ment in common to our heritage will lead most of us along at least parallel educational paths and to scientific findings that eventually reveal a cohesive and cumulative effect and provide a substantial basis for a professional form of practice.

Progress via this route will be very slow, if it comes at all. Certainly a deliberate, relatively widespread emphasis on the necessity for theory development for more than two decades has yielded little in the way of a circumscribed body of nursing knowledge. In fact, in only two schools in the country do faculty and students seem to share a common research orientation and whose reports reveal orderly, even sequential progress in theory development. There probably are not more than a dozen nurse scientists whose work reveals a central focus and an effort to build. Nonetheless, many nurses appear to think this is the most desirable route and perhaps the only route. When reasons are given, they often include the difficulties in obtaining a faculty consensus on nursing's reasons for being (and this is very real); a strongly held belief that a scientist should be "free" to follow his own destiny (as if any scientist is really free of some kind of mental image to guide empirical research, or as if he did not have the "right" to change his images); and an insistence that we already know what we are about and where we are going (and no rational counterargument serves any purpose here).

A second alternative is to follow medicine's path, a route nursing has used in the past often without overt recognition of the significance and the consequences of doing so. Moreover, it is a route that today is increasingly sanctioned and well rewarded. A number of nurses have chosen this path willingly and deliberately —some because they do not think nursing has a destiny of its own and that the occupation's identity rests on a specialized competence within medicine; some, because they are simply seeking greater intellectual challenge and personal responsibility than is currently available in most practice settings today; and some, motivated largely by altruistic aims, because they want to bring better medical care to the poor and to the geographically isolated.

The proportion of nurses who would willingly

"give up nursing" entirely to follow the medical path is very small, it seems, for most nurses who have taken this route in practice or in research are attempting to maintain identification as nurses while adopting actual practice or scientific orientations that vary on a scale of mixed orientation from partly nursing to largely medical. These nurses can be found in hospitals, often in intensive care units, and in outpatient clinics and other community settings. In the latter setting, they sometimes operate under the guise of providing "health care" as a synonym for nursing care. Nurse scientists who use medicine's research orientation in empirical investigations tend to study problems rather directly related to nursing activities in the diagnosis and treatment of disease. Others, many of whom claim the laissez faire attitude, appear to use the medical model indirectly to determine the appropriateness or significance of a particular problem area, but actually identify and study the problem from the orientation of one of the basic sciences, both the natural and social sciences being involved.

Progress toward a theoretical body of *nursing knowledge* via this route is inconceivable to anyone who envisions a distinctive professional identity for nursing. And without such an identity, there is little reason to be concerned about theory development at all. If nursing represents simply an area of specialized competence in medical practice, then whatever theoretical contributions nurse scientists, who do not have a medical education, might make to medical science are likely to be restricted along much the same lines as would hold for the basic scientist, or to be limited to technological advances. This is, however, a safe and rewarding option for nurses in practice, and it appears to have certain benefits for patients. For investigators, it provides clear direction and does not require a great deal of risk-taking in research. And, certainly, there is no guarantee that the other options available will lead to a circumscribed body of knowledge that can be called the science of nursing and support an increasingly well-defined and distinctive professional service.

The third alternative does involve risk-taking, a good deal of it; it also requires another choice among still other options. It is, of course, to accept as a premise that nursing has a distinctive professional service to offer and to attempt to answer the question posed in that light. Available to assist in making such a decision are nursing's history, observations drawn from current practice, and the ability to analyze the kind of service patients require that nursing might provide. History suggests that the nurse's primary concern has been for the person who is ill, rather than the illness itself, and that in particular her concern has been for the part played by the ambient environment in fostering illness or in preventing recovery (Nightingale, 1860). That same concern appears prevalent today, although it is perhaps less evident in practice at times than in clinical and research reports in the literature. It is a concern that is expressed in the attention given to patient adjustments and adaptations under the changed circumstances of illness, to coping abilities and strategies, to personalized care and patient comfort during illness, to the development of life styles and behavior patterns conducive to a sense of physical, psychological, and social well-being, and the like. And, most significantly, reason suggests that within the organization of relationships and the way of life found especially in today's society, patients require precisely that which nursing, by heritage and current interest, seems uniquely qualified to give: concern for the person and assistance in living and coping with his circumstances and his environment in such a way that illness may be prevented or recovery may be facilitated.

Building the Conceptual System

The majority of nurses today probably hold to this view of nursing's general purpose. Moreover, this purpose represents a significant social responsibility and, when formulated as an explicit ideal goal, the service will make a valuable and valued difference in the lives of people. Implicit in this last sentence is the rub, however, for nursing's difficulty is not eased appreciably by acceptance of this general statement. There remains the necessity of building a focused and cohesive conceptual system of the person to be served and of deriving from that system an abstract model for practice that will allow such a purpose to be fulfilled. We must proceed in much the same fashion as was the case in medicine, when physicians, focused on bodily ills, both sought in the basic sciences and helped to create a conceptual system which explains the person to be served as a biological system, subject to inefficiencies and disorders in operation as a consequence of internal difficulties or environmental forces. From this they were able to project medical practice as consisting of the recognition and treatment of biological system problems.

Any number of individuals in nursing now are attempting to do just this. Some are focused primarily on practice and are working on more goal directed approaches to nursing diagnosis and treatment by developing diagnostic protocols and typologies of nursing problems (Gebbie & Lavin, 1974; McCain, 1965). Others, concerned with curriculum development and revision, have attempted to formulate theoretical frameworks that would give clear direction to the selection and organization of courses and learning experiences and provide a diagnostic and treatment orientation for practice (Lum & Kim, 1967; McDonald & Harms, 1966; Vaillot, 1970). A growing number of expositions of practice models, both published and unpublished, are becoming available as well. Since these have been more completely developed and are accompanied by the underlying rationale, and since they also are more general and more abstract, they may well be nursing's greatest source of assistance.

Most, if not all, of these individual efforts to conceptualize the consumer of nursing service appear to have started from about the same point of view of nursing's general purpose. Nonetheless, if the various routes were followed to their logical conclusions not only would practice and the nature of curriculum offerings differ now, but, at some future point the research undertaken to support different forms of practice would provide differing bodies of knowledge also. For example, the two most common types of models now available are developmental models and system models. If the person is conceptualized as a developmental process of some kind, and nursing's goal is seen as the maximization of development along specific lines, then the research task is to identify and explain potential problems in that course of development and to develop the theoretical and technological means of preventing or controlling these problems or of otherwise fostering developmental progress. On the other hand, if the person is conceptualized as some kind of system, and nursing's goal is seen to be the maximization of effective system operation, then the research task is to identify and explain potential problems in the functioning of the system and to develop relevant rationale and means of management. Clearly these two different classes of approaches to understanding the person who is a patient, not only call for differing forms of practice toward different objectives, but also point to different kinds of phenomena, suggest different kinds of questions, and lead eventually to dissimilar bodies of knowledge.

Conceptual Models

The conceptual models now utilized or discussed include, among the developmental models, models based on the developmental theories of Erikson (1963), Freud (1949), Maslow (1954), Peplau (1952), C. Rogers (1959), Sullivan (1953), and of the behaviorist school (Bijou & Baer, 1961). Among the system models are found the adaptation system model of Roy (1970), the triad system of Howland and McDowell (1964), the life process system of M.E. Rogers (1970), and Johnson's behavioral system model (1968). There are no doubt others in each of these general categories; and still others might well be developed since man's development proceeds along many dimensions, and it is possible to conceptualize man as a number of different kinds of systems. Then, in addition, there is another type of model for nursing practice, called an interaction model, since its conceptual system in dependent upon symbolic interaction theory. The most well-known model in this group is that of Orlando (1961) and Wiedenbach (1964).

A number of these specific models have been used as a guide to practice and as a basis for curriculum development. Several—specifically the M.E. Rogers and Johnson system models, Peplau's developmental model, and the Orlando-Wiedenbach model—have been used as a framework for theory construction. Most are commensurate with the general purpose of nursing but are far more specific, clearly goal-related, and reducible to concrete terms. None of these models can be judged at this point in time as the best model, or the right one for nursing. In this regard, it is particularly important to emphasize that as long as the conceptual system for understanding the person is reasonably sound, 'scientifically, the question of "truth" plays no part in judging a model for nursing practice, education, and research based on that conceptual system. The question of whether any model is right or wrong *for nursing* is a social decision, and criteria extrinsic to the substance of the model must be utilized.

Criteria for Evaluation

Three criteria may be helpful in evaluating models. The first is *social congruence;* that is, do nursing decisions and actions which are based on the model fulfill social expectations or might society be helped to develop such expectations? The last phrase here is included in full recognition that current nursing practice is not entirely what it might become and that society might come to expect a different form of practice, given the opportunity to experience it. The second is *social significance;* that is do nursing decisions and actions based on the model lead to outcomes for patients which make an important difference in their lives or well-being? This criterion recognizes that a professional service is a highly valued one because it is critical to people in some way. The third criterion is concerned with the value of the model for the profession, its *social utility;* it asks whether the conceptual system on which the model is based is sufficiently well-developed to provide clear direction for nursing practice, education, and research.

The task for the nurse scientist, practitioner, or educator who chooses the third alternative is to select one of the options now available or to develop another that will provide answers to such questions as: practice toward what goals? knowledge and skills for what purpose? theory about what? It is for the theory developer and postbaccalaureate educator that answers are most urgently needed, however, since both practitioners and basic service educators can continue to get along for a while, just doing what has always been done. The scientist in nursing has no past and she faces many difficulties in this old occupation, newly awakened to the need for a sound scientific basis for professional practice. Without the self-confidence and scientific respectability granted by parentage or ancient heritage, newcomers in the world of science—most often with research training not in their proposed field of study but in various other fields—our scientists, our founding parents, if you will, cannot share a common identity with one another, nor can they identify with nursing as a science. This in a time and in a world which does not look kindly, either professionally or scientifically, upon new founding parents, particularly if they are mothers, and illegitimate themselves, have questionable educational backgrounds, appear to share scientific interests loosely if at all, and seem to be encroaching on the boundaries of other disciplines. The best anchor for this group, as well as others in nursing, acting either individually or collectively, is self-conscious reflection, and decision about the purpose for which theoretical knowledge is intended. Only this will provide a rationale and open the door to a rational course in the development of theory.

The scientist in nursing also faces the exciting challenge of influencing nursing's direction and progress as a profession and a scientific discipline. Purposeful and goal-directed development of the theoretical knowledge of an emerging profession is a rare opportunity and one to be cherished all the more because of its unusual demands.

References

Bijou, J.W., & Baer D.M. (1961). *Child development I: A systematic and empirical theory.* New York: Appleton-Century-Crofts.

Bullough, B., & Bullough, V. (1964). *The emergence of modern nursing.* New York: Macmillan.

Cogan, M.L. (1953). Towards the definition of profession. *Harvard Education Review, 23*(1), 33–50.

Dickoff, J., & James, P. (1968). A theory of theories: A position paper. *Nursing Research, 17,* 197–203.

Erikson, E.H. (1963). *Childhood and society* (2nd ed.). New York: Norton.

Freud, S. (1949). *An outline of psychoanalysis.* New York: Norton.

Gebbie, K., & Lavin, M.A. (1974). Classifying nursing diagnoses. *American Journal of Nursing, 74,* 250–253.

Goode, W.J. (1960). Encroachment, charlatanism, and the emerging professions. *American Sociological Review, 25,* 902–914.

Greenwood, E. (1961). The practice of science and the science of practice. In W.G. Bennis et al. (Eds.), *The planning of change* (pp. 73–82). New York: Holt, Rinehart and Winston.

Howland, D., & McDowell, W.E. (1964). Measurement of patient care: A conceptual framework. *Nursing Research, 13,* 4–7.

Johnson, D.E. (1968). One conceptual model of nursing. Lecture given at Vanderbilt University, Nashville, TN.

Lum, J.L., & Kim, H.T. (1967). A faculty undertakes a major curriculum revision. *Journal of Nursing Education, 6,* 19–21, 24–25.

Maslow, A.H. (1954). *Motivation and personality.* New York: Harper & Row.

McCain, R.F. (1965). Nursing by assessment—not intuition. *American Journal of Nursing, 65,* 82–84.

McDonald, F.J., & Harms, M.T. (1966). A theoretical model for an experimental curriculum. *Nursing Outlook, 14,* 48–51.

New, P.K.M. (1965). Another approach of professionalism. *American Journal of Nursing, 65,* 124–126.

Nightingale, F. (1860). *Notes on Nursing.* New York: Appleton.

Orlando, I.J. (1961). *The dynamic nurse-patient relationship.* New York: Putnam.

Peplau, H. (1952). *Interpersonal relations in nursing.* New York: Putnam.

Rogers, C. (1959). A theory of therapy, personality, and interpersonal relations as developed in a client-centered framework. In J. Koch (Ed.), *Psychology: A study of a science* (Vol. III). New York: McGraw-Hill.

Rogers, M.E. (1970). *An introduction to the theoretical basis of nursing.* Philadelphia: F.A. Davis.

Roy, C. (1970). Adaptation: A conceptual framework for nursing. *Nursing Outlook, 18,* 42–45.

Sullivan, H. (1953). *The interpersonal theory of psychiatry.* New York: Norton.

Vaillot, M.C. (1978). Nursing theory, levels of nursing, and curriculum development. *Nursing Forum, 9,* 234–249.

White, L. (1963). Humanism and the education of engineers. *Studies of courses and sequences in humanities, fine arts, and social sciences for engineering students* (EDP Report No. 7–63). Los Angeles: Humanities Subcommittee, Education Development Program, College of Education.

Wiedenbach, E. (1964). *Clinical nursing: A helping art.* New York: Springer.

Reactions

Nursing Research, January-February 1975, 24(1), 63.

To the Editor:

I was pleased to see the publication of Dorothy Johnson's article, "Development of Theory: A Requisite for Nursing as a Primary Health Profession," so that a greater number of members of the nursing profession can obtain knowledge similar to that which I received in graduate study at the University of California, Los Angeles. Miss Johnson and other members of the UCLA faculty encourage the utilization of a conceptual nursing model for continued development of a theoretical body of nursing knowledge.

I have utilized the Johnson behavioral system model for nursing as a graduate student, practitioner, and educator. This model serves as an excellent framework for the nursing process and meets the criteria for evaluation. I encourage *Nursing Research* readers to utilize the Johnson model in their areas of expertise. . .

Miss Johnson conceptualized her model from the general systems theory. This task alone is a remarkable achievement and an important contribution to the nursing profession. Because no single nursing educator, researcher, or practitioner could begin to adequately define, operationalize, and evaluate every facet of this model into the various patient settings, I believe it is the responsibility of every individual utilizing the Johnson model to operationalize this conceptualization and apply it to various research studies and patient care settings. Future publication and correspondence of the results of these applications will provide further evaluation of the Johnson behavioral system for nursing.

MAE PAULFREY, M.N., R.N.
Instructor, Department of Nursing
San Jose State University
San Jose, California

Nursing Research, July-August 1975, 24(4), 308.

To the Editor:

I am overdue in writing my appreciation of Dorothy E. Johnson's thoughtful article, "Development of the Theory: A Requisite for Nursing as a Primary Health Profession.". . . Professor Johnson's criteria for the evaluation of theoretical models are also pertinent for the evaluation of health related, and in particular, nursing research. Increasingly, scientists are obliged to consider the social relevance of their research, and this is no less true in nursing than in other fields. Professor Johnson's point that the basic biologic and behavioral sciences may profit more than nursing from the contributions of nurse scientists who have taken their major doctoral preparation in one of these basic fields may hold for theory development, although some will disagree. This observation does not hold, in my opinion, for advancements in research in nursing, particularly with regard to design and procedures. We have noted an unmistakable increase in rigor in the research grant applications submitted to us for review, which we feel is due to the investigators' methodological training as well as research experience. Of interest, too, is the choice of problems for study: Many deal with clinical concerns, and not a few would receive approbation as dealing with issues that are socially as well as scientifically congruent, significant, and potentially useful.

SUSAN R. GORTNER, Ph.D., R.N.
Chief, Nursing Research Branch
Division of Nursing
Bureau of Health Resources Development
Health Resources Administration
Public Health Service
U.S. Department of Health, Education and Welfare
Bethesda, Maryland

Epistemologic Constraints to the Development of a Theory of Nursing. Nursing Research, March-April 1978, 27(2), 128–129.

To the Editor:

Despite frequent attempts at the development of a theory of nursing, there seems to be little satisfaction with the efforts exhibited thus far. Indeed, each new theory proposed seems only to complicate the matter with new terminologies and perspectives. Although this may be viewed as part of the dialectic process of truth-seeking, a more realistic and perhaps more disturbing reason for the lack of consensus may have been ascertained by Dorothy E. Johnson (1974) when she suggested that the various nursing theory models now being evaluated are all viable, ultimately depending on a social decision for validation. The implication, then, is that any conceptual model is valid insofar as it is reasonably sound with regard to the particular anthropology employed (i.e., man as developing, adapting, interacting).

Unfortunately, the criteria for evaluation of these conceptual models present an added complexity in terms of determining the suggested parameters of social congruence, significance, and utility. Further, no guidance is given for determining the direction of the models since, according to Johnson, "truth" plays no part in judging a model—thus relegating the entire question to social pragmatism (Johnson, 1974, p. 376). To allow this to happen would require nursing to give up its self-determination as a profession, as well as its concomitant voice of expertise. Yet the logic of Johnson's position is flawless: Given the consistency of a theorist's scientific conceptual framework, there is no intrinsic criterion for validational judgment.

Scientific Epistemology

Insofar as nursing deals with the patients as a whole, there are as many theories as there are scientific conceptions of man. The problem, then, does not lie within the province of nursing, but in the sciences which describe aspects of man's reality according to their individual frames of reference. This is to say that each scientific discipline explains reality in terms of its own a priori biases. Thus, the physicist, biologist, psychologist each has his own perception of the world. Usually, these perceptions exhibit themselves as extensions of idiosyncratic principles into a wide variety of phenomena commonly considered under the rubric of reality. How to assimilate these logical but disparate conceptions has been a concern for thinkers for centuries. Not until the modern era, however, with its expansion of knowledge, has this concern been given significant attention under the banner of "holism" and other similar derivative ideas (Alexander, 1920; Bergson, 1907; Morgan, 1923).

The Noetic Problem

Although many holistic theories exhibit a certain seductive attractiveness, practical application reveals confounding difficulties, as nursing has discovered. Such a situation suggests a closer examination of the process of holistic knowledge. To do this it might be useful to examine a simple holistic theory.

One such theory, developed in outline form as philosophical anthropology, was proposed by William Kelly (1967). It is holistic in that it seeks to understand man's total reality by examining every experience he is capable of having.

Kelly's philosophic anthropology is organized around four philosophic "habits of thinking" in viewing man's nature: (a) the empiriological-experiential (scientific research coupled with significant intrapersonal experience), (b) the empirical-metaphenomenal (hypothesis, theory, and law), (c) the philosophical-metaphenomenal (human contingencies of man's existence viewed with a regard to a space-time axis), (d) and the philosophical-transcendental (formalities which embrace being with precision from the space-time axis). This schema attempts to organize knowledge on the basis of a concrete versus abstract continuum. The logicality of such an approach is convincing, yet Kelly himself admits to a difficulty not immediately apparent. Specifically, depending on the a priori psychologic conditions concomitant with the interpreter of the facts, it is possible to construct a wide variety of philosophies of human nature (Kelly, 1967, p. 55). This problem of relating the interpretation of facts to truth has been widely discussed, yet never adequately resolved (Russell, 1929).

Another difficulty requires further elaboration. Kelly's first three habits of thinking are related in a cumulative way. Thus, scientific data give rise to hypotheses and laws, which, in turn, give rise to analyses of human behavior and existence. At this point, however, the interpreter may face a series of disquieting problems: In recalling the first three habits, an important factor has always been the observer and his cognition—a knowing subject stands over against an object which is known or to be known.

A subject is always necessary to the act of knowing: It is he who enacts the noetic process, but his knowledge cannot be dissolved simply into a product of the subject. The subject must distinguish what is reality, yet still realize that there is a subjective limitation which must either be eliminated or appropriately utilized (e.g., those objects which might be known only if they are participated in). As a result, the cognitive process tends to remain inconclusive and somewhat relative.

Under the aspect of the second habit, this fact is revealed by the difficulty of modern physics to understand certain phenomena completely and has given rise to the quantum theory and its concomitant controversies (Heisenberg, 1958).

Under the aspect of the third habit, the problem of the "self" and the totality of the object world presents another difficulty. It becomes apparent that the self which initiates cognition cannot "see" itself, because the self becomes what it will by the way it understands itself. The object world, on the other hand, is an object of knowledge, partially and only in certain aspects. Attempts to resolve these questions lead to the fourth habit.

At this point the topic of faith (not necessarily in the religious sense) is crucial. With a realization that he is faced with a discrepancy in his knowledge (i.e., with regard to self and being), an observer can follow one of two paths: accept a blind faith in his cognition   even with the admission of its *lacunae;* or seek to understand these *lacunae* as perhaps experiences of cognition in a different form. Much contemporary research has suggested the latter alternative (Gurwitsch, 1966; Heidegger, 1949). Specifically, the knowledge of the discrepancies of knowledge regarding the self and being is knowledge of a special sort: It provides no new information, but does change the understanding of what the observer does know—it is a qualitative change of knowledge.

The realization that understanding of self is conditioned by a constant becoming within the totality of being confronts the observer with what has been termed the "naught" of his *lacunae* (Heidegger, 1949). It reveals a certain frailty, and, at the same time, perhaps, a certain responsibility toward his knowledge as a subject of a being which can produce anxiety within him by indicating the naught of death. Faith may then be considered an act of the subject becoming aware of his posture toward the "naught." This is not a rational process in the normal sense, although it can be clarified only in the realm of rationality; i.e., factual experience. This situation can be further complicated by positing the existence of a supernatural world which would then be mediated by a "supernatural" faith.

Theoretical Implications

As can be seen from this brief discussion of a paradigm for experiential knowledge, several subliminal considerations are operative either to enhance or to attenuate the efficacy of a particular model. On the molecular level, atomistic facts can be interpreted in a variety of ways, while on the transcendental level, gaps in knowledge can lead to a theory of the supernatural. Indeed, on the basis of certain physical principles, some scientists have attempted to justify the notion of free will (Wald, 1965).

A major determinant for the direction a particular model takes is the way the theorist views relationships between the various levels of a model. Essentially, the question of relationships and ordering is an ethical one. In everyday experience this question is most often encountered as "What ought I to do?" Such a question implies on the part of the "I" a negative judgment with regard to its existing situation. This is to say there is a need for a change in some specific direction. Viewed this way, the ethical proposition might be considered as (a) a relationship *quantitatively* between an agent, his means, and his end, and (b) a relationship *qualitatively* in terms of good, bad, or neutral. Thus, if a particular theory is to be really useful, it must provide some exposition of its relationships; moreover, it must determine the quality of those relationships. Such exposition should include the theorist's understanding of (a) theory of knowledge, (b) logic, and (c) the congruence of science and philosophy.

In terms of a theory of knowledge, clear delineations of a priori and a posteriori reasoning should be made. The limits and conditions of knowledge need to be considered, as well as the capabilities of the experimental and observational methods of empirical science.

In terms of logic, "atomistic" versus "organistic" views need to be elucidated. The organic opinion views everything being affected in its intrinsic nature by its relations to everything else. Thus, a knowledge of a single thing would induce knowledge of a multitude of other things. To the contrary, atomism maintains that the intrinsic character of a thing does not enable anyone to induce logically its relationships to other things. This is not to say that there are no relationships, rather than these relationships cannot be known a priori.

Finally, correspondence between science and philosophy requires evaluation. Does science exhibit a special knowledge apart from philosophy, or are they totally congruent, ultimately mediated by a mathematical logic? The answer to this question can rebound significantly upon a discipline such as psychology. This is to say that if the concomitance of science and philosophy obtain within psychology, the concept of "mind" may be viewed as some form of an epiphenomenalism of neural processes. It would then be necessary to reconsider the traditional conative aspects of man's existence, i.e., ideals and motivations.

Implications for Nursing Theory

In suggesting possible reasons for the current and continuing confusion regarding nursing theory, what has been inferred is that much disagreement is based not so much on the overt expression of a particular theory as on the unexpressed a priori biases which motivate the theory. This situation is not remarkable, considering the conflicting trends of our culture: Existential and idealistic philosophies motivate our lives and professions, while positivistic philosophies motivate our science and scholarship. Fortunately, however, nursing is not alone in its theoretic confusion. The very disciplines which seek to understand man scientifically are reconsidering their theoretic presumptions (Chomsky, 1967; Heelan, 1976; Mayr, 1974; Stent, 1975, 1976).

In view of this ongoing reappraisal, it might be proper for nursing to abandon the development of a theory of nursing, and concentrate its efforts on the development of a methodology of nursing. By this meant the development of a structure with appropriate criteria for the integration of new concepts of man. This structure could function analogously to a Hegelian dialectic; i.e., it would be both a doctrine and a method, which is to say the method is the formulation of the doctrine, and the doctrine is the expression of the method (Mure, 1940, 1950). The nursing process, then as the practical apparatus, would use the structure as a resource for the elaboration of goals. Following upon this, the nurse researcher's task would be to integrate evolving knowledge into the structure. In this way, nursing could avoid the Procrustean bed of reactionary dogmatism, and insert itself into the academic and professional community as a dynamic discipline.

JOSEPH P. ZBILUT, Ph.D.

(The author of this letter was a nursing student at St. Francis Hospital School of Nursing, Evanston, Illinois, when this letter was written.)

REFERENCES

Alexander, S. (1920). *Space, time, and deity.* New York: Macmillan.

Bergson, H. (1907). *L'evolution creatrice.* Paris: Felix Alcan.

Chomsky, N. (1967). The formal nature of language. In E.H. Lenneberg (Ed.), *Biological foundations of language* (pp. 397–442). New York: John Wiley & Sons.

Gurwitsch, A. (1966). *Studies in phenomenology and psychology.* Evanston, IL: Northwestern University Press.

Heelan, P. (1976). Medical praxis and manifest images of man. In H.T. Englehardt & D. Callahan (Eds.), *Science, ethics and medicine* (pp. 218–224). Hastings-on-Hudson, NY: Institute of Society, Ethics and Life Sciences.

Heidegger, M. (1949). *Was ist Metaphysik?* Frankfurt am Main: Verlag Klosterman.

Heisenberg, W. (1958). *Physics and philosophy.* New York: Harper Brothers.

Johnson, D.E. (1974). Development of theory: A requisite for nursing as a primary health profession. *Nursing Research, 23,* 372–377.

Kelly, W.J. (1967). Towards a humanistic anthropology. *Continuum, 5,* 50–60.

Mayr, E. (1974). Teleological and teleonomic, a new analysis. *Boston Studies in Philosophy of Science, 14,* 91–117.

Morgan, C.L. (1923). *Emergent evolution.* New York: Henry Holt.

Mure, G.R.G. (1940). *An introduction to Hegel.* Oxford: Oxford University Press.

Mure, G.R.G. (1950). *A study of Hegel's logic.* Oxford: Oxford University Press.

Russell, B. (1929). *Our knowledge of the external world.* New York: Norton.

Stent, G.S. (1975). Limits to the scientific understanding of man. *Science, 187,* 1052–1057.

Stent, G.S. (1976). The poverty of scientism and the promise of structuralist ethics. *Hastings Center Report, 6,* 32–40.

Wald, G. (1965). Determinancy, individuality, and the problem of free will. In J.R. Platt (Ed.), *New views of the nature of man* (pp. 16–46). Chicago: University of Chicago Press.

The Author Comments

The title of this paper came to me when I was invited to speak at the University of Minnesota. If I remember correctly, the purpose of the lecture was to encourage and perhaps assist faculty members who were developing research programs and proposals. For me, it was yet another opportunity to make a plea for rational decision making and actions in building nursing knowledge and to point out some of the difficulties inherent in the process. I decided to submit for publication a paper based on the presentation because I wanted to offer a revised, reframed, and further developed viewpoint about the nature of nursing as a profession and about its scientific future. Having just reread the paper preparatory to writing these remarks, I am somewhat surprised to find that it contains little that I would change; moreover, I believe the content is nearly as relevant to the current nursing world as it was to the world of 1974. While I have made other contributions to the nursing literature since 1974, insofar as theory development is concerned, this paper might be said to represent my swan song.

—DOROTHY E. JOHNSON

Chapter 33

Theory Construction in Nursing: An Overview

Ada K. Jacox

How scientific knowledge is developed and organized into theories; how theories describe, explain, or predict events as they take place in the real world; how models describe the relationships that may exist among concepts in a developing theory; and how theory has application in nursing practice are discussed.

Professional nurses profess that their practice is based largely on science. This claim has implications for how the knowledge used by nurses is to be developed, organized, and tested. The aim of this paper is to pull together and relate various aspects of theory construction in a brief overview.

The Nature of Scientific Knowledge

The term "science" has what is called process-product ambiguity in that it refers both to an activity or process and to the outcome or product of that process (Rudner, 1966–1967). Science as process is concerned with the methods or research strategies by which knowledge is developed and tested. It refers to that which scientists do—observing, critical thinking, experimenting, measuring, and so forth—when they are developing knowledge. When speaking of science as product, we mean a body of accumulated knowledge that purports to describe some selected aspects of the universe. Thus, we speak of the science of astronomy, or the science of physics, or of psychology, meaning the accumulated body of knowledge of those fields.

Scientific knowledge can be contrasted with nonscientific knowledge by the method in which the knowledge is gained. Scientific knowledge claims must be capable, at least in principle, of being confirmed or disconfirmed by anyone with the necessary intelligence using the technical devices of observation and experimentation (Feigl, 1953). Claims of knowledge by revela-

About the Author

ADA K. JACOX is currently a Professor of Nursing at the Johns Hopkins School of Nursing, Baltimore, Maryland. She has taught nursing for more than 20 years at the graduate and undergraduate levels and has held faculty appointments at the Universities of Kansas, Iowa, Colorado, and Maryland. A basic nursing graduate of the Genesee Hospital School of Nursing in Rochester, New York, Dr. Jacox has also studied at Columbia University (B.S.), Wayne State University (M.S.), and Case Western Reserve University (Ph.D. in Sociology).

An active professional, Dr. Jacox is involved in research, writing, and various professional organizations. She has authored or coauthored three books that each won *American Journal of Nursing* Book-of-the-Year Awards. She has served as a research consultant to several universities and institutions and has been principal investigator on eight projects funded by the U.S. Department of Health and Human Services (formerly Department of Health, Education and Welfare). She has served as President of the American Nurses' Foundation and First Vice-President of the American Nurses' Association (1982 to 1984). In addition, she serves as an associate editor of the *Annual Review of Nursing Research*, a member of the editorial boards of *Nursing Administration Quarterly* and *Nursing Economics*, and as a member of the review panels of *Nursing Research* and *Nursing Outlook*.

tions or visions, which cannot be independently verified by others, fall outside the domain of science.

The main business of science is the discovery of truths about the world. "Truths state facts, either individual, like 'Smith is bald,' or general, like 'Dogs are carnivorous.' The truth of either is ascertained by observation. . . .Statements of fact convey knowledge about the world" (Brodbeck, 1968, p.600). Facts deal with the empirical world. "Empirical" refers to that which can be perceived or experienced through the senses, and is open to verification by others who can perceive it in the same way. This sensory experience is what is known as scientific observation. A major assumption of all modern science is that there is a knowable empirical reality (Denzin, 1970). Scientific knowledge, then, is knowledge about the empirical world.

Because isolated facts are of little interest to scientists, they try to put the knowledge of their respective fields together in such a way that the various events or phenomena with which they are concerned are systematically related to one another. A biologist, for example, wants to know not only about cells, species, and adaptation, but also how all of these are related to each other and to other biological phenomena. Scientific knowledge is systematically organized into "theories." The purpose of a scientific theory is to describe, explain, and predict a part of the empirical world.

For example, suppose a social psychologist is interested in constructing a theory to describe and explain the productivity of members of small groups in response to various types of leadership. He develops a theory so that there are empirical referents in it—that is, at least some of the words or terms that he uses in his theory must have reference or correspondence to the empirical world. He states what he means by "small group," what specific kinds of observed behavior indicate "authoritarian" leadership, "democratic" leadership, or whatever kinds of leadership he is dealing with in his theory, and specifies how "productivity" can be observed and measured. He can then conduct experiments using small groups with different types of leaders and observe the productivity of the group in response to the leadership types. If he finds that members of small groups do not behave in the way proposed in his theory, he modifies the theory to correspond with empirical reality. If his theory did not contain terms that had empirical referents, he could not test whether the theory accurately describes and explains the empirical reality with which it is concerned.

In developing the theory of leadership behavior in

small groups, the investigator might begin his observations using college students organized into small groups and responding to different types of leaders. Since he is interested in explaining not just the behavior of college students, he will go to other kinds of people, or "populations," such as industrial workers, nursing teams on hospital units, or perhaps teams of basketball players. He will most likely find it necessary to revise his theory with each new group, until he is able to make statements in his theory about how the productivity of small groups in general is related to various types of leadership. When his theory has been sufficiently tested and revised so that it accurately describes and explains small group productivity in response to leaders, he should be able to predict what will happen in small groups he has not yet tested. To the extent that his theory is accurate, his predictions will be accurate. Thus, theories are used not only to describe and explain what is observed, but to predict new situations with varying degrees of accuracy.[1]

While an aim of scientists is to relate facts systematically into theories, not all facts in any given science are so organized. If the science is a relatively new one, such as the social sciences, there may not yet be a large body of well-developed and well-tested theories. A mass of empirical data, or facts, however, may have been established about the field, with some beginning efforts to develop theories that will systematically relate the facts. In general, theories in the physical and biological sciences such as chemistry, physics, and biology are well developed and capable of explaining and predicting the phenomena with which each of these sciences deals. The behavioral and social sciences, which have shorter histories than the physical and biological sciences, have less well-developed and well-tested theories. The theories of applied fields such as nursing, social work, and urban planning only recently concerned with theory construction are even less developed and tested.

In the attempt to develop a theory, efforts may proceed through various levels or stages. These levels are identified differently by various writers (Brodbeck, 1968; Dickoff, James, & Wiedenbach, 1968; Dubin, 1968; Merton, 1968; Parsons & Shils, 1959; Rudner, 1966–1967; Turner, 1967; Wallace, 1971; Wooldridge, Skipper, & Leonard, 1968), but generally include:

1. A period of specifying, defining, and classifying the concepts used in describing the phenomena of the field.
2. Developing statements or propositions which propose how two or more concepts are related.
3. Specifying how all of the propositions are related to each other in a systematic way.

Concepts and the Empirical-Theoretical Continuum

All sentences or statements of a theory consist of arrangements of words.[2] Words that describe objects, properties, events, and relations among these are called descriptive terms or *concepts*. The things or phenomena to be studied are classified and analyzed according to the characteristics they have in common. Groups of concepts may also be formed into "higher-level" concepts that describe a wider range of things. For example, "professional nurse" is a concept that stands for nurses who have certain characteristics in common. "Practical nurse" denotes another kind of nurse. The concept "nurse" may in turn include both professional and practical nurses as well as all other kinds of nurses. In this sense, it is a "higher-level" concept. "Health

---

[1] As the phrase, "with varying degrees of accuracy," implies, it may be possible in some circumstances to predict only in a general way what will happen. This is especially true with regard to human behavior, in which many contingencies may operate to produce a specific behavior. While it may be possible, in retrospect, to explain why that behavior resulted, it may not have been possible to predict it ahead of time (Kaplan, 1964, p. 347).

[2] More precisely, theoretical statements are composed of two kinds of words: concepts and logical words. The latter are words such as "and," "or," "if. . .then," which in themselves denote no specific thing. They connect the descriptive terms or concepts that do describe. While concepts differ from science to science, logical words are common to all sciences (Brodbeck, 1968).

practitioners," which would include nurses, physicians, dentists, psychologists, social workers, and others, is a still higher-level concept.

Concepts indicate the subject matter of a theory. For instance, concepts in a theory of psychology might be "personality," "intelligence," and "cognition." A theory in biology might include such concepts as "protoplasm," "cell," and "species." A nursing theory might be composed of concepts such as "patient," "health," "interaction." Concepts can be thought of as a symbolic or abstract way of referring to empirical reality. Without this symbolic way to refer to an instance of an empirical "thing," we would have to point to a specific, concrete example whenever we want to refer to an object or event. Concepts are abstract representations of reality.

In forming concepts to use in a theory, it is important to define precisely what is meant by each concept. In everyday, nonscientific language, the same word may have several meanings which can cause confusion and lack of consensus and precision in what we are trying to communicate. The same situation can occur in the development of scientific concepts unless care is taken to define them precisely.

A major task in the definition of concepts is to specify the part of the empirical world that they are intended to represent. Although scientific theory is grounded in or rests upon the empirical world of events, many of the concepts used in the theories are only indirectly related to sensory experience. In other words, there is not a specific, concrete "thing" that can be observed for every concept that is developed. Many concepts depend on what can be only indirectly observed or defined in terms of their relationship to other concepts. The relationship between empirical reality and the theoretical terms used to describe and explain that reality can be viewed in terms of what Kaplan referred to as the "empirical-theoretical continuum" (Kaplan, 1964, p. 7). At one end of the continuum are those concepts that have a directly observable empirical referent. These are concepts for which the empirical referent can be easily seen, heard, felt, or otherwise

perceived. We can see a chair; we can point to something which exemplifies the color red; we can hear someone tell us that he is experiencing pain.[3]

A move up the continuum is when we indirectly observe an event and infer its presence; i.e., draw a conclusion based on certain evidence. A newborn infant cannot report verbally that he is in pain, so we cannot directly experience an infant pain report. We can, however, observe the infant behaving in a particular way (evidence) and infer (conclude) that he is in pain. The pain has been indirectly observed. In another kind of indirect observation, we may use special instruments to observe the existence of something. Consider a genetic pattern, for example. We cannot see the pattern directly with the naked eye, but with a high-powered microscope particular arrangements of chromosomes in the tissue can be observed. Thus, an empirical event is scientifically observed, indirectly. When conducting research, major effort is made to try to define concepts in terms of what can be observed or experienced, either directly or indirectly.

Moving along the continuum, still further from empirical referents, we encounter concepts that are not clearly observable, either directly or indirectly, but may be defined in terms of observables. "Personality," "role," and "society" are examples of concepts that are not directly or indirectly observable, in the way that "chair" is directly observed and "pain" is inferred or indirectly observed. A concept such as "society" is called a "construct" and is *constructed* of concepts that are directly or indirectly observable. We do not "observe" a society, although we can observe the people in a society. The concept of "society," however, means more than the individuals who compose it. It also includes, for instance, relationships that exist among the people, and norms that influence how these people relate to one another. People, relationships, norms, and other concepts included in the higher-level concept (or

---

[3] We have not "seen" pain; we have heard a report of pain. How we interpret or what we do with that report is another question, but we have directly observed a "pain report."

construct) or "society" can be directly observed or inferred, and, therefore, the concept "society" is in principle definable in terms of observables. To specify precisely all the empirical referents for the concept "society," however, would be a hopelessly complex, if not logistically impossible, task. Another kind of concept falling into this category of "construct" is one in which some values of it are not, even in principle, observable. Examples of this kind of concept are "length," "volume," "age," and "mass" (Rudner, 1966–1967, p. 23). To specify how "maximum length," for example, would be indicated, is impossible when "length" could conceivably go on into infinity, but such concepts are important in developing scientific theories capable of describing and explaining empirical events.

A final point on the empirical-theoretical continuum is the theoretical term which has no meaning apart from a particular theory. Concepts (constructs), such as "society" and "personality," are used in a variety of theories and have somewhat similar meanings, even though how they are defined in one theory may differ slightly from their definition in another theory. The concepts "superego" and "Oedipus complex," in contrast, have no meaning apart from psychoanalytic theory. They are interpreted in terms of their relationship to other concepts within that particular theory.

These, then, are the points along the empirical-theoretical continuum. It is difficult and, perhaps, impossible to say clearly at what point along the continuum each concept falls, but it should be possible to comprehend in general that there are significant differences in the degree to which various concepts are related to observable reality. As Kaplan pointed out, the first two levels (directly and indirectly observable) sometimes are combined and referred to as "observational" and the last two (constructs and theoretical terms) combined as "symbolic," but ". . .however the lines are drawn, it is important to recognize that drawing them is to a significant degree arbitrary. The distinctions are vague, and in any case a matter of degree" (Kaplan, 1964, p. 57).

A scientific theory in its entirety rests upon an empirical base. Even the most abstract and high-level concepts have some reference to the empirical world.

Propositions and the Process of Induction

A proposition[4] is a statement of a constant relationship between two or more concepts or between two or more facts. The statement, "The more anxious a patient is preoperatively, the slower will be his recovery rate from a surgical procedure," expresses a relationship between the concepts "anxiety" and "recovery rate." If the proposition asserts that a change in one thing causes a change in another thing—i.e., if there is a change in "a," it will produce a change in "b"—it states a *causal* relationship between the concepts. Note that nothing has been said about the truth or falsity of the statement, but only that a proposition *asserts* a relationship between two or more concepts or facts. All scientific propositions are based on empirical generalizations that may be proved false in the future.

To "generalize empirically" means that particular phenomena or events have been observed to occur regularly in the same way and we thus infer or conclude that this is the way in which they generally occur. To pursue the example given above, suppose that a nurse who observes 40 or 50 preoperative patients and notes that they are all anxious concludes that all preoperative patients are anxious. This is an empirical generalization which she may think is true until she encounters or learns about a preoperative patient who is *not* anxious. The nurse (along with others interested in the same phenomenon) will then try to observe under what conditions patients are anxious preoperatively and to make empirical generalizations about what kinds of conditions regularly are associated with preoperative anxiety in patients. The nurse might also expand her observations about anxiety in preoperative patients to include

---

[4] The term, "proposition," in this paper, refers to universal propositions of those that apply to all cases analyzed. This is contrasted with conditional propositions, which apply only to a subclass of events observed (Denzin, 1970).

the effects of preoperative anxiety on the postoperative recovery period, as suggested in the proposition stated at the beginning of this section. This would involve a more complex proposition than the one linking being "preoperative" with being "anxious," since it introduces another concept, that of "postoperative recovery."

The process by which empirical generalizations are established is known as "induction." Induction is a type of argument in which one argues from the particular to the general, or from the individual to the universal. That is, one observes empirical events and generalizes from these specific events to all similar events. By the process of induction basic propositions are initially established.

Some propositions are called "laws." A law states an empirical regularity among phenomena that as far as is known is invariable under the conditions stated in the law. An example of a law is Newton's second law of motion: "The force acting upon a body is proportional to its change in momentum (mv), and determines the direction in which the change in momentum occurs." That is, "F = ma" (Turner, 1967, p. 323). The point at which a regularly occurring relationship can be said to be a law is a difficult and often arbitrary matter. Some authors speak of "law-like generalizations," a term which well expresses the difficulty of specifying when scientific laws have been established, and how tentatively they may be held. Even in an old and well-developed science, such as physics, what has been accepted as a law for a long period of time may be modified when new evidence indicates that not all of the specified phenomena behave in the way proposed by the law. In the social sciences, there are innumerable propositions, but few can be classified as "laws."

It may be that a relationship between two or more concepts or facts has been asserted but enough data or empirical evidence have not yet been gathered to support the assertion strongly. When a proposition has this very tentative and inconclusive nature, it is referred to as "hypothesis." The primary notion in a hypothesis is the tentativeness of the proposition. The hypothesis is the conventional way of stating the relationships

among concepts that a scientist is seeking to establish when he conducts research. There is no clear cut point at which a proposition can be said to have sufficient empirical evidence supporting it so that it is no longer a hypothesis. A proposition can be disproved by finding only one instance in which the proposed relationship does not hold. There is, however, no given number of times that the relationship must be shown to hold in order to say that it will always hold in the future.

"Principle" is a term often used in nursing to refer to a universal (or near universal) proposition, although there is little discussion of the term "principle" in literature of theory construction. Nurses have long used "principles" as a basis for their practice, or to "explain" or "predict" what kind of action will produce a given effect. An example of this is the principle (proposition) relating lack of oxygen to the tissues (X) to tissue break-down (Y). "If prolonged decreased circulation to a part occurs (X), a decubitus ulcer will form (Y)." This principle (proposition) can be used either to explain why a decubitus ulcer occurred or to predict that one will develop if prolonged decreased circulation to a part is allowed to occur. The question "Why did 'Y' occur?" may be answered by referring to the principle, "Whenever 'X' occurs, 'Y' will result." If it can be shown that X occurred in this case, the occurrence of Y is said to be "explained." The question "What will happen if 'X' occurs?" may be answered by referring to the same principle. "Whenever 'X' occurs, 'Y' will result." In this way, "Y" or the formation of a decubitus ulcer is "predicted." Both explanation and prediction are based on propositions relating facts or concepts.[5]

While nurses have made wide use of principles (propositions) on which to base nursing action, there has been little attempt to relate these principles systematically to one another. This systematic organization of propositions comprises the third level of theory construction.

---

[5] For an opposing viewpoint on the relationship between propositions that are part of a theory and principles, see Lorraine O. Walker's "Toward a Clearer Understanding of the Concept of Nursing Theory." *Nursing Research, 20,* 428–435.

Theory and the Process of Education

When concepts have been well defined and related by propositions, a theory may be developed. "A theory is a systematically related set of statements, including some law-like generalizations, that is empirically testable" (Rudner, 1966–1967, p. 10). The notion of "law-like generalizations" and the necessity to test theory empirically have been discussed earlier; a final important aspect of a theory is that there be a "systematically related set of statements" composed of the concepts discussed earlier.

An understanding of the process of deduction is essential to comprehend how statements are systematically related in a theory. Deduction is another type of argument in which one reasons by taking one or more premises or statements assumed to be true and deriving or deducing other statements or conclusions. For example, if it is known that A is larger than B and B is larger than C, then it can be deduced or concluded that A is larger than C. Those who are familiar with Euclidean plane geometry will recall that theorems are deduced from axioms and postulates. The axioms and postulates are propositions which state the more general case, and by combining them in a certain way, theorems are derived.

Consider the following example of deduction:

Premise (Proposition): All patients who are anxious preoperatively will vomit postoperatively.
Premise (Proposition): All cardiac surgery patients are anxious preoperatively.
Conclusion (Proposition): All cardiac patients will vomit postoperatively.

In this example, a nurse-researcher may have stated two propositions (the premises) that she believes have sufficient empirical support to consider that they are true. She then deduces that, if the first two statements (premises) are true, then the third (conclusion) will be true. The investigator may conduct a study to see whether all cardiac patients vomit postoperatively. When empirical evidence is found that some cardiac patients do *not* vomit postoperatively, the conclusion

and at least one of the premises is proved to be false. Further research may then be done to test the two premises that were initially thought to be true. This example illustrates not only the process of deduction (taking statements assumed to be true and deriving other statements) but also how such deduced statements are tested by research.

Part of the definition of a theory is that it is a systematically related set of statements or propositions. This means that the propositions are *deductively* arranged—some basic propositions are assumed to be true. This assumption is based on what the theorist considers to be adequate empirical evidence to support the assertions made by the propositions. These basic propositions are called "axioms." From them, other propositions called "theorems" are deduced. Well-developed and well-tested theories that identify axioms and theorems are found most commonly in the older sciences. Few fundamental propositions have been established in the behavioral and social sciences, and few well-developed and well-tested theories relate these propositions. More commonly, in these new sciences broad propositions that summarize existing knowledge are established, other propositions are deduced from them, and they are used as hypotheses in conducting research. If a hypothesis is disproved, at least one of the propositions from which it was deduced is false. An effort is then made to determine which propositions are false by subjecting them to further empirical testing.

An example of an attempt to do this is provided by a social psychologist who developed a theory of influence processes in small groups, using five concepts and 15 propositions relating these concepts. Nine propositions were identified as axioms, from which six others were derived (Hopkins, 1964).[6] Following are three of the propositions that relate three of the concepts dealing with small groups (rank, centrality, and observability).

For any member of a small group:

---

[6] Also see H.M. Blalock's *Theory Construction* (Englewood Cliffs, NJ: Prentice-Hall, 1969), pp. 21–26, for a discussion of Hopkins' work.

1. The higher his rank, the greater his centrality (axiom).
2. The greater his centrality, the greater his observability (axiom).
3. The higher his rank, the greater his observability (derivation or theorem). (Blalock, 1969, p. 22)

All three statements are propositions; the first two are identified as axioms from which the third (theorem) is derived. Other social scientists may, of course, argue with the claim that the first two propositions have sufficient empirical evidence to be treated as axioms. This extreme theoretical tentativeness for social scientists (and members of applied disciplines such as nursing and social work) who attempt to construct theories is well expressed in the following comment by Blalock, a sociologist: "For a considerable period of time, social scientists will have to settle for highly tentative theories based on axioms that are really nothing more than rather plausible assumptions" (Blalock, 1969, p. 11).

Construction and testing of a theory to describe, explain, and predict a selected aspect of empirical reality necessitates use of both deduction and induction. A set of deductively connected propositions could be developed apart from induction; but, without empirical testing (and empirical generalizations), there would be no satisfactory way of knowing how accurately the propositions fit empirical reality. Conversely, many separate empirical generalizations could be made and cataloged without attempting to relate them in a comprehensive theory. Use of this approach exclusively can be wasteful of energy and resources since each scientist-investigator may be narrowly concerned with a very limited part of reality, and not with how his own observations relate to the findings of other scientists. Science is cumulative, meaning that one scientist's work builds upon, extends, and modifies the body of knowledge developed by other scientists. This cumulative nature of science is facilitated when each researcher tries systematically to relate what he is doing to what others have learned, through the use and modification of theories.

The definition in this discussion of a scientific theory as "a systematically related set of statements, including some law-like generalizations, that is empiri-cally testable" clearly implies the close relationship between theory construction and research.[7]

Models

In the construction of a theory, scientists frequently make use of a "model" to describe more clearly the relationships among concepts that they think may exist in the theory they are developing. A model is an analogy or example that is used to help visualize and understand something that cannot be directly observed or about which little is known. It is a heuristic scientific device used to guide research and exploration into new areas of inquiry.

Most nurses are familiar with one type of model from anatomy classes, in which plastic replicas of organs and cells are used to help in explaining the structure and functioning of the human body. The model of the heart, of course, is not an actual heart, but an imitation of one. To the extent that it does accurately imitate a human heart it is useful in increasing understanding of the heart after which it is modeled.

When a thing and a model of it are similar in certain respects they are said to be "isomorphic"(Brodbeck, 1968, p. 580). There are degrees of isomorphism. Complete isomorphism occurs when:

1. There is a one-to-one correspondence between the parts of the model and the parts of the thing (e.g., every blood vessel, muscle, and so forth of the real heart is represented in the model).

---

[7] Another term that is sometimes used in connection with theory construction and research is "conceptual framework" which refers to identification of the concepts with which the research is concerned. It is a way of indicating that the concepts and propositions that relate them are not yet systematically organized into a theory. For example, a nurse-researcher who is interested in studying the effects of preoperative teaching on postoperative recovery will identify and define all concepts with which the study is concerned. This might include such concepts as "teaching," "anxiety," "level of illness," "recovery," and any other concepts thought to be relevant. Some attempt would be made to relate these concepts to one another by reviewing the literature, including empirical findings of similar studies. The concepts and propositions linking them would constitute the conceptual or theoretical framework for the study. Such frameworks are more than isolated concepts and propositions, but do not yet meet the requirements of a theory.

2. The relationships among the parts are preserved (e.g., the aortic valve is in the same position in relation to the sino-atrial node in the model as it is in the real heart and, further, the model is constructed to scale).
3. The model "works" on the same principle as the original thing (e.g., the heart muscle contracts and expands, and blood is pumped through the model heart).

A picture or diagram of a heart is also a model, although there is obviously little isomorphism between the real heart and a picture of it. The same limited isomorphism is true of other pictures, graphs, or drawings of boxes, circles, and lines intended to illustrate relationships among various concepts in a theory. The term "model" is not restricted to visual models but also refers to verbal or other symbolic representations. A theory in one field may be used as a model for a theory in another field if the elements of the original field are believed to behave in the same way as those in the field for which the model is developed. Some sociologists, for example, have developed theories of society based upon biological theory of a human organism with various parts of society said to correspond with organs, tissues, and systems of the body. Another example of an attempt to use theory about one aspect of the empirical world to help in understanding behavior of other aspects of that world is the use made of stimulus-response or behaviorist learning theory. Early experimental psychologists developed elaborate and precise theories to describe, explain, and predict how rats and other nonhuman animals learn by responding to stimuli. The concepts and interrelated propositions developed and tested with rats were then used as a model for explaining how human beings learn. To the extent that rats and human beings are similar in factors influencing the learning process, the model is a useful one. In those areas of learning where rats and human beings differ (for example, the ability of the human to reflect on his own behavior, a characteristic absent in subhuman animals) the exclusive use of the rat model could be grossly misleading.

Very often, when knowledge about a given area is limited, this kind of attempt is made to use a theory that has successfully described and explained another part of empirical reality. If the two areas are highly isomorphic, the effort can stimulate numerous productive insights about the new area. If there is little or no isomorphism, an inaccurate, incomplete, and sometimes ridiculous description and explanation of the new phenomena will result.

One highly abstract kind of model is a mathematical model. Here, a theory of mathematics is used as a model to express the interrelationships among persons, actions, and events in numerical form (Theodorson & Theodorson, 1969). For example, consider the proposition that in the concept "cost of hospitalization," (Y) is equal to the sum of several factors such as "cost of equipment and supplies" (A), "salaries for personnel" (B), "cost of maintaining buildings" (C), and all other factors contributing to costs (D). Each of the concepts identified as "Y," "A," "B," and "C" could presumably be defined in terms of actual dollars over a certain period of time. If the statement of their relationship to each other can be correlated to some truth of mathematics, a mathematical model for that proposition can be formed. However, the mere act of assigning numbers does not assure that a mathematical model can be found. Use of this kind of model is common in economics, where prices, wages, costs, and so forth can be precisely specified. In other social and behavioral sciences translating behavioral concepts into precise mathematical formulations is much more difficult. Sometimes, in an effort to make an area about which little is known appear more comprehensible, a mathematical model will be used. As long as no one is fooled into prematurely believing that the model accurately and simply describes and explains the new area, little harm may be done and new insights may be produced.

Mathematical models are also used when statistics, based on the theory of probability, are used to describe and make inferences about empirical phenomena. The assumptions that underlie the use of any given statistical test relate to the need for isomorphism between the statistical model and the empirical situation in which it is used. When statistical assumptions are not met, the statistic does not accurately represent rela-tionships among empirical phenomena, and, like any poor analogy, can be misleading.

Construction of Practice Theory

In recent years, members of a variety of disciplines have concerned themselves with the construction of "practice" theories, or theories to be used in practice (Dickoff & James, 1968; Dickoff, James, & Wiedenbach, 1968; Ellis, 1968; Gouldner, 1957; Greenwood, 1961; Wald & Leonard, 1964; Wallace, 1971; Wooldridge, Skipper, & Leonard, 1968). Philosophers, sociologists, and others have focused on the construction of practice theory in nursing (Dickoff & James, 1968; Dickoff, et al., 1968; Wald & Leonard, 1964; Wallace, 1971). These writers have distinguished between theories de-veloped in the "basic" sciences and those developed in practice or "applied" fields. "Basic" scientists develop theory for the purpose of defining, explaining, and pre-dicting behavior; professionals or those in "applied" sciences develop theories for the purpose of guiding their actions toward some desired goal. Wooldridge, Skipper, and Leonard have called theory that is used to predict the effect of practitioner activities on clients "practice theory," a "theory used to guide a practi-tioner in selecting the most effective means for obtain-ing his ends" (Wooldridge, Skipper, & Leonard, 1968, pp. 10–33). That is, the theory guides the nurse-practitioner in meeting her goals for the patient. Writ-ing in a similar vein, Dickoff and James described nurs-ing theory as situation-producing theory; that which guides action to produce a certain kind of situation: "Situation-producing theories . . . attempt conceptual-ization of desired situations as well as conceptualizing the prescription under which an agent or practitioner must act in order to bring about situations of the kind conceived as desirable in the conception of the goal" (Dickoff & James, 1968, p. 200). Thus, nursing theory is not just theory that describes and explains phenomena. It is theory that says given this nursing goal (producing some desired change or effect in the patient's condi-tion), these are the actions the nurse must take to meet the goal (produce the change). For example, a nursing goal may be to prevent a postoperative patient from becoming hyponatremic. Nursing practice theory states that, to prevent hyponatremia, a particular set of ac-tions must be taken. This kind of theory presupposes and is built upon theory that explains, describes, and predicts, but is not limited to these. It must enable the investigator to go beyond these levels and say, "If I want to produce this condition in the patient (or con-versely, to prevent another condition), this is what I must do." This is practice theory or situation-producing theory.

Another example of this kind of theory used as a guide to the nurse's action might be: When a nurse approaches a patient to carry out a relatively minor treatment or procedure ordered by the physician, the nurse observes that the patient looks anxiously at the equipment to be used for the treatment. Guided by a theory of cognitive structuring which states the proposi-tion that when a person has an understanding of antici-pated events, he will be less anxious concerning them, particularly when the event holds little risk, the nurse provides the patient with an explanation of the treat-ment. The nursing goal in this case is to reduce in the patient anxiety produced by having to have a treat-ment; the means chosen is explanation of the event. The nurse has been guided by practice theory that states "to produce this situation (decreased anxiety), take these actions (explain)." Nursing theory, or at least nursing practice theory, is that which guides the nurse's actions in attaining nursing goals in patient care. It is not theory about nurses, such as how well are nurses, as compared with other groups, able to differ-entiate cognitively among categories, nor is it theory that describes how pain is differentially experienced by various sociocultural groups. However, either or both of these theories may form the basis for a practice theory that states: "When patients experience pain, these kinds of approaches will produce the effect of reducing the pain." A theory of pain alleviation would prescribe when a sympathetic, supportive approach by the nurse, combined with administration of an analgesic might be most effective and when an explanation of the cause of the pain, with or without medication, might be more functional. It would be built upon knowledge of the physiology of pain as well as on behavioral science theory that explicates how, for example, Italian-Americans and Jewish-Americans perceive and respond to painful stimuli differently. The practice theory would be based on the assumption that the nurse had the cognitive skills necessary to be able to discriminate accurately among several patients who are experiencing pain, and to take the action that would most effectively alleviate it for each. As this example illustrates, it is not only the nurse's knowledge of physiological, psychological, and sociocultural factors in the production of pain that is nursing theory. It is the prescribed use that the nurse must make of that knowledge to attain certain nursing goals, such as alleviation of pain, that constitutes nursing practice theory.

Two sociologists, Glaser and Strauss (1967), supported by a grant from the Division of Nursing, National Institutes of Health, described an approach for developing theories in practice fields. They identified four requirements to be met by the practice theory. The theory must:

- Closely fit the area in which it is to be used.
- Be understandable to practitioners using it.
- Be general enough to cover many diverse practice situations and not just a few specific ones.
- Allow the user of the theory (practitioner) control over the everyday situations as they change.

These requirements point clearly to some of the important factors to be considered by those developing nursing practice theory. They refer to the concepts selected for the theory (they must fit the empirical nursing reality) and the necessity to generalize about situations. In addition, they underscore the need for the theory to be couched in terms which can be readily understood by practitioners, in this case nurses. Finally, they recognize the need for the theory to include specific guidelines for control in the practice setting.

The need to recognize and make explicit values implied in the theory is also important (Ellis, 1968). As practitioners, nurses try to promote certain types of conditions in patients. It is important to make clear that nurses place a negative value on some kinds of behavior and a positive value on other kinds. In this sense, the goals in patient care are not "value free," and these values will be reflected in the kinds of theory developed. Although the goals are not "value free," the question of the most effective way to attain these goals is empirical, and testable by research. A value is expressed in saying, "The goal is to relieve the patient's pain." How to achieve that goal most effectively is the empirical question.

Blalock, discussing scientific theories in general, cited some of the desirable features of a theory. A theory must "combine the features of being sufficiently general and complex, explicitly formulated with the direction of causal influences specified, and with a small number of well-defined concepts" (Blalock, 1969, p. 21). For a theory to be "sufficiently general and complex" it should fall somewhere between explaining a very small part of the empirical world and trying to explain everything about a particular science or discipline with a single theory. If attempts to construct nursing theory were placed along a continuum of generality, at one end would fall those theories based on the global definitions of nursing that state that nursing is concerned with anything related to man. Such theory has been called "grand theory" by C. Wright Mills (1959) and is characterized as explaining everything while explaining nothing. The practitioner is given a collection of all-purpose, all-inclusive concepts and propositions that offer few clear or relevant guides for practice. It is little wonder that in such situations the gap between theory and practice is wide. One positive function that such theories can serve is to suggest what Blalock refers to as "sensitizing concepts" which alert the researcher to concepts that may be important ones in a theory of more manageable propositions (Blalock, 1970, p. 79).

At the opposite end of the continuum of generality is the situation in which nurses operate on the basis of isolated facts and principles rather than basing practice on theory that has been well articulated and tested. The tendency to separate theory from empirical reality is also evident in much nursing research. Activity studies in nursing, popular a number of years ago, were an extreme example of this approach. Mills (1959) called the collection of facts isolated from a theoretical framework "abstracted empiricism." Underlying this approach to theory development and research is the assumption that, when sufficient data have been accumulated, the relationships among them will become clear. This is analogous to a collection of bricklayers each making a brick in isolation from other bricklayers and with no blueprint to follow. They throw these bricks together into a large pile, confident that, somehow, a house will emerge.

Robert Merton (1968) suggested development of "theories of the middle range" to avoid the disadvantages of both grand theory and abstracted empiricism. Middle-range theories include a limited number of variables and focus on a limited aspect of reality. Propositions that are not all inclusive can be derived and submitted to empirical test. This kind of development of "middle-range" theory seems particularly well suited to the development of practice theories.

The Debate on Nursing Theory

In the academic division of labor, there are often boundary disputes concerning the proper focus of a discipline that claims to be a science. The older physical sciences have well-defined areas of the empirical world with which they are concerned and have developed and tested theories about these areas. While there is some overlapping of foci, physics and chemistry can generally delineate their fields from each other. There is less consensus over boundaries in the behavioral and social sciences. Sociologists, psychologists, social psychologists, anthropologists, and others frequently claim the same phenomena and concepts as their own. It is difficult enough to define boundaries in these "basic," essentially academic areas concerned with *production* of knowledge. The difficulties are compounded when trying to specify clearly what part of the empirical world can be "claimed" by disciplines in which the major

concern is *use* of knowledge. Professional boundary disputes are well known to nurses, who for years have been attempting to define what their job is and what knowledge they need to perform that job. Part of the difficulty in practice disciplines is that knowledge is commonly drawn from a variety of basic sciences, rather than only one. By what process does the knowledge of chemistry, biology, physiology, and other sciences become medical knowledge or science? How do nurses transform knowledge from sociology, psychology, and other fields into "nursing knowledge"?

These and similar questions have led to the contemporary debate in nursing that asks, "Can and should we develop *nursing theories?*" Those opposed to developing nursing theories often base their opposition on the contention that there are no phenomena or tasks that are specifically nursing's, and, therefore, nurses have nothing to develop nursing theories about. Some make the distinction that there is no *nursing theory,* but that nurses use theories from other fields in nursing—that is, there are *theories in nursing.* Those who take this position frequently maintain that the research efforts of nurses should be expended in the basic sciences from which nurses draw their knowledge. Their belief is that nurses should not be restricted to researching only those problems which are of immediate concern to nursing as it is now practiced. Rather, they are interested in developing knowledge in basic sciences which may or may not be used by nurses. Scientists, they say, are properly concerned with the expansion of knowledge and not with whether it has an immediate practical use.

Those who believe that nurses should develop nursing theories base their argument on the need for nurses to have a systematically organized body of knowledge on which to base their practice. The proponents of nursing theory maintain that, although there is not high consensus on what most appropriately constitutes nursing, there is sufficient agreement to provide guides for the development of theories. Another assertion of those who take this position is that nurses have great need for knowledge which scientists in other fields may not be interested in developing, and, therefore, nurses must take responsibility for developing this knowledge.[8]

An Opinion on the Issue of Nursing Theory

Those for and against the development of nursing theory have strong arguments to support their respective positions. It would be a mistake to define prematurely nursing's area of practice and thus the foci for research and theory construction. It would be equally wrong to use much of nursing's resources to develop knowledge in areas only remotely or very indirectly concerned with nursing practice. This is particularly so in those basic areas where nonnurses have or are investigating these same phenomena.

There is sufficient consensus concerning the definition of nursing practice to enable the construction of some nursing theories. That these theories may not include concepts unique to nursing is not an important consideration, although such concepts could conceivably be developed. What is important is that the relevant concepts to be included are related by propositions and that the propositions themselves are systematically interrelated. There is no pressing need to develop a "grand theory" that supposedly includes everything that nurses need to know. Other sciences have not succeeded in this effort and there is no reason to believe that nursing can. Rather, theory-building efforts may more realistically be focused on developing "middle-range" theories of limited aspects of nursing, such as a nursing theory of pain alleviation, or one concerned with promotion of sleep, or with teaching health measures, or rehabilitation, or socialization of the patient into the health care system. As the focus of nursing changes, as it unquestionably will in response to societal changes, the concepts, propositions, and nursing theories constructed will need to change. Concepts and

theories in any area are invented by those who attempt to describe, explain, predict, and (in the case of practice theories) control events in the empirical world. If the concepts and theories so invented are no longer useful or accurate, they are modified to fit the known and existing empirical reality.

This overview of theory construction is brief and oversimplifies many issues in the construction and testing of scientific theories. Its purpose is to pull together and relate various elements of theory construction which, unless considered together, can be confusing. A related purpose is to begin to bring theory construction out of the ivory tower and into the realm of the practitioner. It is, after all, the experienced practicing nurse who is in the best position to make the empirical observations basic to the construction of relevant nursing practice theories.

Nursing's concern with theory construction is very new. It has been said of the social sciences that they are "infants" in the area of theory construction. If this is so for the social sciences, it is doubly so for nursing, in which theory construction is still a gleam in the proverbial eyes of its would-be founders.

References

Blalock, M.H. (1969). *Theory construction.* Englewood Cliffs, NJ: Prentice-Hall.

Blalock, M.H. (1970). *Introduction to social research.* Englewood Cliffs, NJ: Prentice-Hall.

Brodbeck, M. (1968). Models, meaning, and theories. In M. Brodbeck (Ed.), *Readings in the philosophy of the social services* (pp. 579–600). New York: Macmillan.

Denzin, N.K. (1970). *Research act.* Chicago: Aldine.

Dickoff, J., & James, P. (1968). A theory of theories: A position paper. *Nursing Research, 17,* 197–203.

Dickoff J., James, P., & Wiedenbach, E. (1968). Theory in a practice discipline: Part 1. Practice-oriented theory. *Nursing Research, 17,* 415–435.

Dubin, R. (1968). *Theory building.* New York: Free Press.

Ellis, R. (1968). Characteristics of significant theories. *Nursing Research, 17,* 217–222.

Feigl, H. (1953). The scientific outlook: Naturalism and humanism. In H. Feigl & M. Brodbeck (Eds.), *Readings in the philosophy of science* (pp. 8–18). New York: Appleton-Century-Crofts.

Glaser, B.G., & Strauss, A. (1967). *The discovery of grounded theory.* Chicago: Aldine.

---

[8] This brief discussion has only touched on the major points of the nursing theory issue. For elaboration, see the papers and discussion of issues in the reports of a series of three conferences held on nursing theory (Norris, 1969–1970).

Gouldner, A.W. (1957). Theoretical requirements of the applied social sciences. *American Sociological Review, 22,* 92–102.

Greenwood, E. (1961). The practice of science and the science of practice. In W.G. Bennis et al. (Eds.), *The planning of change* (pp. 73–83). New York: Holt, Rinehart and Winston.

Hopkins, T.K. (1964). *The exercise of influence in small groups.* Totowa, NJ: Bedminster Press.

Kaplan, A. (1964). *The conduct of inquiry.* San Francisco: Chandler.

Merton, R.F. (1968). *Social theory and social structure.* New York: Free Press.

Mills, C.W. (1959). *The social imagination.* New York: Oxford University Press.

Norris, C.M. (Ed.). (1969–1970). *Proceedings of the first, second, and third nursing theory conferences.* Kansas City: Department of Nursing Education, University of Kansas Medical Center.

Parsons, T., & Shils, E.A. (1959). *Toward a general theory of action.* Cambridge, MA: Harvard University Press.

Rudner, R.S. (1966–1967). *Philosophy of social sciences.* Englewood Cliffs, NJ: Prentice-Hall.

Theodorson, G.A., & Theodorson, A.G. (1969). *A modern dictionary of sociology.* New York: Crowell.

Turner, M.B. (1967). *Philosophy and the science of behavior.* New York: Appleton-Century-Crofts.

Wald, F.S., & Leonard, R.C. (1964). Towards development of nursing practice theory. *Nursing Research, 13,* 309–313.

Walker, L.O. (1971). Toward a clearer understanding of the concept of nursing theory. *Nursing Research, 20,* 428–435.

Wallace, W.L. (1971). *The logic of science in sociology.* Chicago: Aldine-Atherton.

Wooldridge, P.J., Skipper, J.K., & Leonard, R.C. (1968). *Behavioral science, social practice and the nursing profession.* Cleveland: Case Western Reserve University Press.

Reactions

Nursing Research, July-August 1974, 23(4), 355.

To the Editor:

My compliments for the very illuminating, concise, and helpful article by Ada Jacox. . . . Dr. Jacox put into an understandable perspective the building materials which are required for theory construction and the directions which appear both desirable and practical for nursing and nurses to pursue in the development of the "relevant nursing practice theories."

I shall recommend this article to my colleagues who are deeply involved with giving guidance and assistance to nurses engaged in the practice of nursing.

LAURA C. DUNSTAN, Ed.D., R.N.
Assistant Commissioner for Nursing Services
New York State Department of Health
Albany, New York

To the Editor:

I have just read Jacox's article on "Theory Construction in Nursing." I see it as a good, basic overview and would like to make it required reading for a course I teach in nursing theory. . . .

ROSALEE C. YEAWORTH, Ph.D., R.N.
Acting Director
Graduate Programs in Nursing
College of Nursing and Health
University of Cincinnati
Cincinnati, Ohio

Nursing Research, January-February 1975, 24(1), 63–64.

To the Editor:

Jacox's article . . . needs to be commended for the clarity and precision it demonstrates in discussing theory in nursing. However, it contains several errors which are recurrent within the nursing literature.

The first difficulty lies in Jacox's notion of inductive reasoning. She states: "Induction is a type of argument in which one argues from the particular to the general, or from the individual to the universal" (p. 7). The equation of induction with logical movement from the particular to the general (and the frequent companion assertion that deduction is a logical movement from the general to the particular) is inadequate, however, Irving Copi in his (1972) text, *Introduction to Logic,* clearly addresses this problem:

"Deductive and inductive arguments are sometimes characterized and distinguished from one another in terms of the relative generality of their premises and conclusions. . . . Thus the classical example of deductive argument

> All men are mortal.
> Socrates is a man.
> Therefore Socrates is mortal.

indeed has a *particular* conclusion inferred (validly) from premises the first of which is a general or universal proposition. By contrast, a fairly standard form of inductive argument is illustrated by

> Socrates is a man and is mortal.
> Plato is a man and is mortal.
> Aristotle is a man and is mortal.
> Therefore probably all men are mortal.

in which a general or universal conclusion is inferred from premises all of which are particular propositions. There is some merit to this method of distinguishing between deduction and induction, but it is not universally applicable. For valid deductive arguments may have universal propositions for conclusions as well as for premises, as in

> All men are animals.
> All animals are mortal.
> Therefore all men are mortal.

and they may have particular propositions for their premises as well as for their conclusions, as in

> If Socrates is a man, then Socrates is mortal.
> Socrates is a man.
> Therefore Socrates is mortal.

And inductive arguments may have universal propositions for premises as well as for conclusions, as in

> All cows are mammals and have lungs.
> All horses are mammals and have lungs.
> All men are mammals and have lungs.
> Therefore probably all mammals have lungs.

and they may have particular propositions for their conclusions, as in

> Hitler was a dictator and was ruthless.
> Stalin was a dictator and was ruthless.
> Castro is a dictator.
> Therefore Castro is probably ruthless.

So it is not altogether satisfactory to characterize deductive arguments as those which derive particular conclusions from general premises, or inductive arguments as those which infer general conclusions from particular premises" (Copi, 1972, pp. 24–25).

While Jacox correctly characterizes deduction as a process by which one may infer with certitude a conclusion, given premises, her characterization of induction contains the difficulties which Copi has pointed out above. Induction might be better characterized as a process of making inferences based on observation which are subject to revision given further empirical evidence, i.e., the certitude present in deduction is absent in induction.

The second difficulty occurring in this article is Jacox's treatment of practice theory. After a painstaking explication of the concept of theory, Jacox seems to stumble when she turns to practice theory. Instead of building on her preceding discussion of theory, she introduces practice theory as a distinct type of theory, unlike scientific theory, which "guides the nurse practitioner in meeting her goals for the patient" (p. 10). It is my contention, however, that what is called "practice theory" is not a distinct form of theory, but rather the application of propositions derived from a theory or set of laws to the explanation of clinical practices and events. As such, practice theory is more akin to scientific explanation than to a theory. When using such explanations in the practice domain, it is more typical to call them the "rationale" or "principles" which underlie a practice or procedure. The examples Jacox gives in her article seem to be consistent with my contention that practice theory is the rationale for practice; e.g., the selection of propositions from a theory of cognitive structuring is used to guide the nurse's action in producing the effect of lowering a patient's anxiety as the latter faces a minor treatment (p. 10). If my appraisal is correct, then practice theory is not a distinct type of theory but the use of theory, just as a scientific explanation is not a type of theory but the use of theory. The difference between the use of scientific theory in a scientific explanation and in a rationale for practice appears to be the nature of the event which provokes the use of theory. In the case of an explanation, it is a puzzling event; in a rationale it is a puzzlement about the means by which an effect may be or is achieved. If my analysis of practice theory is correct, nursing might best be served by abandoning the terms "practice theory."

I hope *Nursing Research* will continue to publish articles on nursing theory of commensurate quality to that of Jacox. In so doing, perhaps the mystery of the role of theory in nursing will be solved.

LORRAINE WALKER, Ed.D., R.N.
Associate Professor, School of Nursing
University of Texas at Austin
Austin, Texas

REFERENCE
Copi I. (1972). *Introduction to logic.* New York: Macmillan.

The Author Comments

When I finished my doctoral program and began to teach nursing research to master's students, there was nothing in the literature on the philosophy of science in nursing that I considered to be sufficiently accurate or at a level appropriate for nursing graduate students. Most of the material was either too superficial or just plain wrong. I drafted and redrafted a paper and used it with three classes of students who provided valuable criticism.

Unfortunately, I was unaware of the revolution taking place in the philosophy of science while I was writing the article and depended on what was in the philosophy of science literature at the time. I now view this article as outdated—although its inclusion in this anthology does serve a historical purpose. In my subsequent writing on theory construction in nursing (Suppe & Jacox, 1985; Webster & Jacox, 1985; Webster, Jacox, & Baldwin, 1981), I have worked with philosophers to ensure that the ideas expressed are current.

—ADA JACOX

REFERENCES
Suppe, F., & Jacox, A. (1985). Philosophy of science and the development of nursing theory. In H.H. Werley & J.J. Fitzpatrick (Eds.), *Annual review of nursing research* (Vol. 3 pp. 241–267). New York: Springer.

Webster, G., & Jacox, A. (1985). Toward the liberation of nursing theory. In J.C. McCloskey & H.K. Grace (Eds.), *Current issues in nursing* (2nd ed.). Boston: Blackwell Scientific.

Webster, G., Jacox, A., & Baldwin, B. (1981). Nursing theory and the ghost of the received view. In H.K. Grace & J.C. McCloskey (Eds.), *Current issues in nursing* (pp. 26–35). Boston: Blackwell Scientific.

Chapter 34

Competing Theories of Science

Ada K. Jacox
Glenn Webster

The purpose of this paper is to explore the relevance of several alternative conceptions of the nature of science to competing theories in nursing. During the past 25 years, two sets of activities have been occurring simultaneously but not in close relation to each other: theory development in nursing and a revolution in the philosophy of science. Since the Renaissance, about four hundred years ago, there has been intellectual turmoil about what science is and how theories are developed. This turmoil seemed to have been resolved by the positivistic philosophy of science of the 1930s. However, in the past 25 years a revolution has occurred within philosophy of science proper.

During the same 25 years nurses began to give attention to theory construction in nursing. Such people as Martha Rogers, Hildegard Peplau, and Dorothy Johnson were among the first in the early 1960s to write about what kind of theory nurses need. During the late 1960s there was a series of conferences at Case Western Reserve University that dealt with the ideas of theory in nursing. Later, at the University of Kansas, under the direction of Catherine Norris, those of us who were beginning to develop an interest in theory came together to learn more about theory construction and the implications for nursing. In those conferences held in 1969 and 1970, forty nurses were involved; during that period eight finished their doctoral degrees. Most of us who were finishing at that time got our degrees in sociology or education. Our notions of what science is were developed in those disciplines and were what we brought to nursing in writing and teaching about theory construction.

Unfortunately the revolution that was occurring in philosophy of science was not reflected in the developing nursing theories. The work of most nurse theorists during the 1960s and 1970s was rooted firmly in pre-1960 notions of science. The 1980s are beginning to see some notable exceptions—at least at the level of

This chapter was written for this volume. The quote on page 338 is reprinted with permission from Current Issues in Nursing.

writing about science. The old ideas of theory construction are well reflected in the paper published in 1974 and reprinted in this volume (Jacox, 1974; see Chapter 33). That paper and the literature from which it was drawn are overly rigid and narrow accounts of what theories are and how they are developed. We would like to identify some of our concerns about this view of science and theory and its effects on nursing activities.

The first is that the constricted view of theory represented in that approach is incompatible with the philosophy of nursing that the majority of nurses espouse. Our philosophy of science does not match our philosophy of nursing. A second related concern is that the research methods reflecting this notion of science have restricted our research. Nursing research has overemphasized precision, quantification, and numbers. We tried so hard to study the trees in precise isolation that we often missed the forest.

The third consequence of the domination of this view of science is that some nurses continue to spend their time and energy in pursuit of activities that appear to be scientific in their attempts at precision, but that require far too much time and energy for the results achieved. A prime example is nursing's preoccupation with behavioral objectives. The heavy emphasis on behavioral objectives that has characterized nursing education is dysfunctional for the creative development of nursing knowledge.

A fourth consequence is reflected in some of the recent attempts to develop taxonomies in nursing. Classification is useful; it has heuristic value and is needed for purposes such as communication and computer access. An overly rigid approach can waste time and be grossly misleading. The belief that categories should be mutually exclusive creates confusion and frustration when, for example, one attempts to separate fatigue from anxiety and depression. These phenomena are not clearly separated in humans, and it is difficult to develop category definitions and measurements that clearly differentiate them. For heuristic purposes, it may be necessary to say that for the time being we will somewhat *arbitrarily* categorize a behavior in this way. As long as no one forgets that the classification is some-

what arbitrary and temporary, little harm is done. If, however, people act as if those categories really do represent human behavior, misleading conclusions will be drawn. It is when this reification of concepts or categories occurs that we get into trouble. It is not useful to develop classifications that we know do not represent reality and then act as if they do. Nursing theory and concepts are reticulate; they interact, they are related to each other. Those phenomena that we deal with in patients are very much interrelated. They cannot be separated except for heuristic purposes, and the notion that they can be separated should be discouraged. It is also dysfunctional to develop nursing classification systems that do not overlap with medicine. What nurses do in practice overlaps tremendously with what physicians do, and to develop theories that do not acknowledge this overlap is not a useful enterprise.

We would like to insert the caveat here that we do not mean to include all nurse researchers or theorists in this criticism. There have been and are many exceptions. Neither do we intend to suggest that quantitative scientific methods as we know them have no use. Certainly they do, but they are far too narrow and dogmatic to reflect nursing reality completely, or any other reality for that matter.

Changes in Philosophy of Science

One of the persons who has had major responsibility for some recent changes in philosophy of science is Thomas S. Kuhn. In 1962 he published a book titled *The Structure of Scientific Revolutions,* in which he proposed a different view of science. In studying the history of science, he noticed that science did not develop in the very systematic and rational manner that has been generally supposed. Rather, its actual development was quite different from the typical "textbook" picture. He said that there are three stages of science: The first is the preparadigm stage of "immature science." The second stage is "normal" science—the stage of rational puzzle solving on the basis of shared metaphysical and methodologic assumptions about how the part of the world being studied operates and how it should be studied. This is called a paradigm. Numerous specific theories are generated and abandoned within the context of the same paradigm, all on the basis of the common assumptions. "Normal science" is the condition of most of the recognized or "developed" sciences. The third stage of science Kuhn calls "revolutionary" science. It is the stage of abandonment of previously shared assumptions, of challenge from new potentially shared assumptions, often introduced by those "improperly" socialized in the beliefs of the older paradigm. Kuhn's most troubling doctrine is his contention that such shifts take place for largely noncognitive reasons, i.e., for social, political, or economic concerns.

It is not clear precisely what Kuhn meant by the concept of a paradigm. Margaret Masterman (1977) has identified at least 21 different ways in which Kuhn uses the term "paradigm" in his first book. One of the major definitions is that it is the general theory that a normal science shares. (Kuhn has moved away from the discussion of paradigms and now talks about disciplinary matrices, which are very similar to the meaning of paradigm noted above.) In his second major use of the term "paradigm," Kuhn refers to a key historical occasion of success within the discipline: the event itself becomes the exemplar of how science ought to be done in the field—e.g., Newton's *Principia.* This meaning of the term paradigm is interesting because of its philosophical significance for the problem of relativism or subjectivism in Kuhn's view of science. Viewing the paradigm as the exemplar event provides a basis for historical realism. But the issue of why one exemplar is recognized rather than another is still to be settled.

Kuhn says that professional education consists of socialization, a kind of brainwashing of students, in which they are taught to think about the world in the manner in which the intellectual leaders of their discipline believe that scholars ought to think about it. Teachers transmit a set of conceptual boxes from the dominant phage group of the discipline to the students of the discipline. A *phage group* is a group of frequently communicating scholars, usually not more than a hundred in number, who share common beliefs and goals through their network of communication and are thus much more effective and coordinated politically than are smaller groups and isolated scholars. The dominant phage group provides the actual social and political support for the common assumptions that are the paradigm of a normal science. The dominant phage group usually controls the presentations at scientific meetings and publications in professional journals. They also dominate the key university departments of their discipline, and by their common agreement, determine which departments are recognized as essential or outstanding. Thus it is through a dominant phage group that a paradigm controls a discipline, and the control is largely social and political rather than cognitive and rational.

A paradigm is rejected when a number of anomalies or unsolved empirical problems accumulate, requiring an increasing number of *ad hoc* explanations, which in turn undermine the plausibility of the basic assumptions of the paradigm. But the paradigm is not refuted. Rather the process of socialization of students breaks down, and an increasing number of young scholars in the discipline begin to explore solutions to problems outside of the accepted assumptions of the old paradigm. This is the stage of revolutionary science, which is largely nonrational in nature, with persuasion and politics playing as large a role in determining the nature of the new normal science as cognitive or rational considerations. From among the alternative paradigms that emerge to challenge the old, one is made to seem more empirically successful than its alternatives —in fact, a new phage group coalesces and comes to dominate the discipline, and it is the new phage group that selects and enforces the new paradigm.

The Received View Theory of Science

Kuhn's ideas of science provide a good background for understanding the "Received View" theory of science that has dominated nursing and science generally. This paradigm dominated our understanding during the early part of this century and into the 1960s.

The "Received View" is a label that was adopted in the recent literature of the philosophy of science. One of the major persons responsible for the label is Frederick Suppe (1977), a philosopher at the University of Maryland. The Received View is the name given for the theory concerning the nature of science that dominated the philosophy of science through the 30s, 40s, and 50s. Advocates of the theory had no label for it since they thought it was simply the truth about science. The Received View is a somewhat sarcastic and unfriendly label adopted by its critics who chafed for several decades under the prescriptions and prohibitions of what was a very powerful and dogmatic orthodoxy, controlling the key journals and departments in philosophy of science.

Ironically and to their credit, it was the advocates of the Received View, in their attempt to refine it and make it more adequate, who did the most to loosen its hold on the philosophy of science. Almost every one of its fundamental doctrines was modified or rejected by its later supporters. Another irony of history was that news of the modifications and rejections was slow to reach the external imitators and followers of the Received View, so that by the mid-1960s, strong supporters of the original Received View existed only outside of mainstream philosophy of science in such disciplines as sociology. The insiders had changed the Received View to something only recognizable as a distant descendent of the original, and to something that was obviously not *the* truth about science but only *a* truth.

The Received View developed out of the seventeenth century world view, including the notions that the world was like a clock or simple machine and only God understood fully the laws by which it operated. The business of science was to discover those laws and to learn enough about them to achieve perfect predictability. There has been much intellectual turmoil over the past few centuries while those ideas have changed, with a clear intellectual division emerging in the nineteenth century. This intellectual bifurcation influenced the development of the Received View. The near consensus concerning the basic nature of the world that dominated much of the seventeenth and eighteenth centuries gave way to two competing world view level traditions: the philosophy of nature, taking its cues concerning the basic nature of reality from the physical sciences, especially mathematical physics; and the philosophy of mind, concerned with the nature of human experience, represented by such traditions as German Idealism, phenomenology, and existentialism. Positivism, both nineteenth-century Comptian positivism and twentieth-century logical positivism, is part of the philosophy of nature in the nineteenth-century sense.

Science became dominated by those focusing on physical reality and the philosophy of nature. The core group responsible for developing what we now call the Received View of science was composed of philosophers who gathered in Vienna in the 1930s and labeled themselves Logical Positivists. Logical Positivism was most well known for its advocacy of Hume's Fork (the notion that statements are either analytic or synthetic and never both); its interest in formal logic and formalization issues; and its rejection of metaphysics or theory of reality, since the only reality was physical reality and the physical sciences were the only appropriate disciplines for its study. Implicit in this position is the view that mind is either not an appropriate subject for science or that it is reducible to physical reality. As we said above, those who developed the Received View later criticized, refuted, and abandoned it.

The following tenets or doctrines were hallmarks of the original Received View of the nature of science as it was developed by Vienna Circle Logical Positivism in the 1930s:

> One doctrine was that a theory is either true or false and it's very important to determine which. This comes partially from the heavy emphasis that was placed on mathematics and the notion that formal languages are the basis for expressing science. In a formal language such as mathematics it is possible to set up rules such that truths are possible. Two plus two, is four, under the rules developed, is true; two plus three is four, is false. The notion that was appropriate for the part of science which is mathematics was taken as a basis for all scien-

tific knowledge. It gave rise to the notion that theories themselves must be either true or false, and there was no room for degrees of truth or adequacy.

The second doctrine was that the more mature or developed theories must be formalized—that is, they have to be developed and expressed in formal languages.

Third, they must also be axiomatized, although this doctrine was rejected very early as the result of work done in formal logic. They found very soon that almost any set of necessarily true well formed formula in logic could be used as an axiom set, with all of the rest of the necessarily true well formed formula being derivable, in accordance with inference rules, as theorems. In logic, the choice of an axiom set was completely arbitrary. Worse, general arithmetic could not be successfully axiomatized.

Another characteristic was that the physical sciences are basic, especially physics. Physics is top dog in the sciences and is the model that all sciences ought to follow.

A fifth doctrine was that observational terms or language should be distinguished from theoretical terms or language, and that the two can be clearly separated. Correlated with that was the notion that a scientific theory should contain correspondence rules for the exchange of theoretical and observational terms. That is, it was possible to separate clearly the theoretical from the empirical. Again, there is absence of the idea of degree. Whereas in reality, some concepts and theories are more theoretical and some are more empirical, but the belief that they can be completely separated is false.

Another characteristic is that the purpose of science is to predict the occurrence of events by combining descriptive laws with statements of initial conditions. This was the way in which perfect predictability could be achieved.

A seventh characteristic of the Received View is that science has nothing to say about value. It is value free and completely objective, and value is not a proper subject of its concern. Yet another doctrine was that science progresses by reducing earlier theories to later theories, with all previous theories being incorporated into the most recent. And science also progresses by reducing less basic to more basic sciences; i.e., sociology is reducible to psychology, which in turn is reducible to physiology, and so forth.

Finally, the doctrine that there was a single scientific method was espoused (Webster, Jacox, & Baldwin, 1981, pp. 29–30).

None of these tenets is unequivocally true. All have been rejected or seriously modified by recent philosophers of science. The rejection of several of these doctrines has important implications for nursing. Two related doctrines were that physical sciences are basic, especially physics, and that less basic sciences can be reduced to more basic sciences. The holistic view of persons espoused by nursing is incompatible with those ideas. The idea of body-mind dualism, that experiences of the mind are reducible to physical explanations, is antithetical to nursing and to the development of its scientific knowledge. For instance, Socrates the man cannot be reduced to George the electron. The rejection of this doctrine and acceptance of the interrelatedness of the body and mind are crucial for nursing. The study of the mind and mind-body relationships are intellectually respectable pursuits and must be accepted as such for the sake of the advance of nursing science.

Unfortunately, the respectability of the study of mind and mind-body relationships is still news to many. Those who sit on interdisciplinary research committees know that biological scientists, and most committees that include them, are still dominated by the Received View theory of science, a domination that may continue for some time, due in part to recent successes in microbiology. However, the general scientific community is gradually accepting the idea that it is intellectually respectable to study the mind and mind-body relationships and to recognize the fact that people are experiencing entities as well as physiological systems. The fact that the general scientific community is beginning to accept the validity of the claims of behavioral scientists should have a positive effect on nursing research.

Another Received View hallmark, the refutation of which has positive implications for nursing, is the tenet that theoretical and observational terms can be clearly separated. This is not possible; there is no such thing as a theory free observation. A researcher always works back and forth between the theoretical and the empirical. Sometimes the work is more theoretical and sometimes it is more empirical, but in research and theory development it is necessary to move back and forth.

The argument whether theories are or should be deductively or inductively developed also is a false argument, based on a false dichotomy. Some attempts may use a more deductive or a more inductive approach than others, but all theory construction includes both. It is a question of more or less.

Another refuted doctrine of the Received View is that science has nothing to say about value. Science is value laden from the very beginning. What is accepted as normal science is the result of evaluation; our ideas about science are value laden; the choice of problems to study is value laden; how we study them, how they are interpreted, and who accepts them are all the results of valuation. Science is not value free. Neither is nursing value free. Nursing places positive value on health, human well-being, and similar states and processes. It is better to try to understand how our values influence the science and the theories that we construct rather than to continue with the notion that science is value free. The refutation of these and other doctrines of the Received View is important for nursing. Newly developing alternative views are much more consistent with the development of a relevant knowledge base for nursing practice than is the outdated Received View of science and theory.

Alternative Theories of Science

During recent years a dozen or more alternatives to the Received View have been proposed, in addition to the theory of T. S. Kuhn, which we have already considered. A more extreme form of "historicism" than Kuhn's is that represented by Paul Feyerabend (1977). "Historicism" is the general label for historical relativism and skepticism made popular by Karl Popper's title, *The Poverty of Historicism* (Popper, 1944, 1945/ 1976). Where the Received View believed that the meaning and truth of scientific theories were absolute, historicism holds that both meaning and truth are relative to the social and historical context within which the theory is developed and asserted. Feyerabend (1977) recommends methodologic anarchy—the only truth about scientific method is that "anything goes."

He says that theory and observation are so interrelated and dependent on historical context that it is impossible to compare one theory with another. According to Feyerabend, there are no neutral rules or terms for comparing across theories; and fact is so theory laden that there are no neutral facts. The theory one chooses is a matter of taste, social convenience, or political expediency; whatever works is fair game. He writes:

> To start with, it seems to me that an enterprise whose human characteristics can be seen by all is preferable to one that looks "objective," and impervious to human actions and wishes. The sciences, after all are our own creations, including all the severe standards they seem to impose upon us. It is good to be constantly reminded of the fact that science as we know it today is not inescapable and that we may construct a world in which it plays no role whatever. (Such a world, I venture to suggest, would be more pleasant than the world we live in today.) What better reminder is there than the realization that the choice between theories which are sufficiently general to provide us with a comprehensive world view and which are empirically disconnected may become a matter of taste? That the choice of our basic cosmology may become a matter of taste? (Feyerabend, 1977, p. 228)

Feyerabend is a little too extreme; though he represents one of the current views of science, nursing needs a more realistic and nonrelativistic view of science. Stephen Toulmin (1977), Dudley Shapere (1977), Imre Lakatos (1977), Larry Laudan (1977), and others are somewhere between the Received View and Feyerabend's extreme historicism. All of the above, except the Received View theorists, agree that observation is theory laden; and they all focus on the larger contexts of specific theories, denying independent meaningfulness to specific theories. Lakatos, reacting against Kuhn and Feyerabend, says that mature science is concerned with "research programs" (Lakatos, 1977, pp. 39–47). These are similar to Kuhn's disciplinary matrices. But contrary to Kuhn, Lakatos says that it is possible to assess progress within a research program because of the manner in which the later theories within the program contain some of the earlier theories of the same program. Though theories are constantly changing, it is possible to rationally evaluate the efficacy and progress of a research program from within the research program. Kuhn, in contrast, allows only for the rational evaluation of individual theories within a disciplinary matrix, but not for the evaluation of the disciplinary matrix itself. Where all of these philosophers differ from Feyerabend is in greater degree of rationality that they are attempting to find within the scientific endeavor.

Shapere (1977) talks about the "scientific domain," again focusing on the broader context of the specific theories. He suggests that as knowledge is added the domain is changed. He denies that there are any fixed canons of rationality, saying that the canons of rationality themselves are changed as a result of new knowledge. He does not throw out rationalism, but he does not say that reason provides us with a rigid, unchanging set of rules either. Toulmin (1977) talks about "scientific disciplines" in much the same way that Shapere talks about scientific domains and Lakatos talks about research programs. All of these authors share the notions that observation is theory laden, science is progressive, and that rationality plays a part in that progression, but they disagree on the part that rationality plays. They all focus on the board context within which specific theories are developed.

Larry Laudan (1977) is one of the philosophers whose work is particularly helpful to those outside philosophy of science. He is very readable and operates from a pragmatic base, which is useful for a practice discipline such as nursing. Laudan says his concern is to offer objective criteria for determining when progress has occurred in science. He tries to develop in a systematic way how and when to judge that progress has occurred. The particular kind of progress with which Laudan is concerned is cognitive progress, which is nothing more than progress with respect to the intellectual aspirations of science. Cognitive progress is progress in deepening of understanding. It has both an empirical and a conceptual dimension. Progress in the empirical dimension is achieved by generating new specific theories allowing for the coverage of new facts in a manner that relates them to old facts and theories.

Progress in the conceptual dimension is achieved by more adequately placing specific theories and their supporting research programs within the body of scientific knowledge as a whole. Cognitive progress neither entails nor is entailed by material, social, or spiritual progress.

Science, for Laudan, is a problem-solving activity. Problems are the focal points of scientific thought and theories the end result. Theories are cognitively important insofar as they provide adequate solutions to problems. Problems constitute the questions of science; theories constitute the answers. The function of a theory is to reduce ambiguity, to reduce irregularity to uniformity, and to show that what happens is somehow intelligible or predictable. The first test for any theory is whether it provides acceptable answers to interesting questions or satisfactory solutions to important problems.

There are two major points with respect to Laudan's work that have particular interest for nursing. First:

> What is crucial for evaluation of theory in any cognitive assessment of a theory is how it fares with respect to its competitors. Absolute measures of the empirical or conceptual credentials of a theory are of no significance; decisive is the judgment as to how a theory stacks up against its known contenders. Much of the literature in the philosophy of science has been based upon the assumption that theoretical evaluation occurs in a competitive vacuum. By contrast, I shall be assuming that assessments of theories always involve competitive modalities. We ask: is this theory better than that one? Is this doctrine the best among the available options? (Laudan, 1977, p. 71)

Another important aspect of Laudan's work for nursing is his delineation of two classes of what are usually called scientific theories, or two different kinds of propositional networks. He says that theory is used in scientific literature in at least two different ways. In the first way, theory refers to a very specific set of related doctrines, such as Marx's labor theory of value and Freud's theory of the Oedipal complex. In contrast, the term theory is also used to refer to much more general, less easily testable, sets of doctrines or assumptions. The atomic theory or the theory of evolution each refers not to a single theory, but to a whole spectrum of individual theories. Laudan suggests that the ways of evaluating these two different kinds of theories are radically different, and that "until we become mindful of the cognitive and evaluation differences between these two types of theories, it will be impossible to have a theory of scientific progress which is historically sound or philosophically adequate" (Laudan, 1977, p. 71).

The notion that there are two types or levels of theories is not unique to Laudan. All of the philosophers we mentioned have some name for this more general collection of theories that have common metaphysical and methodologic assumptions. Acknowledging this distinction between the two types of theories would make moot the question often raised within nursing: should there be one theory or many? The answer, of course, is "There should be several traditions and numerous theories within those traditions." Viewing theories in this broader context would free us to become more creative in the development and evolution of nursing theories.

In this discussion we have only touched the surface of the vast literature that has developed over the past 25 years. It is not clear that any single theory of theories will emerge as another dominant view of what normal science is. The richness in choice of theory and of theory of science should enable the development of more relevant and useful nursing theories and research.

References

Feyerabend, P. (1977). Consolations for the specialist. In I. Lakatos & A. Musgrave (Eds.), *Criticism and the growth of knowledge.* London: Cambridge University Press.

Jacox, A. (1974). Theory construction in nursing: An overview. *Nursing Research, 23*(1), 4–13.

Kuhn, T.S. (1962). *The structure of scientific revolutions.* Chicago: University of Chicago Press.

Lakatos, I. (1977). Falsification and the methodology of scientific research programs. In I. Lakatos & A. Musgrave (Eds.), *Criticism and the growth of knowledge* (pp. 39–47). London: Cambridge University Press.

Laudan, L. (1977). *Progress and its problems: Towards a theory of scientific growth.* Berkeley, CA: University of California Press.

Masterman, M. (1977). The nature of a paradigm. In I. Lakatos & A. Musgrave (Eds.), *Criticism and the growth of knowledge* (pp. 58–89). London: Cambridge University Press.

Popper, K. (1976). *The poverty of historicism.* London: Routledge & Kegan Paul. (Originally published as The poverty of historicism, I, II, III in *Economica, 11,* 86–103, 119–137, and *Economica, 12,* 69–80.

Shapere, D. (1977). Scientific theories and their domains. In F. Suppe (Ed.), *The structure of scientific theories* (2nd ed.) (pp. 518–565). Urbana, IL: University of Illinois Press.

Suppe, F. (Ed.). *The structure of scientific theories* (2nd ed.). Urbana, IL: University of Illinois Press.

Toulmin, S. (1977). Does the distinction between normal and revolutionary science hold water? In I. Lakatos & A. Musgrave (Eds.), *Criticism and the growth of knowledge* (pp. 39–47). London: Cambridge University Press.

Webster, G., Jacox, A., & Baldwin, B. (1981). Nursing theory and the ghost of the received view. In J.C. McCloskey & H.K. Grace (Eds.), *Current Issues in Nursing* (pp. 29–30). Boston: Blackwell Scientific.

Chapter 35

Theories: Components, Development, Evaluation

Margaret E. Hardy

The roles of concepts, statements of relationship, and models in theory development are examined. Criteria for evaluating theories are outlined, and the tentative nature of theories is discussed.

Although nurses in their everyday work are expected to evaluate health conditions of persons under their care, usually little thought is given to evaluating the soundness of the theory and knowledge which guides their action. If the theory is poorly suspended by evidence (i.e., the theory is not "true"), the health of the persons for which nurses are responsible may be severely jeopardized. As health professionals, nurses need to be able to make sound judgments about the rationale for various treatments, therapies, and care. It is often assumed that because an idea is in print (particularly if in a textbook or professional journal), it must be true. Many of the theories on which health professionals base their activities, however, are open to severe criticisms. With the speed with which new ideas are published, nurses now more than ever need to keep abreast of the development of relevant knowledge and be able to evaluate that knowledge in order to make informed judgments.

Unless nurses can assess the knowledge generated in such diverse areas as stress, systems, decision making, leadership, self-concept, body image, family, groups, body systems, they cannot use that knowledge wisely and constructively. Failure or inability to assess knowledge relevant to her area of work means the nurse must function as a technician, depending on others to interpret the knowledge-base which guides her actions. If nurses intend to direct their own actions in a responsible manner, they must become well informed on developing knowledge, they must be able to evaluate critically the knowledge developed, and they must make informed judgments based on this knowledge. They also must learn to function optimally as generalists. A competent practitioner really does not have the luxury of concentrating her efforts in a restricted area (psychiatry is currently under attack for the narrowness of its activities), but must take into account a wide variety of phenomena which have bearing on her clients.

Our comprehension of the world around us is based on the use of concepts, hypotheses, and theories. Nurses, as practitioners in the health field, apply and use knowledge generated from theories. In spite of the pervasiveness of theories in guiding and controlling our everyday life, the literature on theory development is diverse and confusing, and it generally is little related to the activities of practitioners. This article attempts to identify the structure of theory, to differentiate between different types of theoretical statements, and to identify criteria for evaluating theories.

Concepts

Concepts are labels, categories, or selected properties of objects to be studied; they are the bricks from which theories are constructed. Concepts are the dimensions, aspects, or attributes of reality which interest the scientist. Patients, illness, cardiovascular diseases, nurses, or physicians are examples of concepts used in health-related fields on which research may be based. The scientist constructs theories in his domain of interest by linking concepts of one class or attribute to concepts of other classes or attributes. When he has a set of interrelated statements or hypotheses concerning the relationships between concepts (i.e., when he has filled between the bricks with mortar), he has a theory. Concepts are the basic elements of theory. A major part of the evaluation of a theory is the identification and assessment of the concepts.

Components and Structure of Theory

A theory may be viewed from a variety of perspectives. For the purpose of exploring the structure of a theory, one may view theory as a language (Rudner, 1966). Like any language, theory consists of elements, formu-

lations, and a set of definitions, i.e., it is comprised of syntax and semantics. When an investigator studies a scientific theory, he is interested in the logical structure or the relation between the elements (concepts) of the theory (the syntax) and the meaning given to the elements (the semantics). Syntax, then, is concerned with the occurrence of concepts in the axioms, postulates, or hypotheses of a theory and the relationship between the concepts and between the hypotheses of a theory, while semantics is concerned with the specific meaning attributed to the concepts. When a theory is made explicit or is formalized, one can examine the syntax and determine if the structure of the theory is consistent with the rules of logic.

The Semantics of Theory

Theories consist of two types of elements or terms. One set, the *derived* terms, are specifically introduced through definition whereas the other set, the *primitive* terms, remain undefined (Hempel, 1952). The primitive terms (or concepts) are the primary building blocks of theories from which new terms are derived. Both primitive and derived terms appear in a theory's axioms and postulates and give meaning to an otherwise uninterpreted or formalized system.

Concepts are defined and their meanings are understood only within the framework of the theory of which they are a part. Much conceptual confusion exists in theoretical areas upon which nurses draw. Concepts are often vaguely defined; the same concept may be defined and described many different ways (each writer providing his own definition). For example, within the area of role theory the concepts of role, status, and role behavior overlap and are often used interchangeably. Concepts develop as part of theory and are altered and refined as a body of knowledge grows. The concern for clarifying concepts involves a dilemma of trying to achieve consistency in meaning without premature closure of theories. Conceptual confusion and vagueness in theories appear to be a necessary and an important condition for creativity in science as elsewhere. Persons in the more applied professions often find this state of confusion difficult to cope with.

The refinement of concepts (improving the bricks) is a continuous process which involves not only sharpening of theoretical and operational definitions, but also modification of existing theory. Theories and concepts are reformulated by relating the theoretical world to the empirical, by organizing a great many concrete items into a small number of classes (regrouping the bricks), and by relating diverse concepts within a more general system of concepts.

General or Abstract

Concepts may be ordered on the basis of their level of abstractness. A specific occurrence, such as a patient's chest pain, is treated as a special case of a more general condition, such as heart disease. Heart disease, in turn, is a special condition of the more general area, the circulatory system.

Concepts are also appraised for their degree of generality; they are assessed according to the extent they change or vary. Concepts which refer to classes or categories of phenomena may be called *nonvariable* (Hage, 1972). Such concepts are found in typologies in which classes are clearly defined; an observation either fits or does not fit into a given category, depending upon the presence or absence of the property of interest, e.g., male, female. Concepts which are used to order phenomena according to some property or concepts which refer to dimensions of phenomena are called *variables* (Hage, 1972). When the results of observations fall on a continuum, the property being observed is a variable concept, e.g., 27 years, 82 years. It has been argued (Hage, 1972) that concepts that have a continuum should be utilized more frequently in conceptualizing and theory construction because such concepts facilitate theory development, are not restricted to time and place, and are more subtle for description and classification. The following illustrates the difference between nonvariable and variable concepts: Schizophrenia, manic depression, phobic reactions, and passive-aggressive traits are nonvariable concepts; they are bound by culture. The following general variable con-

cepts are not so bound: anxiety, the degree of depression, intensity of affect, extent of contact with reality, frequency of phobic reactions. These general variable concepts may be utilized to describe the specific mental disorders listed above as well as other normal and abnormal mental states, whereas the nonvariable concepts (disease entities) are specifically either-or types of abnormal phenomena. By using both abstract and variable concepts, the scientist is able to develop laws and theories which have a wide range of applicability.

Theoretical or Operational

Concepts, whether nonvariable or variable, may have both a theoretical definition and an operational definition. The theoretical definition gives meaning to the terms in context of the theory and permits any reader to assess the validity of that definition. The operational definition tells how the concept is linked to concrete situations. An operational definition, which is used in the process of giving experiential meaning to the concept of a theory, describes a set of physical procedures which must be carried out in order to assign to every case a value for the concept. For example, the concept of level of aggression may be operationally defined as the number of times a child hits another child during an hour of play. How adequately the operational definition reflects the theoretical concept is another matter for consideration. That is, not only do concepts need operational definitions but the operational definition must be a valid reflection of the theoretical meaning of the concept. In this example, the operational definition certainly permits an observer to assign a level of "aggression" to each child observed. The level of aggression score for a child, however, may not reflect the theoretical meaning of the concept. The operational definition does not take into account the intent of the child, aggressive acts other than hitting, or the intensity of the act. The dilemma encountered in trying to link observable events to theoretical constructs is that the more concretely concepts are defined, the more restricted is the scope of the theory and the less useful is the theory. In spite of the difficulty in developing operational definitions, it is necessary to define theoretical terms in a way that the concepts can be measured. Only through developing measurements of concepts can hypotheses and, in turn, theories be tested.

Operational definitions are a necessary part of theory construction. Operational definitions permit the validity of concepts to be assessed. They permit hypotheses to be tested and the empirical relevance of a theory to be assessed. They also permit other scientists to replicate the study. Operational definitions, which form the bridge between the theory and the empirical world, are modified over time as both theoretical and technological knowledge grow.

Theoretical concepts only make sense when considered within the framework of the theories of which they are a part. Such concepts may be examined on the basis of the degree of observability of their referent. Observable concepts (concepts that refer directly to observable objects) are likely to be found in derived theorems which are to be tested, whereas nonobservable concepts are found in axioms. Nonobservable concepts —intervening variables or hypothetical constructs— are derived on the basis of inferences from observable referents. Intervening variables are concepts that are based on inferences from observations. To illustrate this point, consider the following: A state of anxiety is often inferred on the basis of observations of increased heart rate, sweaty palms, and nausea. Anxiety per se is not observable.

Hypothetical concepts are more abstract than intervening variables. Belief in their existence is based primarily on theoretical support, and only indirectly on supporting empirical data. The id and the unconscious are examples of hypothetical constructs. The distinctions between intervening variables and hypothetical constructs are not at all clear. In one theory, a concept may be a hypothetical construct; in another theory, the same concept may be an intervening variable.

Attributes of Concepts Utilized for Evaluation

Concepts are abstractions from concrete events; concepts themselves can have a varying degree of abstraction. As one moves up the level of abstraction in order to develop systematic explanations of general phenomena, one is faced with the problem of relating back from the symbolic concepts to concrete phenomena. Part of the difficulty in doing this is dependent on the adequacy of the rules of correspondence (or the links one is able to make) between the theoretical concepts and their empirical referents. The generality (abstraction) of concepts and the relationship between the concepts and the empirical referent (testability) are criteria used to evaluate a theory. Examinations of the semantics of a theory provides another means for evaluation. This may, in part, be examined by assessing the intersubjectivity of meaning. The intersubjectivity of the meaning of concepts refers to whether the concepts are given a meaning similar to the meaning used by other scientists in related areas (Reynolds, 1971).

Statements of Relationships Between Concepts

Syntax of Theory

If a theory is formalized or made explicit, the syntax, or relationship, between concepts can be examined and the logical adequacy of the theory can be assessed. In assessing a theory's logical structure, the meanings of the concepts themselves are not taken into consideration. That is, symbols may be used to represent the concepts. This facilitates the examination of the logical structure without confusing the issue by considering the explicit meaning of the concepts. For example, the statement that social stress results in heart disease can be expressed symbolically. If social stress is represented by X, heart disease by Y, and results in by $\rightarrow$, then the statement social stress results in heart disease can be expressed by $X \rightarrow Y$. A formalization of statements like this and other interrelated statements in a theory facilitate the examination of the structure of a theory.

Types of Relationships

To analyze the structure of a theory it is necessary to identify the relationships between concepts. Some types of relationships and their meanings are summarized in Figure 35-1. Relationships listed are not mutually exclusive. Some of the relationships between concepts may be illustrated by using Selye's (1956) theory of stress. This stress formulation indicates that stressors result in a physiological syndrome identified as the General Adaptive Syndrome (GAS). If in this formulation the relationship between stressors and GAS is determinate, then this implies that the concepts are *time-ordered* (stressors occur prior to the development of GAS), *sufficient* (if stressors occur, then GAS occurs regardless of anything else), and *necessary* (if stressors and only if stressors occur, then GAS occurs). The determinate relationship between stressors and GAS is asymmetrical (if stressors occur, then GAS occurs; if no stressors occur, then no conclusions may be reached about the occurrence of GAS) rather than symmetrical (if stressors occur, GAS occurs; if GAS occurs, then stressors occur). It is possible, however, that the relationship between stressors and GAS is not determinate but probabilistic (if stressors occur, there exists a 90 percent chance that GAS will occur) or conditional (if stressors occur, then GAS occurs, but only if specific physiological condition W exists). For clarity in theoretical formulations, it is necessary to specify the type of relationships between concepts. Although the in identification of causal relationships in the health sciences is the reason for considerable success in disease prevention, relationships which are stochastic and relationships which are conditional are valuable in the prediction and control of disease-related events and hence should be identified rather than ignored.

Sign of the Relationship

An additional characteristic of the relationship between concepts is the sign (±) of the relationship. Concepts may be either positively (+) or inversely (−) related. The sign of relationships, though being discussed here in the context of theory development, really relates to the concept of measures of association or correlation. Thus, in the postulates—the greater X, the greater Y, and the greater Y, the greater Z—a positive relationship is implied between concepts as measured by some measure of association. Knowing that Y increases with X and Z increases with Y, it can be logically deduced that Z increases with X. The sign of the relationship between X and Z depends upon the sign of the relationships between the concepts X and Y, and Y and Z in the postulates. The sign rule has been summarized from work by Zetterberg (1963); Costner and Leik (1964) stated that the sign of the deduced relationship is the algebraic product of the signs of the postulated relationships. If Y is positively correlated with X and Z is positively correlated with Y, then it can be concluded by deduction and the sign rule that Z is positively correlated with X. This process of deduction may be expressed as:

$$\text{If} \qquad X \xrightarrow{+} Y$$
$$\text{and} \qquad Y \xrightarrow{+} Z$$
$$\overline{\text{then} \qquad X \xrightarrow{+} Z}$$

It is still an empirical question as to whether this logically deduced relationship actually exists. A relationship which is true according to logic is not necessarily true empirically.

Formalizing and Examining a Set of Statements

This discussion has emphasized that the evaluation of a theory's structure is facilitated if the concepts and the relationships between the concepts are formalized. The following stress formulation will be utilized

Nature of Relation[1]	Meaning
Symmetrical	If A, then B; if B, then A
Asymmetrical	If A, then B; but if no A, no conclusion about B
Causal	If A, always B
Probabilistic	If A, probably B
Time order	If A, later B
Concurrent	If A, also B
Sufficient	If A, then B, regardless of anything else
Conditional	If A, then B, but only if C
Necessary	If A and only if A, then B

[1]The relations are not all mutually exclusive

Figure 35-1 *Relationships between Concepts*

to illustrate ways of assessing the syntax of theory: Social stress results in emotional tension whereas cognitive dissonance and social stress are inversely related; emotional tension results in somatic dysfunctioning. These statements may be formalized and displayed diagrammatically or in a matrix (Figure 35-2a and b). The matrix used here is an adaptation of a data correlation matrix. The visual representation of the formalized model makes it relatively simple to examine the theory's structure. The diagram shows the relationship between the concepts while the matrix readily displays the completeness and logical consistency of the formulation. Discontinuities in the stress formulation are evident in both the diagram (lack of connections between the concepts) and the matrix (empty cells). Deductions can be made from the postulates stated. Using the sign rule and the deduced relationship, we may conclude that A and C are positively associated. That is, an increase in social stress is associated with an increase in somatic dysfunctioning. From this deduction the formulation is made more complete; no logical inconsistencies exist. The formalization of a theory to facilitate an evaluation of it will be discussed later.

Types of Statements

Although "postulates," "proposition," "hypothesis," "axiom," "laws," "principles," and "empirical generalizations" refer to different types of statements, they have a common characteristic in that they link together two or more concepts. A theory is made up of a set of interrelated propositions, theorems, or hypotheses derived from axioms, initial hypotheses, or postulates. Hypotheses refer to facts that are as yet unexperienced; they are corrigible in view of fresh knowledge. Principles and empirical generalizations are statements about data and are generally believed to be true. The distinguishing characteristic between empirical generalizations and hypotheses is that a hypothesis may be formulated in the absence of data, while an empirical generalization summarizes empirical evidence. Statements differ in their degree of generality and degree of empirical support. Empirical generalizations, since they summarize data, are closer to reality than are hypotheses. However, hypotheses, because they are at a higher level of generalization, are invaluable in aiding our understanding of events which have not yet been systematically tested.

Scientific hypotheses are more or less *grounded* on previous knowledge, i.e., they are partially supported (or at least not refuted) by empirical evidence and by theory. Hypotheses are developed from a rationale; they are not wild, groundless guesses. They should show reasonable conjecture—not fly in the face of existing knowledge.

Laws are well grounded; they have strong empirical support. They state a constant relation among two or more variables, each representing (at least partly and indirectly) a property of concrete systems. An example of a law is $E = Mc^2$. In the psychosocial area few, if any, laws exist. Laws are propositions that assert universal connections between properties.

Statements on the highest level of generality are

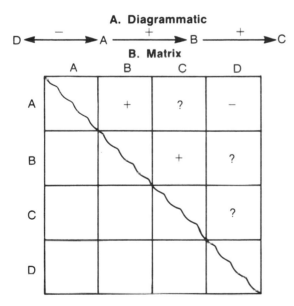

Figure 35-2 *Diagrammatic (a) and Matrix (b) Representation of Stress Formulation: Concepts and Their Relationships*[1]

[1] Concepts: Social stress, A; emotional tension, B; somatic dysfunctioning, C; cognitive dissonance, D. Sign of the relationship: Positive, +; inverse, −; unspecified, ?
Relationships between concepts: Symmetrical, ↔; asymmetrical, →

laws and axioms. Statements on a lower level of generality (propositions, theorems, hypotheses) can be deduced from laws. The purpose of deduction is to test the general statements. In a deductive system, high-level statements can be falsified by the falsification of lower-level (deduced) statements. In any hypothetico-deductive theory, the less universal statements or lower-level statements are themselves still, strictly speaking, universal statements; they are empirical generalizations and must have the character of hypotheses. Postulates, axioms, and laws are primitive statements about an infinite universe, whereas hypotheses and empirical generalizations are statements about a finite universe.

The following examples may illustrate the difference between laws and hypotheses: A law in physiology is: Cardiac output = heart rate × stroke volume. This statement is true under all conditions (i.e., for all human hearts regardless of time or culture and also for nonhuman hearts). An hypothesis in physiology is: Resting potentials in nerve and muscle cells depend only on the difference in potassium ion concentration across the cell membrane. The statement has not reached the status of a law. Although there is reasonable evidence to support this statement, experimental evidence suggests that other ions may affect resting potentials. The generalization holds true for most muscle and nerve cells rather than for all cells. An hypothesis in social psychology is: In any task-oriented group, inequality in task activity among group members occurs and results in role differentiation. This generalization has mixed empirical support. Some experimental studies corroborate this hypothesis, while other experimental studies identify conditions under which role differentiation in task-oriented groups does not occur. The generalization may only apply under specific conditions and only in the American culture.

Models

Although a scientific theory is considered to be a deductive system, the relationship between variables may best be expressed in terms of a model. That is, an investigator may formalize a theory, identify its postulates, identify or derive the remaining propositions, and then decide that the problem of relationships is best represented by a model. A model is a simplified representation of a theory or of certain complex events, structures, or systems. Constructing a model forces the theorist to specify the precise relationship between components.

Models, like theories, are isomorphic systems; they are selective representations of the empirical world with which the scientist is concerned; crucial aspects of the phenomena are identified and aspects not considered important are ignored. Models are descriptive; they simplify the area of concern and can help the scientist grasp key elements and the relationships between these elements. The distinction between theories and models is not always clear. For example, what is considered a well-established theory in one academic area may be used as a model to represent phenomena in another area. Modeling is a technique used to describe and explain as well as to generate ideas and predictions.

Types

One type of model is an *analog* model, or an analogy. This model directs attention to resemblances between theoretical entities and familiar subject matter (Kaplan, 1964). For example, a nurse may use the analogy of a mechanical pump to explain to a patient the workings of his heart. In doing this, the nurse is using properties of the pump (an entity with which the patient is familiar) to explain characteristics about the heart (an entity with which the patient is unfamiliar). A problem which is difficult to understand may be made more comprehensible by the use of an analogy. The study of social organizations has been based on an organic model, e.g., Parsons' (1951) description of social systems, and social interactions have been described in terms of economic exchanges (Blau, 1964). Because the model is "true" in one area of science, however, does not mean that it will be true or hold up on another area. The model must be tested for its validity in each area of application. Although many characteristics of the organic model are inappropriate for describing social systems, the organic model has been a useful starting point for the study of social phenomena.

Iconic models are used if a direct representation of the subject is wanted (DiRenzo, 1966). The model may vary as to the number of properties represented and the level of abstraction. A kidney machine, for example, although it does not resemble the kidney in appearance, does represent relatively accurately some of the kidney processes. A model of the heart (built to scale), a scaled model of a DNA molecule, an organizational chart of a hospital, and a miniature social system depicting the hierarchical structure and communication processes in an organization are examples of iconic models. These models represent the original phenomena but in another form. Such models are useful to the extent that they increase our sense of understanding of the entity. This type of modeling has been utilized more perhaps in the physical sciences than in the social sciences. The usefulness of iconic models for understanding social phenomena may be directly related to our ability to identify key variables and to abstract these characteristics. For many persons it is easier to accept a plastic model of the heart as a useful model than it is to accept a three-person decision-making network as a useful model of a social organization. The value of models is dependent upon the extent to which they increase understanding, explain phenomena, or give us a sense of what is going on and why.

Another type of model is the *symbolic* model which represents phenomena figuratively (DiRenzo, 1966). A set of connected symbols, objects, or concepts may be used to represent a problem of interest. The relationship between concepts may be represented diagrammatically to facilitate conceptualization and understanding.

Use

Although models have proved to be extremely helpful in theory construction, they should be used carefully. Models have no truth value themselves. There is no guarantee that a model that has been successfully used in one area of study will be useful in another area. A major question to consider is the extent to which the model faithfully represents the phenomena of interest. There may be a tendency to overlook the differences between the phenomena of interest and the model since the scientist is more interested in the similarities. The differences, however, may completely negate the usefulness of the model. Models are tools for understanding reality which should be used judiciously and be replaced or modified when outmoded or inappropriate.

Criteria for Evaluating Theories

Theories are sets of interrelated hypotheses which are subject to reformulation and refinement. The development of adequate theories to describe, explain, predict, and control phenomena is a slow process and requires the cooperative effort of many persons. Knowledge is not acquired by one person in isolation but results from the cumulative efforts of many persons over a long period of time. Various writers, primarily philosophers, have suggested criteria to assist in the evaluation of theory. A theory may be evaluated in terms of its logical adequacy, abstractness, testability, empirical adequacy, and pragmatic adequacy (Schrag, 1967). These criteria are not meant to hinder the development of theories but to provide guidelines.

Theories are developed to help describe, explain, predict, and control phenomena in the world around us whether the theory is concerned with the area of astronomy, genetics, physics, chemistry, psychology, sociology, physiology, or biology. Implicit in the discussion of theories is the assumption that a theory can be evaluated according to certain universal standards. Regardless of the content of the theory, an investigator examines the underlying assumptions, the validity of the concepts and of the general perspective, the degree of generality of the theory, the soundness of the reasoning, the testability of the hypotheses, the empirical support for the hypotheses, the ability to control and manipulate the phenomena, and the degree of accuracy with which predictions can be made.

Meaning and Logical Adequacy

That few theories successfully meet all these criteria does not mean that theories should not be evaluated. A first step in evaluating theory is to identify basic assumptions (these may not be stated), the concepts, and the relationships between the concepts and to consider the validity of the assumptions, the validity of the meaning attributed to the concepts (are the concepts defined in a manner similar to that used by other scientists in the area?), and the logic of the theoretical system.

When an investigator has reached a conclusion about the validity of the concepts and proposed theory, he can assess the logic of the argument. In doing this, the scientist is concerned with the reasonableness of the argument. The logical adequacy of a theory can be evaluated by formalizing the theory and examining it for discontinuities, discrepancies, and contradictions. In the example cited earlier (Figure 35-2a and b), discontinuities in the theory were evident. When the theory was formalized, it was apparent that nothing was said about the relationship between social stress and somatic dysfunctioning or about the relationship between cognitive dissonance and emotional tension and cognitive dissonance and somatic dysfunctioning. From the postulates and using the sign rule, it was deduced that A and C are positively associated. Since D is related (inversely) only to A, nothing can be said about its relationship to B or C. Because the relationships between A and B and B and C are asymmetrical (A → B, B → C), the conclusion that A is positively correlated with and results in C is logical. Had the relationship between the variables been symmetrical (A ↔ B, B ↔ C), then the conclusion that A is related to C might not hold up. The relationship between A and B, for example, says that A and B vary together; the relationship is not necessarily causal. A and B may be related because of their common relationship to another variable, i.e., the relationship could be spurious.

Likewise, the symmetrical relationship between B and C might be spurious. If either or both of the rela-tionships in these postulates are spurious, then the relationship between the concepts in the deduced proposition is open to question. No contradictions were evident in the stress formulation. Formalizing a theory increases the probability that discontinuities and contradictions will be identified.

Operational and Empirical Adequacy

Next, the theory can be assessed for its testability. To be testable, a theory must have operationally defined concepts. Since Bridgman's (1927) introduction of the phrase, "operational definition," scientists in all areas have been concerned with identifying adequate operational definitions for their concepts. When operational definitions for theoretical concepts have been established, the theory can be tested. Assessing the operational adequacy of a theory requires consideration of (a) whether the concepts can be measured and (b) how accurately the operational definitions reflect the theoretical concepts.

In testing a theory, it can be subjected to falsification (be found false) rather than to confirmation (Popper, 1959). If a sincere attempt is made to refute a theory and the theory stands up, the theory is considered supported or tentatively confirmed. Terms such as "confirmation," "verification," "support," "corroboration," "disconfirmation," "falsification," "failure to support," relate to the empirical base for a theory. Hypotheses may not be proved true, verified, or falsified by limited evidence, but evidence gathered over time from a variety of sources may tend to support, bear out, corroborate, or be in accord with an hypothesis, and thus be confirming evidence. If the evidence does not support the hypothesis, the evidence may be viewed as disconfirming rather than falsifying; the hypothesis is not "proved false." The use of the term "evidence" and the terms "disconfirming," "supporting," and "corroborating" suggests that one recognizes the status of the hypothesis as tentative—awaiting further testing. An hypothesis is not an absolute statement or a truth statement; it should be stated in a way that it can be tested and refuted. For data from any one study and for cumulative evidence from numerous studies, the question of the empirical adequacy of the theory is raised, i.e., how well does the evidence support the theory?

Over time, evidence that both supports and fails to support a theory accumulates. When the relative strengths of the evidence are evaluated, some conclusion about the empirical adequacy of a theory may be reached. Assessing the empirical adequacy of a theory requires the determination of the degree of congruence between the theoretical claims and the empirical evidence.

Generality

Another criterion used to evaluate a theory is the degree of generality or the degree of abstractness which characterizes it. The more general a theory, the more useful it is. A theory of the grieving process which can be applied to persons of all ages, to persons in any culture, and to losses of any object is more useful than a theory of grieving which can be applied only to middle-aged persons who lose a spouse.

Contribution to Understanding

A theory may be assessed as to how much it increases understanding. Does it describe the phenomena and give a sense of insight? Does it suggest new ideas and a new way of looking at the phenomena? The scientist constantly looks for theories that will increase his understanding of phenomena, which are relatively simple explanations, and which suggest new lines of reasoning and new avenues of exploration.

Predictability

Another criterion used to assess theory is the extent to which predictions can be made. A theory may describe a process, may increase the understanding of the process, but it may not assist in making any predictions about the outcomes of that process. A theory, for example, may permit a description and explanation of a process after it has occurred; i.e., it is possible to look at a family which has suffered a "loss" and describe the family behavior in terms of adjustment to a crisis, but it may not be possible to predict accurately the behavior of family members in response to this crisis before the crisis occurs.

Pragmatic Adequacy

Since the purpose of a theory is to explain, predict, and control, the ability to control phenomena of interest is one means for assessing a theory. This criterion is pragmatic adequacy (Schrag, 1967). A theory may permit explanation and accurate prediction, but the theory may not permit the scientist to control the phenomena of interest.

The business of the applied professions (nursing, engineering, social work, medicine, architecture, political science) is to make *use* of existing theory to predict certain processes or outcomes and to control "events" in such a way that desired outcomes are achieved. The usefulness of a theory (pragmatic adequacy) for changing conditions is of major importance to the health professions. In the biological sciences many theories enable scientists or professionals to control outcomes; e.g., disease control, control (prevention) of degenerative process in the body, and control or replacement of defective body parts. Although it is recognized that science has as its goal the production of knowledge for predicting and controlling phenomena, the ethics of using this knowledge is only now being examined in detail. Some of the decisions as to whether man should use the knowledge he has generated to control and alter the forces around him are being questioned more in some areas than in others, i.e., few question the use of vaccines to prevent disease, but the use of abortions to prevent overpopulation has been severely attacked by some segments of the population. Although there are relatively few theories (particularly in the area of social behavior) which permit the scientist to control phenomena, the development of such theories is likely to increase. The problems associated with the use of these theories by the applied professions will also increase.

Tentative Nature of Theories

Although rules and guidelines can be postulated to aid in the development and evaluations of theories, theories are tentative. With new knowledge, old facts are subject to different interpretations, and different data are brought to light. The development of theory is man's attempt to establish structure and meaning in his world. In assessing existing knowledge, one needs to take into account the culture of the scientific community as well as the values of society in general. The values of both communities come into play in many aspects of the process of establishing knowledge. The selection of problem areas and the development and use of concepts involve arbitrary choices. The theories that develop reflect the interests of the scientific community and of society and do not necessarily represent the areas that are in most need of examination.

References

Blau, P.M. (1964). *Exchange and power in social life.* New York: John Wiley & Sons.

Bridgman, P.W. (1927). *The logic of modern physics.* New York: Macmillan.

Costner, H.L., & Leik, R.K. (1964). Deductions from axiomatic theory. *American Sociological Review, 29,* 819–835.

Di Renzo, G.J. (Ed.). (1966). *Concepts, theory and explanation in the behavioral sciences.* New York: Random House.

Hage, J. (1972). *Techniques and problems of theory construction in sociology.* New York: John Wiley & Sons.

Hempel, C.G. (1952). Fundamentals of concept formation in empirical science. In *International encyclopedia of unified sciences.* Chicago: The University of Chicago Press.

Kaplan, A. (1964). *The conduct of inquiry.* San Francisco: Chandler.

Parsons, T. (1951). *The social system.* Glencoe, IL: Free Press.

Popper, K. (1959). *The logic of scientific discovery.* New York: Basic Books.

Reynolds, P.D. (1971). *A primer in theory construction.* Indianapolis: Bobbs-Merrill.

Rudner, R.S. (1966). *Philosophy of social science.* Englewood Cliffs, N.J.: Prentice-Hall.

Schrag, C. (1967). Elements of theoretical analysis in sociology. In L. Gross (Ed.), *Sociological theory: Inquiries and paradigms* (pp. 220–253). New York: Harper & Row.

Selye, H. (1956). *The stress of life.* New York: McGraw-Hill.

Zetterberg, H. (1963). *On theory and verification in sociology (A much revised edition).* Totowa, NJ: Bedmeister Press.

The Author Comments

My interest in comparing theories that address similar phenomena began in graduate school when I read Karen Horney's publications and found them to be a viable alternative to Freud's theory. During my first position as an instructor of nursing at the University of Washington, I became more aware of the need for a rational basis for selecting the "best" theoretical approach to a clinical problem, and my interest in comparing theories expanded. At this time, I was preparing for my first teaching assignment, a graduate level course on application of biopsychosocial approaches to care of adult medical patients. The course had a clinical component that augmented the need for the theory component of the course to be relevant and useful. In reading the literature, I was absolutely amazed by the diversity of approaches to anxiety, stress, crisis, and adaptation; by the lack of empirical support for most theoretical notions; and by the continued dominance of some ideas despite the generation of research that did not support them. I wondered on what basis (other than personal preference for a theoretical approach) a clinician decided which theoretical approach to use. I felt that an eclectic approach was not useful: it not only did not contribute to knowledge development but also tended to be a superficial acknowledgment of some theoretical ideas rather than a serious guide to action.

In preparing for the second course I taught, which was for nursing administration students, I found that although the theories for this course had to do with leadership and job satisfaction, rather than anxiety and stress, the same problem in theory selection existed—with an added dimension. The nursing literature tended to present ideas as "true" and seldom acknowledged or presented the diversity of theory and research that actually existed. The *scientific* work on organization and group processes was not used in the nursing literature. Furthermore, the nursing sources tended to draw fairly heavily on someone else's interpretation of this scientific literature and to present these interpretations erroneously as well-established generalizations. I found the literature in the basic social sciences a fascinating source for teaching and felt compelled to let students know about various research strategies for studying social structures and processes. My approach of reading widely in diverse disciplines for class preparation probably began in this period.

My doctoral work in sociology increased my awareness of the importance of theory, the presence of diverse perspectives, and the historical development of social theory. I also became aware of the understanding and skill necessary for carrying out research—the necessary variables had to be controlled, manipulated, and measured in order for there to be clear-cut research findings that had a direct bearing on theory.

During my period of doctoral study at the University of Washington, the value of much of the social psychological research was being questioned as the operant psychology approach began to be used successfully to look at sociological phenomena. The validity of symbolic interaction theory and cognitive processes was being questioned in light of principles of operant psychology, which made it possible to explain a great deal with a handful of concepts. Multivariate analysis was being used by some faculty to develop theory while others studied the same concepts using a handful of subjects in a small group laboratory. For example, Richard Emerson, who had an appointment partially funded by the nurse-scientist program and accordingly influenced the thinking of many nurse-scientists, was consciously attempting to construct a theory of social exchange that was based on operant principles but went beyond them to explain social processes and social structure. Some theoretical predictions on exchange and cooperation were being researched using a small computer to "run" the experiments. In the room next door, hard-wired operant-psychology-type studies (with button pressing) were being conducted on the same theoretical notions. Diversity in theory and methodologic strategies were the order of the day. The diversity of approaches in the sociology department were tied together by a total commitment to the value of sound empirical work. Methodologic issues and problems were the focus of discussion, teaching, publishing, and research of faculty (and doctoral students).

Another concept affecting theory was being introduced at this time. In my last 3 years in the department (1968 to 1971), equality for women (students and faculty members) was becoming a major departmental issue, and much consciousness-raising occurred. However, the possible importance of gender as a significant variable worthy of study had not yet become a subject of discussion. In 1970 and 1971, I had to make a conscious decision whether to use males or females as subjects for my dissertation. It was very apparent in the research studies of cooperation and coalition that patterns of behaviors for males varied under identifiable conditions but that females, on the other hand, did not have identifiable or predictable patterns of cooperation or competition. To control variance and obtain clear results I used male subjects. The notion that gender may be a significant concept within a theory, the focus of a theory, or in altering existing theory had not yet been articulated.

My first teaching position after doctoral work involved developing and teaching a core graduate-level course on stress, crisis, and adaptation. It readily became apparent to me that if graduate students were to do more than regurgitate information on an objective exam, they needed to know more about theories, how to examine them, how to distinguish among theories in the same theoretical domain (e.g., stress theories), and how to weigh the soundness and value of existing theory. The abstract nature of this approach was initially, in early classes, difficult for students to grapple with and understand. Student anxiety was high and I became aware of many students using tape recorders and others trying to take down "exactly" what I said or what was written on an overhead projection. I knew that what I was teaching was important and also valuable to students. Several semesters later in their clinical program students would drop by and comment on how very valuable the course had been to them in subsequent course work, how it had changed their way of thinking. It is difficult to convince new students of this when their anxiety is high over the content and when there are few good library sources (let alone textbooks) for a course. I decided to write out my ideas for students to read and condensed 24 hours (what had evolved from one class in the first set of lectures to six lectures three years later) of solid, referenced lectures into an article titled "The Nature of Theories." I distributed this to students and received a favorable response. I felt that learning was occurring with much less anxiety than before. For the purpose of maximizing student learning, and to lessen their frustration and mine, I spent the summer putting together the book *Theoretical Foundations of Nursing* (New York: MSS Information Corp., 1973). The following year I submitted the article to *Nursing Research,* and it was published in 1974 as "Theories: Components, Development, Evaluation."

It should be noted that many faculty members themselves did not feel comfortable with teaching theory, so I—a naive, energetic new graduate—took on classes of 180 students. In teaching a summer offering of this course in seminar style, the ambiance was totally different—not one of anxiety but one of challenge, intrigue, excitement, and insight. I have often wondered whether I would have written the article had I not had large classes in which students expressed such a need to have information on theory pulled together for them. However, I realize I probably would have because students still need that same type of information.

I found last year that, regardless of the subject matter of a course, if I spent the first couple of classes talking about theory, concepts, and evaluation of theory before moving into the substantive content of the course (e.g., role theory), students' learning of substantive content markedly increased and the intellectual tone of the class increased. This seemed to occur whether or not students had already taken a theory course or any courses at the master's level.

In retrospect, the article probably should have been broken into two parts—one dealing with components of theory an the other with evaluation of theory. In rewriting a chapter that included a section on theory evaluation for *Role Theory: Perspectives for Health Professionals* last summer I found the basic ideas still germane. The evaluative criteria can be more clearly prioritized but are basically sound. Perhaps I have emphasized the theoretical embeddedness of concepts more, but the importance of logical adequacy and empirical adequacy of a theory is still utmost importance for those planning to implement a theory-based change—whether for a client, family or community. The growing interest in working with the "revised view of science" does not invalidate the evaluation criteria and process but circumscribes the criteria that are likely to be of value.

To summarize, my motivation for writing the article can probably be identified as responding to students' frustration in dealing with abstract and new ideas, to the lack of sound writings in the literature to which students could turn, and to my commitment to the importance of theory in nursing and the use of a rational base for selecting theory. The focus of my work evolved from an ongoing dialogue with students on the one hand and, on the other, continuous work with the ideas in the literature.

—MARGARET E. HARDY

REFERENCE

Hardy, M.E. (1973). *Theoretical foundations of nursing.* New York: MSS Information Corporation.

Chapter 36

Nursing Systems and Nursing Models

John R. Phillips

Since the primary goal of nursing theory is the generation of knowledge specific to nursing, the process of theory building must be couched in a nursing frame of reference. Otherwise, the obtained knowledge will not be nursing knowledge which can be used to build or expand nursing science or be used for nursing education, practice, or research.

The evolution of nursing science as any young science is dependent upon knowledge borrowed from other disciplines. There will always be a core of knowledge which will be used by all the sciences. However, the process of borrowing theories and models from other disciplines has hampered nurses in learning how to ask questions which are of specific concern to nursing or in conceptualizing how the borrowed knowledge is to be used to generate theory to expand nursing science.

The creation of nurse scientist programs was an attempt to avoid the pitfalls of borrowing knowledge from other disciplines. One would wonder how effective these programs have been in the testing of theory to obtain knowledge to advance nursing science. Newman (1972), in reference to nurse scientist programs, points out that the testing of theory in another discipline's framework relates the data more to that discipline than to nursing. Nurse scientists may contribute to the general knowledge of order in man, but it will continue to be borrowed knowledge (Johnson, 1968). As long as nurses continue to borrow theories and models and test theory in other disciplines and not relate the data to nursing, the evolution of nursing science will be slow. Borrowed knowledge from other disciplines must be synthesized into conceptual systems and models of nursing; otherwise, the focus of nursing will remain within the conceptual systems and models of other disciplines.

Nursing practice is another method nursing uses to discover theory (Wald & Leonard, 1964). The lack of

About the Author

JOHN R. PHILLIPS is currently an Associate Professor in the Division of Nursing at New York University. A Virginian by birth, Dr. Phillips considers New York City, where he has lived and worked for more than 30 years, to be home. After serving for 4 years in the U.S. Air Force, Dr. Phillips moved to New York and began his nursing education at Bellevue School of Nursing. He continued to work at Bellevue after graduation and at the same time continued studies leading to a B.S.N. from Hunter College in 1968. Dr. Phillips has received a M.A. and a Ph.D., both in Nursing, from New York University. Before joining the N.Y.U. faculty in 1977, Dr. Phillips taught at Hunter College for 7 years.

Dr. Phillips has a wide variety of professional interests and has written on numerous subjects, including faculty abuse, health care provider relationships, and perceptions and care of the elderly. He comments, "My interests in the arts and humanities enhance my understanding of the human predicament. Readings in contemporary science, philosophy and science fiction help me to understand and theorize about the 'unexplainable' in the man-environment mutual process."

When asked to consider the future of nursing, Dr. Phillips responded "Will nursing continue to rely primarily on the scientific method whereby human beings are seen only as machines, rather than whole persons? There is a greater need to integrate the arts and humanities into the education and research process. The development of the scientific body of nursing knowledge will occur only if research is done within a nursing conceptual frame of reference. Finally, the survival of nursing will occur only if nurses take a proactive role rather than a reactive one in the shaping of the profession."

success of this method in building nursing knowledge is related to nurses practicing within borrowed conceptual models and theoretical frameworks of other disciplines. In other words, the gestalt for practice is not uniquely nursing because of inadequate synthesis of theories and models from other disciplines into nursing systems and models. The advancement of nursing science will occur only when nursing systems and models are created which nurses can use to construct theories from practice and from which principles and theories can be evolved to explain, describe, and predict phenomena of man. When this inductive and deductive approach to nursing theory becomes more of a reality, nursing will have a "ground" for education, practice, and research.

The method of borrowing theories and models from other disciplines has been of benefit, but the point in the evolution of nursing has arrived where nursing must be more productive in the creation of conceptual systems and models of nursing. One needs only to analyze some of the models borrowed from other disciplines to understand why the advancement of nursing science has been stymied. The analysis will help to clarify why nursing has had difficulty in differentiating

itself from other disciplines and in identifying the boundaries which are unique to nursing.

The Medical (Disease) Model

The most pervasive model borrowed by nursing is the medical model. The medical model forces nursing to view health-illness manifestations as organic phenomena where emphasis is upon disorders in the structure and function of the body. With this disease-oriented approach to clients, the nurse is concerned with underlying defects or structural aberrations—changes in organs, tissues, and cells—which "must be identified, prevented, removed, counteracted, neutralized, or corrected" (Wu, 1973). The medical model framework of signs and symptoms, cause, pathology, course and prognoses, and treatment is used by the nurse to plan care. The utilization of the medical model compels a person to view disease as the failure of the body as a physiochemical machine, and patients are helped by interventions in bodily processes (Engel, 1970). As long as nurses use the medical model, chronic illnesses will present a difficult problem. To treat a person as sick rather that impaired gives rise to discouragement of normal behavior (Shagass, 1975).

The process of nursing education within the medical model has its theoretical base derived primarily from the biological sciences. A look at nursing textbooks which are medically oriented reveals principles directed toward minimization or elimination of disease processes. Nursing interventions are directed toward causal factors or pathology. The medical model purports also that mental disorders are illnesses like any other illness. Nursing educators who held this view taught this belief to students under the assumption that there is an underlying cause for the individual's behavior. Thus, the educational process focused on the causes of abnormal or maladaptive behaviors rather than the behaviors themselves. Nursing is not medicine but nursing!

The medical model posits a dichotomy between mind and body which is not congruent with the philosophy of nursing in its concern with the whole person. Not only is nursing concerned with the structure and function of the body but also with human experience, behavior, feelings, and the influence of social forces upon the body—manifestations of the man-environment interaction, whether they be termed normal or abnormal. As nurses became dissatisfied with the medical model with its focus upon the body, the psychologic model was borrowed to look at the health-illness of man.

The Psychologic Model

The psychologic model concerns itself with normal human growth and development and deficits which occur with the maturation process. Emphasis is placed upon disruptions in the individual's development and the undesirability of certain states of mind, feeling, or conduct (Leifer, 1970–1971). Using the psychologic model nursing added theories of psychodynamics, interpersonal relations, crisis intervention, and ego development and defense mechanisms to its repertory of borrowed knowledge. The use of the word "added" can

be understood after an examination of nursing texts is carried out. The importance of understanding the psychological component of man is stressed; yet, the content of the texts deals with alterations in physical structure and function of the body. Here, specific reference is made to the medical-surgical nursing texts where interest is shown in the mind and behavior of man for the purpose of understanding and altering bodily mechanisms.

When one looks at the psychiatric texts, there is still mention of alterations in physical structure and function. But, when mention is made of physical and structural disruptions, it is for the purpose of understanding their effect on mind and behavior. However, the borrowing of the psychologic model enabled the nurse to begin to move away from a disease orientation to one whereby the psychologic meaning of events, feelings, and behaviors could be explored and incorporated into nursing interventions. The psychologic model gave nurses an opportunity to teach patients how to experience their feelings. The model also gave nurses the opportunity to explore with clients how to bear feelings which appeared to be beyond bearing.

The medical and psychologic models place a dichotomy between mind and body which is built into nursing curricula where separate courses in medical-surgical nursing, parent-child nursing, psychiatric nursing, psychosocial aspects of nursing, and interpersonal relations in nursing are presented. Fortunately, the inadequacy of such curricula has been recognized, and integrated curricula have been and are being developed. The proposed success of these curricula will remain a myth, however, as long as they remain under the aegis of models borrowed from other disciplines. To be successful, the borrowed knowledge must be synthesized into nursing systems from which conceptual models for curricula can be created.

The medical and psychologic models are oriented toward individuals, but man does not exist as an entity unto himself but interacts with his environment. The medical and psychologic models do not deal with the relationship of man to his environment. The borrowing of the ecologic model was one attempt by nursing to gain a better understanding of the interaction of man with his environment.

The Ecologic (Public Health) Model

The ecologic model is an extension of the medical model (Pasewark & Rardin, 1971). Disease in this model is postulated as not being caused by disruptions in the structure and function of the body but by multiple factors both within the outside man. In other words, an ecological relationship between the host (man) and the environment where illness is a function of genetic man and the total effects of his environment (E. S. Rogers, 1960).

The effects of the ecologic model upon nursing can be seen with the addition of public health nursing and epidemiology into nursing curricula. The ecologic model gave rise to the concept of prevention which is one of the prime foci of nursing today. There is movement away from tertiary and secondary prevention (medical model) to primary prevention. Even though the ecologic model is an extension of the medical model, it helped to open paths for nurses such as primary care and independent nurse practitioners in their attempt to move away from the constraints of the medical model. The passage of new Nurse Practice Acts was a tremendous impetus toward independent practice in nursing.

Nursing's rejection of the medical model and movement toward more autonomy has the medical profession in an uproar about the role and function of nursing. The physician still "tries to legislate out of existence those who would cure human ills" (Nemiah, 1970–1971), even nursing. As long as the physician can enforce the medical model, only he will be able to confer the sick role through his diagnoses (Shagass, 1975). As long as nurses continue to function within the medical model, only the physician will be allowed to make diagnoses and prescribe treatment for manifestations of illness.

The Social Model

The social model explicates further the influence of the environment upon man since the primary assumption of the model is that the manifestations of an individual are essentially the consequence of cultural variables that impinge upon him. These forces upon the individual come directly from the culture or from such cultural groups as the family, social institutions. and agencies (Pasewark & Rardin, 1971).

The social model enables the nurse to have concern for individuals as they exist in a group of meaningful others and to have better understanding of how groups of individuals influence each other. However, the social model is not a specific frame of reference for nursing. Manifestations of illness in the social model are viewed as "an impairment of capacity to perform one's social roles and/or valued tasks relative to his status in society" (Parsons, 1958). Within this frame of reference, illness is defined in terms of the social position or role a person is expected to occupy or play (Wu, 1973).

Nursing borrowed from the social model theories of group dynamics and group socialization and theories concerning the development of various role patterns. The borrowed knowledge helped the nurse to focus on the ways individuals function in social systems. But, the frame of reference for nursing still remained within another discipline. Theories constructed within this frame of reference are tainted by another discipline's views of the health needs of people.

The analysis of the models borrowed by nursing in its attempt to expand nursing knowledge elucidates two major questions with which nursing is concerned. Will the process of borrowing knowledge make nursing unique from the other disciplines? What are the boundaries of nursing? It is hoped that the present conceptual systems and models of nursing will provide answers to these questions. However, the use of some of the models cannot be successful in providing the answers. Some nursing theorists have simply taken theories and models from other disciplines and transposed them into what is called a "nursing" model. The dangers of this method of model construction are that the theories and models borrowed may not have been supported in the other disciplines, and the theories and models may not be generalizable to nursing. If the borrowing method is to be used by nursing, the theories and models must be supported from a nursing frame of reference before being synthesized into conceptual systems and models for nursing. Other nursing models have great potential in providing answers to the questions. Theories and models from other disciplines were not borrowed; instead, concepts were used to construct the nursing model. With the nursing models constructed from concepts, it is possible to build theories to generate knowledge unique to nursing. This knowledge in turn might be borrowed by other disciplines to expand their knowledge!

The discussion of the models which nursing has borrowed to advance nursing science makes clear the fact that not one of the models views man in his totality in his interaction with the environment. Some of the nursing models constructed from borrowed theories and models perpetuate this dichotomy of man and environment. The more abstract nursing models constructed from concepts and not from borrowed theories and models look at the complementarity of the man-environment interaction. Two examples of the more abstract nursing models are the *Rogers life process* model (M.E. Rogers, 1970) and the *Johnson behavioral system* model (Auger, 1976; Riehl & Roy, 1974). These models can be used as a framework for theory construction which can generate nursing knowledge—knowledge which can be used for nursing education, practice, and research. Nursing must continue to construct systems and models which are truly nursing so theory can be developed to generate nursing knowledge. Nursing can no longer afford to have its frame of reference couched in the systems and models of other disciplines.

References

Auger, J.R. (1976). *Behavioral systems and nursing.* Englewood Cliffs, NJ: Prentice-Hall.

Engel, G.L. (1970). Sudden death and the 'Medical Model' in psychiatry. *Canadian Psychiatric Association Journal, 15*, 527–37.

Johnson, D.E. (1968). Theory in nursing: Borrowed and unique. *Nursing Research, 17*, 206–209.

Leifer, R. (1970–71). The medical model as ideology. *International Journal of Psychiatry, 9*, 13–21.

Nemiah, J.C. (1970–71). The myth of mental illness. *International Journal of Psychiatry, 9*, 26–29.

Newman, M.A. (1972). Nursing's theoretical evolution. *Nursing Outlook, 20*, 449–453.

Parsons, T. (1958). Definitions of health and illness in light of American values and social structures. In E.G. Jaco (Ed.), *Patients, physicians, and illness.* New York: Free Press.

Pasewark, R.A., & Rardin, M.W. (1971) Theoretical models in community mental health. *Mental Hygiene, 55*, 358–364.

Riehl, J.P., & Roy, C. (1974). *Conceptual models for nursing practice.* New York: Appleton-Century-Crofts.

Rogers, E.S. (1960). *Human ecology and health, Part III.* New York: Macmillan.

Rogers, M.E. (1970). *An introduction to the theoretical basis of nursing.* Philadelphia: F.A. Davis.

Shagass, C. (1975). The medical model in psychiatry. *Comprehensive Psychiatry, 16*, 405–413.

Wald, F.S., & Leonard, R.C. (1964). Towards development of nursing practice theory. *Nursing Research, 13*, 309–313.

Wu, R. (1973). *Behavior and illness.* Englewood Cliffs, NJ: Prentice-Hall.

The Author Comments

In reviewing the literature in preparation for the creation of a theory development course for a master's curriculum, I was surprised to find how sparse the nursing theoretical underpinnings were. A survey of nursing texts indicated that much of what was being taught in nursing schools was based on knowledge from other sciences. There also was little substantive nursing research to be found to indicate that this knowledge was appropriate for nursing.

Thus, I felt a need to write about the evolution of the theoretical base for nursing and to postulate how the science of nursing should be developed through the use of nursing systems and models. More important, I believed that nursing students had to be taught theory development from a nursing perspective if the science were to develop at a more rapid pace. Even today, however, some nursing schools are still developing theory and doing research primarily from the perspective of another discipline. Too, some of the recognized scholars and leaders of nursing are questioning the use of nursing systems and models.

Today, some of my colleagues use "system" and "model" synonymously—in other words, they see no difference between the two terms. One colleague commented that there was no need to create any more confusion in nursing by making such a distinction. Maybe further clarification of the terms is needed to show how they are involved in theory development and to point out the interconnections between and among various nursing systems and models.

The outlook, however, is optimistic. Nursing texts are appearing that present a *nursing* approach based on nursing science. In some of these texts, a major portion of the book has been devoted to the process of theory development. Our future graduates will expand the science of nursing through testing of theory developed within a nursing perspective.

—JOHN R. PHILLIPS

Chapter 37

A Model for Theory Development in Nursing

Peggy L. Chinn
Maeona K. Jacobs

The development of theory is the most crucial task facing nursing today. Theory, because of its predictive potential, is the major means by which identified goals of the nursing profession will be reached. Theory development is the means by which nursing will establish a defined area of concern. While this is not the only goal or justification for theory development in nursing, delimitation of an area of concern will ultimately be a significant outcome. Through precise, guided and theoretically based investigations, nursing can begin to clarify areas of expertise. It is reasonable to expect that if nursing acquires expertise in areas of specified concern, nurses will become more effective in dealing with phenomena in these areas than persons with other types of knowledge and expertise. Subsequently, nursing can exercise responsibility and control in relation to phenomena within its areas of expertise.

Conceptualization of Theory

Theory is more than the mere description of events. It is *an internally consistent body of relational statements about phenomena which is useful for prediction and control.* Although some authors Dickoff, James, & Wiedenbach, 1968; Hage, 1972; Hearn, 1970; Jacox, 1969 conceptualize varying levels of theory which include descriptive and explanatory statements as levels of theory, such statements are excluded from the definition of theory proposed in this article. Using our definition, it is only when events can be predicted, based on testing and application of the theoretical statements, that theory has been developed. As opposed to "theory," statements that provide descriptions and explanations of phenomena, or that have undeveloped potential for prediction and control untested in a labora-

From Advances in Nursing Science, *October 1978, 1(1), 1–11. Copyright © 1978 by Aspen Systems Corporation. Reprinted with permission from Aspen Systems Corporation.*

tory or natural setting, may be labeled "conceptual frameworks." Our purpose in labeling theoretical types of statements differentially according to their level of development is to focus attention on the ways in which they can or should be used in research and practice. A theoretical statement which we label "conceptual framework" may be used for such purposes as categorizing data and investigating simple relationships between isolated phenomena, or may serve as a foundation for proposing and testing more complex interrelationships in research and practice. Theory, as we have defined it, already has this background of initial development. It can be used to verify in laboratory or natural settings the more complex interrelationships set forth, and can be applied in practice with a greater degree of confidence to achieve the outcomes desired.

It is recognized that the description and explanation of events are not easily accomplished. Further, differentiating between the description of events, their explanation and their prediction is exceedingly difficult. Prediction of an event generally requires more complex relational statements than does explanation. Simply stated, events may be explained by relating them to fewer phenomena. If an event is to be predicted, several explanations must be incorporated into a consistent, parsimonious statement. Thus the distinction between statements of explanation and prediction is often arbitrary and somewhat ambiguous.

The existence of predictive knowledge, or theory, in relation to events and phenomena does not ensure control over them since there are events which, despite prediction, cannot be controlled. However, if predictive knowledge does exist, some measure of control can usually be exercised in relation to the event predicted.

Traits of Systems for Theory Development

A theory development system may be thought of as a guide used in evolving theory, or a set of operations to be applied in developing theory. There are several such systems, each having more commonalities than differences (Brodbeck, 1970; Jacox, 1969; Murphy, 1971; Piotrowski, 1971; Simon, 1971). First, most systems for theory development are circular in nature, in that as soon as one operation is completed, another is begun and the process of moving among and between operations within the system continues indefinitely. In addition to circularity, theory development systems usually embody operations that are intimately interrelated. The operations at any given point in time will determine how subsequent operations are carried out.

Second, information about the system does not provide prescriptions regarding those phenomena or events to which the system is applied. In addition, once theory is developed from system application, the decisions of when to apply it are made on the basis of the practitioner's values, rather than on the basis of system prescription.

Third, the application of scientific systems requires a specific kind of research approach. Research which is not, at some point, incorporated into theory is less useful than research which is. This is not to say that research aimed at explicating and setting forth facts cannot, or will not, fit into such a framework. However, unless research is undertaken with the ultimate aim of incorporation into theory, it is likely to remain a mere compilation of isolated facts. If research is to be useful to theory development, there must be recognized and planned circular interrelationships between the two.

Finally, the use of systems for theory development requires not so much completely new thought patterns as the reorganization of existing patterns to ensure that scientific investigation is controlled and rigorous. For example, everyone has concepts about phenomena and events which occur in everyday life and interrelates events accordingly. What has not been accomplished in most thinking and problem solving is the critical analysis of ideas, their systematic organization into relational statements and their validation in empirical reality. Everyday thought patterns do not require the precise determination of whether ideas represent reality, but scientific thinking does; this determination is what systematic theory development processes accomplish.

The Model for Theory Development in Nursing

The operations within this theory development system are: (a) concept examination and analysis, (b) formulation and validation of relational statements, (c) theory construction, and (d) practical application of theory. Taken together, the four operations embody the elements of description, explanation and prediction of phenomena. The model is depicted in Figure 1 as a circle divided into four quadrants. Each quadrant represents a system operation. The model is bounded, signifying system limits, and there is a historical core of events from which the theory development process emerges. The whiplines emanating from this central core represent significant historical, and present, influences on application of such systems. The whiplines are curved to convey the idea that use of, and influence on, the system is dynamic. The overall morphology of the model is meaningful and will be explained further, following an explanation of each of the system operations. An operation is simply defined as a series of actions that include both "thinking and doing" processes. These operations can be thought of as occurring on a continuum of completeness.

Examination and Analysis of Concepts

The first operation is the examination and analysis of concepts. In applying the system, relevant concepts must be at least examined; for many purposes, they require analysis as well. Concepts are the complex ideas underlying, and determining, the direction of inquiry. Concepts are defined as *complex mental formulations of events, objects or properties which are derived from an individual's perceptual experience.* They are somewhat paradoxical in that they may appear to be deceptively simple ideas which are easily explained. The operation of concept examination and analysis provides the beginning examination of phenomena important to the area of inquiry. Through this operation, the system user begins to generate ideas about what must be described and analyzed and the relative diffi-

culty of the task, as well as the nature of relational statements to be set forth. Basically, concept examination and analysis demands refinement of the image of reality being dealt with. In this system, concept examination and analysis is probably the most important, yet most frequently neglected, operation. It is crucial in that it underpins and directs each of the other operations. Without careful concept examination and analysis, the effectiveness of the system is significantly weakened.

The operation of concept examination and analysis is paradoxical in that it requires great rigor and precision, but leads to a tenuous, inexact kind of end product. This operation requires much effort and work which can appear to yield few returns. Therefore it is often not understood and is generally neglected. Examination of concepts requires careful analysis rather than a superficial scan. A successful concept analysis requires abandoning the notion that one understands what she or he thinks. When ideas are rigorously examined through concept analysis, the reality which reflects those ideas and the ramifications of choosing one reality over another are better understood. There are many such techniques, including Wilson's (1969) method, which has been useful in our work. In addition, descriptive research may be required to fully delineate and refine the nature of a concept.

Formulation and Testing of Relational Statements

The next operation within the system, formulation and testing of relational statements, embodies three main subcomponents: (a) formulation of the relational statement, often in the form of a hypothesis,; (b) determining empirical referents necessary to validate the relational statement, and (c) validation of relational statements through application of systematic methods of research. This operation requires an interrelating of ideas accruing from concept examination and analysis in a specific form—that of relational statements. In the empirical sciences, and in nursing, the naming of empirical referents is necessary to validate relational statements. Empirical referents are observable phenomena which are selected to qualify or quantify each of the concepts under investigation. The selection of empirical referents begins during concept analysis as an "educated guess," and referents are tentatively confirmed with testing of relational statements. The analysis of the concept determines its reality representation. If, for example, anxiety were conceptualized in a study as a primarily physiological phenomenon, empirical referents chosen to represent "anxiety" would be physiological events observable in reality. Similarly, if "anxiety" were conceptualized as a behavioral phenomenon, the referents would be behavioral ones.

Relational statements are verified by comparing actual, observed relationships among referents of concepts with the proposed relationships set forth in the statements. In other words, the scientist determines whether objective, "out-there" reality is harmonious with hypotheses. This operation determines whether proposed relationships "hang together" and "make sense" when the statements of relationship are represented by a specific, objective reality; empirical referents. Mathematical models are often employed when carrying out this system operation. These can be thought of as devices to help the scientist judge whether relational statements, when represented by reality, are consistent enough to be considered valid.

Theory Construction

The third operation of the system is theory construction. This operation, like that of concept analysis, is primarily a cognitive function. Theory construction requires that validated hypotheses or relational statements be compiled into coherent theoretical formulations. Although the theory construction operation is discussed as if it followed the two operations already outlined, it can conceivably take place anywhere in the series of operations. Certainly, how theory development actually proceeds is determined by the nature of the phenomena of concern. Because many phenomena in nursing directly or indirectly affect life and health, it seems particularly hazardous to develop nursing theory without empirical validation of proposed relationships,

especially if the definition of theory used in this article is accepted.

Practical Application of Theory

The fourth and final operation within the system has been labeled practical application of theory. It can be thought of as a "final" testing, where theory is applied in the setting of intended utilization. In this operation, the relationships proposed and determined to exist are applied as a second check of the theory's utility. Practical application of theory seems crucial for nursing. It is this operation which will allow nursing to determine whether a theory is sufficiently predictive to allow for control in natural settings. It is in natural settings that control is required to meet professional nursing goals. Theoretical statements and formulation must therefore, at some point, be applied in such settings to determine, and ensure, their utility for nursing practice. Moreover, through application of this final operation, further refinements in theory are made.

Application of this series of operations in nursing will generate ordered and valid knowledge about reality which is useful for prediction and control. Illustrations from nursing practice have not been incorporated into this article. However, a detailed discussion (Chinn & Jacobs, n.d.) of system applications utilizing examples from nursing is available.

System Morphology

The dividing lines between the quadrants depicted in the model (see Figure 37-1) are particularly meaningful. The lines represent the separateness of the operation in each quadrant. They are broken to indicate the mutual influence each operation has on the other. The operations are considered separate because each one represents an independent set of activities. For example, the system user cannot know what has been generated from concept analysis (Quadrant 1) simply by knowing the status of relational statements (Quadrant 2). Moreover, if concept examination and analysis is imprecise, it cannot be improved by generating more or different relational statements. At the same time, the operations

Quadrant 1

Quadrant 3

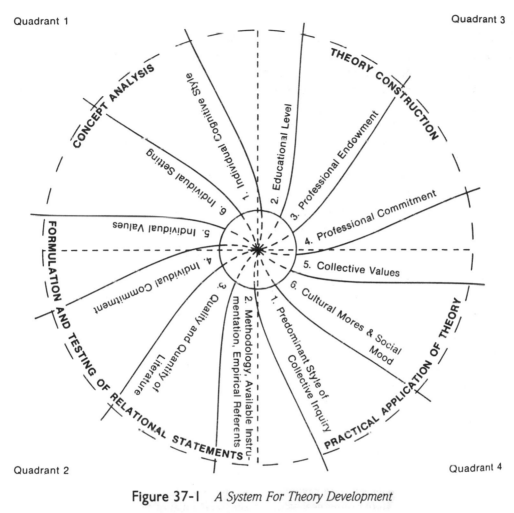

CONCEPT ANALYSIS

THEORY CONSTRUCTION

1. Individual Cognitive Style

2. Educational Level

3. Professional Endowment

4. Professional Commitment

6. Individual Setting

5. Individual Values

4. Individual Commitment

3. Quality and Quantity of Literature

2. Methodology, Available Instrumentation, Empirical Referents

1. Predominant Style of Collective Inquiry

6. Cultural Mores & Social Mood

5. Collective Values

FORMULATION AND TESTING OF RELATIONAL STATEMENTS

PRACTICAL APPLICATION OF THEORY

Quadrant 2

Quadrant 4

Figure 37-1   *A System For Theory Development*

are mutually interrelated because each one is influenced by activities carried out in the others. For example, concept examination and analysis determines the nature of relational statements formulated.

Placement of the quadrants represents additional important ideas. The horizontal broken lines separate the primarily cognitive operations of concept examination and analysis and theory construction from the more empirically based operations of formulation and testing of relational statements and practical application of theory. Theory development in general can proceed only when the upper two operations of the system are utilized. For the empirical sciences and for nursing,

the adequate development of theory also depends on the empirically based functions of the system represented by the bottom two quadrants. Bypassing the lower two operations requires a priori development of predictive relationships. In so doing, one takes a rather significant risk that these statements will indeed represent reality.

The vertical broken lines separate the primarily descriptive and explanatory functions of the system from its predictive and controlling functions. Thus concept examination and analysis, as well as the formulation and testing of relational statements, is viewed as providing descriptive and explanatory knowledge, while the operations of theory construction and the practical application of theory provide predictive knowledge useful for the control of phenomena.

Within the system, there is a free flow of influence among and between all operations. Each operation has the common feature of utilizing systematic and rigorous methods of inquiry, but the nature of these methods is quite different for each operation. There has been no attempt to represent the direction and strength of influence of one operation upon the other since these depend on the purpose of the system's user.

The broken lines bounding the system symbolize that every empirical science has limits on its areas of inquiry. Although the entire system is bounded, there is a free exchange of content and processes among and between sciences; this exchange is conceptualized as occurring at the boundaries. As a potential science, nursing influences and is influenced by activities in other sciences.

The boundary lines symbolize that the concerns of a science must be limited, for no discipline can realistically or effectively carry out scientific endeavors in a broad array of areas. In seeking to endlessly extend boundaries and encompass the whole of reality, a discipline weakens the power of its scientific endeavors. Areas of overlap among disciplines are significant and represent mutual areas of concern, but areas where overlap does not occur are also important. For example, both the nursing and medical professions deal with certain human responses to illness. However, each discipline recognizes the enormity of the range of responses and concentrates its efforts on generating knowledge about those which seem most related to the discipline's particular goals. There is nothing good or bad about including a particular phenomenon as an object of scientific study. Inclusions or exclusions are determined by the potential benefits to the particular profession.

The solid central core represents the historical past of any science. The historical core is conceptualized as continuous with system operations and is a significant influence on them. For example, nursing's history determines to a great degree its present use of scientific systems. Moreover, its history determines its areas of concern—past, present and future—and affects the nature of exchange at the system's boundaries. The historical past changes in a cumulative manner. That is, it is added to but never subtracted from. Factors contained within the historical core are more or less important, depending on the phenomena and events being dealt with in system application.

The present-day use of scientific systems in nursing will influence and determine the evolving historical core of nursing, in that what happens today influences the direction nursing takes in the future with regard to theory development. Some historical factors seem more important than others in determining the use of scientific systems in nursing. It is these factors that are represented in the model as whiplines emanating from the historical core. As previously stated, the whiplines are curvilinear to convey the idea of movement through time and the changing nature of their influence.

In the model, an attempt has been made to label each whipline according to the importance a certain factor may have in relation to one system operation as opposed to another. Labels which correspond to each other have been given the same number. One label with number 5, for example, refers to an individual trait, while the other number 5 refers to a group or collective trait. These numbers, as they are placed in the model, indicate that individual traits more heavily affect the upper quadrants, while the group traits more heavily affect the lower quadrants.

The designation of system influencers in the model will vary according to the discipline using the system. The whiplines should be envisioned as extending beyond the boundaries of the system into areas that are tangential to scientific systems of other disciplines. Thus the historically derived factors influencing the application of scientific systems within one discipline will have reciprocal influences on scientific system application within other disciplines.

Value and Use of the Model

The model is a valuable heuristic device which has been demonstrated to be of significant benefit in understanding the theory development process. Orientation to the system allows individual research and study to be seen in relation to theory development as a whole rather than as an isolated effort. It also enhances the scientist's appreciation of the value of diverse scientific approaches. Nothing is more detrimental to the development of science than the illusion of individual scientists that their own particular approach is the "right" one. Study of the model results in a working knowledge of how different types of research yield varying types of products, each contributing to the total development of the science. The model assists in conceptualizing different scientific talents and styles and their respective values. In order to achieve the overall goal of developing the science, it is important that a sense of mutual respect exists between scientists whose styles may be very different. Finally, the model helps to conceptualize differences between possible goals and the development of explanatory and predictive systems which will be useful in reaching those goals.

The problem of which phenomena should be selected for the development of nursing theory has been well debated. The *process* of developing theory, and not a specific outcome, should be emphasized. That is, the *process* has greater value for nursing than the *product*. This is not to imply that scholars should freely develop theories about just any phenomena, but arguing fine points about the nature of theory to be developed is often misplaced emphasis. Theory development efforts should be concentrated in areas that can be reasonably assumed to be of central concern to nursing. The aim of theory should always be prediction and, ultimately, control in relation to the phenomena which are affected by nursing actions. This emphasis gives impetus to refining the definition and concept of nursing. Describing and explaining nursing practice activities do not necessarily require delineating the event to the predicted; hence understanding the nursing process does not promote practice definition as effectively as do those activities that lead to prediction of events with which nursing is concerned.

It is necessary to make judgments about the events and phenomena to which theory-building efforts will be related, and its is recognized that these cannot encompass all of nursing. Concentration of efforts will certainly vary with the background and interests of the scientists concerned. It is important, however, that all theory-building activities in nursing be cemented by common concepts other than process. It is doubtful that these commonalities should be, or even can be, agreed upon at present. They will emerge as theory development proceeds within the profession. As long as there are differences of opinion about what constitutes common concepts and events of concern to nursing, there will also be disagreement about what constitutes the practice of nursing. Persons who are adequately qualified should go ahead with scientific endeavors in areas that can be justified as being within the domain of nursing. Some attention should be given to desirable areas of emphasis for nursing theory development and how such emphasis can be influenced through allocation of monies, political action or control of admission standards to educational programs. Nursing scientists and clinicians involved in research will shape the concept of nursing to the extent that they attend to critical factors which influence the course of theory development and, consequently, the evolution of nursing science.

Facilitating the Evolution of Nursing as a Science

A system for theory development is one means of facilitating the evolution of nursing as a science. The system embodies operations that are essential to the development of useful theory in nursing. Although presented in this article in a certain sequence, the system is not necessarily applied in that order. However, if predictive knowledge results from application of the system, the person or group of persons applying the system will, at some point, have carefully accomplished each of the system operations. It is through such application of theory development systems and the accumulation of predictive knowledge that nursing will evolve into a science. And it is scientific knowledge that is the basis for continual advancement of nursing practice.

References

Brodbeck, M. (1970). Models, meaning and theories. In L. Netzer et al. (Eds.), *Interdisciplinary foundations of supervision*. Boston: Allyn and Bacon.

Chinn, P., & Jacobs, M. (n.d.) *Theory development in nursing*. Audio cassette tape series available from P. Chinn.

Dickoff, J., James, P., & Wiedenbach, E. (1968). Theory in a practice discipline: Part I, Practice-oriented theory. *Nursing Research, 17*, 415–435.

Hage, J. (1972). *Techniques and problems of theory construction*, New York: John Wiley & Sons.

Hearn, G. (1970). Theory building. In L. Netzer et al. (Eds.), *Interdisciplinary foundations of supervision*. Boston: Allyn and Bacon.

Jacox, A. (1969). Issues in construction of nursing theory. In C.M. Norris (Ed.), *Proceedings of the First Nursing Theory Conference*. Kansas City, KS: Department of Nursing Education, University of Kansas Medical Center.

Jacox, A. (1974). Theory construction in nursing: An overview, *Nursing Research, 23*, 4–13.

Murphy, J. (1971). Introduction. In J. Murphy (Ed.), *Theoretical issues in professional nursing*. New York: Appleton-Century-Crofts.

Piotrowski, Z.A. (1971). Basic system of all sciences. In H.J. Vetter & B.D. Smith (Eds.), *Personality theory: A source book*. New York: Appleton-Century-Crofts.

Simon, H.M. (1971). Logical empirical approach to developing a body of knowledge. In J. Murphy (Ed.), *Theoretical issues in professional nursing*. New York: Appleton-Century-Crofts.

Wilson, J. (1969). *Thinking with concepts*. New York: Cambridge University Press.

The Authors Comment

This article developed as a result of our early experiences teaching theory development to graduate students at the University of Utah. We developed the model as a pedagogical tool to help beginning students comprehend the interrelationships among theory, research, and practice. It also demonstrated to students how their individual efforts contribute to the development and use of science in nursing. The model conveys that various diverse activities are needed to formulate and validate theory in a practice discipline like nursing. Since this article was published, we have revised, refined, and expanded many of the ideas contained herein. Our current thinking related to the model (now termed a *system* for theory development), is contained in our book *Theory and Nursing: A Systematic Approach* (3rd edition) (St. Louis: C.V. Mosby, 1991). A major shift in our thinking is represented by our current definition of the concept "theory." Theory is no longer held to be ". . .an internally consistent body of relational statements about phenomena . . . useful for prediction and control," that can be differentiated from conceptual frameworks. We now view theory much more broadly, and have formulated a definition that includes normative-ethical practice as well as scientific-empirical theory.

—PEGGY L. CHINN AND MAEONA K. KRAMER

REFERENCE

Chinn, P.L., & Jacobs, M.K. (1991). *Theory and nursing: A systematic approach,* (3rd edition) St. Louis: C.V. Mosby.

Chapter 38

Evolving Issues in Theory Development

Gretchen Crawford

Sister Karin Dufault

Ellen Rudy

Theory development in nursing has often been accompanied by controversy. Many issues have emerged, some of which have been addressed directly in the literature and others implied. The purpose of this article is to review some of the major issues in nursing theory development and to redefine these issues in light of the recent article by Donaldson and Crowley (1978). The discussion will attempt to clarify the complex and often overlapping nature of the following issues: (a) whether nursing science is basic or applied and whether nursing theory is borrowed or unique; (b) whether theory is unified or pluralistic—that is, theory *of* nursing or *for* practice; and (c) what paths to knowledge development exist.

Nursing Theory: Borrowed or Unique?

The efforts within nursing to develop a scientific body of knowledge that will guide practice have resulted in dialogue aimed at clarifying what nursing science is and how to develop such knowledge. The following questions have often been debated in such discussions. Do nurses simply take basic scientific knowledge and use it in the practice of nursing, so that they only need knowledge of the basic sciences? Is nursing knowledge being developed about how to apply basic science theories to practical situations? And is the development of nursing science something entirely different from the development of any other science? Historically, nursing practice has mirrored prevailing theories of health and disease, and the growth in nursing knowledge has been inextricably linked with the growth of medical knowledge (Levine, 1966; Wald & Leonard, 1964). Wald and Leonard (1964) noted that nurses have been quick to embrace the scientific underpinnings of other fields such as education and the social and behavioral sciences, only to find that when the knowledge and methods were applied to nursing, they failed to provide the profession with knowledge useful in guiding prac-

About the Authors

GRETCHEN CRAWFORD was born in Richmond, Indiana. She calls herself a "Case product," having received her B.S.N. and M.S.N. degrees from the Frances Payne Bolton School of Nursing at Case Western Reserve University (CRWU). In 1980, Dr. Crawford received her Ph.D. in Nursing from the CWRU School of Graduate Studies.

Clinically Dr. Crawford has specialized in community health, working in a variety of impatient and outpatient settings. After receiving her doctorate, Dr. Crawford held faculty appointments at CWRU, the Ohio State University College of Nursing, and at the University of Connecticut School of Nursing. Currently, Dr. Crawford is Director of Nursing Education for the New York State Nurses Association. She also holds an adjunct appointment and teaches nursing theory in the graduate program at Russell Sage College in Troy, New York.

Led by her research interest in the concept of social support, Dr. Crawford has investigated support in relation to teenage parents, cancer patients, and clients with arthritis. She has published scholarly articles on the concept in *Advances in Nursing Science, Nursing Research*, and *The March of Dimes Nursing Roundtable*. Dr. Crawford is a member of the New York State Nurses Association, National League for Nursing, Sigma Xi (national scientific honor society), and Sigma Theta Tau. In her leisure time, she likes to walk, often for several miles a day. "It gives me time to think about nursing," she says.

KARIN J. DUFAULT was born in Yakima, Washington. After living in Portland, Oregon for most of her professional nursing life, she returned to Yakima in 1987. She received a B.A. and B.S. in Nursing from Seattle University, and a M.S.N. from the Frances Payne Bolton School of Nursing at CWRU in 1976. In 1981, Dr. Dufault received her Ph.D. in Nursing from CWRU School of Graduate Studies.

A Sister of Providence, Dr. Dufault has specialized in the care of cancer patients, elderly persons, and their families, particularly in the acute care setting. After completing her doctoral research (titled *Hope and Elderly Persons with Cancer*), she accepted a position at Providence Medical Center, Portland, Oregon, as Clinical Nurse Specialist/Nurse Researcher. This position enabled her to combine clinical practice, education, and research with patients and families, hospital staff, physicians, the community, and students. In 1984, Dr. Dufault accepted an appointment as Assistant Administrator for Patient Care Services at Providence. In this position, she was responsible for the departments of Nursing, Home Health/Hospice, Social Work, and Pharmacy and had program management responsibility for Oncology and Gerontology. She also was a Clinical Assistant Professor at Oregon Health Sciences University School of Nursing from 1981 to 1987. In 1987, she accepted the position of Administrator at St. Elizabeth's Medical Center, Yakima, Washington. On June 1, 1991, she became full-time Chairperson of the Board of Directors of the Sisters of Providence Health Care Corporations, Seattle, Washington.

Concepts of particular interest to Dr. Dufault include hope, pain hospice, grief, chronic illness, health care ethics, and coping. She is an active member of the Washington Nurses' Association, Oncology Nursing Society, Sigma Theta Tau, Gerontological Society, Western Society for Research in Nursing, and Society for Health and Human Values. She has served as an appointed member of the American Nurses' Association's Committee on Ethics and Cabinet on Nursing Administration.

ELLEN BEAM RUDY is Professor at the Frances Payne Bolton School of Nursing, Case Western Reserve University. She received her education at Ohio State Universtiy (B.S.N., 1958), University of Dayton (M.P.A., 1974), University of Maryland (M.S.N., 1977), and Case Western Reserve University (Ph.D., 1980).

A very successful researcher, Dr. Rudy currently has three funded studies from the National Center for Nursing Research: one involving head-injured adults in critical care, another dealing with an alternative model of care delivery for long-term critically ill patients, and the third exploring the effects of running on the menstrual cycle. She has published widely in both research and clinical journals, has authored two books, and currently is working on a book for critical care nurses.

Dr. Rudy remains active in the American Association of Critical Care Nurses. Recently, she worked with the National Kidney Foundation in developing a video to help critical care nurses approach families about organ donation and was appointed as a member of the NIH Nursing Study Section for the National Center for Nursing Research.

tice. They based their conclusions on the writings of Henderson (1957), McManus (1961), Schlotfeldt (1960), and Simmons and Henderson (1964).

Wald and Leonard rejected the idea that knowledge for nursing practice should be developed by applying principles from other disciplines. They proposed that nursing expend its energies in developing its own theories, its own knowledge base, and in so doing become an independent "discipline." In order to do this, Wald and Leonard urged the development of nursing practice theory.

Later writers (Dickoff & James, 1968, 1975; Dickoff, James, & Wiedenbach, 1968; Ellis, 1968; Jacox, 1974) expanded this idea of "practice" theories, or theories to be used to direct practice. As described by these writers, practice theories do not stop with defining, explaining, and predicting behavior, but go beyond to become prescriptive. That is, practice theories identify practice goals and actions necessary for attaining these goals. Dickoff and James label these as situation-producing theories; Wald and Leonard call them prescriptive cause-effect theories; and Ellis refers to them as giving direction to practice. Whatever they are called, practice theories would guide nurses in meeting goals for patients.

Nursing Science: Basic or Applied?

In spite of the promotion given to the idea of knowledge development in nursing to direct practice, the issue surrounding the use of theories from other disciplines in the development of nursing science was far from resolved. In 1968, a conference was held on the nature of science and nursing in an attempt to understand more fully the issue of pure and applied science as it relates to scientific study in nursing (Crowley, 1968; Folta, 1968; Leininger, 1968).

The writers who contributed to the conference defined the difference between basic and "pure" science and applied science. As they saw it, basic science is usually described as knowledge only for the sake of knowledge, value free, more abstract, and involving research which is dictated by its cognitive significance. In contrast, applied science is defined as knowledge which has practical aims and application, is less abstract, and is developed more for the sake of utility than for cognitive stimulation. They claim that it is impossible to maintain a sharp distinction between a pure and an applied scientific field. Any kind of knowledge, once it is obtained, is used or applied to concrete life situations in various ways.

The 1968 conference addressed the problems involved in nursing research in its endeavor to become a scientific discipline, but did not come to any conclusions about the nature of nursing science. In addition, no reference was made to the idea of nursing science being developed from practice theories.

In a symposium on theory development in nursing, Johnson (1968) examined the distinction between borrowed and unique theories for nursing and presented her views on the appropriate focus for nursing theory and knowledge development. She defined borrowed theory as knowledge that nursing draws on which has been developed primarily by other disciplines. Unique theory was defined as knowledge built on observations of phenomena and the raising of questions which are characteristic of nursing but not of other disciplines. Johnson presented her ideas concerning the nature of knowledge required for nursing practice and referred to the need for knowledge which goes beyond descriptive and predictive levels to knowledge used to control (prescriptive). At a later time, Johnson

(1974) reaffirmed her ideas and stated that because the phenomena of interest to nursing and its perspective differ from those of the basic sciences, a different body of theoretical knowledge which is unique to nursing will be developed.

According to Donaldson and Crowley (1978), the questions of whether nursing knowledge should be basic or applied and whether borrowed or unique theory should predominate in theory development become false issues. In their view, there is a need for development of basic, applied, and prescriptive theories that give direction to practice within a professional discipline such as nursing. There is therefore a need for basic research in nursing to increase understanding of phenomena; for applied research in nursing to demonstrate applicability of basic knowledge in real situations; and for research to generate prescriptive theories explaining how to utilize knowledge in order to achieve goals in practice.

In regard to applied research, Donaldson and Crowley (1978) note that since each discipline's perspective is unique, knowledge per se cannot be borrowed from other disciplines. Knowledge from another science or discipline cannot be adequately understood if it is removed from the context that generated it. For this reason, when one uses borrowed concepts and theories, one must redefine and synthesize them according to the perspective of the borrowing discipline. This supports Johnson's (1968, p. 209) statement that the nature of knowledge required for nursing will foster theory development that is unique to nursing.

Knowledge gained from the types of research noted above (basic, applied, and prescriptive) comprises nursing science, and this knowledge is unique to nursing. In addition to nursing science, Donaldson and Crowley (1978) point out that nurses also utilize knowledge from other disciplines such as medicine, education, and the basic sciences. This knowledge is used in nursing education and practice.

From the foregoing analysis, we suggest that the thinking surrounding theory development in nursing and directed toward the building of nursing knowledge has evolved to a point exemplified by the following statements:

1. All knowledge utilized by the profession of nursing is not nursing knowledge; only those theories and knowledge which have been derived from nursing's perspective comprise nursing knowledge.
2. Nursing knowledge will be developed from nursing's unique perspective by asking questions and viewing phenomena unlike other disciplines.
3. The knowledge base of nursing will be developed from basic, applied, and prescriptive research in nursing.

The urgent task for nursing is to continue to clarify and make more explicit the unique perspective and focus of nursing. Historically, nurses' primary concern has been the ill person—not the illness itself—particularly in regard to the influence of the "ambient environment" in enhancing his susceptibility to illness or in preventing recovery (Johnson, 1974, p. 375). More recently, nursing has studied the wholeness or health of humans, recognizing that humans are in continuous interaction with their environments (Riehl & Roy, 1974; Rogers, 1970). As Donaldson and Crowley note, "Nursing's perspective evolves from the practical aim of optimizing of human environments for health" (Donaldson & Crrowley, 1978, p. 119). Nursing's perspective will be defined by the phenomena it chooses to study and the purpose for studying these phenomena. Nurse researchers must continue to strive to maintain nursing's perspective so that it is the underlying focus of their research.

Theory of Nursing, or for Practice?

Another issue that has recurred in nursing literature on theory development has been whether nursing theory is a single theory or many theories. This is a two-faceted question. The first facet focuses upon whether attention in theory development should be directed to a single unified nursing theory or diverse and multiple nursing theories. The second facet focuses upon whether to begin by developing a theory (or theories) *of* nursing or *for* nursing practice. In general, theory *of* nursing refers to a delineation of the definition and scope of or about nursing and the nursing process; and theory *for* nursing practice refers to conceptualizations guiding nursing action toward desired goals.

Early nursing theory literature did not make a clear distinction between nursing theory or theories. Wald and Leonard (1964) have presented their case for nursing practice theory. They argue for causal theories of nursing practice based on empirical reality with the aim of improving practice. However, the authors also allude to the importance of "building a coherent practice theory" which might be interpreted as advocating a unification or synthesis of nursing practice theory (Wald & Leonard, 1964, p. 311). Dickoff, James, and Wiedenbach (1968) suggest that nurses should look for the unity factor in the structure of all nursing practice theory, but add that they should also recognize that there may be more than one good nursing theory. On the other hand, when Putnam addressed nursing theory, she did so not with nursing practice theory in mind, but rather with the understanding of theory as "a generalized theory capable of supporting an overall concept of a process of nursing" (Putnam, 1965, p. 430).

At the 1967 Symposium on Theory Development, Ellis (1968) called attention to the various ways in which the term, theory, was being used. She distinguished between the prepositions used to connect the words "theory" and "theory development," to the word, "nursing." Ellis clarified that her paper was concerned with theory development *for* nursing and she presented characteristics of significant theories *for* nursing practice.

The controversies surrounding the issues were made explicit at the series at three nursing theory conferences held at the University of Kansas during 1969–70. In the introduction to the proceedings of the first conference, Norris (1969) stated the issue as "whether we should develop one theory of nursing or whether there should be many theories." She went on to say that "At the same time it was argued that theories *of* nursing are not important; that theories *for* nursing would bring a wider range of knowledge to bear on nursing problems." The various perspectives on the issue were discussed within the context of the presentations and in the discussions. Most participants did not address the issue directly; Jacox (1969) and McLeod (1969) were among those who did.

Quoting from the work of Mills and Merton, Jacox warned against the development of "grand theories" based on global definitions of nursing and the opposite tendency, which involves collecting facts without using a theoretical framework—"abstracted empiricism" (Mills, 1959). Rather, she suggested the development of "middle-range theories" (Merton, 1957), which "include a limited number of variables and focus on a limited aspect of reality" (Jacox, 1969, p. 16). She used a theory of pain alleviation and a theory about care of dying patients as examples of middle-range theory. Integration of these middle-range theories into an all-encompassing theory was viewed as a possible future venture, although she questioned the desirability of such a task.

McLeod (1969) identified an attempt on the part of the conference to develop nursing theory that would define the nursing profession and form the framework for orderly and comprehensive growth of nursing through research and application of research findings to practice—that is, a *theory of* nursing. She also was of the opinion that a unified and comprehensive nursing theory was unrealistic and would be too vague to offer direction and guidance.

The third and final theory conference exemplified the struggle of participants to deal with both facets of the issue. A variety of ways of looking at synthesis of nursing theory and several levels of synthesis emerged. For example, a synthesis of theories *of* nursing could mean arriving at a *unified theory* by relating and combining theories considered applicable to the nature of nursing. It could also be considered as the development of new theories through the discovery of new relationships among existing theories. On the other hand, the conference participants considered synthesis as a concern in the development of theories for nursing. This synthesis, they believed, should involve articulating or combining research efforts related to a common problem studied from the perspective of several different scientific disciplines. The participants did not resolve the issue although they did rephrase it (Norris, 1970).

At the time of the theory conferences and in the years immediately following them, several books were published that focused on the development of theories or conceptualizations *of* nursing. Among them were the works of Rogers (1970), King (1971), and Orem (1971). In addition, 1971 witnessed attempts to clarify the concept of nursing theory, beginning with Walker's (1971) article and followed by responses from other nursing theory writers—among them Dickoff and James (1971), Ellis (1971), Folta (1971), and Wooldridge (1971). Issues were also reexamined and reformulated. In the introduction to the papers on adaptation in *Theoretical Issues in Nursing,* Murphy (1971) described the position of the contributors as being one in which a variety of approaches to theory construction was proposed, resulting in multiple theories based on observations of the empirical world of nursing. An attempt was made to use "adaptation" as one of the unifying theories which makes sense out of disparate knowledge interests.

More recently, the attention to theories of or about nursing has been redirected to nursing model development and clarification of the concept of nursing. The work of the Nursing Development Conference Group (1973) and Riehl and Roy's (1974) book are representative of this movement. Riehl and Roy discuss nursing model development and the relationship between models and theories. The closing chapter presents the advantages and disadvantages of a unified nursing model and proposes the broad outlines of a unified model of nursing practice that could serve as a structure from which prescriptive theories (theories for nursing practice) could be developed. Johnson (1974) views the growing number of expositions of practice models, both published and unpublished, as being the greatest source of assistance in building a "focused and cohesive conceptual system" in nursing.

Donaldson and Crowley (1978) provide a fresh perspective to the issue of unity versus diversity in theory development in nursing. In their view, the goal is not to identify a single theory of nursing, but rather to be able to place theories within the context of a discipline of nursing. Their important paper makes the elements of the discipline of nursing explicit. Within it, they advocate pluralism of theories as a means to promoting productivity. They point out that depending on which "structural conceptualizations" are utilized, widely different theories can be developed for testing. (This point was further illustrated by Schlotfeldt, 1975.) The theories lead not to different bodies of knowledge but to different aspects of a single body. Donaldson and Crowley (1978) argue that testable theories are more important than proposing in all-encompassing, but untestable theory.

Thus, they moved away from what they viewed as a "quest for *the* definition of the nature of nursing" or theory *of* nursing (Donaldson & Crowley, 1978, p. 113). Instead, they identify relationships and common themes among nursing writers through the ages as a means of determining boundaries for enquiry and theory development within the discipline of nursing. Both descriptive and prescriptive theories are generated and tested from this perspective and utilized to achieve the practical aims of the professional discipline and practice realms that are nursing.

Paths to Knowledge Development

In the 1960s and early 1970s, differences of opinion could be identified in the literature concerning how to develop knowledge in nursing. With a focus on scientific research methodology as the means to development of knowledge, Simon (1971) argues for an inductive approach and Putnam (1965) argues for a rational-deductive approach. The argument as to which method nurses should use to develop knowledge has been pointed out as a false issue by Murphy (1971) and Jacox (1969), who emphasize that both methods are needed and they are complementary.

Currently, rather than limiting the focus to inductive and deductive scientific research methodology as means to develop knowledge, additional paths to knowledge have been identified. For example, Donaldson and Crowley (1978) do not discuss inductive and deductive methods as such; instead, they point out the structure of the discipline of nursing. They define the two dimensions of the structure of a discipline as the substantive structure, consisting of the conceptualizations that fit the discipline's perspective, and the syntactical structure, which is composed of the research methodologies and criteria used to distinguish acceptable (true) findings from those which are not acceptable.

In addition, Donaldson and Crowley (1978) identify two kinds of research: testing theoretically derived hypotheses, and examining the discipline's structural conceptualizations and values. It appears that the first type of research involves testing of theories generated within the discipline in order to develop new knowledge; the second type concerns study of the key elements of the discipline (such as its structural conceptualizations) in order to organize knowledge about the discipline. This view of research suggests that inductive and deductive methods are only some of the ways to develop knowledge and that other methods are also necessary.

In regard to the use of methods other than the scientific ones of induction and deduction, McKay (1977) suggests use of nonscientific methods—for instance, historical and philosophical methods—since not all of nursing's knowledge is scientific in nature. Schlotfeldt (1977) also notes the need for historical and philosophical research in order to examine the history of nursing science; to identify philosophies and conceptualizations that have been a part of nursing knowledge over time; and to study the questions of values, ethics, and social significance in nursing.

In addition, Silva (1977) suggests that the philosophical methods of introspection and intuition should be considered as methods useful to nursing since it is important to be open to all "potential avenues" which might be used to add knowledge. Recalling the types of research noted by Donaldson and Crowley (1978), these methods would seem appropriate to use in order to organize knowledge about the key elements of the discipline. Carper's (1975) dissertation is an example of this kind of research. She analyzes nursing literature using a "philosophic view" to identify the structure of knowledge in nursing.

Donaldson and Crowley (1978) do not identify the syntactical structure of nursing, choosing instead to focus on the substantive structure. However, their definition of syntactical structure raises the following questions: 1) What methods are recognized as appropriate for knowledge development, and 2) What are the criteria used to determine acceptability of findings in nursing?

McKay (1977) notes that syntactical structure may not be unique to a discipline but is pervasive in that members agree about what methods are most appropriate to determine acceptability of findings. However, McKay (1977) suggests that the "dominant syntax" in nursing has not yet developed (p. 29). McKay's comments suggests that we do not yet have answers to the questions, what methods are recognized as appropriate, and what are the criteria for acceptability of findings.

It is interesting to observe that, given the long-standing concern with method in nursing, we do not yet have a dominant syntax. Certainly, the literature has emphasized method and pointed out various methods appropriate for nursing. Perhaps a clue to the reason for nursing's lack of dominant syntax is provided by Stevens:

> The nurse researcher [often] selects a methodology and then seeks a nursing question (however trivial) which lends itself to the given methodology. We challenge the nursing community first to identify significant nursing questions and then to seek out explanations and appropriate research methodologies, however difficult that task may be. (Stevens, 1978, p. 2)

Stevens seems to limit her comments to scientific research methodologies but, as noted above, nonscientific methods may also be appropriate, depending upon the nursing questions being asked. In regard to formulation of significant nursing questions, Donaldson and Crowley (1978) would advocate that questions be asked about the structural conceptualizations in nursing, and they identified some phenomena—for example, holistic functioning versus functioning of parts—which these questions could address.

In conclusion, the issue concerning paths to knowledge development involves two dimensions. On the one hand, an earlier focus on inductive and deductive scientific approaches has been broadened to include nonscientific methods such as philosophical and historical approaches. On the other hand, there seems to be a shift from preoccupation with method to an emphasis on first asking significant nursing questions about nursing phenomena and then finding appropriate methods to study these questions. So, rather than being limited to scientific methods, we have a wide array of methods from which to choose in studying nursing questions.

The emphasis on first formulating significant nursing questions about nursing phenomena provides an organizing focus for study. As nurses study these questions, choosing or developing methods which seem best suited to answering them, the dominant syntax in nursing can be expected to emerge. At present, nursing needs to determine what kinds of questions are significant and about what phenomena they should be asked.

References

Carper, B.A. (1975). Fundamental patterns of knowing in nursing. (Doctoral dissertation, Columbia University Teachers College). *Dissertation Abstracts International, 36,* 4941B. (University Microfilms No. 76-7772).

Crowley, D.M. (1968). Perspectives of pure science. *Nursing Research, 17,* 497–498.

Dickoff, J., & James, P. (1968). A theory of theories: A position paper. *Nursing Research, 17,* 197–203.

Dickoff, J., & James, P. (1971). Clarity to what end? (Commentary on Walker's "Toward a clearer understanding of the concept of nursing theory"). *Nursing Research, 20,* 499–502.

Dickoff, J., & James, P. (1975). Theory development in nursing. In P.J. Verhonick (Ed.), *Nursing Research I* (pp. 45–92). Boston: Little, Brown.

Dickoff, J., James, P., & Wiedenbach, E. (1968). Theory in a practice discipline: Part 1. *Nursing Research, 17,* 415–435.

Donaldson, S.K., & Crowley, D.M. (1978). The discipline of nursing. *Nursing Outlook, 26,* 118–120.

Ellis, R. (1968). Characteristics of significant theories. *Nursing Research, 17,* 217–222.

Ellis, R. (1971). Reaction to Walker's article. (Commentary on Walker's "Toward a clearer understanding of the concept of nursing theory"). *Nursing Research, 20,* 493–494.

Folta, J.R. (1968). Perspectives of an applied scientist. *Nursing Research, 17,* 502–505.

Folta, J.R. (1971). Obfuscation or clarification: A reaction to Walker's concept of nursing theory. (Commentary on Walker's "Toward a clearer understanding of the concept of nursing theory"). *Nursing Research, 20,* 496–499.

Henderson, V. (1957). An overview of nursing research. *Nursing Research, 6,* 61–71.

Jacox, A. (1969, March). Issues in construction of nursing theory. In C.M. Norris (Ed.), *Proceedings of the First Nursing Theory Conference* (pp. 8–18). Kansas City, KS: Department of Nursing Education, University of Kansas Medical Center.

Jacox, A. (1974). Theory construction in nursing: An overview. *Nursing Research, 23,* 4–13.

Johnson, D.E. (1968). Theory in nursing: Borrowed and unique. *Nursing Research, 17,* 206–209.

Johnson, D.E. (1974). Development of theory: A requisite for nursing as a primary health profession. *Nursing Research, 23,* 372–377.

King, I.M. (1971). *Toward a theory of nursing.* New York: John Wiley & Sons.

Leininger, M. (1968). Conference on the nature of science and nursing: Introductory comments. *Nursing Research, 17,* 484–486.

Levine, M.E. (1966). Adaptation and assessment: A rationale for nursing intervention. *American Journal of Nursing, 66,* 2450–2453.

McKay, R.P. (1977). Discussion: discipline of nursing—syntactical structure and relation with others disciplines and the profession of nursing. In M.V. Batey (Ed.), *Communicating nursing research: Optimizing environments for health: Nursing's unique perspective, Vol. 10* (pp. 23–30). Boulder, CO: Western Interstate Commission for Higher Education.

McLeod, D. (1969). Physiological approach to nursing theory. In C.M. Norris (Ed.), *Proceedings of the First Nursing Theory Conference* (pp. 47–57). Kansas City, KS: Department of Nursing Education, University of Kansas Medical Center.

McManus, R.L. (1961). Nursing research: Its evolution. *American Journal of Nursing, 61,* 68–71.

Merton, R.F. (1957). *Social theory and social structure.* Glencoe, IL: The Free Press.

Mills, C.W. (1959). *Sociological imagination.* New York: Oxford University Press.

Murphy, J.F. (1971). Introduction. In J.F. Murphy (Ed.), *Theoretical issues in professional nursing.* New York: Appleton—Century-Crofts.

Norris, C.M. (1969). Introduction. In C.M. Norris (Ed.), *Proceedings of the First Nursing Theory Conference.* Kansas City, KS: Department of Nursing Education, University of Kansas Medical Center.

Norris, C.M. (Ed.). (1970). *Proceedings of the Third Nursing Theory Conference.* Kansas City, KS: Department of Nursing Education, University of Kansas Medical Center.

Nursing Development Conference Group (1973). *Concept formalization in nursing: Process and product.* Boston: Little, Brown.

Orem, D.E. (1971). *Nursing: Concepts of practice.* New York: McGraw-Hill.

Putnam, P.A. (1965). Conceptual approach to nursing theory. *Nursing Science, 3,* 430–442.

Riehl, J.P., & Roy, C. (1974). *Conceptual models for nursing practice.* New York: Appleton-Century-Crofts.

Rogers, M.E. (1970). *An introduction to the theoretical basis of nursing.* Philadelphia: F.A. Davis.

Schlotfeldt, R.M. (1960). Reflections in nursing research. *American Journal of Nursing, 60,* 492–494.

Schlotfeldt, R.M. (1975). The need for a conceptual framework. In P.J. Verhonick (Ed.), *Nursing research I.* Boston: Little, Brown.

Schlotfeldt, R.M. (1977). Nursing research: Reflection of values. *Nursing Research, 26,* 4–9.

Silva, M.C. (1977). Philosophy, science, theory: Interrelationships and implications for nursing research. *Image, 9,* 59–63.

Simmons, L.W., & Henderson, V. (1964). *Nursing research.* New York: Appleton-Century-Crofts.

Simon, H.M. (1971). Logical empirical approach to developing a body of knowledge. In J.F. Murphy (Ed.), *Theoretical issues in professional nursing* (pp. 25–43). New York: Appleton-Century-Crofts.

Stevens, B.J. (1978). Theory, research, and the scholarly paper (Guest editorial). *Research in Nursing Health, 1*(1), 2.

Wald, F.S., & Leonard, R.C. (1964). Towards development of nursing practice theory. *Nursing Research, 13,* 309–313.

Walker, L.O. (1971). Toward a clearer understanding of the concept of nursing theory. *Nursing Research, 20,* 428–435.

Wooldridge, P.J. (1971). Meta-theories of nursing: A commentary on Dr. Walker's article. (Commentary on Walker's "Toward a clearer understanding of the concept of nursing theory"). *Nursing Research, 20,* 494–495.

The Authors Comment

The ideas embodied in the article began to take shape as we completed our second-level doctoral theory course and were studying for candidacy examinations. We had read and studied articles written in the late 1960s and 1970s that argued about the types of scientific knowledge that nursing needed as a profession and ways to develop that knowledge. When Donaldson and Crowley's paper "Discipline of Nursing: Structure and Relationship to Practice" was published by the Western Interstate Council on Higher Education (WICHE) in 1978, we read it and discussed it in class and in our study group. The three of us began to see that this paper altered or resolved many of the issues in theory development that we had studied.

After we took our candidacy examinations, Ellen suggested that we work together on an article to identify the major issues in nursing theory development and to demonstrate the impact of the Donaldson and Crowley paper on those issues. We met together and identified three topics to cover in the article. Each of us took responsibility for one section, then I edited the sections so they flowed together cohesively. Before sending the manuscript to *Nursing Outlook* for publication consideration, we asked Rosemary Ellis, our former teacher, to review and critique it. She offered several suggestions, which we incorporated into the final draft.

—GRETCHEN CRAWFORD

In studying together for doctoral candidacy exams related to nursing theory, we three often challenged one other to identify major issues in theory development and debated the issues as influenced by the authors we had studied. Our discussions were valuable and contributed to our own growth. Ellen's suggestion that we try to write an article expressing our conclusions was welcomed. We agreed that the process would be valuable for ourselves and also for other students of nursing theory, because we had not read a similar article on the subject. It has been rewarding to hear nurses' comments on the article and to know that the article continues to be relevant. Their interest has helped sustain my continued interest in nursing theory and its application to clinical practice and nursing research.

—KARIN DUFAULT

One of the reasons I wanted the three of us to write this article was that I felt others should benefit from what we had gained trying to digest and synthesize the issues involved in developing scientific knowledge for nursing. Also, speaking for myself, I knew that I would never know the subject in the same depth as I did while preparing for the candidacy examinations. Taking a "now or never" approach, it seemed to be the best time to write it!

—ELLEN RUDY

Chapter 39

Models for Nursing

Helen A. Bush

In recent years nurse scientists, as well as other persons concerned with science, have emphasized that knowledge in the field of nursing must be set in order and systematized. General systems science has made a significant contribution in revealing the potential dangers of failure to consider all pertinent factors surrounding a process or event—the most significant being that of drawing false conclusions. The use of "models" has been adopted as a system for observing, ordering, clarifying and analyzing events.

The process of model construction is one by which existing knowledge may be ordered or reordered, or relationships between known objects or events conceptualized and understood; it is a valuable means by which either abstract or unobservable phenomena can be portrayed, taught and observed.

The Concept of "Models"

In order to understand the particular ways in which science uses the term *model*, it is necessary to bring to conscious awareness its broader range of meaning and application. The term has acquired a decided halo effect, and, as Kaplan (1964) has aptly acknowledged, models are considered to be "good things" having great status and value in the scientific endeavor. As a result, the term is often applied loosely, without awareness of the ways in which its unconsidered use confuses the reader.

In common language, the term model refers to a precise replication of the structure of an object—as, for example, a model train or model ship. In other instances, the term is used to describe an ideal version of

From Advances in Nursing Science, *January 1979, 1(2), 13–21. Copyright ©1979, Aspen Systems Corporation. Reprinted with permission of Aspen Systems Corporation.*

About the Author

HELEN A. BUSH currently is a Professor of Nursing at Texas Woman's University, Denton, Texas, where she has been on the faculty since 1977. Besides her teaching responsibilities at TWU, she has worked administratively as Dean ad interim, Assistant Dean of Graduate Studies, and Coordinator of Curriculum for the College of Nursing. Dr. Bush is a graduate of Mercy Hospital School of Nursing in Baltimore, Maryland. She continued nursing studies at the University of Arizona and Texas Woman's University and earned B.A., M.A., and Ph.D. degrees in Education from Arizona State University. Before coming to TWU, Dr. Bush held faculty appointments at Northwestern State University in Shreveport, Louisiana; Arizona State University; and Mesa Community College in Mesa, Arizona.

Dr. Bush's research interests focus on various aspects of theory development in the care of older persons. Besides her research activities, she also serves as curriculum development consultant to colleges of nursing. She is a member of the American Nurses' Association, National League for Nursing, American Gerontological Society, Pi Lambda Theta, and Sigma Theta Tau.

something, usually an abstract ideal. Examples of such usage are "model child" or "model city" or "model hospital unit." Here, for instance, a model hospital unit may or may not exist; or it may be constructed according to the abstract ideals conceptualized in advance, in order to demonstrate the feasibility or possibility that such an ideal might exist. The critical feature in each of these common usages is isomorphism; that is, the model is constructed in such a way as to be structurally "true" to the object for which it is a model.

Brodbeck (1969) emphasizes the importance of isomorphism in scientific models, stressing that it must be maintained in two distinct ways. First, the reality represented must determine the form of the model. Second, the relations between the parts of that reality must be maintained in the model.

The Study of Structural Relationships

Models in both general and scientific usage provide a means of exhibiting, examining, observing and teaching the structural relationships of a selected reality in a way that is not possible in reality. For example, a planetarium provides a model of the universe as viewed from the planet Earth, and the structural entities in the planetarium may be caused to move in a way that is analogous to the reality we observe in the heavens. However, in certain critical ways the model of the heavens does not correspond to reality. The forces that move the

heavenly bodies are contrived, and the speed with which the movement occurs may be altered according to the purposes of the person working with the model. Further, the model heavenly bodies themselves do not replicate the organic substances or energy complexes which exist in reality. Thus, while the model has great value in teaching, observing and studying various movements of the heavens, it does not explain or predict these movements, nor does it demonstrate certain functional or causative phenomena which are recognized or speculated to exist.

Fuller has stated that "how we think is epistemology, and epistemology is modelable; which is to say that knowledge organizes itself geometrically, i.e., with models" (Fuller, 1975, p.487). Models therefore provide an important means of communicating what a scientist has in mind when speaking of an abstract entity, or a structure or process that cannot be directly observed. For example, a structural model of an atom or a molecule may be presented to students or colleagues to visually represent a scientist's conceptualization of an entity not yet observed directly. The traits of the atom are deduced from certain events that have been demonstrated in the laboratory, and the scientist constructs a model to depict its inferred structural properties.

Similarly, a model might be used to depict a behavioral process or structure that exists in reality, but that can only be observed through the indirect behaviors of those engaged in the process or structure. Thus an organizational structure model pictures otherwise intangible ways in which the persons in the organization relate to one another.

An example may be found in Claus and Bailey's (1977) model of power and influence which depicts elements that are conceptualized as being essential to the abstract, but real, phenomenon of power. Because of the obvious difficulties of representing them pictorially, abstractions—such as "authority"—are expressed in words and abstract relationships by arrows. In a model, the word "authority" in a box does not represent real authority in the same sense that a sail on a model boat represents an actual sail on a real ship. However, the building of a model is always a logical activity, in which a group of perceptions of reality is symbolically or otherwise represented (Meadows, 1957).

Cognitive Styles

Kaplan (1964) presents six cognitive styles used by scientists to accomplish their scientific goals. They are: (a) literary, (b) academic, (c) eristic, (d) symbolic, (e) postulational, and (f) formal.

The literary cognitive style is generally used in sciences concerned with human behavior, and emphasizes the perspective of the people who are being studied rather than the scientist's own explanatory scheme. The discipline of anthropology often uses this style. The academic cognitive style—used by sociologists such as Parsons—is much more abstract and uses a technical vocabulary to express ideas. The events studied tend to be highly ideational rather than observational, and are interpreted from a theoretical or speculative standpoint. The eristic style focuses on proof of specific propositions, and makes much use of experimental and statistical data. Behavioral psychologists such as Pavlov have worked in this mode.

The symbolic style conceptualizes its subject matter mathematically. The probabilistic study of learning theory has utilized this style, for example. The postula-

tional style is related to the symbolic style, but differs from it as logic differs from mathematics; i.e., the focus is on the validity of proof, rather than on the content of the propositions. Validated postulates, or axioms, serve as the basis for deriving theorems, which are verified in the empirical reality of the subject matter being studied. The study of kinship systems is conducted in this manner.

The formal cognitive style is based on the postulational style, but differs from it in that the mathematical terms are not defined in relation to any empirical content. The relationships between the mathematical symbols themselves are deemed to be consistent regardless of the subject matter to which they are applied. Euclid's geometry is one such system: the "points" to which it refers can be interpreted as ordered pairs of real numbers or its "lines" as linear functions of real numbers. This style is relatively rare in behavioral sciences.

Kaplan (1964) states that the term *model* and the scientific process to which it applies are most accurately used in conjunction with the formal, postulational and perhaps the symbolic style. In such applications the term model comes closest to its classic scientific meaning: a theory established in one field but transferable to another. The laws connecting concepts in the first field can be shown to connect corresponding concepts in the newer field—that is, the laws are isomorphic, obviously symmetrical and can be demonstrated to remain the same regardless of the subject matter. With such a "transfer," an established theory becomes a "model" for understanding, explaining and predicting the relationships of the newer field to which it is applied. An example is applying a theory of epidemiology of disease to the transmission of social information.

Common Features

Though concepts and styles of modeling vary, all models have certain features in common. A model represents some aspect of reality, concrete or abstract, by means of a likeness which may be structural, pictorial, diagrammatic or mathematical. A model focuses attention on the structure of a model itself rather than on properties of its subject matter. Where structural or functional relationships are depicted or implied, the *nature* of such relationships is not inherently a part of the model.

Functions or structural relationships may be defined in quantifiable terms, but not in causative, or explanatory, terms applied to the nature of the subject matter. In other words, the richness of the underlying phenomena and their relationships are not explained by the model. A model does not undertake to determine *why* a certain structure or relationship occurs. What a model accomplishes is the precise structural expression of a scientist's thinking. A model orders, clarifies and systematizes selected components of the phenomena it serves to depict.

The Relationship Between Models and Theories

In order to fully appreciate the nature, function and value of models, it is necessary to examine their relationship to theory. Often the terms *model* and *theory* are used interchangeably; this is confusing and blurs the precision which science seeks to attain.

Kaplan (1964) believes that the practice of regarding all theories as models had its beginning in language and meaning at a time when a true proposition had the same structure as the fact it validated. Today the building of models is only one technique the scientist uses and is not to be considered *the* important work of the scientist.

Nevertheless, scientific models, by virtue of exhibiting a structure, do simplify a complex system or properties of a system, selecting certain components deemed necessary for the conceptualization of the object of study and consciously omitting certain other related phenomena. For example, a planetarium, which may be conceptualized as a model of the heavens, does not include an accounting of the real physical forces which cause the heavens to rotate as they do. A model may exhibit, in simplified form, the structure of reality,

but the feature or relative simplicity is not what causes it to be a model.

Appropriately Relating Models to Theories

How then are models appropriately related to theories? While a model primarily expresses structure, a theory provides substance in addition to structure. Kerlinger defines theory as follows:

> A theory is a set of interrelated construct (concept) definitions, and propositions that present a systematic view of phenomena by specifying relations among variables, with the purpose of explaining and predicting the phenomena (Kerlinger, 1973, p. 9)

The logical units of a theory are several. A set of concepts is needed which will permit a description of a situation. Basic assumptions and certain definitions must be stated. A set of operations is needed to develop the concepts. Relationships between and among the concepts must be shown. Propositions or deductions must be set forth. In order to verify the concepts and the hypotheses that are stated or implied by the theory, empirical indicators are needed. As conceptualized by Weber (1969), theory construction requires that the interdependence of concrete phenomena be shown, and the causes of the conditions (variables) and their significance be presented.

Three Types of Relationships

Three types of relationships between models and theories may be identified. First, models may be constructed for *theories.* A physical model (e.g., a model of an atom or a molecule) may be used to display certain structural and functional relationships that are inherent in a specific theory. Similarly, a diagrammatic model may portray certain features of a theory of group dynamics.

In these instances, the model is offered to represent aspects of the theory that cannot be easily or completely communicated in descriptive language alone. Such a model is "tied to" a particular theory and serves to examine or explain certain of its structural features.

The model's meaning is limited to the terms of the theory which it represents, and is viewed from a perspective offered by that theory alone.

A second type of relationship exists when theories are used to explain certain features of an independently constructed model—that is, one that is not tied to a particular theory. Thus, in the planetarium example, theories of physical phenomena may be used to identify the causes of celestial movements displayed in the model and the unusual or out-of-the-ordinary events that occur, and to predict future occurrences in the universe. Different theories, sometimes not compatible with one another, may be offered and studied for their validity and reliability in explaining and predicting the movements of the universe. The model serves a useful purpose in that it presents a manipulatable exhibit of the reality being studied, and stimulates development of possible scientific explanations.

The Claus and Bailey (1977) power and influence model exemplifies this type of model-theory relationship. Their model has been constructed to exhibit a structural relationship between various behavioral phenomena. The authors have made certain observations and drawn on the validations of other scientists in order to offer the model as an acceptable isomorph of the relationships perceived to exist in reality. However, the degree of isomorphism between this model and the reality it represents is not as easily validated as that which can be demonstrated between planetarium and universe. Various theories are used to explain the nature of the relationships, and to offer alternate explanations of "why" these relationships exist.

The third type of relationship is a formal model of a theory. (See the previous discussion of the formal cognitive style.) Such a model, usually mathematical in nature, exhibits certain "true" relationships that are independent of subject matter. The model can thus be applied to any number of different phenomena, and the relationships inherent in it will be demonstrated to be constant. The model exists independent of subject matter, though its theoretical expression may vary considerably according to the nature of the subject under

consideration. In each theory derived from the model, however, the relationships of the model remain consistent.

Utilization of Models for Nursing

Research

Models can be used in two different ways in relation to the process of nursing research. First, the research process itself may be conceptualized by means of a model such as the one described by Chinn and Jacobs (1978) in "A Model for Theory Development in Nursing." Such a model brings to conscious awareness each structural component of the research process as conceptualized by the authors, and exhibits certain features of relationship among and between these components. The model may help to define and guide specific research tasks; it also makes it possible to maintain a focus on the overriding goals or intended outcomes of the research effort.

In another sense, the researcher may use a model to facilitate thinking about concepts and relationships between them. The model selected depends on the nature of the research. It may have any of the three types of relationships to theory described above, although the formal model-theory relationship is probably nonexistent in nursing at present. The researcher may use an existing model or may construct one specifically for the research at hand.

The model simplifies, and by so doing it assists in ordering, clarifying and analyzing concepts and thinking processes. It brings together crucial elements of knowledge economically—providing structure while minimizing the fullness of the substance. Caution is needed, however, to avoid oversimplifying the phenomena under study. To view phenomena conceptually by means of a particular model is to put on mental "blinders." These may prevent the recognition of certain critical variables excluded from the model or may enhance inaccurate preconceived notions about possible reality.

Batey says of the guiding or "mapping" function within the conceptual phase of research:

> . . . the substance for the map is the background knowledge that delineates the present knowledge state about the problem. The mapping process yields the theoretical statement through which the investigator attempts to construct as accurate an image of the phenomenon of study as existing knowledge and her logical interrelation of that knowledge will permit (Batey, 1978, p. 326).

The model may thus be seen as providing the structure or map which enables theory to take form in relation to the research under way.

Education

Educational models can generally be used in three ways: in guiding the student-teacher interaction, in planning the curriculum and in selecting materials for instruction. In nursing education, as in nursing research and nursing practice, a model serves to unify, to give direction and to simplify. By using a model, the nurse educator can identify focuses and rationalize them within an appropriate frame of reference.

Nursing education uses two major types of models: general models for the teaching-learning process and models developed specifically for nursing. In the first category are models of learning processes, motivation, human interaction and human development. Examples of nursing-specific models used in nursing curricula are: Rogers' model of unitary man, Neuman's total person approach to patient problems, the Roy Adaptation model and the Johnson Behavioral System model. Some models are designed for very specific purposes, while others have wider applications.

Practice

Nurse practitioners have special concerns relating to the day-to-day problems and situations they deal with. Where changes are needed in these areas of concern, there must be objectives for change—and in order to achieve objectives or outcomes of care, the practitioner must have some thoughts on direction and evaluation. It is here that a model or models may be of assistance. Chin (1969) states that the practitioner has a style of

thinking about situations which utilizes concepts to sort out events, and that behind the conceptualization lie assumptions. By building or utilizing a model the practitioner "becomes at once the observer, analyzer and modifier of the system of concepts he is using" (Chin, 1969, pp. 297–312).

A comparison of various conceptual models for nursing practice reveals likenesses—which is logical, since nursing generally attends to human behavior and its environment. Major models used in nursing practice are the system model, the developmental model and the interactionist model. System models have been generated by Johnson, Roy, Neuman and Rogers. This type, the system, is a universal. Interdependencies and interactions are inherent. There are structure, organization and stability in a system, which is itself a model. Developmental models have been derived from the theoretical works of Freud, Erikson, Maslow, Sullivan and Rogers. The central theme of this type of model is growth and change to meet certain stated goals, and movement takes place from one level or state to the next. Selected factors are responsible for this movement, and it is these natural or environmental forces which practitioners work to predict and control.

King, Orem, Orlando and Wiedenbach have created interactionist models which have their basis in the Gestalt principle of the whole being greater than the sum of its parts. Wholeness is the major construct, and integrity of the person is the goal of nursing. The categories of terms which form the essence of this type of model are social systems, interpersonal relationships, interactive process, perceptions and health.

Models Stimulate Scientific Process

Building and using models is a logical activity in which a group of perceptions is represented— symbolically or otherwise—so as to clarify them and communicate them more effectively. Models provide analogues to reality and stimulate the scientific process by identifying new possibilities for explanation, prediction and control of phenomena. As with the use of other types of analogies, the limitations of the likeness must be recognized and understood. The selection of a model or models to be used depends on the discipline, the particular purposes of the research at hand and the personal preference of the nurse-artist-scientist. Whatever model is chosen, it would represent reality as precisely as possible.

For nurses, the model or models constructed or chosen must represent the ordered reality of nursing's focus—persons, their environment, their health and nursing itself. As nurse practitioners collaborate with nurse scholars in viewing outcomes of nursing care, through the use of clearly represented models, nursing's actions will become precisely and consistently specified.

References

Batey, V. (1977). Conceptualization: Knowledge and logic guiding empirical research. *Nursing Research, 26,* 324–329.

Brodbeck, M. (1969). Models, meanings and theories. In M. Brodbeck (Ed.), *Readings in the philosophy of the social sciences.* London: Macmillan/Collier-Macmillan Limited.

Chin, R. (1969). The utility of system models and developmental models for practitioners. In W.G. Bennis, K.D. Benne, & R. Chin (Eds.), *The planning of change.* (pp. 297–312). New York: Holt, Rinehart and Winston.

Chinn, P.L., & Jacobs, M.K. (1978). A model for theory development in nursing. *Advances in Nursing Science, 1*(1), 1–11.

Claus, K.E., & Bailey, J.T. (1977). *Power and influence in health care: A new approach to leadership.* St. Louis: C.V. Mosby.

Fuller, R. (1975). *Synergetics, explorations in the geometry of thinking.* New York: Macmillan.

Kaplan, A. (1964). *The conduct of inquiry.* New York: Crowell.

Kerlinger, N. (1973). *Foundations of behavioral research.* New York: Holt, Rinehart and Winston.

Meadows, P. (1975). Models, systems and science. *American Sociological Review, 22,* 3–9.

Weber, M. (1969). Ideal types and theory construction. In M. Brodbeck (Ed.), *Readings in the philosophy of the social sciences.* London: Macmillan/Collier-Macmillan Limited.

The Author Comments

In the summer of 1977, Peggy L. Chinn taught a course called "Practice-Oriented Nursing Theory" to a group of master's-level graduate nursing students. Later, a group of faculty members led by Peggy taught the course. As is typical, each faculty member selected several concepts to develop for the class. Among several other topics, I selected "Models for Nursing."

In preparation for the class, the faculty discussion led us to at least three major content areas:
1. The idea of similarities and differences between a model and a theory
2. The use of models in nursing and in the three areas of research, education, and practice
3. The various models developed by nurses as well as those developed by others but being used by nurses.
This article was based on the lecture that I developed around these major ideas.

Currently, I believe that models and theories are better understood but still are underutilized by nurses as tools to support better nursing care. As a natural part of the thinking process, the individual nurse has available a world model to assist in dealing with the environment. Within the world model are those major models that the nurse uses on a day-to-day basis: a decision model, an interpersonal relationships model, an adaptation/change model, a communications model, and a nursing model.

Because nursing is very complex, the conscious use of models to abstract from reality is most advantageous. Modeling does not negate using intuition, and in fact there may be a reciprocal relationship between the using models and intuitive thinking. If the nurse does not use models and theories, the nurse has a collection of concepts without relationships. With relationships constructed, implications can be derived and predictions identified. The necessary analysis is made easier by the order provided by the model. Thus, models and theories can help the nurse change knowledge into knowledgeable action.

—HELEN A. BUSH

Chapter 40

Areas of Agreement in Nursing Theory Development

Jacquelyn Haak Flaskerud

Edward J. Halloran

Progress in developing nursing theory has slowed considerably since the flurry of work done in the late 1960s and early 1970s, which generated advances now evident in required nursing theory courses at the graduate level and in continuing nursing theory conferences. Many practitioners either have not heard of nursing theory or find its usefulness abstract; educators circumvent or argue about it; and researchers use frameworks from other disciplines.

There are several reasons for the slow progress of nursing theory development, including the propensity of nurses to downgrade themselves, their services, and their products. While nurses do not hesitate to term the formulations from anthropology, sociology, and psychology as "theory," they cautiously warn that their attempts at theoretical formulations are "models" or "conceptual frameworks." Nurses continue to believe that theories from other disciplines are better developed than their own. The use of outside theories in research is encouraged and taught to nursing students. Schlotfeldt (1975) and Johnson (1974, 1978) warn of the fallacy of this belief and its detrimental effects on nursing theory development.

Many of the theoretical formulations in both the nursing and social science disciplines do not meet the rigorous criteria of narrow boundaries, specificity, and explicit interrelationships required of a theory (Johnson, 1974). Yet the social science disciplines do not waste time in controversy over whether their attempts at theory are "models" or "theories" but concentrate on developing them into theories. Nursing, however, seems to have reached a plateau in theory development, concentrating on the differences between models and theories, which deters theory development, rather than concentrating on content analysis and testing of theories.

The downgrading of nursing theory and the emphasis on differences have led to the widespread belief

About the Authors

JACQUELYN HAAK FLASKERUD was born in and grew up in Indiana. After high school, she lived in the Greater Chicago area for 18 years, then moved to California in 1978, where she has lived ever since. She is a graduate of Chicago Wesley Memorial Hospital and Northwestern University (B.S.N., 1964) and received both a M.S.N. in Psychiatric Nursing (1972) and a Ph.D. in Nursing (1978) from the University of Illinois at the Medical Center, Chicago. She currently is a professor at the UCLA School of Nursing. Before accepting a faculty appointment at UCLA in 1980, Dr. Flaskerud taught at California State University and the University of Illinois.

Dr. Flaskerud currently devotes considerable attention and research to two major areas: AIDS and low income women, and culture and mental illness. She describes herself as a social, political, and professional activist, and states that her political outlook ". . .has influenced my approach to nursing—to energize it, work for change, self-respect, and self-esteem for nursing and nurses."

When asked about the future for theory development in nursing, Dr. Flaskerud responded "I recently gave the keynote address at the first National Nursing Theory Conference at UCLA. Five of the original nurse theorists were there. It was an exciting and historical occasion. I was impressed by the work being done in the areas of research, clinical practice, and curriculum development using the models developed by these pioneers in nursing theory."

EDWARD J. HALLORAN was born in Waterbury, Connecticut, and grew up in New Britain in central Connecticut. After graduating from a diploma nursing school, he studied for a bachelor's degree in night school for 7 years. He later completed full-time study for a master's degree in Public Health at Yale in 1975, then received his Ph.D. in Nursing from the University of Illinois at the Medical Center, Chicago, in 1980. He was taught by his mentor, Professor John D. Thompson of Yale University, to appreciate the historical context of health care matters. Since 1970, he has practiced nursing administration in a rural hospital in northwestern Connecticut, in a suburban Chicago hospital, and in an urban teaching hospital in Cleveland. He now teaches nursing in the undergraduate, registered nurse, masters, and doctoral programs at the University of North Carolina School of Nursing.

Dr. Halloran has been actively involved in the affairs of the American Assembly for Men in Nursing, on the premise that men and boys in this country need visible role models to encourage their consideration of nursing as a career. He has convinced himself, through study, practice, and research, that nursing is a highly valued societal service.

among nurses that theory is useless and that there is little agreement among nurse theorists. The strong disagreement among nurses about the apparent lack of agreement on what is uniquely nursing leads to discouragement, frustration, and inattention to theory development. However, a closer examination of theory development work indicates that disagreement is more imagined than real.

Although there are differences in interpretations of what constitutes a theory, most nurses agree that concepts are labels or categories of objects, persons, and events to be studied in a field (Fawcett, 1978; Hardy, 1978; Jacox, 1974; Stevens, 1979; Yura &

Torres, 1975). Theory can exist at a descriptive- or concept-naming level, an explanatory- or concept-relating level, and a predictive or causal level, any of which can be normative (Stevens, 1979).

Concepts Central to Nursing

Nurses generally agree on the central concepts which have been identified in nursing. Yura and Torres (1975) reported on a National League for Nursing (NLN) survey of baccalaureate nursing programs. The major concepts in nursing were identified as man (sic), society, health, and nursing. Fawcett (1978) considered these concepts to be the essential units of nursing but substituted the word *person* for *man* to avoid sexism and *environment* for society to express this concept more fully.

In addition to identifying the major concepts, Yura and Torres (1975) provided some descriptions of these concepts from the NLN survey. However, Stevens (1979), in her criteria for analyzing nursing theories, gives some direction for what each of these concepts must encompass to be useful to nursing. Environment is not included. Stevens points out that *persons* must be defined in two ways: first, in their entirety as human beings, and second, in their role as patients or candidates for nursing. Nursing must be defined as something the nurse does that is unique. The concept of *health* is treated as *health-illness* because nursing actions occur in this aspect of a person's life. Health and illness must be defined in terms of the limits of nursing intervention in a person's life. The relationships of nursing actions to person, nursing actions to health-illness, and person to health-illness are included in Stevens' criteria for analyzing nursing theory. Stevens (1979) advocates that these criteria be sought in any nursing theory.

Further support for the centrality of these concepts to nursing science can be seen in the theories themselves. An analysis shows that these concepts are addressed in each of the theories. (Each of the theories chosen illustrates our point in each case. They were chosen to represent variety and quantity. A theory used at a particular point could illustrate another point, or additional theories not referenced could be used.)

Person as an entirety is addressed holistically (Levine, 1971; Rogers, 1970) or as having parts broadly identifiable as biologic, psychologic, and sociocultural (Johnson, 1980; Orem, 1980; Roy, 1980). Person as a patient or candidate for nursing actions is defined as ill, healthy, or both healthy and ill (Levine, 1971; Orem, 1980; Rogers, 1970; Roy, 1980). Nursing actions are defined as what nurses do for and with the person as patient (Henderson, 1966; Orem, 1980; Orlando, 1961). Environment, interacting with the person (Johnson, 1980; Orlando, 1961; Roy, 1980) or coex-

tensive with the person (Levine, 1971; Rogers, 1970), is defined as a source of or an influence on the health or illness of the person (Johnson, 1980; Neuman, 1980; Roy, 1980.)

There is a consensus among nurses on the importance of these concepts, but this area of agreement needs greater emphasis and recognition, so that it can be taken as a stepping-off point in theory development. For example, it is now possible to pull these four concepts from a particular nursing theory and use them as part of a framework to structure a curriculum. The concepts thus become more clearly defined.

One clarifying note should be made. Fawcett (1978) raised the issue of whether a theory, to be considered a nursing theory, must include all four of the essential units or concepts. Fawcett argued that the most sophisticated nursing theories would do so but that theories including one or more of these concepts could also be considered nursing theories. However, in any nursing theory the concept of nursing as an activity must be included. Theories on the nature of the person, health and illness, and environment help explain nursing's basic concepts and relationships. However, these theories are also useful to other social and health sciences. Nursing theory must include the concept of nursing and, at higher levels of development, must explain and predict how nursing actions affect or interrelate with other concepts to produce a desired patient outcome.

The Concept of Nursing

Although nurses give some attention to differing interpretations of person, environment, and health and illness, nurses are most acutely aware of supposed differences in conceptualizing the nursing role or what nurses do that is unique. In this area, too, the differences are more imagined than real. There is basic agreement among nursing theories concerning the role and unique qualities of nursing.

Florence Nightingale (1860/1946) described nursing action as the provision of an environment conducive to healing and health promotion. In her time and with her authority in the emerging field of nursing, clearly this action was uniquely nursing. Since that time, explanations of which actions are uniquely nursing have ranged from "maid's work" to "junior doctoring" to "doing everything." The lack of a clear explanation of what actions are uniquely nursing has resulted in conflicting guidelines for practice within schools of nursing, complaints that new graduates do not know how to practice, and too few studies by researchers of the effect of nursing interventions. The blame has been placed on a lack of agreement. However, there is a consensus among nursing theorists on what nurses do, and it has not changed dramatically since Nightingale defined it.

Most nursing theories agree that nurses manage the interaction between the patient and the environment to promote healing or health. Nursing activity consists of constantly and immediately regulating, promoting, modifying, maintaining, and monitoring the interaction between the patient and the environment and communicating that interaction. This is the activity for which other health professionals and the public rely on nurses. There also is agreement on the process by which nursing activity is carried out—through assessment, planning intervention, and evaluation (Johnson, 1980; Nueman, 1980; Orem, 1980; Roy, 1980).

Partial Focus on Person-Environment Interaction

The attention given in nursing theories to managing the interaction between the person and the environment can be categorized on two levels; theories with a partial focus on the interaction and theories that focus nursing activity entirely on this interaction.

Some nursing theories (Henderson, 1966; Orem, 1980; Orlando, 1961) view the nurse's role as substituting for patients in meeting health-related needs when patients are unable to do so for themselves. These theories state that the nurse assumes responsibility for patients' health and daily living needs until they are able to reassume this responsibility. For example, after defining self-care as the practice of activities that individuals initiate and perform to maintain their life,

health, and well-being (Orem, 1980), Orem indicates that nursing action compensates for patients' self-care limitations and fosters and protects their self-care abilities. However, Orem recognizes the relationship between human beings and their environment and acknowledges that the ability to perform self-care can be influenced by a change in environment. Nursing techniques include, but are not limited to, managing the patient's social, physical, and psychological environment.

In a closely related explanation of nursing activity, Henderson (1966) saw the function of the nurse to be identifying and substituting for what patients lack to be independent in their will, physical strength, and knowledge of health. Many of Henderson's 14 components of basic nursing care or activity involve assisting the patient in interaction with the environment; for example, assisting with breathing, eating, drinking, eliminating, maintaining body temperature, avoiding danger in the environment, and communicating with others (Henderson, 1966, pp. 16–17).

Orlando (1961) also views nursing activity as a response to health-related physical and mental needs that patients cannot provide for themselves, including physical limitations caused by developmental factors, disability, or environmental restrictions; adverse reactions to the setting or environment; and inability to communicate. In at least two of these categories, nursing activity consists of assisting the person in interacting with the environment.

Total Focus on Person-Environment Interaction

Many nursing theories focus nursing activity completely on the interaction between the person and the environment. As mentioned earlier, Nightingale (1860/1946) described nursing activity as providing the environment in which healing could occur or optimal health could be recovered. The environment was viewed as the external conditions of ventilation, warmth, effluvia, noise, and light that the nurse could regulate to enhance recuperation of the patient. In this context nursing activity would consist of managing the interaction between the patient and the environment by providing a physical environment conducive to health.

For Levine (1971), nursing action is the conservation of unity or integrity presented as the nursing problems of conserving patients' energy and structural, personal, and social integrity. The nurse accomplishes this conservation through supporting or promoting the patient's adaptation to the environment (the particular situation of the patient defined as perceptual, operational, and conceptual). Adaptation in this context can be viewed as a form of interaction.

Rogers' (1970) concepts of complementarity, helicy, and resonancy describe the individual and the environment as inseparable and coextensive (Falco & Lobo, 1980; Rogers, 1970). Change in one is inseparable from simultaneous change in the other. Nursing intervention aims at the interaction between the individual and the environment by simultaneously promoting change in the environment, the life processes of the individual, and the rhythmic patterns of their interaction.

Roy (1980), too, bases her theory on the constant and changing interaction between the person and the environment. The environment appears to be the source of stimuli to which the person must adapt to remain healthy. Nursing intervenes to maintain or promote the person's adaptation by manipulating the stimuli within the environment. Roy identifies three classes of stimuli and four modes of adaptation.

Neuman's (1980) theory includes nursing activity in interventions attempted by all health workers. This theory views the patient as an open system with lines of defense and resistance in interaction with stressors, viewed as intrapersonal, interpersonal, and extrapersonal; interpersonal and extrapersonal stressors are environmental. The nurse (or health care worker) intervenes on one of three levels of prevention to strengthen the line of defense or deal with the stressor. Intervention occurs at the point of interaction between the patient and the stressor.

Johnson's (1980) theory describes the whole person as a behavioral system consisting of interrelated and interdependent subsystems, each with certain needs to maintain health. These needs come from the environment, as do the stimuli that initiate subsystem response. Nursing regulates the environment to provide or maintain supplies or to control response.

Although each nursing theory develops the concept of nursing by bringing in other and, in many cases, different concepts, each begins with the basic notion that nursing as an activity in management of the patient-environment interaction. Thus theorists appear to have accepted a unified beginning point. Riehl and Roy (1980) give examples of other concepts (recipient of care and goal of nursing) that show a common structure in the nursing theories. Johnson (1974) points out the effectiveness for nurses, other health professionals, and the public of a unified approach to developing nursing theory. Thus nursing theorists agree on the nursing role, nursing actions, and the nursing process. Now what can be done to further this focused development?

Future Directions

Current nursing theories stress developing the concept of the person, as shown by specific descriptions of the person in nursing curricula. Courses in anatomy, physiology, biochemistry, psychology, and sociology emphasize aspects of the person, as do person-oriented nursing courses (newborn, child, adult, maternal, and geriatric).

In comparison, nursing theories or nursing curricula give little attention to developing the concept of environment. Yet development of the concept of nursing seems to hinge on an interaction and an equal development of the concepts of person and environment. It is difficult to determine from many of the nursing theories what the theorists believe to be the environment.

Questions that need to be raised and answered include: Of what does the environment consist? Where does environment end and person begin? Are persons part of the environment and indistinguishable from it? Are they shells encasing environment? Is the environment or the person deterministic? The answers to these questions will affect nursing management of the patient-environment interaction. Development of the concept of environment as it relates to a person's health or illness seems to rely on study and attention by nurse educators, researchers, and practitioners. If managing the person-environment interaction is uniquely a nursing activity, then nursing students should begin studying the environment as it relates to the person's health or illness. From this study, techniques for managing that relationship should emerge.

Development of one concept is related to development of the others. The health and illness concept also needs development because it establishes the parameters of nursing activity. It should be developed congruent with the development of the other concepts.

In American culture the concepts of person and illness have been developed according to a philosophy that sees the person as distinguishable from the environment and illness as a disease or disorder specific to the person: the person has been developed as a whole system composed of interacting subsystems. Illness has been conceptualized as a disease or disorder of a subsystem that affects the whole as well as other subsystems. To remain recognizable to the public, other health professionals, and our own practitioners, it would probably not be useful to study environment as subsuming the person but rather as distinguishable from and interacting with the person.

The areas of agreement in nursing theory development and in the nursing theories are both important and apparent. Emphasizing the controversies and disagreements to the exclusion of consensus in nursing theory leads away from its development. It is time to identify and develop the areas of agreement. Guideline's for development become clear as the areas of agreement are recognized.

In addition, recognizing the areas of agreement leads to recognition of the usefulness of current theoretical formulations in nursing. In education, nursing curricula can be structured using the four concepts central to nursing as a framework. In education and practice, skills and technologies of nursing can be selected and developed based on management of the patient-environment interaction. These nursing interventions can be extended using theories of the person, environment, and forms of management and then tested in research for their effect on patient outcomes.

References

Falco, S.M., & Lobo, M.L. (1980). Martha E. Rogers. In Nursing Theories Conference Group (Eds.), *Nursing theories: The base for professional nursing practice* (pp. 164–183). Englewood Cliffs, NJ: Prentice-Hall.

Fawcett, J. (1978). The what of theory development. In *Theory development: What, why, and how* (pp. 17–33). (NLN Pub. No. 15-1708). New York: National League for Nursing.

Hardy, M. (1974). Theories: Components, development, evaluation. *Nursing Research, 23,* 100–106.

Henderson, V. (1966). *The nature of nursing.* New York: MacMillan.

Jacox, A. (1974). Theory construction in nursing: An overview. *Nursing Research, 23,* 4–13.

Johnson, D.E. (1974). Development of theory. *Nursing Research, 23,* 372–377.

Johnson, D.E. (1978). State of the art of theory development in nursing. In *Theory development: What, why, and how* (pp. 1–10). (NLN Pub. No. 15-1708). New York: National League for Nursing.

Johnson, D.E. (1980). The behavioral system model for nursing. In J. Riehl & C. Roy (Eds.), *Conceptual models for nursing practice* (2nd ed.) (pp. 207–215). New York: Appleton-Century-Crofts.

Levine, M. (1971). Holistic nursing. *Nursing Clinics of North America, 6,* 253–263.

Neuman, B. (1980). The Betty Neuman health-care systems model: A total person approach to patient problems. In J. Riehl & C. Roy (Eds.), *Conceptual models for nursing practice* (2nd ed.) (pp. 119–134). New York: Appleton-Century-Crofts.

Nightingale, F. (1946). *Notes on nursing.* Philadelphia: J.B. Lippincott. (Originally published in 1860.).

Orem, D. (1980). *Nursing: Concepts of practice* (2nd ed.). New York: McGraw-Hill.

Orlando, I. (1961). *The dynamic nurse-patient relationship: Function, process and principles.* New York: Putnam.

Riehl, J., & Roy, C. (1980). A unified model of nursing. In J. Riehl & C. Roy (Eds.), *Conceptual models for nursing practice* (2nd ed.), (pp. 399–403). New York: Appleton-Century-Crofts.

Rogers, M.E. (1970). *An introduction to the theoretical basis of nursing.* Philadelphia: F.A. Davis.

Roy, C. (1980). The Roy adaptation model. In J. Riehl & C. Roy (Eds.), *Conceptual models for nursing practice* (2nd ed.) (pp. 179–192). New York: Appleton-Century-Crofts.

Schlotfeldt, R. (1975). The need for a conceptual framework. In P.J. Verhonick (Ed.), *Nursing research I* (pp. 3–24). Boston: Little, Brown.

Stevens, B. (1979). *Nursing theory.* Boston: Little, Brown.

Yura, H., & Torres, G. (1975). Today's conceptual frameworks within baccalaureate nursing programs. (NLN Publication No. 15–1558, pp. 17–25). New York: National League for Nursing.

Reactions

Advances in Nursing Science, July 1981, 3(4), xi.

To the Editor:

I can appreciate the intent and contribution of Flaskerud and Halloran's article (*ANS* 3:1), but I believe they falter in their discussion of "future directions" for nursing theory development.

First, health and illness are depicted as a single concept. I do not believe this to be true, and to continue with this conceptualization of two distinct phenomena will not contribute to the further theoretical development of health as a central and significant concept basic to the science of nursing.

Second, when considering the criteria of external consistency of a theory, I do not agree that nursing must necessarily perpetuate the conceptualization of a dichotomous person and environment. This perspective adds nothing that is unique to nursing. Furthermore, I think the authors underestimate the ability of people to understand the notion of "environment as subsuming the person."

Finally, I do not understand the statement "emphasizing the controversies and disagreements to the exclusion of consensus in nursing theory leads away from its development." What is meant by "its development," a single theory in nursing or perhaps nursing as a science? To the first possibility, I must state that the more theories we have in nursing to order and explain diverse phenomena, the better. Also, I do not believe there to be "a theory in or of nursing" toward which we strive.

BARBARA CHADWICK
Doctoral Student
Wayne State University
Detroit, Michigan

Response

1. I'm not sure whether Ms. Chadwick is saying we depicted health/illness as a "single concept" or conceptualized it as "two distinct phenomena." To clarify our meaning, health/illness was depicted in the foregoing fashion to convey the notion that health and illness bear some relationship to one another. Some theorists have conceptualized a continuum; others have conceptualized levels. However, there seems to be plenty of room in nursing for further conceptualizations of health/illness.

2. My personal bias is that the environment subsumes the person. But I think it's unrealistic at this point to project that other health professionals and the public share this bias. My fondest wish is that this explanation will become widely accepted. I see only fringe evidence of it at present.

3. "Nursing theory" is used in a plural sense. I also believe in many nursing theories for the science of nursing.

JACQUELYN H. FLASKERUD
Associate Professor
University of California
Los Angeles, California

The Authors Comment

This article was written to give a boost to nursing theory development and nursing theorists—to help move us along. It was meant to say "look, we're making progress and we've come a long way." It was written at a time when I thought nursing theory development had bogged down and nurses were despairing of ever developing "theory." We wanted to encourage us to continue by summarizing what had been done and by suggesting future directions. Although I realize that we now have a nursing journal that focuses on the development of the extant nursing models, my belief currently is that these models are viewed by the profession as having historical but not scientific value. The energy in theory development recently has been on the nursing diagnoses and theoretical modeling. I am not optimistic that either of these approaches will contribute to the development of nursing theory.

—JACQUELYN HAAK FLASKERUD

As members of the first class in the Ph.D. program in nursing at the College of Nursing, University of Illinois, we had numerous discussions on the nature of nursing. Our initial discussions led to some systematic observations of what was written about nursing and how it differed from the reality of nursing practice. This early discussion led to the publication of a paper entitled "Avoidance and Distancing—A Descriptive View of Nursing" (Flaskerud, Halloran, Janken, Lund, & Zetterland, 1979). We continued this discourse throughout our time together on the Chicago campus. Although our backgrounds differ greatly, Dr. Flaskerud's and I both found that many papers written about nursing used very different language but were making similar points. We set forth these observed commonalities in this article.

I continue to be impressed today by the common language used by nurses in speaking about their patients and their work and by how this language differs from how physicians and hospital administrators characterize nursing activities. Few, if any, theoretical descriptions of nursing describe the procedures or tasks that nurses are observed doing, nor do they describe the medical condition of the recipients of nursing care. In essence, it continues to be of great importance to identify the unique contributions that nurses make in the care of their patients. In a letter to Sir Henry Aukland, written in 1869, Nightingale wrote: "Nursing and medicine must never be mixed up—it spoils both." Nurse theorists have given us a golden opportunity to think of nursing as making a separate contribution to patient well being.

—EDWARD J. HALLORAN

REFERENCES

Fitzpatrick, J.J., & Whall, A.L. (1983). *Conceptual models of nursing: Analysis and application*. Bowie, MD: Brady.

Fitzpatrick, J.J., Whall, A.L., Johnston, R.L., & Floyd, J.A. (1982). *Nursing models: Applica-* tions to psychiatric mental health nursing. Bowie, MD: Brady.

Flaskerud, J., Halloran, E.J., Janken, J., Lund, M., & Zetterland, J. (1979). Avoidance and distancing, a descriptive view of nursing. *Nursing Forum, 18*, 158–174.

Chapter 41

A Framework for Analysis and Evaluation of Conceptual Models of Nursing

Jacqueline Fawcett

Conceptual models are important in guiding the development of the discipline of nursing. Yet the difference between these abstract schemes and substantive theory is often confused. This article defines and describes both types of knowledge and offers a framework for analysis and evaluation appropriate for nursing models.

Nursing knowledge is rapidly organizing around and developing from several abstract conceptual models. Among the best known are the Roy Adaptation Model (Roy, 1976), Orem's (1971) Self-Care Model, the Johnson Behavioral Systems Model (Grubbs, 1974), M.E. Rogers's (1970) Life Process Model, and King's (1971) Social Systems Model. If nursing is to continue to emerge as a distinct discipline, nursing educators must define and explore semantic and substance issues surrounding these models and their relation to other forms of knowledge. Even if we can't agree on major points, we should clarify language usage and terminology.

This article seeks to provide a clear definition of conceptual models, to delineate the particularly confused distinction between conceptual models and theories, and to develop an appropriate framework for analysis and evaluation of conceptual models. Educators must understand this material before they can effectively incorporate conceptual models into nursing program curricula. The framework presented here will permit educators and students to fully examine several models before adopting the one most congruent with their philosophy. It will also help those who prefer a more eclectic approach to choose those bits and pieces from several models that can be combined into a mean-

About the Author

JACQUELINE FAWCETT is a Professor at the University of Pennsylvania School of Nursing in Philadelphia, having joined the faculty in 1978. She makes her home in Storrs, Connecticut, and commutes to Pennsylvania. She is a graduate of Boston University (B.S., 1964) and New York University (A.M., 1970; Ph.D., 1976).

A prolific writer, Dr. Fawcett has published more than 40 articles in scholarly journals, 20 chapters in books and monographs, and 3 books. She also has been an associate editor of *Nursing Research*. Dr. Fawcett comments that she has derived great satisfaction from contributing to the advancement of nursing through her writing and publishing activities.

Besides being an accomplished writer, Dr. Fawcett is an active nurse researcher. Her research projects have investigated concepts related to the experience of pregnancy, such as spouses' body image changes, physical and psychological symptoms before and after pregnancy, and functional status. She also has conducted a series of studies dealing with reactions to and preparation for cesarean birth. She is a member of the ANA's Council of Nurse Researchers and of Sigma Theta Tau, and has served as Chairperson of Sigma Theta Tau's National Research Committee. She has helped to develop nursing theory through her writing and research activities, and as a member of the Nursing Theory Think Tank. In 1979 Dr. Fawcett was elected a Fellow in the American Academy of Nursing, in recognition of her contributions to the profession.

ingful and logical whole. Moreover, this material may be used as an organizing structure for courses focused on conceptual models.

Definition of Conceptual Model

The term conceptual model, and synonymous terms such as conceptual framework, system, or scheme, refer to global ideas about the individuals, groups, situations and events of interest to a science. These phenomena are classified into concepts, which are words bringing forth mental images of the properties of things. Concepts may be abstract ideas, such as adaptation and equilibrium, or concrete ones, such as table and chair.

Concepts are linked to form propositions stating their interrelationships. These statements constitute the basic assumptions of the science. An example of this kind of relational statement is: "People and their environments are open systems."

A conceptual model may therefore be defined as a set of concepts and those assumptions that integrate them into a meaningful configuration (Nye & Berardo, 1966). Each model, then, specifies certain phenomena

by identifying relevant concepts and by describing the connections among them. Thus, a conceptual model might outline the environmental forces or stressors acting on a person to create adaptative change, as well as the resources available to help the person maintain equilibrium while coping with these stressors.

The concepts in a conceptual model are highly abstract and usually not directly observed in the real world. Similarly, the assumptions linking the concepts are abstract generalizations that are not immediately testable. By identifying relevant phenomena, a conceptual model provides a perspective for scientists, telling them what to look at and speculate about. By describing these phenomena and their interrelationships in general and abstract terms, *the model represents the first step in developing the theoretical formulations* needed for scientific activities.[1]

---

[1] Theoretical Formulations, as used here, refers to ideas ranging from loosely constructed conjectures to fully developed, widely accepted theories. The substantive knowledge of a discipline is made up of these untested or partially validated speculations, as well as of established principles and laws.

It is not unusual to find that more than one discipline or school of thought is interested in the same concepts. What distinguishes these fields of inquiry are different definitions and measures of the concepts, and different assumptions tying them together. For example, while sociologists explore social origins of language, psychologists may examine genetic influences on the ability to communicate.

Conceptual models usually evolve from the intuitive insights of scientists, often initially within the frame of reference of a related discipline. The synthesis that occurs in the development of a new conceptual scheme, however, results in a product unique to the field. Conceptual models may also represent deductive systems that creatively combine propositions from several areas.

Conceptual models can clearly specify the phenomena of interest to nursing science, encompassed by four essential concepts: person, environment, health, and nursing (Yura & Torres, 1975). Existing nursing models define and describe person and environment and their interrelations. Most conceptualizations view the person as a biopsychosocial being who interacts with family members, the community, and other groups, as well as with the physical environment. However, each scheme presents these essential concepts in such unique ways as adaptive systems, behavioral subsystems, or complementary four-dimensional energy fields. The models further provide a definition of health, often describing both the well and ill person and environments conducive or detrimental to health. They also identify the goals of nursing, which usually derive directly from the definition of health. For example, a nursing goal might be to assist the person to attain, maintain, or regain health as defined by that conceptual scheme. Finally, each model spells out its version of the nursing process, frequently in great detail.

The several conceptual models of nursing represent various schools of thought within the discipline of nursing. As such it is not surprising that each operationalizes the four essential concepts differently and links these concepts with diverse assumptions.

Distinctions Between Conceptual Model and Theory

A conceptual model is *not* a theory. A theory is formally defined as "a set of interrelated constructs (concepts), definitions, and propositions that present a systematic view of phenomena by specifying relations among variables" (Kerlinger, 1973, p. 9). It postulates specific relations among concepts and takes the form of a description, an explanation, a prediction, or a prescription for action. Any theory presupposes a more general abstract conceptual system; the concepts, definitions, and propositions of the theory are derived from the concepts and assumptions of the model.

The literature contains many different routes from model to theory, but there is little agreement as to which path is the best. A discussion of these diverse theory-building strategies, using inductive, deductive, or retroductive thought is beyond the scope of this article (Burr, 1973). Two points, however, may be made here. First, whichever path is chosen, reaching its end requires imagination, knowledge of the subject matter, and logical thinking. And second, this road must be a rocky one, since so few conceptual models ever lead to theories.

The crucial distinction, then, between a conceptual model and a theory is the level of abstraction. As noted earlier, a conceptual model is a highly abstract system of related global concepts. A theory, in contrast, contains more concrete concepts, along with their definitions and the propositions linking them. A theory also provides greater specification of phenomena and more detailed explanations of postulated relationships than does a conceptual model. A conceptual model embodies the "world view," the paradigm, of a discipline or school of thought. Each theory derived from the model explains some or all of the paradigm's phenomena but only within a limited range. A theory is both more precise and more limited in scope than its parent conceptual scheme. For example, a nursing model might suggest that the individual's health status is a function of total environmental influences. A theory of mental health nursing might then postulate that certain patterns of family interaction foster psychological dysfunction in a given family member and explain the reasons for this outcome.

Although some people consider conceptual models to be what Merton called "grand theories"—global orientations that attempt to explain a totality of events—the position taken here is that conceptual schemes are too abstract to be considered any type of theory. As used here, theory refers to Merton's "theory of the middle range"—speculations concerned with relatively narrow ranges of data (Merton, 1957, pp. 5–6).

With these distinctions in mind, we can define a nursing theory. Nursing theories are most appropriately derived from the conceptualizations of nursing. They are characterized as sets of interrelated propositions and definitions that present systematic views of the essential concepts of nursing—person, environment, health, nursing—by specifying relations among variables derived from these ideals (Fawcett, 1978a).

Theoretical model, theoretical framework, and theoretical rationale are essentially synonymous terms frequently seen in the nursing literature. These terms refer to networks of theoretical ideas and research results from which we can deduce empirically testable hypotheses. In some articles, two or more specific theories may be connected to form a more general theory that is still sufficiently concrete to permit testing. In other articles, the rationale may rest upon generalizations from a series of observations and descriptive research findings that do not comprise a formal theory.

By now we can see that conceptual models are not specific enough to provide more than general guidelines for scientists' endeavors. Therefore, theoretical formulations must accompany the model if definitive directions for action are needed. The function served by a model determines the type of speculations required to further explain events. In nursing, conceptual frameworks act as general guides for practice, research, curricula, and administrative systems. The particular practice situation, research problem, educational program, or management setting will dictate the explanations

needed to flesh out the skeleton provided by the model. To date, we have borrowed most of these theoretical ideas from other disciplines, including psychology, sociology, biology, physics, and chemistry. Nursing theories probably will amplify or replace this borrowed knowledge as scholars succeed in their efforts to establish a body of nursing knowledge.

Some examples will help to clarify this point. Conceptual models and related theories are beginning to be used in clinical practice. For instance, Roy's assessment scheme has been applied by a family nurse clinical in her practice. Intervention strategies for this nurse's clients were guided by the model and by knowledge of physiology. In this case, we expect that the nurse's accrued observations will eventually lead to nursing theories (Roy & Obloy, 1978).

Similarly, models are now being used in development of nursing research projects. A study of body image changes of pregnant women and their husbands was derived from Rogers's conceptualization of person-environment complementarity. Since this model is highly abstract, it was necessary to base the research hypotheses on the more concrete tenets of body image theory. The study findings of similar alterations in spouses' body images during and after pregnancy lent support to both specific aspects of body image theory and global assumptions about person-environment interactions. The next step in this research program will be to develop a unique nursing theory to explain these and other aspects of the experience of pregnancy as shared by family members (Fawcett, 1977, 1978b).

Educational programs have employed conceptual frameworks to organize content for several years. Indeed, so many articles have documented this process that further elaboration is hardly required here.

Finally, conceptual models are also useful in administrative situations. For example, a hospital or community health agency could arrange nursing care plans according to the categories of a particular model's nursing process. Or, as one author suggested (C.G. Rogers, 1973), areas of clinical specialization could be developed from categories outlined in a model. In each case, additional detail would follow from relevant theories now borrowed from other sciences. However, as we accumulate observations in each category, the building blocks of nursing theories will emerge.

Analysis and Evaluation of Conceptual Models

Clearly, the distinctions between conceptual models and theories are sufficiently great to warrant different frameworks for analysis and evaluation. The nursing literature contains such excellent presentations of criteria for theories that further effort in that direction seems unnecessary (Ellis, 1968; Hardy, 1978; Torres & Yura, 1975).

The literature also includes evaluative schemas that reflect the confusion between conceptual models and theories. The one proposed by Riehl and Roy (1974) used the Dickoff and James (1968) survey list for

situation-producing theory, and therefore, from our position, is too concrete for abstract conceptualizations.

Conversely, two other review systems claimed to be designed for theory evaluation but were applied to conceptual models. Both the Duffey and Muhlenkamp (1974) and the Stevens (1979) plans include some questions appropriate to a model's level of abstraction, but like the Riehl and Roy schema, offer other items more germane to concrete theories.

Two additional schemas are appropriate for conceptual model evaluation but seem too limited for comprehensive reviews. Johnson's (1974) criteria are focused solely on social decisions while Peterson's (1977) questions lack necessary scope and detail. However, taken together, these several plans provided some building blocks for construction of the analytic and evaluative framework presented in Figure 41-1.

This framework separates questions dealing with analysis from those more appropriate to evaluation.

Questions for analysis

- What is the historical evolution of the conceptual model?
- What approach to development of nursing knowledge does the model exemplify?
- How are the four essential concepts of nursing explicated in the model?
  How is person defined and described?
  How is environment defined and described?
  How is health defined? How are wellness and illness differentiated?
  How is nursing defined? What is the goal of nursing?
  How is the nursing process described?
- What statements are made about the relationships among the four concepts?
- With what problems is the conceptual model concerned?
- What is the source of these problems?

Questions for Evaluation

- Are the biases and values underlying the conceptual model made explicit?
- Does the conceptual model provide complete descriptions of all four essential concepts of nursing?

- Do the basic assumptions completely link the four concepts?
- Is the internal structure of the conceptual model logically consistent?
- Does the conceptual model reflect the characteristics of its category type?
- Do the components of the model reflect logical translation of diverse perspectives?
- Is the conceptual model socially congruent? Does the model lead to nursing activities that meet social expectations or do the expectations created by the model require societal changes?
- Is the conceptual model socially significant? Does the model lead to nursing actions that make important differences in the client's health status?
- Is the conceptual model socially useful? Is the model comprehensive enough to provide general guides for practice, research, education, and administration?
- Does the conceptual model generate empirically testable theories?
- Do tests of derived theories yield evidence in support of the model?
- What is the overall contribution of this conceptual model to the body of nursing knowledge?

Figure 41-1   *A Framework for Analysis and Evaluation of Conceptual Models of Nursing*

The former queries permit nonjudgmental, detailed examination of the conceptual model, including its philosophical base, content, and scope. In contrast, evaluative questions allow one to draw judgmental conclusions by focusing on internal validity of a model, although not on external comparisons among various conceptualizations. This important distinction implies "that any conceptual model is valid insofar as it is reasonably sound with regard to the particular anthropology employed (i.e., man as developing, adapting, interacting)" (Zbilut, 1978, p. 128). Indeed, it is imperative that the reader understands on what level conceptual models may be compared. Since models explain the phenomena of district disciplines or schools of thought, we cannot make direct comparisons. Reese and Overton cautioned that "because of basic lack of communication, the partial overlap in subject matter, and the difference in truth criteria, (each model) must be evaluated separately, and in obedience to its own ground rules" (Overton, 1970, p. 122). Thus, judgments must be limited to the adequacy of each conceptual scheme as it stands alone.

In sum, the framework for analysis and evaluation leads to a decision to retain, modify, or discard the model, and also provides an answer to the pragmatic question of whether I can use the conceptual model for *my* nursing activities.

Questions for Analysis

A conceptual model is derived from an author's personal philosophy and scientific orientation. This philosophic base and the method of model development (usually inductive but sometimes deductive) are often revealed in the author's earlier writing and in preliminary versions of the conceptual system. The first aspect of analysis, then, asks the questions:

• What is the historical evolution of the conceptual model?
• What approach to development of nursing knowledge does the model exemplify?

Earlier we established that a conceptual model comprises a set of concepts and linking assumptions, and that the essential concepts of any nursing model

are person, environment, health, and nursing. These components lead to the second aspect of analysis. The questions are:

• How are the four essential concepts of nursing explicated in the model?
• How is person defined and described?
• How is environment defined and described?
• How is health defined? How are wellness and illness differentiated?
• How is nursing defined? What is the goal of nursing?
• How is the nursing process described?
• What statements are made about the relationships among the four concepts?

The final aspect of analysis derives from the fact that any model must be limited in scope; it cannot deal with *all* things in the universe. Although most authors start with the same view of the general purpose of nursing, in final form nursing models reflect different perspectives of the essential concepts and hence lead to considerations of different problems in the person-environment interactions related to health. Moreover, the source of these problems may vary from, for example, dysfunctional internal factors to hostile environmental factors. Borrowing from Duffey and Muhlenkamp, the questions to be raised are:

• With what problems is the conceptual model concerned?
• What is the source of these problems?

Questions for Evaluation

The first aspect of evaluation concerns the philosophic underpinnings of the model. The question is:

• Are the biases and values underlying the conceptual model made explicit? The next aspect of evaluation deals with the content of the model and relates back to the answers supplied by the second aspect of analysis. Here the questions to be posed are:
• Does the conceptual model provide complete descriptions of all four essential concepts of nursing?
• Do the basic assumptions completely link the four concepts?

This portion of the evaluation must also consider the logic of the model; its internal structure must be evaluated for congruity. Internal consistency also takes the classification of models into account. Nursing models have been categorized according to the discipline or anthropology from which they were derived and are most often labeled developmental, interaction, or systems models. Each of these "world views" has distinct characteristics that shape organization of knowledge and methodologies for application.

Internal consistency is especially important if the model incorporates more than one view of any of the essential concepts, since each has different criteria for determining the truth of statements. A synthesis that mixes perspectives also mixes truth criteria.

However, we can translate viewpoints by redefining them in a consistent manner. Translation represents the construction of a brand-new, unmixed model that is logical (Reese & Overton, 1970). The questions to be raised, then, are:

- Is the internal structure of the conceptual model logically consistent?
- Does the conceptual model reflect the characteristics of its category type?
- Do the components of the model reflect logical translation of diverse perspectives?

Johnson's evaluation criteria represent another aspect for consideration. She maintained that conceptual models are validated by social decisions. The first is *social congruence,* and the question is:

- Does the conceptual model lead to nursing activities that meet social expectations or do the expectations created by the conceptual model require societal changes?

The second decision is *social significance,* and here the question is:

- Does the conceptual model lead to nursing actions that make important differences in the client's health status?

The third decision is *social utility,* and the question to be raised is:

- Is the conceptual model comprehensive enough to provide general guides for practice, research, education, and administration?

The next part of evaluation reflects the relation between models and theories. As was noted earlier, theories are derived from models; thus, the theory-generating contributions of the model should be judged, as well as the result of empirical tests of any theories derived from the model. The questions to be posed are:

- Does the conceptual model generate empirically testable theories?
- Do tests of derived theories yield evidence in support of the model?

The final aspect of evaluation is as general as the models themselves. This question judges the contribution of the model to nursing knowledge, asking:

- What is the overall contribution of this conceptual model to the body of nursing knowledge?

Conclusion

This article sought to distinguish between two forms of knowledge—general conceptualizations and specific theoretical formulations. Further, in light of the current expansion and elaboration of nursing models, a framework for analysis and evaluation appropriate to their level of abstraction was developed. This plan can assist nurses in comparing various methods before choosing one to guide their activities. My own work in applying these questions to individual conceptual schemes indicates that gaps and logical inconsistencies are identifiable and readily corrected. Moreover, my experience in teaching nursing science courses shows that the framework greatly facilitates students' comprehension and fuller use of the models as bases for nursing practice, research, education, and administration.

References

Burr, W.R. (1973). *Theory construction and the sociology of the family.* New York: John Wiley & Sons.

Dickoff, J., & James, P. (1986). A theory of theories: A position paper. *Nursing Research, 17,* 197–203.

Duffey, M., & Muhlenkamp, A.F. (1974). A framework for theory analysis. *Nursing Outlook, 22,* 570–574.

Ellis, R. (1968). Characteristics of significant theories. *Nursing Research, 17,* 217–222.

Fawcett, J. (1977). The relationship between identification and patterns of change in spouses' body images during and after pregnancy. *International Journal of Nursing Studies, 14,* 199–213.

Fawcett, J. (1978a). The 'what' of theory development. In *Theory development: What, why, how?* (NLN Pub. No. 15–1708). New York: National League for Nursing.

Fawcett, J. (1978b). Body image and the pregnant couple. *The American Journal of Maternal Child Nursing, 3*, 227–233.

Grubbs, J. (1974). An interpretation of the Johnson behavioral system model. In J.P. Riehl & C. Roy (Eds.), *Conceptual models for nursing practice* (pp. 160–197). New York: Appleton Century-Crofts.

Hardy, M.E. (1978). Evaluating nursing theory. In *Theory development: What, why, how?* (pp. 82–86) (NLN Pub. No. 15–1708). New York: National League for Nursing.

Johnson, D.E. (1974). Development of theory: A requisite for nursing as a primary health profession. *Nursing Research, 23*, 376–377.

Kerlinger, F.N. (1973). *Foundations of behavioral research* (2nd ed.). New York: Holt, Rinehart and Winston.

King, I.M. (1971). *Toward a theory of nursing.* New York: John Wiley & Sons.

Merton, R.F. (1957). *Social theory and social structure* (Rev. ed.). New York: Free Press.

Nye, F.I., & Berardo, F.M. (1966). *Emerging conceptual frameworks in family analysis.* New York: Macmillan.

Orem, D.E. (1971). *Nursing: Concepts of practice.* New York: McGraw-Hill.

Peterson, C.J. (1977). Questions frequently asked about the development of a conceptual framework. *Journal of Nursing Education, 16*, 22–32.

Reese, H.W., & Overton, W.F. (1970). Models of development and theories of development. In L.R. Goulet & P.B. Baltes (Eds.), *Life-span development psychology* (p. 122). New York: Academic Press.

Riehl, J.P., & Roy, C. (Eds.). (1974). *Conceptual models for nursing practice.* New York: Appleton-Century-Crofts.

Rogers, C.G. (1973). Conceptual models as guides to clinical nursing specialization. *Journal of Nursing Education, 12*, 2–6.

Rogers, M.E. (1970). *An introduction to the theoretical basis of nursing.* Philadelphia: F.A. Davis.

Roy, C. (1976). *Introduction to nursing: An adaptation model.* Englewood Cliffs, NJ: Prentice-Hall.

Roy, C., & Obloy, M. (1978). The practitioner movement—Toward a science of nursing. *American Journal of Nursing, 78*, 1698–1702.

Stevens, B.J. (1979). *Nursing theory: Analysis, application, evaluation.* Boston: Little, Brown.

Torres, G., & Yura, H. (1975). The meaning and functions of concepts and theories within education and nursing. In *Faculty-curriculum development, Part III: Conceptual framework—Its meaning and function* (NLN Pub. No. 15–1558) (pp. 5–6). New York: National League for Nursing.

Yura, H., & Torres, G. (1975). Today's conceptual frameworks within baccalaureate nursing programs. In *Faculty-curriculum development, Part III: Conceptual framework—Its meaning and function* (NLN Pub. No. 15–1558) (pp. 17–25). New York: National League for Nursing.

Zbilut, J.P. (1978). Epistemologic constraints to the development of a theory of nursing [Letter to the Editor]. *Nursing Research, 27*, 128.

The Author Comments

Doctoral course work with Martha Rogers at New York University sensitized me to the differences between conceptual models and theories. I began developing the framework for analysis and evaluation of conceptual models of nursing in a graduate seminar conducted at the University of Connecticut School of Nursing during the fall semester of the 1976–1977 academic year. I was dissatisfied with evaluative schemes found in the literature, which either reflected the confusion between conceptual models and theories or were too limited for a comprehensive analysis and evaluation. I have revised the framework since the publication of this article in *Nurse Educator*. The most recent revision appears in Chapter 2 of the second edition of my book *Analysis and Evaluation of Conceptual Models of Nursing* (Philadelphia: F.A. Davis, 1989).

—JACQUELINE FAWCETT

REFERENCE

Fawcett, J. (1989). *Analysis and evaluation of conceptual models of nursing* (2nd ed.). Philadelphia: F.A. Davis.

Chapter 42

Models and Model Building in Nursing

Wade Lancaster
Jeanette Lancaster

Nursing education has historically focused on knowledge related to practice skills. However, in recent years increasing emphasis in the classroom has been placed on research and theory. Nursing has moved from an applied art borrowing theories from the behavioral and physical sciences to explain its practice to a profession actively involved in the delineation and development of nursing theory. Few topics are receiving more attention in the nursing literature than the need for a refined and clearly articulated theoretical base.

Nursing educators and practitioners generally agree that nursing theory, practice, and research are intimately interdependent. Theory can only be derived from research in nursing practice. Chinn and Jacobs maintain that "the development of theory is the most crucial task facing nursing today" (Chinn & Jacobs, 1978, p. 1). If nursing is to gain power and prestige within the health care system it is increasingly impor-

tant that practitioners have theoretical bases for their practice.

As one way of moving toward the development of a theoretical base for practice Chinn and Jacobs (1978) have set forth a four-stage set of operations for a theory development system: (a) concept examination and analysis, (b) formulation and validation of relational statements, (c) theory construction, and (d) the practical application of theory. While there is no argument with their position that nurses must become increasingly involved in the development of theory, the mastery of each step in this four-stage process needs careful attention. Chinn and Jacobs emphasize that concept examination and analysis is probably the most important, yet most frequently overlooked, operation in the theory development system.

A model is a device to facilitate the examination and analysis of concepts. Unfortunately not enough

About the Authors

WADE LANCASTER is Director of Marketing at the University of Virginia Health Sciences Center and holds faculty appointments in both the School of Medicine and the School of Commerce. Before joining the University of Virginia in 1989, he held faculty appointments at Wright State University, the University of Alabama in Birmingham, and Texas Christian University. His educational background is in business administration; he has studied at Kent State University (B.B.A., 1970), Texas Christian University (M.B.A., 1971), and the University of Oklahoma (Ph.D., 1983). Dr. Lancaster believes that his marketing background meshes well with his interest in health care and nursing. He writes that "writing and lecturing about the application of marketing and consumer behavior concepts in the health care arena has always been a satisfying experience because the appropriateness of the applications forces me to critically examine the assumptions underlying the concepts. Working with nurses and writing about nursing has given me a broadened interdisciplinary perspective which, in turn, stimulates new ideas and a whole host of related questions to be investigated."

Along with his writing, research, and teaching activities, Dr. Lancaster finds time to run. He comments that "running provides an opportunity to escape into an environment that is conducive to exploring new ideas, sorting out complex problems, and thinking about anything and everything."

JEANETTE LANCASTER is Dean and Professor at the University of Virginia School of Nursing. She has been a nurse educator for more than 20 years, teaching at Case Western Reserve University, Texas Christian University, and the University of Alabama in Birmingham and serving from 1984–89 as Dean and Professor at Wright State University–Miami Valley School of Nursing. She received her basic nursing education at the University of Tennessee, earning a B.S.N. in 1966. She continued her education at Case Western Reserve University (M.S.N., 1969) and the University of Oklahoma (Ph.D., 1977).

Dr. Lancaster has written on various aspects of community mental health nursing. Many of her published articles have been co-authored with Dr. Wade Lancaster and incorporate marketing principles with concepts of nursing practice. Besides her journal articles, Dr. Lancaster has written six published books and chapters in six other nursing texts.

Interest in models and theory development is also reflected in Dr. Lancaster's writing and research. She comments "I have enjoyed being able to learn with students as they question nursing models, and debate whether a theory of nursing exists. Students with bright, inquisitive minds who wish to explore varied issues in nursing and health care challenge me to continue my own work. This challenge makes me ask: What will nursing in the year 2000 really be like? Will the practice models currently being developed serve us well in the future?"

attention has been devoted (either in the classroom or in the literature) to the development of models. Students seem intimidated by the prospect of developing and using models in either practice or research. The purpose of this article is to define and classify models, outline the model building process, and discuss the advantages and disadvantages of models. The position taken here is that a basic understanding of both models and their development is a first step in the process toward theory development.

What are Models?

Most people tend to view a model as any structure which purports to replicate, reproduce, or represent something else. While this notion of a model is consistent with the scientific view of a model, it ignores the use to which the model is put. Hence a key distinction between the common view of a model and the scientific view is in the use to which the model is put.

In the scientific sense a model may be used to

define or describe something, to assist with analysis of a system, to specify relationships and processes, or to present a situation in symbolic terms that may be manipulated to derive predictions. There seems to be only one common characteristic of the various usages of scientific models. According to Kaplan, "we may say that any system A is a model of system B if the study of A is useful for the understanding of B without regard to any direct or indirect causal connection between A and B" (Kaplan, 1964, p. 263).

In various branches of science, engineering, and industry models are used to solve both simple and complex problems by concentrating on some portion or some key features instead of on every detail of real life. This approximation or abstraction of reality, which may be constructed in various forms, represents the scientist's idea of a model. As Hazzard (1971) points out, no one segment of the human universe is so simple and easy to understand that it can be grasped and controlled without the use of abstraction. Consequently, models do not, and cannot, represent every aspect of reality because of the innumerable and changing characteristics of the real world to be represented. Because models use abstraction, attention is focused only on the details of reality that are received to have the greatest relevance to the situation. This feature is an intrinsic part of the scientific model.

Relationship Between Models and Theories

The term *model* has often been used as a synonym for theory. While many authors use these terms interchangeably, the substitution of one term for the other has led to their misuse. As Rudner notes, the term *model,* like the term *theory,* shows a "melancholic lack of uniformity in the vocabulary of scientists and others who talk about science" (Rudner, 1966, p. 23).

The position taken here is that all theories are models, because all theories purport to represent some aspect of real world phenomena. However, the converse is not true; all models are not theories because

many models will not have all the requisites of theoretical construction. To qualify as a theory, the phenomena under consideration must be precise and limited, and the concepts need to be clearly defined (Williams, 1979). Theory also includes the capability for prediction and control regarding the relational statements set forth about the phenomena which constitute the theory (Chinn & Jacobs, 1978). Hence, according to Rudner, "a theory is a systematically related set of statements, including some lawlike generalizations, that is empirically testable. The purpose of theory is to increase scientific understanding through a systematized structure capable of both explaining and predicting phenomena" (Rudner, 1966, p. 10).

While a model describes the structure of events or systems, a theory moves beyond description to the level of prediction by stating relationships among components. Models provide useful mechanisms for depicting the relationships which exist among the variables of the theory. The construction of a model allows theorists to graphically illustrate and explain relationships. In this context model building is viewed as an early step in the more time-consuming and complex process of theory development.

Although certain characteristics distinguish models and theory from one another, they also share certain common qualities. Both vary in their degree of abstractness, and both are isomorphic systems. Isomorphism refers to the similarity between a thing and model of it (Brodbeck, 1969, p. 580). For a model to be maximally useful, it must accurately depict the object which it purports to represent. Isomorphism requires a one-to-one correspondence between the model or theory and reality. While models are an important tool for theory construction, not all models are designed for this purpose. Therefore, to more fully understand the nature of models, they need to be classified.

Classification of Models

Any model can be classified and described in different ways. However, the task of categorizing models is com-

Mental Image Models	Symbolic Models	Physical Models
(Highly abstract)		(Concrete, specific replicas)

Figure 42-1   *Models Classified According to Level of Abstraction.*

plicated by the lack of a uniform terminology. A comprehensive review of the literature revealed a considerable variety of terms used to distinguish among various types of models. When several terms are used to describe the same type of model, confusion rather than clarification results. In the classification schema which follows, the basic types of models are identified and, where possible, synonymous terms are noted.

Classification According to Level of Abstraction

Models are frequently described according to their level of abstraction, which essentially refers to their composition or manner of presentation. When models are classified according to their level of abstraction, they can be arranged along a continuum with *mental models* at one polar end and *physical models* at the other. In this context mental models represent the highest degree of abstraction. In contrast, physical models are specific, concrete replicas of their real-life counterparts. Symbolic models are positioned between pure mental models and physical models. Thus by starting with mental models and moving toward physical models, all models can be positioned on a continuum in which the manner of presentation becomes less abstract (Figures 42-1 and 42-2).

Mental Models

Mental models, sometimes called images or implicit models, are the pictures of the world held in the mind. Mental models consist of though patterns composed of words and concepts arranged to constitute a meaningful image of reality. These thought patterns can be formulated into language, which ultimately allows people to communicate and describe abstractions to others.

A mental model is a simplification of the situation it portrays, consisting of a few incomplete and abstract concepts which are considered integral to forming a meaningful image of reality. It is fortunate that mental models reduce the full scope of the situations which they portray. This enhances their usefulness by not overwhelming the individual with the complexities of reality. The real value of mental models comes from their not corresponding precisely to the complexity of the phenomenon under scrutiny. Instead the model

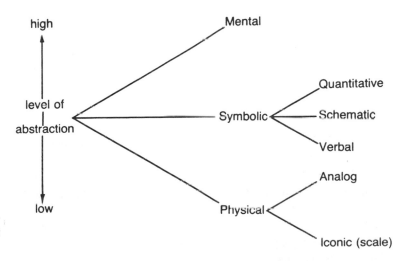

Figure 42-2   *Classification of Models According to Level of Abstraction and Including Subcategories.*

focuses on the details of reality which have the perceived greatest relevance to the situation.

Physical Models

Not all phenomena can be understood by the use of mental models. Consequently highly abstract models may become explicit in the form of physical models.

Iconic Model.   One type of physical model is the iconic model. An iconic model looks like what it is supposed to represent; it is a physical representation of some real-life object, either in a somewhat idealized form or on a different scale. Some iconic models are exact replicas of the entities they are designed to represent, whereas others deviate from reality in the number of properties represented. Iconic models are sometimes referred to as scale models. While not all iconic models involve a change in size, many are designed to be either smaller or larger than the entity being depicted.

Iconic models are frequently used by engineers and designers. For example, they are used in the design of ocean liners, bridges, water supply systems, and various products, ranging from automobiles to stage scenery. Aeronautical engineers use miniature models of airplanes to represent full-sized planes in wind tunnel tests. Iconic models are also used by nurses as replicas of various body organs, such as the heart, kidney, or brain, used for instructional purposes.

Analog Model.   When a model ceases to look like its real-life counterpart, thus becoming more abstract, while simultaneously retaining physical properties, it is referred to as an analog model. In contrast to iconic models, in analog models properties are transformed. One property is used to represent another. There is a substitution of components or processes to provide a parallel with what is being modeled.

A topographic map in which the property color is substituted for height above sea level is one common example of an analog model. Another example is a graph, such as an electrocardiogram (ECG), in which a unit distance along alignments used to represent a unit of time or speed. The ECG is realistic in behavior, re-flecting what is occurring in the heart, but it does not have characteristic features of any aspect of the processes producing the data displayed.

Symbolic Models

When a model no longer has a recognizable physical form and takes on a higher level of abstraction it becomes a symbolic model. In this type of model, phenomena are represented figuratively by using a set of connected symbols, objects, or concepts (Hardy, 1974). Symbolic models can be either verbal, schematic, or quantitative.

Verbal Model.   A *verbal* model is any worded statement indicating the important aspects of a phenomenon. It is either written or spoken in a language that is familiar to those who seek to understand the model.

An important characteristic of this type of symbolic model is that it is easily constructed and communicated. For example, in medicine effective verbal models that describe the transmission of disease have been useful in the eradication of many epidemic diseases. Similarly, Harvey's model of the circulatory system and the various models of the reaction of the human body to invading organisms have influenced the development of the modern treatment of diseases.

Schematic Model.   Another type of symbolic model is the schematic model, which represents a useful next step in the process of symbolizing a verbal model. Many diagrams, graphs, drawings, pictures, and similar schemata are schematic models. This type of model is more abstract than the analog model mentioned earlier. It is generally descriptive, but it cannot be easily tested for representativeness and may lack precision. However, schematic models often provide an effective way to communicate with nonexperts and can bring together ideas that will be used in formulating other types of models.

One common example of a schematic model is the communications map of an organization, such as a hospital, which uses arrows to show how messages and other means of communication are transmitted. The map does not show anyone talking to anyone else and yet one can easily determine from the map which persons communicate with each other.

Quantitative Model.   A final type of symbolic model is the quantitative model, which uses mathematical symbols to represent a phenomenon or certain aspects of a phenomenon. Such a model possesses many useful and desirable characteristics. Quantitative models are concise and add the potential for certain kinds of precision. Moreover, they are not easily misconstrued. Mathematical symbols are easier to see and manipulate than words because tools of logic and mathematics may be used with quantitative models. Finally, quantitative models are easier to test and replicate than other types of models.

There are various types of quantitative models, some of which are relatively simple while others are extremely complex. One example of a quantitative model is the health belief model, developed by Becker (1974), which has been expressed in the form of several equations as well as being depicted verbally and schematically.

Classification According to Purpose

Not only can models be distinguished from one another in terms of their level of abstraction, but one model can be contrasted with another by considering its purpose. The intent of the model brings into focus a variety of factors which have been used to distinguish various types of models. By using a series of bipolar adjectives, models can be categorized according to their purpose (Table 42-1). More specifically, models can be classified as being physical or behavioral, static or dynamic, macro or micro, comprehensive or partial, and descriptive or decision.

Physical Versus Behavioral Models.   When models are classified as being either physical or behav-

Table 42-1
Classification of Models According to Purpose

Category	Subcategory	Purpose
Physical		Represent structure
vs		
Behavioral		Depict performance
or		
Static		Portray phenomenon at a given point in time
vs		
Dynamic		Show time as an independent variable
or		
Micro		Focus on individual units and detailed linkages between variables
vs		
Macro		Use varying levels of aggregation and gross relationships between variables
or		
Partial		Limited to a few variables, developed in detail
vs		
Comprehensive		Identify many variables, developed in detail or linked with gross relationships
or		
Descriptive		Describe things as they are or as they act
	Communicative	Describe structural arrangement
	Explanatory	Describe causal relationships
vs	Predictive	Forecast future behavior or events
Decision		Find problem solutions
	Optimization	Find best solution
	Heuristic	Find a satisfactory solution

ioral, the distinction is based on whether the purpose is to replicate the structure of a phenomenon or to duplicate its performance. For example, one purpose of using a model skeleton in an anatomy class is to show the structural relationship of the various bones in the skeletal system. In contrast, the purpose of two faculty simulating a nurse-patient encounter in the classroom is to demonstrate a behavioral phenomenon and illustrate to students a variety of intervention strategies.

Static Versus Dynamic Models.

A similar distinction can be made to differentiate between static and dynamic models. The purpose of a static model is to portray a phenomenon or group of phenomena at a given point. Static models do not readily portray change, although by using several or even a series of static models, change can be depicted. In contrast, dynamic models have time as an independent variable and emphasize the process by which change occurs (Lazer, 1962). For example, the life cycle concept is a dynamic model of human growth and development. In contrast, an organizational chart illustrates a static model. A set of photographs of a child at different ages represents a series of static models that could be viewed as a comparative dynamic model.

Micro Versus Macro Models.

Because models can be built at various levels of detail and complexity, another way of distinguishing among them is based on whether they are macro or micro. Models may be more or less aggregated in terms of the variables on which they build. The micro model is the least aggregated. Its purpose is to focus on individual units as well as to postulate detailed linkages between dependent and independent variables (Kotler, 1980). In contrast, the variables in macro or aggregated models may be of different kinds. Sometimes macro models use aggregated variables which are measured at the individual level, whereas other macro models use variables which have no counterparts at the individual level. While the micro model focuses on detailed linkages between variables, the purpose of macro models is to postulate two or more variables and link them with a gross set of relationships without explaining the specific mechanisms operating within each variable.

An example of a macro model would be a description of the behavior of various population groups with regard to health care service utilization. In contrast, a micro model would focus on the health care service utilization behavior of an individual rather than an entire group.

Comprehensive Versus Partial Models.

Closely associated with macro and micro models are comprehensive and partial models. While these terms are occasionally used interchangeably, there appears to be a substantive difference between them. More specifically, comprehensive models attempt to identify and relate most or all of the variables involved in a phenomenon. These variables are then linked with a gross set of relationships, as is the case with macro models, or the variables are linked with more detailed relationships, as is the case with micro models.

Whereas comprehensive models attempt to identify most of the variables, partial models are limited to a few variables, but these variables are developed in detail. For example, a comprehensive model might examine individual health service utilization behavior by considering all possible variables such as demographic characteristics, and sociopsychological variables. In contrast, a partial model would be limited to the examination of selected variables such as attitudes toward health care services. Once again this examination might take place in either a micro or a macro context.

Descriptive Versus Decision Models.

Another way of classifying models, according to their purpose, is based on the distinction between descriptive and decision models. This distinction is frequently noted in the literature. However, terms such as *positive, systems, behavioral, empirical* and *concrete* have been used to refer to descriptive models. Similarly, terms such as *analytical, normative, goals, optimization, theoretical,* and *hypothetical* are often used to refer to decision models.

The general purpose of descriptive models is to

describe things either as they are or as they work. Descriptive models can be broken down into three subgroups; communicative, explanatory, and predictive models. A communicative model describes the structural arrangement of the various elements or components in a system. An explanatory model describes the causal relationships among the elements in a system. The purpose of a predictive model is to assert or describe the causal relationships among the elements in a system before the events take place. Hence descriptive models either communicate, explain, or predict some phenomenon (Kotler, 1980). Freudian psychology and Maslow's hierarchy of human needs are examples of descriptive models.

In contrast to descriptive models, decision models propose how things should be. Decision models can be grouped into two categories: optimization models and heuristic models. Optimization models may have computational routines for finding the best solution to a stated problem. Examples of optimization models are differential calculus, mathematical programming, statistical decision theory, and game theory. Heuristic models are designed to evaluate alternative outcomes associated with different decisions and to find the best decision when optimization routines are not available or cost effective. Some heuristic models are referred to as rule-of-thumb approaches (Kotler, 1980).

Model Building

Model building allows for complex, real-world problems to be depicted visually, verbally, or quantitatively to assess relations among events, things, or properties. Some of these relational statements made possible by models are of a cause-and-effect nature.

Most real-world problems are complex and have an array of variables which effect their outcome. As a first step in systematically solving any problem, an individual should be able to describe, explain, or predict the pertinent part of reality through the use of abstractions such as thought processes, language, or pictures. Thoughts about any specific problem or situation are merely abstractions from reality. The abstractions which are made about a segment of reality are influenced by past experiences, perception, and the parameters of the current situation.

Thoughts or abstractions about a real situation may seem like three-dimensional moving pictures of the part of the real world that was perceived. The pictorial abstraction of reality frequently represents only a part of the total situation. Just as a photograph cannot capture the total range of hidden thoughts and beliefs, perceptions of reality are limited. Often the most critical and influential part of any mental image is that part which does not correspond to the concrete physical aspects of the situation. Model building and the process of abstraction allow part of reality to be represented at a given time by depicting complex events in a form which deletes extraneous factors and only portrays essential components of the situation.

Because model builders are concerned with phenomena with occur in the real world, the model builder must clearly describe the system which is to be analyzed. To describe the system that the model hopes to replicate, the model builder must clearly state the assumptions and values implicit in the model as well as in the society which comprises the environment for the model. For example, in a communications model, likely assumptions would include honest, straight-forward interaction among participants, and the ability to hear as well as to understand the spoken or written word. Certain mechanisms for interchange would be implicit, including face-to-face contact, telephone, or the written mode of communication.

The model builder needs to maintain an awareness of the degree of congruence between the model and society at large or at least that segment of society which is in close influential proximity. For example, a model for open communications among all levels of an agency's hierarchy would be doomed to failure if the agency value was: "never talk to other departments or they will steal your ideas."

Next the model builder must be able to "observe and analyze a system of real events in order to isolate the determining variables that are operating in the system" (Stogdill, 1970, p.8). The major components of the model must be clearly defined and must also be identified as separate, observable units that can be related to one another.

To clearly and logically discuss the units of any given model the ultimate goal or outcome of the model must be described. Each variable or subset should be described in clear, easily understood terms which others can recognize and interpret. Next the actors in the model need to be noted as well as their expected roles and activities. For example, in a nursing situation the caregiver and recipient comprise the actors in the model; their roles, goals, and expected outcomes must be enumerated.

The next step is for the model builder to describe the goals and actual process of the steps taken or activities selected. The activities should relate to the problem statement, the expected outcome, and the characteristics of the actors. The choice of activities includes ongoing awareness both of the model's structure and its functioning because any alteration in one part of the model is likely to affect all other parts. The last skill for the model builder is clearly stating a set of defined concepts and statements which describe them as well as a set of statements which discuss the relationship between the concepts and constituent parts of the model.

Lippitt (1973) elaborates on this last step when he purports that any model builder must describe thoroughly and accurately the situation, problem, or system by identifying the essential variables, components, or subsystems and then ask the following questions about each variable:

1. Relevance: Is each variable relevant and necessary for a clear assessment and understanding of the situation?
2. Relationships: How are the variables related to one another, to the total situation, and to characteristics external to the situation being scrutinized?
3. Relative importance: What is the weight of each variable according to the magnitude of its significance to the total situation?
4. Outside constraints: What boundaries exist for the situation? What forces can exert an influence?
5. Internal constraints: What limits exist within the situation under consideration?

Advantages and Disadvantages of Models

Positive and negative results can ensue from the use of models for depicting aspects of a practice-oriented profession such as nursing. The following advantages of models are set forth by Lippitt (1973) and have transferability to nursing practice. First, models allow experimentation without risk. By using model building techniques a wide range of alternative interventions for any given problem can be addressed without actually altering the status quo. Such an approach takes a "what if" orientation. The model builder might initially set forth the current situation and then experiment with a variety of variables by considering: "What would be most likely to happen if I did _____?" The range of human reactions and responses to any change in the status quo cannot always be accurately predicted, but some ideas can be gleaned by considering the responses of the persons involved to previous change events.

A second advantage of using models, especially as a preliminary stage in the change process, is that models are good predictors of system behavior and performance. Models are more accurate as describers than as predictors. Any attempt at prediction must consider the wide range of human variables which could easily influence the outcome of the process.

A further advantage of model development for nursing practice is that models promote a higher level of understanding of the system than may have been previously held. To construct a model of a real world situation, careful attention must be paid to looking at each element as well as the relationships between them. By providing a careful assessment of the situation under consideration the model-building process promotes heightened awareness of the relative significance of each component. For example, if any change in A would most likely affect B, C, and then D, then A is central to the situation or problem being considered. Moreover, model building may often indicate where missing data exist. If a situation is being graphically depicted and there suddenly appears a gap in information, then the process has been useful.

The disadvantages inherent in model development may include a tendency to overgeneralize in an attempt to fit all the information available into a preestablished set of categories. The model builder may be tempted for the sake of simplicity and convenience to make the situation fit the model rather than trying to fit the model to the situation. Models have no truth in and of themselves; their accuracy lies in how well they describe reality. The lack of readily available evaluative tools also may be a disadvantage in model building. Once the model is built there may not be a clear-cut way to evaluate its effectiveness.

Summary

There is considerable value in the nursing profession furthering its understanding of models. Nursing models are currently widely applied by both practitioners and academicians. The use of analogies, constructs, verbal descriptions of systems, idealizations, and graphic representations is widespread. As nurses become increasingly skillful at developing practice approaches based on sound theoretical information, the usefulness of models will increase.

References

Becker, M.H. (Ed.). (1974). *The health belief model and personal health behavior.* Thorofare, NJ: Charles B. Slack.

Brodbeck, M. (1969). Models, meanings and theories. In M. Brodbeck (Ed.), *Readings in the philosophy of the social sciences* (pp. 579–600). London: Macmillan/Collier-Macmillan Limited.

Chinn, P.L., & Jacobs, M.K. (1978). A model for theory development in nursing. *Advances in Nursing Science, 1*(1), 1–11.

Hardy, M. (1974). Theories: Components, development, evaluation. *Nursing Research, 23,* 100–107.

Hazzard, M.E. (1971). An overview of systems theory. *Nursing Clinics of North America, 6,* 385–393.

Kaplan, A. (1964). *The conduct of inquiry.* Scranton, PA: Chandler.

Kotler, P. (1980). *Marketing management* (4th ed.). Englewood Cliffs, NJ: Prentice-Hall.

Lazer, W. (1962). The role of models in marketing. *Marketing, 26,* 9–14.

Lippitt, G.L. (1973). *Visualizing change: Model building and the change process.* La Jolla, CA: University Associates.

Rudner, R. (1966). *Philosophy of social science.* Englewood Cliffs, NJ: Prentice-Hall.

Stogdill, R. (1970). Introduction—The student and model-building. In R. Stogdill (Ed.), *The process of model-building in the behavioral sciences* (pp. 3–13). Columbus, OH: Ohio State University Press.

Williams, C.A. (1979). The nature and development of conceptual frameworks. In F.S. Downs & J.W. Fleming (Eds.), *Issues in nursing research* (pp. 89–106). New York: Appleton-Century-Crofts.

The Authors Comment

The aim of this article was to simplify what was becoming an increasingly popular yet confusing topic—the process of model building. Many disciplines in recent years have sought to develop a more sophisticated theoretical basis for practice. In seeking to do so, the assumption has been that somewhere in the academic process people were acquainted with the fundamental concepts pertaining to models, including the use and development of models. Actually, however, until recently either this basic information was not consistently provided in courses or the dissemination of such information was not widespread.

The scheme for model building, as outlined in the article, continues to be useful as an explanation and clarification of the model building process. Model building still is viewed as an integral part of theory development and a technique useful for nurses. Since the article was published, doctoral students have expressed appreciation for the simplistic way in which we described a potentially complex process. Colleagues have reported value in using the article with both graduate and undergraduate students.

The article was developed to provide a primer, not a definitive statement regarding models and model building. The scope of the article could be expanded to include higher levels of model building.

—WADE LANCASTER AND JEANETTE LANCASTER

Chapter 43

Conceptual Issues in Nursing

Rosemary Ellis

In recent decades much attention has been given to developing nursing theories, models, and conceptual frameworks within the nursing community (Lancaster & Lancaster 1981; Reynolds, 1971). While the main purpose of these constructs is to effectively develop, organize, use, and transmit knowledge that explains nursing and its goals, many terms are used interchangeably, loosely, or vaguely. Take, for example, the terms theory and model. Conceptualizations such as these should be recognized for what they are and for the purposes they serve regardless of the terms that different authors use, or misuse, to label them.

To illustrate, one mental construction of theory comprises a systematic set of propositional statements that expresses relationships between concepts. It is from the set of statements, which are designed to explain, predict, or understand phenomena, that testable hypotheses can be derived. Such sets of statements are what the term theory means when used by scientists in the phrase scientific theory.

Another type of mental construction describes a distinctive focus on, or orientation to, phenomena of interest to a field of study and has no counterpart in the empirical world. It is not observable; it is an abstraction useful for ordering or developing knowledge or for selective ordering of facts. It describes the key elements or concepts that in combination create a perspective that defines the phenomena that are of interest for some purpose such as practice or research and theory development. Some nursing conceptualizations are of this order such as most current nursing theories.

Both sets of propositional statements, which may include hypotheses and an orienting perspective, are essential for organizing and developing knowledge, but rational development of sets of statements cannot proceed except from a specific perspective and toward a specific purpose. A per perspective is what leads to a knowledge system. It identifies the phenomena of interest, defines the knowledge to be organized or developed, and serves to identify the key concepts that characterize a field of knowledge. Nursing models and theories are statements of belief about an appropriate or essential perspective for nursing. They are "searchings" for nursing knowledge systems.

It is important, therefore, to understand the commonalities as well as some of the issues that arise when comparisons are made between existing nursing models. Before proceeding, a brief recap of older conceptualizations of nursing and the contrast between medical and nursing perspectives will serve as a general orientation.

Historical Perspective

Nightingale (1859) conceptualized nursing as the science of health and described nursing (the verb) as primarily directed toward improving and managing the physical environment so that nature could heal the patient. Her disciples engaged in teaching household and environmental hygiene with the aim of helping women create healthy environments for their families and communities (Nightingale, 1977). These two mainstreams in nursing—the care of the sick and the promotion of health—are identifiable in nursing to this day. In spite of her orientation to a science of health, when Nightingale established the nursing school at St. Thomas' in London in 1860 she resorted to a task analysis of what nurses were actually doing in hospitals to design the curriculum. Consequently, a list of procedures and tasks became the general description of nursing until advances in medical science shifted both medicine and nursing to a focus on disease.

In the United States, tasks and procedures remained important elements in the conceptualization of nursing, but specific diseases or body systems often served as prominent factors in organizing frameworks for nursing curricula until 1950. Note that it was the disease that was to be nursed in a 1940 course "Nursing of Diseases of the Eye, Ear, Nose and Throat."

Rejection of the disease or body-systems perspective for nursing was forced by the identification of a burgeoning list of specific disease entities, the recognition of the import of psychological and social factors in

disease or in response to it, and by discovery or, at least, affirmation of the obvious: patients are people. Therefore, nursing activity is concerned with human interaction and with people's feelings, beliefs, knowledge, and behavior, not just with disease.

Henderson's definition of nursing was a major shift from the task-procedure perspective and one of the earliest, widely used definitions to present a conceptualization of nursing that included the idea of function and goal. According to Henderson (1960), nursing is "to assist the individual, sick or well, in the performance of those activities contributing to health or its recovery (or to a peaceful death) that he would perform unaided if he had the necessary strength, will or knowledge. And to do this in such a way as to help him gain independence as rapidly as possible." This widely accepted conceptualization of nursing served the profession in the U.S. during the 1950s and 1960s, and internationally through its adoption by the International Congress of Nursing. Since the 1970s, it has competed with the conceptualizations of nursing by theorists such as Rogers (1970), King (1971), Orem (1980), Roy and Roberts (1981), Johnson (1980), Schlotfeldt (1975), and others who have influenced our conceptualization of nursing today.

Disease vs Health Perspective

Nursing, nevertheless, has been strongly influenced by the medical perspective or paradigm that is focused on disease rather than health. Although efforts have been made to humanize medicine by seeking to include such concepts as *personhood* and *life-style* within its perspective, the dominant structure of medical thinking is centered on diagnosis and cure. Baron (1981) argues that to achieve these ends the focus is on signs and symptoms, which implicitly has the consequence of separating the patient from the disease. According to Baron, disease then becomes the organizing, centering concept for medicine so that the physician's clarifying diagnostic view can result in exorcising the disease or trying to get the patient and the disease to live together in peace. Therefore, personhood and life-style are to be understood only as they affect the onset, manifestations, and often treatment and course of an illness.

The emphasis in nursing is different. Disease or health problems are not the dominant focus, rather they are to be understood or considered because of their effect upon or consequences for personhood and life-style. Nursing and medicine may include identical elements in their orienting perspectives or knowledge systems, but focus, emphasis, goals and therefore bodies of knowledge, models, theories, and research will differ, as will many of the activities of the professional practitioners in the two fields.

Focus on Health Promotion

Health promotion, an aspect that has always existed in modern nursing, has become increasingly dominant in recent years. As a consequence, a major conceptual issue for those concerned with organizing and developing nursing knowledge is to resolve the question: Should health or some alternative such as illness, disease, or problem be the dominant concept in the nursing perspective? The choice will have far-reaching consequences. It will identify the population of reference for nursing. Is it the helpless, the weak, the sick, the vulnerable as Harmer (1922) noted? Is it only those with problems or at risk? Or is it people in general, including the well? Henderson clearly included the well in her definition. A health focus in contrast to a problem or illness focus also affects the context, milieu, and reasons that bring about the initial contact between nurse and client. Few current models of nursing adequately conceptualize the initiation of a nursing relationship, though some focus on the nature of that relationship. As nursing has moved from doing *for* patients to working *with* patients, helping people to care for themselves and involving them in their care and decisions about their health, the modes of nursing are increasingly those of educating, guiding, or motivating not only the identified patient or client but his family and/or community.

Health promotion has long been a major activity of public health nurses and school nurses and is the goal of prenatal classes and child development or well-child clinics. It is also emphasized in rehabilitation nursing and in nursing the elderly. Although it is not a new idea, two quite different terms—prevention of disease and health promotion—are used to label it. Conceptually, promotion of health is health centered; prevention is disease centered. If one defines health as the absence of disease, and nurses have rejected that limited meaning, prevention and promotion are conceptually quite distant and focus on quite different phenomena. Can nursing's knowledge system accommodate such divergent centerings?

What meaning should health have in a nursing knowledge system—health and well-being or their opposites, health problem, illness, or disease?

Health has been considered an all or nothing concept; one either has it or one doesn't. Such a view is evident in folk sayings such as, "Thank goodness I have my health." Health is also viewed by comparative categories such as "good health," "poor health," or "failing health." The nursing literature discusses a health-illness continuum in which health is polar to illness or disease along a single continuum, two extremes of one thing. But if health is more than just the absence of disease as many assert, the single continuum idea is invalid by simple logic.

Other questions also arise. Is health a state of being—a value rather than an empirical phenomenon; an abstract idealized goal; a general characteristic of humans that is alterable? Or is it a label for a general domain in human enterprise in which nursing functions? All of these possibilities come to mind as one reads the nursing literature.

Defining Health

The late theologian Tillich (1961) claimed health is not an element of man's essential nature, rather it is an element added to it. For him, the meaning of health is related to two basic elements of the life processes—self-identity and self-alteration. Since these are simultaneously ongoing elements in living, they may have import for nursing in considering the meaning of health.

While nurses have rejected the view of health as the absence of disease, they have not solved the conceptual vacuum created by this move nor have they adequately provided empirical referents for the abstraction, health. This creates problems for nursing in developing and transmitting knowledge among nurses and between nurses and society when they attempt to describe their professional purpose to others.

Smith (1981) has provided a useful resolution to the "seemingly unrelated, multiple, and ambiguous views of health" by offering four models of alternative views of health. These are (a) the clinical model based on the absence of signs or symptoms of disease, (b) the role performance model wherein adequate role performance is the common sense criterion of health, (c) the adaptive model in which health is a condition of effective interaction with one's physical and social environment, and (d) the eudaemonistic model that extends the meaning of health to general well-being and self-realization. However, it remains to be seen how health can be defined as a concept in the nursing perspective.

In a retrospective study of nursing texts and journals from 1964 to 1974, Carper (1975) found that health was one of the five key or representative concepts of nursing. The other four are man, nursing, patient/client, and behavior. The inclusion of the words patient and client reflects the evolution of nursing, which expanded its perspective to include other than clinical populations as recipients of nursing services. Newman (1983) used four concepts—health, client, nursing, and environment—to discuss and illustrate the history of nursing science. While Carper did not single out environment, she included it in her discussion of the concept, man. Analysis of Donaldson and Crowley's (1978) article on the structure of the discipline of nursing provides support for these concepts as major ones in a knowledge structure or system of nursing. Although the issues concerning the concept of health are readily identifiable, there are equally challenging issues surrounding the other key concepts.

For example, consider the concept man or human, or specific types identified by the labels patient or client. Humans or human-environment interactions are unequivocally accepted as focal in all models for nursing, yet the conceptualization is often vaguely expressed as man or man in interaction with the environment. More is needed than general knowledge of man or of people or persons. What is needed is a description of humans that is oriented to nursing as an activity that has something to do with people and that expresses the characteristics of humans that are focal for nursing. Such description must not violate values long held by nurses, values that are expressed in nursing actions and concerns that strive to maintain patient or client dignity and individuality in situations, conditions, and systems that threaten dignity and personhood. Nurses strive to convey that persons are valued, have worth, in spite of confused, inappropriate, or antisocial behavior or in the circumstances of deficits in normal functioning. From a nursing perspective humans are viewed as persons not objects, though we are woefully far from articulating what we mean by the concept, person.

An example of a general description about man that appeared in a recent article states "man is an omnivorous, bimanous, and bipedal, almost erect terrestrial mammal" (Dart, 1980). That is an accurate statement about man, but it was written by a scientist whose perspective relates man to the animal kingdom. To every nurse it is immediately apparent that no nurse wrote that statement and also that it is not very useful for nursing purposes. To be useful, it must be cast from a nursing perspective.

Nursing conceptualizations of man are evident in current models of nursing but some fail to convey the dignity, the humanity, the sense of person that has been characteristic of nursing views of humans. Conceptualizing man as an energy field or some set of behavioral systems, or treating an individual's thoughts or feelings as internal environment, for example, fails to connote clearly the meaning of person, let alone humanity. In this they fail as nursing descriptions of humans. Conceptualizations of humans in terms of needs do not violate the sense of dignity or humanity, but too often they are inadequately stated, selected, and ordered to be adequate vis-à-vis nursing. An orientation somewhat analogous to an expanded list of activities of daily living could perhaps provide a more adequate beginning if whatever is connoted or intended by terms such as "self-actualization," "reaching or realizing one's potential," could be expressed and incorporated. Whether humans are to be viewed as beset by stress, shoring up defenses in a hostile environment or for the purpose of maintaining stability or equilibrium, or are envisioned as developing, seeking beings capable of learning, choosing, and relating constructively with other humans and the environment is unclear in nursing literature. It is, however, a major conceptual problem.

Nurses tend to view people as on some trajectory or path. They want to know their remembered pasts, the focal present, and the imagined or projected possible futures. They conceptualize living as both process and state. It would seem that views of humans acceptable to nursing would recognize and express human resilience; human striving, sometimes ineffectively but often successfully; and human bonding. Nursing has much to do with supporting, maintaining, or enhancing human capacities for living or meeting life crises. It can increase abilities to get or use special resources; it can serve to augment knowledge for healthful living; and it can even enhance strength or will. These possibilities are far beyond problem solving. So also is the giving of emotional support or what really is given currently by nurses but misnamed with the vacuous label "emotional support."

Nurses stimulate cognitive development for understanding and coping with critical life processes and experiences; they augment perceptions or try to correct misperceptions. They strive to help persons preserve a functionally useful concept of the self and the body in the face of threat, change, decline, or impairment. These actions are not directed by a focus on disease or from knowledge of disorder; they are not centered on problems but are directed from a focus on human capabilities and strengths. Such a focus is self-evident in rehabilitation nursing. It also pervades most of nursing, although this is not recognized, addressed, or strengthened. We cannot settle for the abstractions: man, patient, client. We must attach meanings that are congruent with nursing and health.

The Meaning of Nursing

But what do we mean by the term nursing? A usual meaning is some set of actions or functions for some expressed goal, but what are these functions, processes and goals? Reading nursing literature raises the following questions: Is nursing simply caring? Is it some sort of therapy or healing? What are the indications for nursing? Is nursing assessment an art or a science? Is the action or function focused on persons, or on the environment, or on some interface or interaction of human and environment? Nursing models vary. Goals stated as equilibrium, adaptation, repatterning or, vaguely, health, if accepted need much more explication and delineation of indicators before they can be used to explain what nursing is or determine the effectiveness of nursing. They must also be reconciled with, and communicated in terms congruent with, societal expectations. Goals of self-care or enhancement of self-care agency that of enhancing people's health seeking abilities are easier to understand. They are also more amenable to evolution of goal achievement.

Whether to conceive of nursing as process or in terms of product is another conceptual issue in nursing. Process without goal conceptualization is vacuous. Masson has commented on the limitations of process and the hazards by asking "can it be that our tendency to conceive of nursing as process rather than product is responsible for the confusion between means like status, respect, security, and turf and the ends they will permit us to attain?" (Masson, 1979, p. 783).

Conceptualizations of nursing that focus on interpersonal process or the human-to-human relationship have preserved a traditional view of nursing as human-to-human helping relationship, but they have not adequately formulated or described specific goals or the contextual space that enlighten us about nursing as a distinctive type of helping or human relationship.

Finally, if environment is a key concept in nursing's knowledge system, how is it conceptualized? Nightingale meant physical environment. Nurses now would include psychological, social, or cultural elements in a full meaning of environment. But what do we really mean? Is everything environment? How do we deal with environment in nursing models? A modern version of Nightingale's meaning is reflected in part by the conceptualization of environment in terms of its stimulus properties (Roy & Roberts, 1981). More abstract meanings focus on stress or stressors, viewing the environment as somehow hostile and human-environment interaction negatively. A much more positive symbiotic relationship is also a prevalent nursing view (Rogers, 1970). Environment can be viewed as an energy field with which man as energy field is in rhythmic patterned synchrony.

Environment might also be considered as the contextual space in which nursing is called for, initiated and carried out. The contextual space of the hospice is considerably different from that of a hospital, school, and other community agency in which nursing takes place. Contextual space would include the patient or client and that person's reasons for being in contact with a nurse for the purpose of initiating and continuing a client-nurse relationship. Is such contact initiated by the client? Does it arise only in the context of some formal, ordered recognized system? Could it be nurse-initiated? Or is the nurse simply responsive in a contact that is initiated or created and perhaps controlled and defined by others? The answers have significant consequences for what meanings one can attach to environment and also other key concepts—nursing, client, and health.

There is agreement within nursing that nurses and their clients are in relationships concerned with health or health problems. While nurses agree on highly abstract and complex concepts, they have many disagreements, much fuzziness, and multiple conceptual problems when they try to use the concepts to create a system for the transmission of knowledge as a rational base for practice or as a perspective for nursing research and development.

References

Baron, R.J. (1981). Bridging clinical distance: An empathic rediscovery of the known. *Journal of Medicine and Philosophy, 6,* 5–23.

Carper, B. (1975). Fundamental patterns of knowing in nursing. (Doctoral dissertation, Columbia University Teachers College). Dissertation Abstracts International, 36, 4941B. (University Microfilms No. 76–7772).

Dart, R.A. (1980, April). Taungs and its significance. *Natural History, 89,* 11, 66ff. (Reprint from May/June 1926 issue, with biographical sketch).

Donaldson, S.K., & Crowley, D.M. (1978). The discipline of nursing: Structure and relationship to practice. *Nursing Outlook, 26,* 113–120.

Harmer, B. (1922). *Methods and principles of teaching the principles and practice of nursing.* New York: Macmillan.

Henderson, V. (1969). *Basic principles of nursing care* (rev. ed.). London: International Council of Nurses.

Johnson, D.E. (1980). The behavioral system model for nursing. In J.P. Riehl & C. Roy (Eds.), *Conceptual models for nursing practice* (2nd ed.) (pp. 207–216). New York: Appleton-Century-Crofts.

King, I.M. (1971). *Toward a theory for nursing: General concepts of human behavior.* New York: John Wiley & Sons.

Lancaster, W., & Lancaster, J. (1981). Models and model building in nursing. *Advances in Nursing Science, 3,* 31–42.

Masson, V. (1979). On power and vision in nursing. *Nursing Outlook, 27,* 783.

Newman, M. (1983). The continuing revolution: A history of nursing science. In N. Chaska (Ed.), *The nursing profession: A time to speak* (pp. 385–393). New York: McGraw-Hill.

Nightingale, F. (1859). *Notes on nursing: What it is and what it is not.* London: Harrison and Sons.

Nightingale, F. (1977). Health teaching in towns and villages. Rural hygiene. In H. Usui & Y. Kominami (Eds.), *Florence Nightingale: Selected writings on nursing.* (pp. 109–127). Tokyo: Gendaisha Publishing.

Orem, D. (1980). *Nursing concepts of practice* (2nd ed.). New York: McGraw-Hill.

Reynolds, P.D. (1971). *A primer in theory construction.* Indianapolis: Bobbs-Merrill.

Rogers, M.E. (1970). *An introduction to the theoretical basis of nursing.* Philadelphia: F.A. Davis.

Roy, C., & Roberts, S.L. (1981). *Theory construction in nursing: An adaptation model.* Englewood Cliffs, NJ: Prentice-Hall.

Schlotfeldt, R.M. (1975). The need for a conceptual framework. In P. J. Verhonick (Ed.), *Nursing research I* (pp. 3–24). Boston: Little, Brown.

Smith, J.A. (1981). The idea of health: A philosophical inquiry. *Advances in Nursing Science, 3,* 53–60.

Tillich, P. (1961). The meaning of health. *Perspectives in Biology and Medicine, 5,* 92–100.

The Author Comments

The genesis of this article grew from the many issues that abound because of multiple terms—theory, model, conceptual framework—and because of such highly abstract concepts as man, health, environment, and nursing.

Too many nurses are naive about the nature of science, the various scientific processes, scientific explanatory theory, and all that is included by nurses in a diffuse common meaning for the term *theory*. Lack of progress in theory development in nursing and general confusion prompted me to write this article.

—ROSEMARY ELLIS

Chapter 44

Research Testing Nursing Theory: State of the Art

Mary Cipriano Silva

The degree to which investigators have tested nursing theory through empirical research is analyzed. The analysis is based on 62 studies in which the nursing model of Johnson, Roy, Orem, Rogers, and/or Newman was used as a framework for the research. The analysis shows that of these 62 studies, only 9 met specified evaluation criteria for the explicit testing of nursing theory. To better understand this finding, impediments and approaches to testing of nursing theory are discussed, as are implications for nursing theory, research, and practice.

The . . . [person] who is swimming against the stream knows the strength of it. —WOODROW WILSON

For over two decades, nurse scholars have stressed the need for developing and testing nursing theory so that nursing's scientific base might be established. Although during this time the development of nursing theory has progressed systematically, little progress has been noted in the testing of nursing theory, an aspect of nursing science that has remained outside the nursing research mainstream. A reason for this situation is a lack of clarity about what constitutes theory testing in general and testing of nursing theory in particular. To address this problem, the following question is raised:

What is the current state of the art regarding research that explicitly tests nursing theory? To explore this question, the author will:

(a) identify the degree to which investigators have conducted empirical research that meets evaluation criteria for testing nursing theory,
(b) summarize exemplars of empirical research in which nursing theory has been tested,
(c) discuss impediments and approaches to the testing of nursing theory, and
(d) discuss implications of the current state of the art for nursing theory, research, and practice.

The approach used herein was an assessment of empirical research based on five conceptual models of nursing: Johnson's Behavioral System Model, Orem's Self-Care Deficit Model, Rogers's Science of Unitary Human Beings Model, and Newman's Health Model. These five models were included in this state-of-the-art review because they have generated more current empirical research than other nursing models (Silva, 1987).

To locate this empirical research, extensive computer searches and hand searches of the literature were necessary. These searches covered the years 1952 to 1985. Computer searches included *Medline* searches using four different key-word retrieval strategies and *Cumulative Index to Nursing and Allied Health Literature* searches. Hand searches included the perusal of every title, author, abstract, and reference within *Nursing Research* (1952–1985), *International Journal of Nursing Studies* (1963–1985), *Research in Nursing and Health* (1978–1985), *Advances in Nursing Science* (1978–1985), and *Western Journal of Nursing Research* (1979–1985). Hand searches were also conducted on known nursing theory and research books and other relevant research documents, such as proceedings from major research conferences. The hand searches and computer searches of the literature yielded 62 empirical studies that used one or more of the five nursing models as a basis for research. (A list of the 62 studies is available from the author on request.)

Studies included in this state-of-the-art review had to be published; their empirical research had to have been related to one of the five models mentioned above; and the research had to be of sufficient depth and breadth to allow an assessment of the degree of theory testing. Abstracts, reviews of the literature, research commentaries, masters' theses, and unpublished doctoral dissertations were eliminated because they did not meet one or more of these criteria.

Research Based on Nursing Theory: Degrees of Testing

A serious misconception too often exists regarding the testing of nursing theory. It is a belief that if a conceptual model of nursing has been identified explicitly as a theoretical framework for research, then this identification with the model in and of itself constitutes theory testing. It does not. Although explicit identification of the model constitutes a necessary condition for theory testing, it does not constitute a sufficient condition. To clarify this point, three ways in which nurse investigators typically have used the nursing models of Johnson, Roy, Orem, Rogers, and/or Newman in the 62 empirical studies are examined.

Minimal Use of Models for Theory Testing

The first way in which investigators have used nursing models in empirical research is by explicitly identifying a particular nursing model as a framework for research and then doing little more with the model in the study. Typically the model is named and briefly summarized but minimally integrated into the rest of the study. When used in this way, the model contributes little to either nursing research or nursing theory. In addition, such use of the model is potentially misleading because it creates an illusion that nursing theory is being used to organize a study or to test a nursing model when it is not. Of the 62 located studies based on the five models, 24 fell primarily into the category of minimal use of the nursing models to organize the study or to test theory.

Insufficient Use of Models for Theory Testing

The second and most common way in which investigators have used nursing models in empirical research is to organize their studies. These studies are frequently descriptive (rather than hypothesis generating), and the nursing model is typically used to structure instruments. For example, the modes of Roy's Adaptation Model are used as frameworks to study instruments.

Although the use of nursing models in this way may serve a valuable organizing purpose, this purpose in and of itself is insufficient to constitute theory testing. This insufficiency arises because investigators using models only to organize their instruments (or to organize some other aspect of their study) are usually making an implicit assumption that the underlying tenets of the model are valid. To use the preceding example, the investigator assumes that the modes of Roy's model or the self-care requisites of Orem's model are valid conceptualizations. Consequently, the investigator conducts the research based on this assumption. Whether the assumption is in fact valid is difficult to assess because of the few empirical studies that have tested underlying assumptions or propositions of nursing models. Nevertheless, to proceed on the assumption could lead to potentially erroneous results or to misinterpretation of the data. Therefore, when nursing models are used primarily as organizing frameworks, the limitations of this approach should be discussed in the research report. Of the 62 located studies, 29 fell primarily into the category of insufficient use of the nursing models to constitute theory testing.

Adequate Use of Models for Theory Testing

The third way in which investigators have used nursing models in research is explicitly to test nursing theory. Studies that fall within this category ideally meet all of the following evaluation criteria for theory testing:

1. A purpose of the study is to determine the underlying validity of a designated nursing model's assumptions or propositions.
2. The nursing model explicitly is stated as the theoretical framework or one of the theoretical frameworks for the research.
3. The nursing model is discussed in sufficient breadth and depth so that the relationship between the model and the study hypotheses or purposes is clear.
4. The study hypotheses of purposes are deduced clearly from the nursing model's assumptions or propositions.
5. The study hypotheses or purposes are empirically tested in an appropriate manner.
6. As a result of this empirical testing, indirect evidence exists of the validity (or lack thereof) of the designated assumptions or propositions of the model.
7. This evidence is discussed in terms of how it supports, refutes, or explains relevant aspects of the nursing model.

Using these criteria, nine of the 62 studies based on the five models fell primarily into the category of adequate use of the nursing model(s) to constitute theory testing.

However, several limitations must be kept in mind regarding the preceding evaluation criteria. First, theory testing is difficult to define; therefore, the identification of necessary and sufficient criteria to measure such testing is difficult to operationalize. Second, the preceding criteria are formative. Nevertheless, an attempt has been made to explicate evaluation criteria for theory testing in more detail than typically has appeared in the nursing literature. Third, because a study has met the evaluation criteria for theory testing does not necessarily guarantee that the study is sound. The evaluation criteria, in addition to those related to theory testing, are important in assessing the overall quality of a study.

Research Testing Nursing Models: Explicit Exemplars

To examine the concept of theory testing in more depth, three recent studies (Quinn, 1984; Harper, 1984; Engle, 1984) are summarized as explicit exemplars of research that, overall, meet the preceding evaluation criteria for theory testing. The purpose of this summary is to highlight how the investigators used the research process to test nursing theory.

Theory Testing Research Based on Rogers's Nursing Model

Quinn (1984), in examining therapeutic touch as energy exchange, clearly stated that she was studying this phenomenon as a logically deduced proposition derived from Rogers's nursing model. She summarized Rogers's model as a conceptual system where persons are viewed "as four-dimensional, negentropic energy field engaged in a continuous, mutual process with the four-dimensional, negentropic environmental energy field" (Quinn, 1984, p. 43).

Quinn then developed her thesis in depth so that the relationships between Rogers's model, her deduced proposition, and her study hypothesis were clear. In Quinn's words:

> Given the axioms of the Rogerian conceptual system, it can be deduced that the effects of therapeutic touch, being a person-to-person interaction, are not related to the physical contact between the healer and the subject

but rather are outcomes of the unique interaction of their energy fields. A testable theorem deriving from this proposition is that therapeutic touch without physical contact will have the same effect as therapeutic touch with physical contact. Since the effect of therapeutic touch with physical contact on state anxiety is known, state anxiety can provide a measure of the efficacy of therapeutic touch without physical contact. Thus, the hypothesis for the study described here was that there will be a greater decrease in post-test state anxiety scores in subjects treated with noncontact therapeutic touch than in those treated with noncontact (Quinn, 1984, p. 44).

Quinn then went on to define operationally key terms in her study. *Noncontact therapeutic touch* (NCTT) was defined as a 5-minute intervention that consisted of all components of therapeutic touch except the actual laying on of the hands (LOOH). Instead of LOOH, four nurses familiar with therapeutic touch placed their hands 4 to 6 inches from the subject's body in the area of the solar plexus. *Noncontact* (NC) was defined as a 5-minute intervention that mimicked the movements of therapeutic touch without attempting to perform therapeutic touch (i.e., to center, to assist the subject, to attune to the condition of the subject, or to redirect energy). Instead, three nurses unfamiliar with therapeutic touch administered the NC intervention while mentally subtracting from 100 by 7s and by counting backwards from 240 to 0. *State anxiety* was defined as a transitory feeling of tension that was measured by form X-1 of the Self-Evaluation Questionnaire of the State-Trait Anxiety Inventory.

The sample was composed of 60 men and women hospitalized on a cardiovascular unit of a medical center in New York City. These persons were randomly assigned to either the experimental (NCTT) group or the control (NC) group. Following the treatments, statistical analyses were done to determine whether the decrease in posttest state anxiety scores was significantly greater in the experimental or the control group. The result showed that the experimental group's scores decreased significantly more than the control group's scores, thus supporting the hypothesis. The result was discussed within the framework of Rogers's model.

In terms of theory testing, what does this result show? First, it shows that a research hypothesis can be deduced from Rogers's conceptual model and empirically tested. Second, it shows that physical contact is not crucial to explain the effectiveness of therapeutic touch. Consequently, the results of this study give preliminary evidence, albeit indirectly, of the validity of that part of Rogers's conceptual system dealing with energy fields.

Theory Testing Research Based on Orem's Nursing Model

Harper (1984), in applying theoretical constructs of Orem's model to self-care medication behaviors in the elderly, clearly stated that Orem's theoretical constructs of self-care and nursing systems laid the foundation for her study. Based on these constructs, Harper explicitly specified the following four propositions from Orem's model as relevant to her research:

1. Self-care systems result from the individual's knowledge and use of technologies known to meet self-care requisites.
2. Self-care is learned within the context of social groups by human interaction and communication.
3. Self-care is deliberate action on the part of the participant, sequentially performed to meet known needs for care.
4. Through the design of nursing systems, the individual's self-care deficits are assessed, valid and reliable nursing technologies for meeting these deficits are selected, and nursing technologies to meet these deficits are implemented (Harper, 1984, p. 33).

From these propositions, Harper then went on to deduce her research hypotheses that 30 black, elderly, hypertensive women who participated in a self-care medication program would show at 4 days and at 4 weeks posttreatment (H1) more knowledge about their medication, (H2) more internal locus of control, (H3) more self-care medication behavior, (H4) fewer medication errors, and (H5) lower levels of systolic and diastolic blood pressure than would a similar group of 30 black, elderly, hypertensive women who participated in a teaching program about hypertension. She then carefully specified the relationship between Orem's theoretical propositions and her research hypothesis by stating: "In this study, hypothesis 1 was deduced from proposition 1. Hypothesis 2 was deduced from proposition 2, and hypotheses 3, 4, and 5 were deduced from proposition 3. Proposition 4 represents the nursing intervention: the independent variable in this study" (Harper, 1984, p. 36).

By stating the relationship between propositions of Orem's model and her research hypotheses, Harper makes clear what general tenets of the model were being tested through empirical research. Although clarity does not guarantee adequacy, clarity was the main criterion in evaluating the study.

Harper's hypotheses were tested using analysis of covariance. Results showed that at 4 days statistically significant changes occurred in the hypothesized direction for all dependent variables except blood pressure; however, at 4 weeks this positive trend did not continue for any variable except knowledge of medication. In her discussion, Harper was able to relate the study results obtained at 4 days to the theoretical propositions of Orem's model previously stated. However, at 4 weeks the relationships between the study hypotheses and the specified propositions of Orem's model were less clear. As a result, Harper recommended further research in the area of self-care and health behavior over time. The results also have implications for modification of Orem's model. That is, Orem's model does not specify explicit propositions that predict or explain the effects of the passage of time on self-care behaviors. Thus, the explanatory power of the model was inadequate to explain Harper's long-term results.

Theory Testing Research Based on Newman's Nursing Model

Engle (1984), in applying theoretical constructs of Newman's model to the measurement of older adults' health, explicitly stated that she was testing propositions derived from Newman's model. (She also acknowledged the contribution of Rogers's model to that of Newman's.) She discussed the basic thesis of Newman's model: that the interrelated concepts of time, space, movement, and consciousness provided guidance for understanding health. In her study, Engle concentrated on Newman's proposition that "time is a function of movement" (Newman, 1979, p. 60) and built her study on research relevant to this proposition previously conducted by Newman (1972, 1976, 1982) and Tompkins (1980). In addition, Engle went one step further and related time and movement to self-assessed health, a concept she found consistent with Newman's model and necessary to study the health of older adults.

Building upon this theoretical background, Engle first operationally defined key terms and then stated her research hypotheses.

Key terms were defined operationally as follows:

1. Personal tempo was defined as cadence, the number of steps walked per minute at the participant's normal or usual pace. The faster the cadence, the greater the movement.
2. Time perception was defined as the participant's perceived duration of a 40-second interval of clock time while walking at a normal or usual pace using the production method. The shorter the perceived duration of time, the lesser the amount of clock time.
3. Self-assessment of health was defined by the score on a ten-rung Cantril Ladder. The higher the score, the better the health (Engle, 1984, p. 28).

Hypotheses were stated as follows:

1. There is a relationship between personal tempo and time perception such that cadence is negatively related to perceived duration of time.
2. There is a relationship between self-assessment of health and personal tempo such that the score on the Cantril Ladder is positively related to cadence.
3. There is a relationship between self-assessment of health and time perception such that [the] score on the Cantril Ladder is negatively related to perceived duration of time (Engle, 1984, p. 28).

Engle's key terms and hypotheses not only were congruent with Newman's model and previous research but also extended them by incorporating the concept of self-assessed health. The sample consisted of 114 white females, aged 60 or over, who lived in subsidized apartment complexes in a large midwestern city.

Engle's hypotheses were tested using the bivariate correlation technique. In addition, a stepwise, multiple linear regression technique was used to assess the independent contributions of control and demographic variables toward explaining time perception, personal tempo, and self-assessment of health. Hypothesis 1, that personal tempo and time perceptions were related, was supported; however, neither hypothesis 2 nor hypothesis 3 was supported. In addition, none of the standardized regression coefficients were significant.

In her discussion, Engle clearly put her results within the framework of Newman's theory when she wrote: "The significant relationship between personal tempo and time perception found in this study of older, white women supports Newman's proposition that time is a function of movement" (Engle, 1984, p. 32). She also stated that support for Newman's proposition was found in studies of college-aged men conducted by Newman (1972) and in studies of college-aged women conducted by Newman (1976) and Tompkins (1980). In addition, Engle discussed the methodological issues that may have interfered with the attaining of statistical significance for hypotheses 2 and 3.

In summary, three research studies in which investigators have tested hypotheses derived from select propositions within Rogers's, Orem's, and Newman's models have been presented. These studies were selected because they represent investigators' efforts to test nursing theory explicitly.

Impediments and Approaches to Testing of Nursing Theory

The process of theory testing is a complex one. Therefore, attention must be paid to impediments that interfere with the testing of nursing theory and to approaches to diminish these impediments.

Lack of Investigator Commitment

Over the past two decades there has been steady pressure on nurse theorists and investigators to test nursing theory. However, the concept of theory testing has remained ambiguous. As a consequence, many studies in nursing have used conceptual models of nursing as frameworks for research, but only a few have explicitly tested these models in the sense of trying to determine the underlying validity of the model's assumptions or propositions. As a result, little progress has been made in the empirical validation of the models. This situation generates the following question: What is the commitment of theorists and investigators to the empirical validation of nursing models? A verbal commitment is clearly evidenced by the frequency with which calls to test nursing theory occur. But beyond this verbal commitment, there is little evidence of a concerted or systematic effort to test nursing theory through empirical research.

What can be done to improve this situation? First, nurse theorists, in communicating their models, must make explicit key assumptions, propositions, and hypotheses that need to be tested. This step is necessary because theory testing is a complex process that can involve the deduction of dozens of hypotheses from theory propositions. By specifying a limited number of key assumptions, propositions, and hypotheses to be tested, the process of theory testing becomes focused and streamlined. In addition, if nurse theorists can spearhead cluster studies that focus on testing of their theories, more systematic approaches to theory testing may occur.

Second, nurse investigators must become clearer on what constitutes theory testing. It is the atypical research study in nursing that tests theory, as the typical nursing research study uses theory primarily as an organizing framework. As noted previously, there is a serious drawback to using nursing theory in this manner. It is the drawback of too often assuming that the model is valid without presenting evidence that supports or refutes the model's validity. Since a primary purpose of theory in research is to explain the study results, the investigator must understand that if the basic tenets of the model are untested or invalid, then the explanatory basis of the results could be questionable. This is a problem that can be lessened by using theoretical models that have at least some empirical or other support.

This leaning toward support is the current state of the art regarding nursing theory. Beginning evidence points more toward support of the nursing models than lack of support. This situation provides nurse investigators with encouragement and optimism to continue pursuing the testing of nursing theory.

Lack of Tolerance of Methodological Imperfections

In addition to lack of commitment, a second impediment to testing of nursing theory is intolerance of methodological imperfections. Two such commonly perceived imperfections are abstractness and imprecision. By its very nature theory is ultimately abstract and imprecise. However, these characteristics do not necessarily constitute methodological weakness in theory testing.

Regarding abstractness, one must remember its virtues. In abstractness one can be creative, one can dare to imagine beyond the bounds of traditional reality. Theory testing cannot occur without theory, despite all its inherent abstractness. Consequently, the degree of creativity, significance, and explanatory power inherent in a theory proper (with all of its abstractness) can affect the degree of creativity, significance, and explanatory power of the hypotheses deduced from the theory. In a methodological sense, then, what goes into a study as a theoretical framework affects what comes out as study results and discussion. Thus, abstractness has power. For out of abstractness often comes the first ingredient of methodological soundness—creative and significant ideas.

Regarding methodological precision, one must remember its flaws. Chinn puts it well:

> The myth of the perfect method results in compulsive orderliness, repetitiveness, and a fixation on minute details. It encourages us toward mental laziness in envisioning alternative methods, alternative approaches, and alternative assumptions. We re-search and re-search to the point that we know less and less about more and more. . . (Chinn, 1985, p. 47).

Because of the process involved in testing nursing theory, one must sacrifice a degree of methodological precision. This precision typically is sacrificed in the conceptual leaps that must be made in the deducing of hypotheses from theory propositions and in the measuring of abstract concepts of the theory. However, this lack of precision does not have to be viewed only as a flaw but can also be seen as a challenging opportunity. Conceptual leaps are a part of many innovative studies that are on the cutting edge of advances in science. Theory testing cannot move forward if every relevant variable must be precisely defined or meticulously controlled. One must live with the imprecisions that cannot be changed, take them into account in interpreting the results, and acknowledge their benefits. These benefits include creativity, serendipity, and wisdom hewed out of openness to experience.

Lack of Systematic Retrieval Strategies

A third impediment to testing of nursing theory is lack of systematic retrieval strategies to locate studies based on nursing models. This problem arises because nurse investigators frequently do not specify the name of the theorist or the nursing model in a study's title or abstract. Consequently, studies based on or testing nursing theory typically do not show up in computer searches. Thus, investigators often are left in a state of limbo about the state of the art on nursing theory-based research.

What can be done to improve this situation? First, systematic compilations of research based on nursing models need to be given high priority. Second, investigators testing nursing models must explicitly refer to the theorist or the model in the study's title and/or abstract. Lastly, investigators using a nursing model as a framework for research should include in their review of the literature those studies that both support and refute the model, so that a state of the art on the model's validity is addressed.

Sixty-two studies involving five nursing models served as the basis for establishing a state of the art on research testing nursing theory. Studies that used nursing models minimally or as an organizing framework for research were differentiated from those that explicitly tested hypotheses deduced from nursing theory assumptions or propositions. Based on select criteria, three studies were presented as exemplars of research testing nursing theory. In addition, impediments to testing of nursing theory and approaches to overcoming these impediments were discussed.

Based on the 62 studies and in response to the question raised in the introduction of this article— "What is the current state of the art regarding research that explicitly tests nursing theory?"—the following two conclusions are drawn:

1. Investigators have conducted few nursing research studies that have explicitly tested nursing theory. Rather, in their research, investigators have tended to use nursing models minimally or as organizing frameworks.
2. Lack of investigator commitment, intolerance of methodological imperfections, and unsystematic retrieval strategies have impeded progress in the testing of nursing theory.

Implications for nursing theory, research, and practice include:

- Criteria for research-based theory testing should be better delineated in both nursing theory and nursing research courses.
- A sense of commitment should be fostered in investigators regarding the need for conducting research that tests nursing theory and the need for developing innovative theory testing methodologies.
- Systematic retrieval processes should be developed for identifying research based on nursing theory.
- Cluster studies should be conducted that systematically test hypotheses deduced from underlying assumptions and propositions of nursing models.
- Health care providers should be readied for the current trend toward implementation of nursing theory into practice settings.

If nurse theorists, investigators, and clinicians incorporate the preceding implications into their practices, they will be in a better position to move research testing nursing theory into the nursing mainstream. Such movement can only serve to advance nursing theory, research, and practice.

References

Chinn, P.L. (1985). Debunking myths in nursing theory and research. *Image, 17,* 45–49.

Engle, V.F. (1984). Newman's conceptual framework and the measurement of older adults' health. *Advances in Nursing Science, 7*(1), 24–36.

Harper, D.C. (1984). Application of Orem's theoretical constructs to self-care medication behaviors in the elderly. *Advances in Nursing Science, 6*(3), 29–46.

Johnson, D.E. (1980). The behavioral system model for nursing. In J.P. Riehl & C. Roy (Eds.), *Conceptual models for nursing practice* (2nd ed.) (pp. 207–216). New York: Appleton-Century-Crofts.

Newman, M.A. (1972). Time estimation in relation to gait tempo. *Perception and Motor Skills, 34,* 359–366.

Newman, M.A. (1976). Movement tempo and the experience of time. *Nursing Research, 25,* 273–279.

Newman, M.A. (1979). *Theory development in nursing.* Philadelphia: F.A. Davis.

Newman, M.A. (1982). Time as an index of expanding consciousness with age. *Nursing Research, 31,* 290–293.

Orem, D.E. (1985). *Nursing: Concepts of practice* (3rd ed.). New York: McGraw-Hill.

Quinn, J.F. (1984). Therapeutic touch as energy exchange: Testing the theory. *Advances in Nursing Science, 6*(2), 42–49.

Rogers, M.E. (1970). *An introduction to the theoretical basis of nursing.* Philadelphia: F.A. Davis.

Rogers, M.E. (1980). Nursing: A science of unitary man. In J.P. Riehl & C. Roy (Eds.), *Conceptual models for nursing practice* (2nd ed.) (pp. 329–337). New York: Appleton-Century-Crofts.

Rogers, M.E. (1983). Science of unitary human beings: A paradigm for nursing. In I.W. Clements & F.B. Roberts (Eds.), *Family health: A theoretical approach to nursing care* (pp. 219–228). New York: John Wiley & Sons.

Roy, C. (1970). Adaptation: A conceptual framework for nursing. *Nursing Outlook, 18,* 42–45.

Roy, C. (1984). *Introduction to nursing: An adaptation model* (2nd ed.). Englewood Cliffs, NJ: Prentice-Hall.

Silva, M.C. (1987). Conceptual models of nursing. In J.J. Fitzpatrick & R.L. Taunton (Eds.), *Annual review of nursing research* (Vol. 5, pp. 229–246). New York: Springer.

Tompkins, E.S. (1980). Effect of restricted mobility and dominance on perceived duration. *Nursing Research, 29,* 333–338.

Clarification

To the editor:

I would like to clarify one small but important point regarding my article "Research Testing Nursing Theory: State of the Art" (*ANS* 9(1), October 1986). In my original manuscript, I wrote that the hand searches covered the period 1952–1985. The article was printed saying the searches covered the years 1952 to 1985. The hyphen usage was different from my past experience and from what I had intended. The search covered the inclusive dates—that is, 1952 through 1985. This makes a 1-year difference in the database discussed in the article.

MARY SILVA, R.N., Ph.D.
Professor
School of Nursing
George Mason University
Fairfax, Virginia

Reactions

Theory Testing Research: Methodological Issues

To the editor:

I read with great interest Silva's article "Research Testing Nursing Theory: State of the Art" in the October 1986 issue of *ANS*. I believe, however, that one methodological decision made by Silva requires some elaboration. "State of the art" is defined in Webster's Dictionary as "the level of development (as a device, procedure, process, technique or science) reached at any particular time." The state of the art of theory-testing research, then, should reflect the level of development of all research that tests theory. Silva decided to include only published research, excluding all unpublished research, particularly doctoral dissertations and master's theses. It seems to me, however, that to obtain a complete perspective, a state of the art view, it is necessary to include both published and unpublished research. A large portion of the research being conducted in nursing is done by graduate students. To exclude their work in a review such as this minimizes their contribution to the knowledge base of the discipline.

One might argue that by including only published research in the review, a minimum standard of scientific rigor and merit is ensured. However, students completing dissertations and theses have departmental and university requirements that must be met and these help to ensure scientific acceptability, i.e., merit and rigor. To me, there is a major difference between *unpublished* research and *unpublishable* research. Unpublishable research (scientifically unacceptable) is a small subset of the domain of unpublished research. Unfortunately, a great deal of scientifically acceptable research never gets into print, for a variety of reasons.

Silva probably realized (and rightly so) that to include unpublished research in her review would have been extremely difficult, if not impossible, to do. I know from personal experience how hard it is to obtain dissertations and theses. Dissertation abstracts are available in *Dissertation Abstracts International,* but acquiring the actual dissertations is expensive and time consuming. As for theses, no compilation of thesis titles exists that I am aware of, so the first step of identifying possible theses for review is essentially impossible. I can understand why Silva made the methodological decision to include only published research in her review. But understanding her decision does not fully address the issues that are apparent as a result of having read this review. Specifically, I think it is important to realize that this review is a limited view of the state of the art of theory-testing research and this should be made explicit. I would even venture that the title state of the art is not completely accurate.

A more generalized issue relates to the process of disseminating and communicating research results. While individual researchers have a responsibility to present research results, both orally and in published form, the larger professional community should focus more attention on how research reports are catalogued and accessed. A regularly published list of thesis and dissertation titles could be a beginning catalogue; easy accessibility could be achieved by establishing a national archive housing copies of all reports of research done by nurses. Sigma Theta Tau is planning a Center for Nursing Scholarship— maybe the center could serve as a central archival location. These are only two ideas—I am sure there are many other possible solutions.

However, while there may be many solutions, the problem remains: Without accurate information about research being conducted in the discipline, can we ever know exactly what is the state of the art?

LESLIE H. NICOLL, R.N., M.S.
Assistant Professor, Nursing
University of New Hampshire
Durham, New Hampshire
Doctoral Candidate
Frances Payne Bolton School of Nursing
Case Western Reserve University
Cleveland, Ohio

Author's response:

I am genuinely sympathetic to Ms. Nicoll's comments about the exclusion of unpublished works (particularly theses and dissertations) in my article, "Research Testing Nursing Theory: State of the Art." However, Ms. Nicoll makes the assumption that the decision to exclude unpublished work was mine, when it was not.

Some background information should help clarify this point. The database for this article (i.e., the 62 studies mentioned therein) primarily came from a manuscript of mine soon to be published in the *Annual Review of Nursing Research* (ARNR). Because the ARNR series are edited volumes with many contributors, the editors have had to establish some basic guidelines to ensure consistency across reviews. One of my guidelines was that the review was to include *published* research; use of unpublished doctoral dissertations was discouraged. Since this was editorial policy that I felt could be legitimately justified, I honored it.

Nevertheless, clarification of this point does not elucidate the conceptual issue of whether unpublished works (in particular, theses and dissertations) should be included in state of the art reviews or other works. The two sides of this issue have been alluded to by Ms. Nicoll. Let me spell them out more explicitly, as I have heard the arguments.

1. *Against use of unpublished doctoral dissertations:* Doctoral dissertations are conducted primarily to learn about research; thus, they contain many more conceptual and methodological problems than research conducted by seasoned researchers. Consequently, few manuscripts based on doctoral dissertations get published in leading research journals because they cannot meet the rigorous standards of scientific merit. Therefore, to include them in written works would jeopardize the validity of the works as the conclusions drawn may be based on invalid data that have not met peer-reviewed scientific standards. However, if data from doctoral dissertations remain unpublished, one is left with one of two unsettling conclusions: The author of the dissertation chose not to publish the results of the dissertation for whatever reasons, thus neglecting a professional responsibility to publish research results, or the author attempted to publish the dissertation data but was unsuccessful, thus raising doubts about the study's scientific merit.

2. *In defense of use of unpublished doctoral dissertations:* Because research is unpublished does not mean it lacks scientific merit. Doctoral dissertation research follows carefully specified university research requirements and is conducted under the auspices of a committee of research experts, thus helping to ensure scientific validity. In addition, the scientific body of knowledge in nursing is relatively new; therefore, we cannot afford to dismiss the research of an increasingly growing number of potential scholars—doctoral students or candidates. To exclude their research from a state-of-the-art review (or

other works) could invalidate the review (or other works) to the degree that the conclusions drawn with the dissertation data would be different from those drawn without the dissertation data.

Because use of doctoral dissertations in manuscripts is a controversial issue, there is not a right or wrong answer regarding their usage. The challenge is to construct rationally justifiable arguments for one's position. I have tried to show both sides of the issue, as well as underscore the point that the decision may neither be easy nor solely in the author's hands.

In this regard, then, whether or not my state of the art review was limited or inaccurate depends on where one stands on the preceding arguments, as the ultimate concern on both sides of this issue is the possibility of invalid conclusions. In my article the criteria for the studies' inclusion or exclusion were clearly identified (see p. 2), and the conclusions were carefully generalized to that database and not beyond (see p. 10).

Ms. Nicoll makes another assumption about my article—that I did not include unpublished studies (in particular, dissertations) because they are hard to locate. She is correct in her assertion that I did not use dissertations in my article (for reasons previously noted); however, she is incorrect in her assertion that I did not locate dissertation content relevant to my topic. Through systematic hand searches, a research assistant and I located all dissertation abstracts in *Dissertations Abstracts International* from 1952–1984 that explicitly cited the nursing models of Dorothy Johnson, Callista Roy, Dorothea Orem, Martha Rogers, and Margaret Newman. I would be happy to share these references with any interested readers, as I was willing to share the 62 studies in the article under discussion.

The last point Ms. Nicoll raises concerns the process of disseminating and communicating research results. On this point, I am in total agreement with her. Collecting data for the article under discussion was a time-consuming and painstaking task because of the extensive hand searches involved. These hand searches were necessary because the vast majority of research based on nursing models contains neither the names of the theorists nor the models in the studies' titles or abstracts. We in nursing do need to improve our strategies for cataloguing and retrieving research studies, especially those based on nursing and related discipline models.

In sum, then, the use of unpublished research in scholarly writings is controversial. To avoid this controversy, the investigator must make every effort to conduct quality research that has the highest probability of being accepted for publication in a leading research journal. Fortunately, in nursing today, several such journals exist and others are on the horizon.

MARY SILVA, R.N., Ph.D.

The Author Comments

The preceding article, published in *Advances in Nursing Science,* was a direct outgrowth of the chapter on "Conceptual Models of Nursing" published in the *Annual Review of Nursing Research (ARNR)*[1] in 1987. The *ARNR* chapter, which critiqued 62 studies based on five conceptual models of nursing, was written prior to the *ANS* article but published after it.

Both the chapter in the *ARNR* and the article in *ANS* were an outgrowth of several observations I made regarding the relationship between conceptual models of nursing and nursing research. First, I observed that several studies identified a nursing conceptual model as a framework for research but there was virtually no link between the model and the subsequent research; that is, no mention was made of the model either prior to or after its introduction into the study. Second, I noticed that the authors of several studies using nursing conceptual models stated that the purpose of their research was to "test" the model. After carefully reading these research articles, I could not see that any testing of the model had

---

[1]Silva, M.C. (1987). Conceptual models of nursing. In J.J. Fitzpatrick and R.L. Taunton (Eds.), *Annual Review of Nursing Research* (Vol. 5, pp. 229-246). New York: Springer.

occurred; instead, in my opinion, the author(s) had used the model primarily to organize their instruments. Although some of these instruments were well developed, they did not empirically *test* the model but rather *applied* it. Third, I observed that whenever a nursing conceptual model was used as a framework, it would be summarized but no subsequent research related to the model would be integrated into the discussion. Thus, the reader had no current state of the science on the validity of the model. Fourth, I noticed that most authors did not include the name of the nursing model in either the study's title and/or abstract. This omission suggested that the model was not seen as an important part of the study. Furthermore, it presented a difficult retrieval problem for those researchers interested in the state of the science on a given nursing model.

The 62 studies previously noted in the *ARNR* chapter served as the basis for the *ANS* article. In contrast to the *ARNR* chapter, in which the goal was to summarize and critique these studies, the *ANS* article had other purposes: (a) to clarify the term, *testing of nursing theory,* by identifying specific criteria of adequacy for theory testing; (b) to highlight studies that demonstrated these criteria; and (c) to discuss impediments to theory testing in nursing.

Despite the large body of expository literature in nursing on the necessity for testing theory, the term essentially remains undefined. Using a combination of my research experiences, background readings, and reasoning, I formulated the seven formative theory testing criteria outlined in the preceding *ANS* article. Based on these criteria, my goal was to differentiate theory testing from other uses of theory. Three empirical studies, each representing a different conceptual model of nursing, were then summarized to give examples of how different authors tested theory. I linked their approaches to the seven formative criteria. Finally, I offered reasons for what I perceived to be the dearth of theory testing articles in nursing. I still believe that lack of investigator commitment (and investigator understanding) is a problem. However, I believe that progress has been made both in tolerance of nonempirical research methods and in authors including the name of the nursing model in both the titles and abstracts of their research.

In my article and letter response, I offered the nursing community a list of the empirical studies I located on the five conceptual models. To date, 62 persons from all parts of the United States, plus Canada, Sweden, and Ireland have requested the list. This is a good beginning pool from which to draw for those of us interested in testing of nursing models.

—MARY CIPRIANO SILVA

Unit Five

Nursing Theory and Nursing Practice

Discussion of theory in nursing is interesting but serves little purpose if it strays too far from the basic realities of nursing practice in society. Unit Five, Nursing Theory and Nursing Practice, begins to address one of the primary elements of professional nursing—the practice component. No matter what a person's primary interest, clinical orientation, or area of research is, the basic, unalterable fact is that nursing exists to provide a service to an identified group of people.

This description of nursing becomes problematic, however, when one moves from the abstract, i.e., "a service to an identified group of people" to a concrete specification of "service" and "people." The nature of nursing, and of nursing activities and roles, and the identification of nursing's clientele have been questioned by the community of nurses and society as a whole in recent years. Even so, it is probably safe to assume that nurses do believe in considerate, thoughtful, knowledgeable actions and that the intent of nursing is not harm but "beneficence to the client," as Ellis has argued.

Theory is one means to validate nursing actions. A structure, as defined by a theory, provides a frame of reference for the nurse in deciding among nursing activities, all of which may appear to be equally attractive at a given moment. Theory provides a mechanism for understanding a situation and if developed fully, allows the nurse to determine and effectively regulate the outcome.

Theoreticians have been accused of moving too far from the reality of nursing practice. Unit Five provides evidence to the contrary. The twelve articles make clear that one purpose of theory is to provide meaning to the nursing experience—an experience that occurs in realistic, identifiable nursing situations.

In Chapter 45, "Closing the Practice-Theory Gap," Conant argues for a two-way interaction between theory and practice. Theory provides concepts and principles; practice provides a means to test the principles and then, in turn, to refine them.

Chapter 46, "Theory in a Practice Discipline Part I: Practice Oriented Theory" by Dickoff, James, and Wiedenbach, presents an eloquent description of the nature of practice theory and the relationship of theory to practice. Many of the principles presented in this article were first identified in "A Theory of Theories" (see Chapter 8). This article is an example of the continuing development of thought on the part of the authors.

Chapter 47, "Theory: The Professional Dimension" by Hildegard E. Peplau, was presented at the First Nursing Theory Conference held at the University of Kansas in 1969. Peplau's first book, Interpersonal Relations in Nursing, is considered by many to be a description of a theory in nursing. When Peplau wrote the book, she did not use the term theory to describe her text. Her practical purpose was to document her perception of nursing as she had experienced it in working with clients. Through this documentation she believed she could assist students in the process of learning and in working with clients using interpersonal communication principles. Chapter 47 is yet another example of Peplau's clarity of thought in her description of nursing theory, developed from her work with clients and students.

Rosemary Ellis, in Chapter 48, "The Practitioner as Theorist," makes the case for the nurse in practice to work to develop theory. Observations, experience, understanding, all contribute to theory development. Without a reference to practice, nurses would not have the observations and experience needed to gain understanding. Chapter 49, "Nursing Science: The Theory-Practice Linkage" by Maeona Kramer and Sue E. Huether, explicates the linkages between nursing science and nursing theory. Utilization of theory in practice is not easy, in part because of the complexity of theory and the nature of traditional science. Kramer and Huether explore some of these issues.

Chapter 50 is a collection of articles by Jan Beckstrand, with a critique by Rosemarie Collins and John Fielder, and a reply from Beckstrand. The articles examine the nature of practice theory and ask the question, "Is there a difference between nursing theory and nursing practice theory, or is nursing theory a practice theory by virtue of the practice component of nursing?"

Chapters 51 and 52, by Dickoff and James represent extensions of their thoughts, presented elsewhere in this text in Chapters 4, 8, 46, and 53. Variations on these two articles were published in the dental hygiene literature, but have been revised and updated to reflect a nursing perspective for this text.

Unit Five differs from the preceding units in that it presents discussion of some concrete applications of theory. Units One and Two provided a general overview of many aspects of theory; Units Three and Four examined specific elements of theory—science, theory development, and critique. Unit Five has introduced a practical referent for understanding some of the purposes of theory. This theme will be continued in the last unit, Nursing Theory and Nursing Research.

Chapter 45

Closing the Practice-Theory Gap

Lucy H. Conant

Nursing is a practice profession. A nurse must know, and she must also know how to do. There has been a tendency to separate knowing from doing—the schism has been apparent in the clinical papers I have read as a member of the American Nurses' Association Advisory Committee on the Clinical Sessions. Papers that integrate knowledge and practice are relatively rare. Some have developed interesting theoretical concepts, with extensive use of the literature in nursing and related areas, but with minimal clinical illustration or discussion of application to practice. Others have consisted largely of case study material with little or no development of ideas and with little generalization from the situations presented.

Historically, the separation of knowledge and practice in nursing is understandable. Former emphasis on experience with little concern for education, nurses' "training" in service rather than in educational institutions, and, more recently, the opposite extreme of removing nursing education from service are all part of the profession's heritage. But education and administration are both aspects of the broader area of nursing practice, and the practitioner has been the forgotten person. Although lip service is given to her importance, in status and in salary, she has been ignored and neglected, with the result that staff nursing experience has served as a jumping-off point—which has meant jumping away from patient care.

There is now growing interest in the development and use of clinical specialists and an awareness that nursing education and service have perhaps drifted too far apart. These may stimulate the examination of relationships and develop the dimensions of nursing without swinging from one extreme to the other.

What Nursing Theory Is

First, it is important to understand what nursing theory is and why the development of theories of nursing practice is important. In any practice discipline the aim

About the Author

LUCY H. CONANT, a Massachusetts native, was born in Littleton, grew up in Southampton, and currently resides in Chester, in the Berkshire Mountains of western Massachusetts. Dr. Conant graduated from Radcliffe College in 1947 and went on to Yale University to study nursing, receiving an M.N. in 1950. She continued her education at the Harvard School of Public Health (M.P.H., 1957) and returned to Yale for doctoral study in sociology, earning a Ph.D. in 1964.

Dr. Conant worked as a public health nurse in Michigan and as a district nurse in Cornwall, England during 1953 and 1954. She returned to Yale in 1957 and held a faculty appointment, as well as a position as a research associate, until 1968, when she accepted the position of Dean and Professor at the School of Nursing of the University of North Carolina in Chapel Hill.

In 1975, Dr. Conant returned to Massachusetts. She comments "Since leaving the deanship at the University of North Carolina in 1975, I have been seeing what I could do with my farm in the Berkshires. After 25 busy years in the nursing profession, I was ready for a change and realized that I had always been a farmer at heart. Now I raise sheep, berries, and vegetables."

is not merely to describe particular phenomena or to predict results, but to ". . .achieve controlled changes in natural relationships by means of procedures that are scientifically based" (Greenwood, 1961, p. 74). Pertinent factors must be isolated and described; their relationships must be specified and ordered to prescribe activity that will lead to the desired goal, which also must be specified.

Prediction is not enough in nursing or any other practice discipline. We must be able to prescribe, to specify and carry out planned activity that will change the natural outcome to the desired outcome. Not only is scientific knowledge needed, but the selection and adaptation of various kinds of knowledge in order to direct one's activity within a particular situation requires its own special knowledge. Principles are not merely applied to practice, because the "how" in practice includes an art and science of its own. The nurse needs to learn much more about both the "whats" and the "hows" of practice.

Theory and practice operate in both directions. Too often the importance of theory to practice is over-emphasized at the price of underestimating the usefulness of practice in developing theory. Theory helps determine practice, but practice is itself essential in developing theoretical concepts in nursing.

The contribution of practice can be illustrated by some examples: Most nurses have had contact with an unforgettable patient who taught them a great deal about nursing. Also, they have all seen a skilled nurse operating most effectively, using some individual combination of knowledge, experience, intuition, and understanding. Frequently, that nurse cannot be explicit on the rationale for her methods, and to explain her talent by calling her a "born nurse" does not help describe the qualities of such practice or teach students how to develop similar abilities. To capitalize on the effectiveness of outstanding nurse practitioners, there is a need to analyze and describe what they do, to see if general concepts can be developed that can then be tested, refined, practiced, and taught. Generalizing from the particular is as important as deriving the particular from the general. In this way, the insights and abilities of individual nurses can contribute to nursing knowledge and improvement of practice. Too often there is a tendency to rely on intuitive knowledge *per se* or, at the other extreme, to ignore experience and rely on knowledge from other disciplines that may not be relevant to nursing. A scientific basis for nursing practice needs both kinds of knowledge—that obtained from experience and that gained from the intellect.

A Complex Activity

Nursing practice is a complex activity. In a way, nurses know much more than they realize and in performing even a simple procedure may use a great deal of judgment as they make decisions and systematically adapt their nursing activity to the patient and the situation. For example, in a recent theory seminar at the Yale University School of Nursing in which we examined some nursing procedures, we selected routine back care as an example of beginning level practice theory. The procedure sounds very elementary but it proved to be difficult and complex to analyze—it really is not back care but maintenance of skin and underlying tissue, with particular attention to vulnerable areas. Involved are not only the patient's nutritional and fluid balance, and physical manipulation of his body, but use of equipment and appliances as well. Whether or not to use massage, choice of cleansing agents, decision as to use of a lubricant or an astringent—all require decision making based on observation and knowledge. Manual skills are vital in such a procedure. Other aspects include the nurse's encouragement of the patient to move and turn on his own initiative, the meaning to the patient of a backrub—its physical comforting and relaxing qualities—and finally, the fact that carrying out such a procedure may facilitate a good relationship between nurse and patient and encourage the patient to communicate with the nurse.

The Nursing Environment

Not only is nursing a complex activity; but it also usually takes place in an extremely complex environment—the hospital. Physicians, other nurses, hospital personnel, patients, family members are all involved. The policies and procedures of the organization, as well as the physical environment, equipment, supplies, and other factors within the setting influence nursing practice. Nursing does not take place in a vacuum, though sometimes it's taught as if it did.

Yet, in a practice profession like nursing, knowledge is incomplete unless its use in practice can be prescribed. Knowledge must be based on reality if it is to direct activity. Doing is not separate from knowing, rather it is a further, more complex step. The activity is important in itself, but from thoughtful practice come new insights and ideas. We need to ask many more

questions about our practice and speculate more freely. What are the similarities and differences in the nursing care of seemingly similar types of patients? What works, what does not work, and how do we know? What factors may explain apparent relationships? There is so much that we do not know. But while the unknown may be a problem, it also presents many possibilities. Not only the successful outcomes should be examined, but also the failures in practice, not with a sense of blame or guilt but out of interest and a desire to learn. After all, to do research one needs a problem.

While there are many problems in nursing, one of the most difficult tasks in doing nursing research is to develop a researchable problem. In the past we in nursing have not been accustomed to analyzing and speculating about the nature of a nursing problem as a challenge from which we could learn and perhaps eventually help provide a solution to it.

One reason that nursing has attracted the social scientist is its interesting problems accessible for study. But, since the problems have been studied from a sociologic or psychologic viewpoint, the conclusions reached are not always relevant for nursing practice. Among the psychologists only the clinical psychologist, again a practitioner, goes beyond the description and prediction phases of knowledge. Others are not likely to be interested in activity, change, and goal attainment as they relate to practice. After all nursing has the responsibility for studying nursing problems in such a way that the findings relate directly to practice.

While social scientists have been studying nurses they, in turn, have been borrowing from the social sciences. The difficulty is that sometimes a borrowed theoretical concept is used in nursing before its relevance to the nursing situation is determined. Although in developing nursing theory, it is justifiable to use existing knowledge one cannot automatically assume that it is appropriate or useful to nursing practice. For example, in my doctoral dissertation in sociology, I used a widely accepted interaction measure, Bales's *Interaction Process Analysis* (Cambridge, MA: Addison-Wesley, 1950) in analyzing nurse-patient interaction. Preliminary work indicated that it would be a useful tool. The assumptions on which Bales based this measure seemed to apply to the public health nursing home visit, the type of nurse-patient interaction I was studying. The result was that while the measure did provide much useful information, it had some definite limitations both as a general measure of interaction and, more specifically, as it described the nursing situation (Conant, 1965).

The value of knowledge from other disciplines for nursing practice cannot be taken for granted. A general theoretical concept must be examined for the validity to the nursing practice situation, and in the process a contribution may be made to the development and refinement of the concept itself. Too often those in nursing have sought to obtain knowledge from other disciplines, without seeing contribution that nursing could make to the general knowledge of human behavior.

The Role of Research

Clinical research provides the means for systematically moving back and forth between practice and theory, whether testing a hypothesis borrowed from another discipline or one developed within nursing. However, nurses doing research have tended to follow the model of the scientists and have stopped with description and prediction of relationships. Little attempt thus far has been made to move from establishing statistical significance to prescribing nursing activities. At present, there is a wide gap between research and practice, particularly in the application of research findings. The researcher has not seen it as his role to use the findings in practice, and the practitioner is not given the knowledge and understanding necessary to change his practice. Yet research findings in a practice discipline are incomplete until they are tested in practice. The gap exists not only in nursing, but in areas such as medicine, where there is a great gulf between medical knowledge and medical practice. Perhaps in nursing, where research is only getting started, the problem can be recognized early, responsibilities clarified, and the channels developed by which researchable ideas can

come from practice, and research findings be tested and incorporated into practice.

To illustrate the point about interdependency of research and practice—several years ago I had an unplanned combination of experiences which demonstrated how essential practice is for research. My dissertation findings seemed to be an interesting hodgepodge of unrelated facts that were difficult to explain. It happened that I was completing the analysis of data and trying to write the dissertation while I was doing part-time clinical practice as a public health nurse with the New Haven Visiting Nurse Association, the agency where I had collected the data for my dissertation. The nursing experience with patients and families was not only stimulating but clarifying. Their comments and reactions helped me to understand and to explain the dissertation findings. After having sorted out the findings, I was able to test the concept developed in the dissertation to see whether it worked in practice. The practice facilitated the research activity, and subsequently I think the research improved my nursing practice. The practice also provided the stimulation of personal and professional contacts needed to offset the tediousness of continued preoccupation with IBM cards, tables of figures and seemingly unrelated results.

What helped to explain my dissertation findings was the concept of Homans (1958) of interaction as an exchange, with what a person receives from another being a reward, and what he gives to another, a cost. It seems to me that this idea is useful, not only in examining interaction between nurses and patients, but also for analyzing relationships between practitioners and researchers. Each needs the other, and each contributes to the other. The potential contribution of practitioners has been underestimated in nursing research. In our zeal to become scientific, we have tended to forget that observation is a type of data collection that nurses perform constantly. We are quick to arrange for consultation in methodology and statistics for our research projects, but we need to consult nurse practitioners too. If theory is necessary for practice and practice is essential in the development of theory, then not only should nurse researchers be concerned with and involved in nursing practice but practitioners and researchers must work together and pool their knowledge and insights.

Basically, we are all nurses concerned with the improvement of practice. We need to be much more knowledgeable about our practice. Yet, however well we develop this knowledge, nursing, because it is a practice discipline, will always retain the need for creative, intuitive activity which may precede knowledge. We obtain knowledge from practice and at the same time use this knowledge to improve practice.

References

Bales, R.F. (1950). *Interaction process analysis*. Cambridge, MA: Addison-Wesley.

Conant, L.H. (1965). Use of Bales's interaction process analysis to study nurse-patient interaction. *Nursing Research*, *14*, 308–309.

Greenwood, E. (1961). The practice of science and the science of practice. In W.G. Bennis, K.D. Benne, & R. Chin (Eds.), *The planning of change*. New York: Holt, Rinehart and Winston.

Homans, G.C. (1958). Social behavior as exchange. *American Journal of Sociology*, *63*, 597–606.

The Author Comments

This article is based on a speech I gave on April 27, 1966, at the Syracuse University School of Nursing for the Anna Dahlem Memorial Lecture, which was sponsored by the Omicron chapter of Sigma Theta Tau. The speech, titled "The Importance of Nursing Practice in the Development of Nursing Theory," evolved from my experiences at the Yale University School of Nursing. As a faculty member, I was greatly influenced by my contacts with Florence Wald, Robert Leonard, James Dickoff, and Patricia James. Certainly, there were many ideas, challenges, and much stimulation circulating among the Yale faculty during the mid-1960s.

Also, I recently had completed my Ph.D. dissertation in Sociology and had studied nurse-patient interaction using small group analysis. I went on to further research in public health nursing practice. In my clinical practice, I found myself informally testing some sociological concepts and finding at the same time that insights gained from practice helped me to refine those same concepts. It was a two-way street, not a simple matter of applying theory to practice.

—LUCY H. CONANT

Chapter 46

Theory in a Practice Discipline Part I: Practice Oriented Theory

James Dickoff
Patricia James
Ernestine Wiedenbach

The article presented here is Part I of a two-part article on the nature and development of theory in a practice discipline. Part I deals with the relation of theory to practice and with the appropriate structure of any practice theory and, more particularly, of nursing theory. Part II, to be published in the November-December issue of Nursing Research, will deal with theory as a common denominator of research and practice.

Nurse as Theorist?

Granted the nurse's traditional role as practitioner and even her more recent role as researcher. Still it may be asked: What is the point of a nurse's becoming a theorist? Reaction to this question often discloses an orientation to nursing as well as to theory. A reader may be frankly contemptuous that a nurse become a theorist; or he may receive the suggestion more generously with a tentative and cautious openness; or even more encouragingly, his response may betoken a serious entertaining of just how and why today's nurse is or should be theorist.

For an appreciation of the discussion presented here the seriously explorative reading is perhaps the most useful. But the importance of feeling and remembering the two less positive reactions must not be overlooked. For the thesis of this paper—that not only is theory relevant to practice but also practice relevant to theory and both relevant to research—is a position susceptible to many misreadings. It is all too easy to go off any one of three deep ends: A nurse can get lost in the business of theory and then never become reoccupied with practice or research *except* as contributor to theory. Or she can engage in research as a self-perpetuating activity done with no thought of an out-

About the Author

ERNESTINE WIEDENBACH lives in Florida. Although retired for more than 20 years, she has continued to maintain an interest in nursing. She comments "In a retirement community such as the one in which I live, the needs of the elderly are very absorbing and quite fascinating. But here too, I have found that the principles of a prescriptive theory apply; when they are applied, the help given is truly helpful!"

Ms. Wiedenbach is a graduate of Wellesley College, receiving a B.A. in 1922. She studied nursing at Johns Hopkins Hospital School of Nursing and graduated in 1925. For 10 years, she worked for the Bureau of Educational Nursing, Association for Improving Conditions of the Poor as a staff public health nurse, social worker, supervisor, and educational director. In 1934, she returned to school and received an M.A. from Teachers College, Columbia University. From 1934 to 1945 she was Secretary of the Nursing Information Bureau of the ANA, National League of Nursing Education (now NLN), and the National Organization of Public Health Nurses.

Ms. Wiedenbach received a certificate in Nurse Midwifery from the Maternity Center Association, New York City, in 1946, and worked as a staff nurse midwife for the Maternity Center Association for 5 years. She notes that she got great satisfaction from performing home deliveries. In 1952, she joined the faculty of the Yale University School of Nursing, teaching maternal and newborn health nursing until her retirement in 1966. Retirement gave her the time and the opportunity to meet with groups of graduate nurses in many parts of the country, conducting institutes on maternal and newborn health nursing and teaching summer courses at such universities as California State University at Los Angeles and the University of Florida in Gainesville. In 1979, she received the Hattie Hemschemeyer Award for distinguished service from the American College of Nurse Midwives.

Ms. Wiedenbach has worked as a nurse for more than 60 years. Her contributions, including six textbooks, are wide-ranging and have influenced nursing in areas other than maternal-child health. When asked about the future of nursing, she commented "It is my firm belief that effective practice, whether nursing or teaching, is founded on the practitioner's clarity of purpose and results when the nurse understands and acts in relation to the meaning to the individual (patient or student) of the behavior being presented. The clearer we are about our own purpose and philosophy (the inner force that motivates each of us to what we do and the way we do it), the more effective will be our actions."

put beyond research itself—though perhaps making use of practice and theory as guides or aids to research. But a third equally unfortunate response for a would-be theorist in a practice discipline is to conceive the necessary dependence of research and theory on practice as an excuse for resting always with the mere particulars of the immediate problem situation and thereby restricting "analysis" of these situations to recording of anecdotes. Beyond urging that nursing theory, nursing practice, and nursing research are mutually interrelated and interdependent, this paper tries to indicate *how* the three are interdependent and suggests the appropriate hierarchy as among the nurse's competing roles as practitioner, researcher and theorist. The contention here is that theory is born in practice, is refined in research, and must and can return to practice if research is to be other than a draining-off of energy from the main business of nursing and theory more than idle speculation.[1]

---

[1] This paper results from the attempt to bring to bear on the nursing question proposed both an awareness of the realities of nursing and also a pair of mental habits that might be deemed philosophic: First, the skill to make and maintain distinctions; second, the demand to see as joined in significant unity whatever finely distinguished and multitudinous details present themselves. Both these skills—the capacity and patience to make and maintain careful distinctions at whatever level of complexity is needed and the persistence to articulate relentlessly the relation of part to part and of parts to the whole and so focus into unity any multitude that presents itself—must be called on again and again in working out a constructive and significant answer to the question of, Nurse as theorist? But these skills—as any others—must be regarded merely as ancillary in the service of nursing, not as dictators to nursing.

From Practice to Problems to Theory

The Worth of a Critical Comment

Theoretically speaking, anyone capable of speech is potentially capable of theorizing. Though we sometimes regard theorizing as an elevated, distant, and inaccessible activity, to see the roots of theorizing in activities commonly carried on and well within our ordinary powers is both useful and salutary. Spoken criticism—a most ordinary endeavor—can be viewed as a potential starting place for theory though, of course, no criticism itself constitutes theory. A skill essential to theory building in a practice discipline is the art of moving from criticism to more constructive reactions to the situations giving rise to the criticisms.

How can critical comment come to have theoretical worth? First, the comment itself must be respected as potentially valuable. Then the interest or energy required to make the criticism in the first place—we do not bother to criticize what is indifferent to us—must be tapped in further exploration. The criticism as an initial verbalization of a problem situation should be probed for clues to greater generality, on the one hand, and hints for resolution of the difficulty, on the other hand. Criticism evinces not only our interest and concern but suggests that we have in mind, at least implicitly, some standard violated by the criticized activity. To move from criticism to theory may involve explicit conceptualization of the norm violated, explicit characterization of the discrepancy, and conceptualization of a practical means for removing the discrepancy. Such means might be constituted by specifying modes of activity that would not fall short of the norm, or else by rendering the norm itself a more practicable one and then supplying conceptualization of avenues to *that* standard. By way of example let us explore a possible path from criticism toward theory.

It would be an extremely passive, stoic, nonsociable nurse who has not in her nursing experience encountered situations which she would be inclined to criticize at a coffee break with her peers: "That new policy is a real straightjacket for nursing personnel."

"The doctors don't give us much freedom on that service." "The aides don't have enough experience for their responsibilities." "We need at least two more nurses on evenings to staff that unit even safely."

To supply artificially a common store of potential grounds for critical reaction, consider the situations sketched out below. What is your reaction to them? Could you find anything to criticize? Exactly what in the situation strikes you as needing change? What direction would you recommend the change take? How would you actually bring about the change?

1. Patient is tense; has not voided for twelve hours; afraid of catheterization; no evidence of bladder distention. Nurse is helping patient relax; thinks continued support may enable patient to void. Head nurse enters; asks whether patient has voided; learns patient has not, says she will report fact to M.D. Head nurse returns; says doctor wants patient catheterized *stat*.
2. Nurse is helping mother breastfeed baby; baby has finally latched on; is nursing well. Nursery nurse enters; says doctor wants to examine baby; takes baby off breast; carries child to M.D. in nursery; neither attending nurse nor mother has opportunity to question or protest action.
3. Mother wants full participation in birth of her baby; with nurse's support mother relaxes and progresses well; when fully dilated is taken to delivery room. The resident—to gain experience—tells anesthetist to "put her under," delivers her with forceps.
4. Nurse is discussing diet with overweight mother; is helping her see need for making adjustments in diet habits. Resident comes in; scolds mother for having failed to follow his instructions for diet.

A common thread—conflict of interest—seems to run through this group of four incidents. In the voiding example, the nurse's informed judgment is in conflict with the doctor's prescription, and so she is torn between her responsibility to follow the doctor's orders and her responsibility to use her knowledge to further the patient's best interests. In the breastfeeding illustration, the investment of time and energy of both nurse and mother in getting the baby to breastfeed—not to speak of what might have been accomplished, even fairly long range, for the infant—has been annulled by the nursery nurse's very prompt action in response to a doctor's need. In the birth example, the nurse's attempt to facilitate the mother's efforts to have a normal birth experience is aborted by the resident's apparently unilateral decision in response to *his* learning need. The diet example suggests that the activity of nurse and doctor may be mutually destructive even at the moment when both are consciously trying to bring about one and the same goal for the patient. Each example seems to mark a conflict of interest as between the professionals involved. To see this common thread—to invent this characterization of the four discrete happenings—is to move beyond that initial, merely negative feeling toward the particular situation.

1. Head nurse insists student nurse carry out "morning care procedure" in exactly the order procedure is given in procedure book.
2. Very alert, perky, and mobile woman of 80 protests sides on her bed; nurse responds that hospital requires them.
3. Sleepless 12-hour mother is convinced her baby has no toes; wants to see her baby. Nursery nurse tells requesting nurse, "Let one mother break our showing schedule and they'll all be doing it."

Upon reflection we may see that each of these occurrences seems to display unquestioned pattern following. Why did the head nurse make so unconditioned a demand for strict adherence to the letter of the procedure book? Is the institution justified in protecting itself against damage suits even at the expense of the elderly person's dignity; might the nurse have followed the policy and still presented the institution as a bit less of an unreasonable tyrant? And finally, is the babies' showing schedule meant to protect the infants, the nurses' time, or the mothers' rest? These examples might lead us to consider whether stereo-typed patterns of response allow the most economical function of the practitioners and the best maintenance of the unity of ward or hospital. And we might be prompted to ask, how do these patterns provide for the individual professional the latitude for creative or even intelligent response to the particularizing features of the patient or situation?

Here is a list of situations:

1. On delivery service in evening maid does not show up; nurse in charge assigns staff nurse to be "maid" for evening. Assignment is accepted; "nurse" spends her evening cleaning instruments, et cetera, although there is on the floor a full complement of mothers in fairly active labor.
2. M.D. does vena puncture and starts intravenous; when through, leaves adhesive, discarded needle holder, paper carton, et cetera, on chair. Later nurse comes in, gathers up "junk," and discards it into waste basket.
3. Briefing report by head nurse to oncoming nursing staff has a total communication: quick rundown on number of admissions, deliveries, discharges, conditions of mothers in labor room, special medical orders, assignments.
4. Charting under "Nurse's notes": Sent to X-ray; brought him special lunch on his return; good day.
5. Mother is in bed on postpartum unit; had stillborn baby; is crying quietly. Nurse in room aware of mother's situation and tears. Nurse leaves and asks another nurse whether or not to say anything to mother.

Notice in the first of these five examples how willingly, or at least without protest, the charge nurse—to take care of a staffing lack—converts one of her staff nurses into a nonnurse; observe too how willingly, or again at least without protest, the staff nurse accepts the nonnurse role. Who will cover for the nurse now that the nurse is covering for the maid? (Or was the staff nurse after all in excess on the floor?) The second incident might prompt us to ask, What aspects of assisting the doctor require a professional nurse? In the example of the changing of the nursing guard, why—except thanks to noncritical following of custom—is there in a briefing of nurses by nurses no special attention to nursing observations, judgments, and suggestions that might offer the particulars in terms of which a continuity of nursing care might be provided patients? And in the charting illustration, if the nurse thought of her notes not merely as routine to be discharged but as a source of information to guide others in caring for *her* patients might she be more inclined to include more pointed and pertinent information relevant to future care rather than giving only historical data? In the final case, we see that a nurse with a grieving mother may fail to function not necessarily from some lack in the environment or from an overly rigid demand made by the institution nor even from a conflict with the environment—she may fail simply from a lack of clarity and confidence in her own role and its consequences for a particular situation.

Considering examples of nursing that might be regarded as less than ideal serves what purpose? Being able to react critically to the situation described indicates both some interest in and some awareness of the nursing realities involved. But an immediate and merely critical reaction as an end in itself is no more than an emotional outlet. Still such critical reactions—especially if made by a seasoned practitioner or by other sensitive individuals—can be highly valuable when exploited intelligently and purposively. But what is there in criticism to be exploited and how can it be exploited?

Mere Criticism or Constructive Thinking?

Two things are to be exploited from a criticism. First of all, the interest—however masked—that gives rise to the critical reaction. We are oftentimes so aware of the unpleasant and negative connotation of criticism that we overlook that a criticism, even a hostile one, is often far more useful than a reaction of mere indifference. The difficult but desirable stance to take is to maintain a critical attitude while investing the energy and interest which provoked the criticism in something beyond a venting of feelings or a mere publicizing of the faults of others.

The second thing to exploit from a criticism is the happy fact that we rarely keep our criticisms to ourselves but rather tend to voice them to appreciative audiences. But of what significance is this tendency? To voice a criticism is to verbalize it; and whereas critical reaction probably starts with a vague, perhaps not fully conscious *felt* discontent, articulating the criticism tends to bring to conceptual awareness at least some striking feature of the "situation" provoking the critical response.

But now how should the interest evidenced by the criticism and the initial characterization that voices the criticism to be exploited toward activity that might terminate at least indirectly in doing away with the faults of the criticized situation? How can we exploit this interest and articulation to begin getting answers to the questions of: Exactly what needs changing? What direction should the change take? and How can this change actually be brought about?

Consider our initial characterization of the particular situations presented here in hopes of arousing your feelings of discomfort or discontent. Observe that the presentations were in fact not situations but were already a *reporting of what somebody took to be the salient features of some situation*. In the discussion of the incidents and in their grouping, an attempt was made to settle on characteristics common to the various happenings within a group. Whatever other features those cited examples incorporate, three central areas of concern presented themselves—interests clash; organizations or routine may thwart the individual working within their bounds or customs; and finally, the nurse seems often to have no face or image of her own.

More particularly, the Group I examples make vivid certain conflicts of interest among professions within a health-service organization—conflicts between nurse and attending physician, among attending nurse, nursery nurse, and physician; between nurse and resident. The activities of one helping professional may make difficult, prevent, or even nullify those of another—even when the two professionals are "helping" the same individual. Moreover, a professional cannot always decide which of many roles or goals should take precedence at a given moment.

Stereotypes or rigidities imposed by "organizations" or customary habits are fairly clearly exemplified in the second group of examples. The procedure book must be respected despite individualizing circumstances; lines of authority cannot be circumvented even when the nurse seems to have privileged knowledge and judgment about the particular situation; what is done daily by routine demand of the organization is performed often without thought of the purpose to be served and thus sometimes continued long after or in such a way that no purpose is served.

The third and last group of examples illustrates the nurse's willingness, on the one hand, to accept or absorb responsibilities of nonnursing personnel and, on the other hand, to relinquish specifically nursing responsibilities or possibilities to answer other, perhaps less appropriate, demands. Moreover, there seems to be some confusion for nurse, patient, doctor, and organization as to what the nurse's image should be.

If criticism is to be productive of positive action, we must be directed not only to pointing out problems but also at suggesting ways of resolving them; and sometimes the very manner in which we characterize the problem makes a big difference in the possibility of resolving the problem. In other words, it is often well to try to see the "problem" in a wider perspective—to see further elements within the problem situation, to see a broader aspect of the problem, or even to see the problem in relation to other pressing problems or as an instance of some more general problem.

But now we are talking about problems rather than criticisms. Whence and why the shift? First, whence the shift? Whereas criticism can give the initial impetus and direction to problem identification, the fuller articulation and pregnant characterization of a problem requires thought beyond initial reaction. For any presenting situation is ambiguous with respect to what are its salient features and what is the significant interrelation among these features. A more simple-minded way of putting this point is to say that *a situation does not dictate its own description.* Or even more pointedly, it is a bit hard to say what a "situation" is apart from some description of that situation. To say a situation is susceptible to many descriptions is not, of course, to say that every description is as good as any other. Some descriptions plainly do not fit. But for any situation there is an infinitely broad range or characterizations or descriptions. And the manner in which a characterization resolves the ambiguity of the presenting situation is determined at least in part by the past experience of the characterizer, by his particular interests, and by his capacity for noticing. The description is likely to be more or less particular accordingly as the characterizer has developed the habit of describing things with respect to their significance beyond the particular moment or location, the habit of seeing things in ever increasing scope, and the habit of unifying things by attending their interconnection and similarities whatever fine or great differences may be detected.

But when does a criticism become a problem? A criticism is at best saying something is wrong. A problem is a sophistication of criticism to the point of being articulate about *what* is at fault *along with* a desire to remove the fault. Thus we say a problem is a director of inquiry. For genuinely having a problem—rather than a mere worry, criticism, or vague discontent—is having both impetus (interest and energy) and direction (initial conceptualization) for using thought to remove the fault identified by the problem. This move from discomfort felt in practice to articulation of the difficulty, and thence to first speculative and then eventual practical resolution of the difficulty epitomizes that theory is born in practice and must return to practice.

But what outcome must inquiry have in order to remove the fault identified by the problem—that is, to accomplish the end for which the inquiry is initiated? Let us speak specifically in terms of nursing-practice problems. The inquiry must terminate in a speculation or invention related to but not entirely dictated by the problem-giving situation. This speculation must be articulated and understandable in such a fashion that if the speculation is entertained by a practitioner (or more generally an agent) who acts in good faith and with the requisite skill with respect to the content of that speculation, then the practitioner (or any other who similarly entertains the speculation) will not be subject in her nursing activity to the criticisms which gave rise to the problem.

Theory for a Practice Discipline

What is Theory?
Theory as a Conceptual Framework to Some Purpose

In some vague way we all "know" what theory is. But if we want to come to closer grips with theory—to say how to build one or of what use one might be—then we need a more explicit agreement as to what will be meant by "theory" at least in the context of this discussion.

Two divergent but popular notions of theory can be cited. The one has a depreciatory, the other earnestly commendatory connotation. The pejorative notion expects nothing from theory; the other demands that which theory can never give. Together, however, the two notions suggest a rather workable conception—useful particularly with respect to the question: What is the relation of a theory to that about which the theory is a theory?

The practitioner who derides the academic for spinning out "mere" theories in an ivory tower holds to the pejorative notion of theory. Here theory is conceived as an idle speculation invented without reference to pertinent reality and made usually to amuse, to busy, or to promote the theorizer. Being theoretical in this sense is diametrically opposed to being practical. Theory in this light is seen as a gossamer web of concepts, lovely to contemplate in idle moments.

The opposing view conceives theory not as mere speculation but as a picture-image of reality. The theory, if true, reveals the facts about reality. The theory gives us a description of reality as it really is, rather than somebody's speculations made about reality. But what would it mean to have *the* description of reality? Once account is given to reality's relation to thought and language as this relation was suggested, for example, by the characterization and recharacterization of the examples presented earlier, this second view of theory becomes tenuous. Is not every situation or presentation of reality ambiguous with respect to possible descriptions—that is, with respect to possible conceptualizations or theories as to its factors and relations.

Still, there is good sense buried in this picture-of-reality notion of theory; for though the presentation allows many descriptions, yet some must be discarded as not appropriate. And to know what is to be discarded, "reality" must be consulted in one way or another. And too, the notion of theory as speculation buries an equally important aspect of theory. For any description constitutes a conceptual invention or speculation that goes beyond what is given to immediate—or even subsequent—direct inspection, at the very least in the selection of those factors deemed as characteristic of the given.

Theory is neither a useless fairy tale nor a picture of the real. More properly, theory is an invention of concepts in interrelation. If such a conceptual inven-

tion be made to some purpose, and not as an idle speculation, then the invention should hardly be called "mere" theory. And if the invention be further subject to an interplay with reality in an attempt to determine the adequacy of the invention for the purpose the theory is designed to fulfill, we may be willing to consider a theory a good one—even after we realize that we have no way of ascertaining whether the theory gives an exact picture of reality (and when we see that some theories have as purpose something beyond describing reality).

Many theories are proposed for the sole purpose of quieting the mind's demand for a conceptual grasp on reality. Terminologies and classifications, theories of causal and other relations are venerable even as merely academic knowledge. But that theory can serve the end of doing away with intellectual chaos and uncertainty —and further that historically theories have been proposed first of all only for such academic interest—does not preclude that theories shall have no further purpose. We call nonacademic any theory proposed for a purpose beyond mere understanding. Customarily such "nonacademic theories" might be termed "applied" as opposed to "pure" theory or "pure" science, or might be called not theory at all but simply application of theory. Such nomenclature incorporates a serious misconception of the boundaries of theory. But the misconception is understandable. For as we shall see, these pure and purely descriptive theories are essential precursors and building blocks for any nonacademic theory.

The Four Levels of Theory

Another limitation in common notions of theory is to view as theory only sets of causal laws—to treat as theory only those conceptual frameworks that allow prediction on their bases. But we suggest below that we can profitably see as the theory conceptual frameworks allowing something less than prediction (theories of classification or more simply systems or even conventions for naming or marking off significant elements) as well as conceptual frameworks going well beyond mere prediction and offering prescriptions for practice or action.

When we focus attention on what constitutes a predictive theory, three things become evident:

1. Predictive theory presupposes the prior existence of more elementary types of theory.
2. Predictive theory is not the only kind of theory dealing essentially with relations between states of affairs.
3. There is a type of theory which presupposes and builds on theories at the level of relations between states of affairs.

What is a predictive theory and what does it presuppose? A prediction is a statement of relations between two states of affairs, a statement saying that if the first occurs then the second occurs. Predictions may be more or less specific about the time relation between the first and second state. But the name prediction is probably most commonly used where there is a definite and noticeable time sequence *from* the first *to* the second. But if we pay less attention to the exact temporal ordering of the two states we tend to speak more generally of causal laws than of predictions. To know a causal law is to be able to predict what would follow on or from bringing about a certain state of affairs.

To announce a prediction or causal law requires characterizing both the initial and the subsequent state of affairs. And such characterization requires conceptualizing the salient or significant factors within the state of affairs, as well as characterizing the relations as among those factors. Both this conceptualization of factors and the conceptualization of relations among factors are modes of theorizing—i.e., conceptualizing—necessarily prior to predictive or causal theory. These presupposed kinds of theory might be called respectively factor-isolating theories and factor-relating (or depicting) theories.

So, conceptualization that is prediction presupposes earlier modes of conceptions. But not only that. Prediction is a statement of causal or consequential relatedness as between two states of affairs. But it is quite possible to conceive relations other than merely consequential or causal as between two states of affairs and possible also to conceive relations as among more than just two states of affairs. Hence, as there are kinds of theories presupposed by predictive theory, so also there could be theories which deal with relations among states of affairs but which are not merely predictive theories. These further theories might be called theories of promotion or inhibition of occurrence of causal connections. Some may prefer to think of such theories merely as subcases or variations of casual theories, but it may be more useful to think of them as theories of inhibitors, catalysts, preventors, maintainers, etc. Such theories would conceptualize both the qualitative and quantitative subtleties of consequential relatedness.

Once given factoring theories, depicting theories, predictive or causal theories (and promoting or inhibiting theories), yet another kind of theory, which presupposes all of these, is prescriptive theory. Prescriptive theories are situation-producing or goal-incorporating theories. They are not satisfied to conceptualize factors, factor relations, or situation relations, but go on to attempt conceptualization of desired situations as well as conceptualizing the prescription under which an agent or practitioner must act in order to bring about situations of the kind conceived as desirable in the conception of the goal.

The various kinds of theories mentioned can be grouped in four levels:

  I. Factor-isolating theories
 II. Factor-relating theories (situation-depicting theories)
III. Situation-relating theories
    A. Predictive theories
    B. Promoting or inhibiting theories
IV. Situation-producing theories (prescriptive theories)

Each higher level of theory presupposes the existence of theories at the lower levels. A situation is depicted in terms of factors already isolated; predictive or promoting theories conceive relationships between depictable situations; and situation-producing theories prescribe in terms of available predictive and promoting theories, and use depicting theories in the characterization of goal-content. Each higher level theory adds a dimension of complexity: The factor-relating theory is distinctive in supplying conceptions of the static relations among factors already isolated, where the simplest case of such a static relation is the mere correlation, conjunction, coexistence, or co-presence of two factors with no notion of temporal or other asymmetry as between the factors. Situation-relating theories introduce the complexity of conceiving dynamic relations as among situations. Dynamic relations as contrasted with static ones specify priority, direction, and, in general, asymmetry as among the situations related.

With this general orientation, let us look more particularly at some salient features of theory at each level, with particular attention to factor-isolating theory, promoting theory, and prescriptive theory as the kinds of theory whose status is most in need of clarification.

First Level or Naming Theory

Consider first theory at the factor-isolating level, a level so basic it is frequently overlooked. Another label for theory at this level is naming theory. Whether or not we agree that we cannot conceive or think without words, still it is hardly disputed that most times words are meant to express concepts. To claim that naming or factor-isolating is a kind of theory is to be mindful that, logically speaking, the first act of the thinking mind is to make for itself its conceptual atoms or ideas. These most primitive concepts tend to be ideas whose function is to allow the mind to point out, denote, or attend to conceptually a factor within mind's consciousness. No presentation dictates its own factors; it is the work of the mind to conceive or invent unities in terms of which to structure the "presented situation." The verbalization of these primitive ideas is often called naming. Much or little can be built into these names and their corresponding ideas. But the essential function of naming is the giving of a tag to enable reference back to, or the pointing to, or communicating about the factor conceived as having the name assigned. For a factor to have a name is for that factor to become mentionable. More precisely, to be conceived as a factor is to have a name.

If we agree that to theorize is to invent a conceptual framework to some purpose, then naming is a theoretical activity. The theoretical activity of naming manifests itself in many ways, some more self-conscious than others. The kind of naming most often recognized as theoretical activity is called classifying or introduction of technical terminology. Classifying may well be the most elaborate kind of naming. For to classify is to sort or categorize—to assign names in terms of belonging to one bin or kind as opposed to another but in such a way that the total collection of bins or kinds constitutes all the recognized sub-kinds of factors of the one given kind. Another way of looking at the matter is to note that to classify is to name a factor and then systematically to name sub-factors of that factor. For example, protozoa is a significant thing or factor biologically speaking, and ciliata, sporozoa, flagellata, and sarcodina are sub-factors of interest within the kind, protozoa.

A less sophisticated kind of naming that is nonetheless theoretical activity is naming things in some planned sequence so that the name given the factor indicates some characteristic more or less external to the factor named. For example, naming particles, alpha, beta, gamma particles is a naming that reflects most likely the order of "discovery" of the particles—or more precisely, the order in which the theorizer conceptualized the particle-factors as noticeable or worthy of note. And sometimes names are assigned in virtue of who first took account of the factor as a factor —e.g., the fissure of Sylvius, a watt, an ampere, a coulomb. Other times factors are named in a way that reflects the shape, function, or some relation of that factor. For example, a lens is so called because a double convex lens resembles the shape of a lentil seed; a tuning fork is named in virtue of its function, and so on.

At times the name accorded a factor is assigned for no reason beyond giving a tag, mode of reference, or a crutch to conceptualization of the factor in question. Such naming usually signals a rather primitive level or theoretical awareness in the area for which the factor is isolated. But this "close-to-ignorance" situation in naming reflects perhaps better than any other kind of naming the important theoretical function of naming: Naming is the verbal counterpart of *creating* or *inventing conceptual unities*. The less informative the name the more it becomes obvious that one function of naming is to constitute these unities. This need to create the factors or elements subsequently to be related conceptually in more advanced levels of theory is sometimes overlooked because the common language we have at our disposal is in a sense a ready-made factor-isolating or naming theory. But unless we take cognizance that naming or tagging or factor-isolating requires or is conceptual invention (i.e., theorizing), no energy will be directed to the important task of creating as well as refining theories in areas old and new. This lack of factor-isolating theory is particularly detrimental in regions where theory is being self-consciously developed for the first time—notably in nursing. A simple-minded way to emphasize the importance of having theories at the level of factor-isolating is to point out that to have such a theory is to have a terminology. And there is no need to labor the importance of usable and known terminology. Working in a discipline self-consciously seeking theory, we may be more willing to invest time and energy at this more basic level of theory once we realize how any progress or development at the level of factor-relating, predictive, or prescriptive theory depends essentially on—and hence is hampered by any lack in—the astuteness (or even logical correctness) of significant factor identification or terminology.

Second and Third Level Theories

The first level of theory deals with factor-isolating. Once factors are identified we can move to the next level of complexity—that is, seeing things not in isolation but rather in relation. Consider theories which depict or give conceptions of interrelations among factors as opposed to among situations. Such theories are composed of statements usually called mere correlations since in the simplest case the statements are comments as to the joint presence or absence or range of variation as between two factors. But more broadly conceived, any so-called "natural history stage" theory is such a theory. For instance, anatomy might be an example of theory at this level. An illuminating way to think of such theories may be as depictions or descriptions without time reference or as depictions at a given

moment of time. So put, again no need to emphasize the importance of well developed depiction-level theory before any grand attempts at predictive theory, since predictive theory can state relationships only between such situations as are depictable. And note that which is depictable is, of course, dependent upon what factors have been identified. Depicting theory need not restrict itself to the simple relations of absence or presence nor to the consideration of only two factors in relation.

Because there is little mystery about the status of predictive theory, let us consider more particularly only those situation-relating theories of the promoting or inhibiting kind. When we say that situation A causes situation B (or make the prediction that B will happen since A has happened) we mean that A precedes B and when A occurs so does B. But we may be interested in such questions as how can B be made to succeed A more quickly, that is, what might be a catalyst to A's production of B. Or we may be concerned as to what inhibits or slows down the production of B by A, or what are the side effects of A's producing B at what speed, or what is the cost in time, energy, goods, pain, etc., of A's producing B at a certain speed or under certain conditions. To conceptualize such relationships is to propose the so-called promoting or inhibiting type theories. Such types of theory are of incredible importance as a prerequisite for an articulate prescriptive theory. That such theories tend to exist, if at all, only inarticulately in the minds of engineers and other practitioners is a signal of the general unawareness of such possibilities for prescriptive—that is, situation-producing—theories.

The Ingredients of Fourth-Level or Situation-Producing Theory

Before looking at the essence and ingredients of situation-producing theory, the contrast between such theory and the familiar predictive theory might be put thus: Roughly stated, predictive theory says if A happens then B happens; prescriptive or situation-producing theory says B is among the things conceived as appropriate to bring into being and so here is how to bring about A, or here is how to facilitate A's production of B, and so on.

A theory is a conceptual framework invented for some purpose, and the purpose of a situation-producing theory is to allow for the production of situations of a desired kind. So what ingredients must such theory have? A situation-*relating* theory which is a predictive theory has as its aim to allow for prediction and hence must have as ingredients causal-connection statements that give a basis for such prediction. But as the aim of a situation-*producing* theory is more elaborate, so too are its essential ingredients greater in number and more complex in kind. The three essential ingredients of a situation-producing theory are: (a) goal-content specified as aim for activity, (b) prescriptions for activity to realize the goal content, and (c) a survey list to serve as a supplement to present prescription and as preparation for future prescription and as preparation for future prescription for activity toward the goal-content.

Very generally speaking the goal-content specifies the characteristics of the situations to be produced; the prescriptions supply the prescriber's directives for carrying out activity that will in fact produce such situations the survey list calls attention to two sorts of things: First, to all those factors, facets, and aspects of activity judged relevant to achieve situations of the given kind but which for reasons of complexity or primitive state of development are not yet conceptually translated into directives for action, and, secondly, to those theories, at whatever level, knowledge of which or taking account of which is deemed to enhance the possibility or realizing the goal of the situation-producing theory.

We introduce the terminology "situation-producing theory" to supply for fourth-level theory a name in terms of purpose. For such fourth-level theory where recognized has a great variety of names, none of which particularly illuminates the theory's purpose. Depending on which of the first two ingredients is being emphasized, a situation-producing theory is variously known as a goal-incorporation theory, or as a prescriptive theory. Even more generally speaking, a situation-producing theory is often called a "normative theory" or even a "value theory" in contrast to theory whose purpose is merely to describe—whether by giving factors, depictions of situations, or relations of situations —rather than to specify how situations of a described kind can be brought about. The goal-content of a situation-producing theory serves as a norm or standard by which to evaluate activity; activity that furthers the goal is, in terms of the theory, valuable or good activity. And so, the specification of goal-contents entails taking them as values—that is, signifies conceiving these contents as situations worthy to be brought about. When a situation-producing theory is regarded as a source not merely of evaluation but of the actual bringing into existence activity evaluated as good by the theory, then the situation-producing theory tends to be called a practice theory.

The survey-list ingredient, unlike the goal and prescriptive ingredients, has given rise to no prevalent alternative label for situation-producing theory; this lack arises not simply because this ingredient contrasts less strikingly with lower level theories but more probably because this ingredient is less widely understood than even the goal and prescriptive ingredients. These remarks will be better appreciated if we look in more detail at the ingredients of situation-producing theories.

The first essential ingredient for a situation-producing theory is the conceptualization of a goal content—that is, both the conceptualization of a content and the conceptualization of that content as desirable of attainment. The insistence on conception both of content and of the valuableness of that content is to emphasize that no mere feeling of reverence to some shadowy high ideal can substitute in theory for the conception of goal as goal. Nor can any less than articulate (that is, less than verbalized or—what amounts to the same—less than conceptualized in communicable form) notion of that ideal's content serve as a conception of goal content.

The conceptualization of prescriptions to the effect that actions should be taken to realize the goal-content as conceived is the second essential ingredient of a situation-producing theory. At the conceptual and hence communicable level there must be articulated the awareness that the goal-content will not be realized without activity and that activity itself is something that takes place in the particular. Three points about any prescription are noteworthy especially for our subsequent discussion of nursing theory: (a) the prescription is a command and so gives a directive, (b) the given directive commands acting toward a specified end, and (c) the command is directed to some specified agent or agents.

A survey list for activity constitutes the third ingredient of a situation-producing theory. Such a survey list is the articulate conceptual awareness that, however particular the goal-content and however particular the prescriptions, still activity under the prescription toward the realization of the goal is not totally determined by goal and prescription taken together. An agent's judgment, in the good sense connotation of that term, is required to produce particular activity in a given-space situation such that the activity is a response to the prescription as an attempt to realize the goal. But what is this mysterious thing called judgment—or alternatively, experience, practical wisdom, or practical insight? Whatever else it may be, a very important feature of "it" is a capacity—usually with the smooth directness of habit and the lightning speed that makes us think of insight as deep rather than broad—to consult all salient features in the particular situation and make the adjustments of a more routine activity in the light of any idiosyncratic (that is, nonroutine) characteristics presented by these salient features in this particular situation.

The survey list emphasized the gap between, on the one hand, particular activity and, on the other hand, any possible specification of a goal-content and prescription. The survey list, however, is no mere announcement of this emphasis nor any mere casual enumeration of some aspects that need to be consulted to act under the prescription. Rather an explicit conception going beyond mere enumeration must guide the content of the survey list. And since the survey list is one for *activity,* an organization on the basis of the salient *aspects* of *activity* is probably most suggestive and helpful. Whether the situation-producing theory be

a nursing theory, a medical, a legal, or ethical theory, activity has six aspects which cannot be denied significance. But significance for what? As we shall see, they are particularly significant for: 1) practical activity in the light of theory, 2) assessment of theory, 3) construction or refinement of theory, and 4) research that tries to explore the validity of theory or even for research geared to stimulate thinking toward theory.

The six aspects of activity to be highlighted in the survey list correspond to these six questions about activity:

1. Who or what performs the activity?
2. Who or what is the recipient of the activity?
3. In what context is the activity performed?
4. What is the end point of the activity?
5. What is the guiding procedure, technique, or protocol of the activity?
6. What is the energy source for the activity?

The questions are not esoteric. They—like the corresponding aspects of activity—are straightforward and almost obvious once articulated. The corresponding aspects of activity, however, can be unfolded in analysis, layer after layer, to whatever degree of specificity desired. Moreover, no attempt is made to ask the six questions so that the answer to one has no relevance for the others. For the corresponding aspects of activity are such that all the other aspects should be taken account of in trying for a fuller exploration of any one aspect.

The aspects of activity corresponding to the six questions are six vantage points from which to survey activity—six ways to look at one thing—in the hope of revealing different features as point of view shifts:

1. Agency (Who or what performs the activity?)
2. Patiency or recipiency (Who or what is the recipient of the activity?)
3. Framework (In what context is the activity performed?)
4. Terminus (What is the end point of the activity?)
5. Procedure (What is the guiding procedure, technique, or protocol of the activity?)
6. Dynamics (What is the energy source for the activity— whether chemical, physical, biological, mechanical, or psychological, etcetera?)

These six aspects of activity can serve as an organizing principle for a survey list that can function along with goal and prescription as the three ingredients of a situation-producing theory. But what beyond the mere articulation of the aspects would be contained within a survey list? The more elaborately developed a situation-producing theory, the richer will be the survey list in variety, scope of content, and depth of detail. But however complex and elaborate the survey list becomes, still the part of the survey list corresponding to any one of the aspects of activity will contain two distinctive kinds of things: (a) indication of realities judged relevant, and (b) indications of sub-theories held relevant. But relevant to what and so deemed by whom? So deemed by the proponent of the theory and relevant— as supplements to awareness of prescription and goal —to conduct of activity under the theory, or to research done toward evaluating the theory, or to theorizing activity aimed at changing or augmenting the theory.

Thus, the ingredients characteristic of a situation-producing theory can be summed up in this fashion:

I. Goal-content
II. Prescriptions
III. Survey list—organized, for example, as follows:
  1. Agency—Explored, e.g., with respect to:
    A. Dimensions of the aspect (here agency) deemed especially significant, say
      a. External resources of agents
      b. Internal resources of agents
      c. Factors of agency proposed as significant in the statement of the theory or for acting under the theory
    B. Theories from disciplines (at whatever level of theory) deemed relevant
  2. Patiency
    A. Relevant dimensions or realities
    B. Relevant theories
  3. Framework
    A. Relevant dimensions or realitiesc
    B. Relevant theories
  4. Terminus
    A. Relevant dimensions or realities
    B. Relevant theories
  5. Procedure
    A. Relevant dimensions or realities
    B. Relevant theories
  6. Dynamics
    A. Relevant dimensions or realities
    B. Relevant theories

Theory for a Practice Discipline

What Is a Nursing Theory?

Our contention is that nursing theory if it is to have impact for practice must be a theory at the most sophisticated level—namely, a situation-producing theory. But, as noted each higher level of theory presupposes the existence of theories at each of the lower levels; in fact, part of the statement of any situation-producing theory—in particular, the survey list—should include explicit reference to those theories deemed by the theorist relevant preparation either for activity under or for supporting activity under the situation-producing theory in question. Though the point urged here is that nursing theory is a theory at the highest or fourth level, there is no objection to using the term "nursing theory" to refer to lower-level theory provided no claim is thereby made that theory at any of these lower levels exhausts nursing theory in the fullest sense.

Our comments here as to what might be expected in a nursing theory are meant *not* to specify some one nursing theory. Quite the contrary, our remarks are directed to suggesting that awareness of the essential ingredients of a situation-producing theory may help a would-be theorist (and so a would-be researcher) to a systematic consideration of features to which attention must be directed in constructing, testing, refining, or using a nursing theory.

The exploration of the goal and prescription ingredients of theory are here markedly brief. Even the somewhat longer exploration of the various threads of theory's survey list is selective and by no means thorough-going—just samples and indications are given. The aim is not to propose a nursing theory but is rather to touch on what can be expected as ingredients or as a structure of ingredients in *any* proposed nursing theory. And perhaps more importantly—since the earlier general consideration of theory could be viewed as in some sense accomplishing this task—our intention here is to liberate the would be theorist from some all too prevalent "orientation stereotypes." Freed from these sets of mind he may be able to take new viewpoints even on old and recognized dimensions of a difficulty, as well as to invent more novel dimensions from which to treat well known problems. Our indications and examples, it is hoped, will encourage thought either by bringing forth a sympathetic recognition of the nursing significance of these avenues or, at the very least, by provoking an adverse critical response to possibilities offered. Such a response may bring a critic to a more articulate awareness of the position from which he levels the objection and thereby to an inspection of his own current set of mind.

And perhaps even more importantly organizing a theory's survey list in terms of the six-fold aspects of activity suggests how such a systematic—even *a priori* —attack of thought on nursing problems and realities may be profitable. This approach encourages a theorist to treat at the articulate level—a level essential for any empirical testing—matters often regarded as beyond or below the purview of nursing theory but matters which, it is here suggested, may be overlooked or ignored only at grave practical costs. Failing to take account of such areas produces a theory that could never be anything but academic, a theory that could not provide as guides to problems that must be faced in practice the strength of articulated and tested conceptualizations. In this section too, some indication will be given that a theorist may well get stimulating clues as to what should be included in a viable theory by a "creative" viewing of particular practice situations.

Goal Ingredient

So then, a nursing theory as a situation-producing theory must have three ingredients—goal-content, prescription, and survey list. More particularly, a nursing theory must specify a goal-content. The theory must render articulate the conception of the kinds of situations that are to be brought into existence as widespreadly as possible. Notice that the very attempt to articulate such a goal provides the basis for one "test" of that goal: for this overt conceptualization is one way

to realize what we dimly grope after or think we long to produce. The very demand to conceptualize these aims or goals may give opportunity for broadening, refining, and surveying the present set of mind with respect to "objectives." Moreover, to see goal as part of theory urges the further point that goal too may be subject to change in the light of "tests" of the theory as initially stated.

A goal-content when achieved may be less palatable than when conceived; moreover, when persistent attempts to achieve a given goal-content fail, we may wish to articulate a goal-content that seems more feasible to achieve given the circumstances displayed in the attempts to achieve the initial goal.

Regarding goals in this two-fold way—on the one hand, as beforehand specifications of situations the theorist deems worthy to produce, and on the other hand, as explicit conceptualizations subject to revision in the light of "test" (cp. Part II—Practice Oriented Research, to be published) makes goals be seen in a light that maintains their focusing and directing capacity without solidifying them into mere prejudice or personal conviction untouchable either by objective thought or by realities of practice.

Prescription Ingredient

The second essential ingredient of a nursing theory is its prescriptions. A prescription is a directive, and the directive must be explicitly conceived as directive of action (not just of thought or wish) and directed toward specified agents. To conceive the prescription as directive is to realize the prescription as an essential ingredient of a theory meant no simply to enable us to name or describe—even if we include prediction among these descriptions—but rather a theory whose function is to allow the creation of reality of certain dimensions. This directive must be conceived, above all, as a directive for activity; for, unlike God, man creates or produces not by fiat, will, or thought, but rather "by the sweat of his brow." Directives that are simply exhortations as to the worthiness of the goal-content are often deficient as prescriptions. Prescription in a practice theory must explicitly articulate reference to activity but, nonetheless, may be more or less specific as to the exact kind or circumstances of activity for which the directive is given. We could move, for example, from the prescription, "Act," to, "Act compassionately," to, "Put a cover over the patient as you bathe him." The demand that the directive be specific with respect to intended agent may be fulfilled in various ways. The prescription may specify the kind of agents very generally or in any other level of specificity. The directive, for example, may be addressed to any nursing personnel, or more particularly to any registered nurse, or alternatively to any licensed practical nurse, and so on.

Appropriate specificity of goal-content and prescription is an important consideration in any practice theory. The goal-content may be exhausted in one very general characterization of situation or may be given by many items of varying degrees of specificity, whether or not these items are further integrated into a generalized characterization. We might have the following as the total specification of the goal-content:

Patients are made independent as soon as possible.

The Accompanying prescription ingredient might be simply:

Nursing personnel, act to speed the return of patient independence.

Or we might have as the total specification of the prescription ingredient this fuller set of directives:

Registered nurses, let the patient take his own medication as soon as he is able.
   Dietary aides, let the patient feed himself as soon as possible.
   Doctors, let the nurse decide whether she or the patient should manage the foot soak.

The degree of specificity of goal-content and prescription are not matters independent the one of the other. Broadly speaking, the more general the goal-content, the more detailed must be any effective prescriptions. But the appropriate degree of specificity of both goal-content and prescription depends too on who are the agents specified by the theory as well as on who is to use the theory for what, be it practice, research,

further theory building, education, administration, and so on. This question of how specific these two ingredients must be to produce a theory that can affect practice is a question that requires much attention in the initial articulation of a theory and a question that is open to empirical test.

In short, goals and prescriptions can be spelled out to any degree of specificity. Within the directives constituting the prescription ingredient of a nursing theory many directives may be related to a single element of the goal-content, and conversely, some directives may cover action towards various elements of the goal-content. Moreover, the directives within the prescription ingredient need not all be directed to agents of the same kind. More particularly, what is being suggested is that although some nursing theories may specify as agents only registered nurses, a viable nursing theory may have to provide directives for agents other than merely registered nurses, both in the sense of directing members of nursing service who are not registered nurses and even directing personnel outside nursing service. That such a suggestion calls for nursing theory differing radically from any that might have been so far proposed does not preclude that still the suggestion might have to be taken quite seriously by anyone wanting to provide ever-expanding nursing care in a context where the supply of registered nurses is not proportionately increasing. The same point can be urged in other terms: Nursing theory is a theory of activity, but the activity guided by the nursing theory for the purpose of meeting the specified goal may have as agents persons who are not nurses or even agents who are not persons.

Survey List Ingredients

These remarks concerning specificity bring us quite naturally to the last of the three essential ingredients of a nursing theory—a survey list. The survey list neither talks about what is worthwhile nor gives directives for action. What the survey list does do is call attention to certain significant aspects of activity and to certain dimensions, knowledges, or other resources relevant to activity. In nursing theory, as in any situation-producing theory, one fruitful organization of the survey list may be the arrangement in accordance with the noted six significant aspects of activity—namely, agency, patiency, framework, terminus, procedure, and dynamics. A nursing-theory survey list would "contain" a section corresponding to each of these six aspects of activities and might contain under each of the six headings, as for example, under "agency," a treatment of, say,

A. Relevant realities
   1. Internal resources of agents
   2. External resources of agents
   3. Factors of agency proposed as significant by the theory given
B. Theories (at whatever level) from other disciplines deemed relevant to agency or factors of agency[2]

Agency

What would it mean to consider for the purposes of nursing theory agency along the dimension, say, of internal resources of agents? Since what constitutes internal resources of agency depends on the nature of the agent, perhaps the first question to occur when such an exploration begins is: Who might be agents of activity that realizes the nursing goal? This question is significant. It jars us from the complacency which simply assumes or stipulates unthinkingly that a registered nurse is the only agent who performs activity towards realizing the nursing goal. To recognize that there is no theoretical reason that all nursing agents must be nurses or even persons may give the creative freedom to look at the kinds of activity required to realize any specified nursing goal so that constructive and feasible suggestions can be offered as to the "proper" agents for such activities. Among those who might theoretically be feasible agents of nursing activity are professionals such as nurses, attending physicians, residents, interns, medical students, consulting physicians, anesthetists,

social workers, ministers, dietary specialists, medical technicians, and even professional hospital administrators or their deputies. Note that this observation about the non-uniqueness of a nursing agent probably reflects what goes on at times quite fortuitously in practice. A relevant case in point is the registered nurse who, on hearing the anesthetist or resident doing an effective job of talking with the presurgical patient, herself does not duplicate the performance but reinforces the maneuver by expressing her satisfaction to the patient that he talked with the doctor or anesthetist and thereby providing opportunity for the patient to discuss any lingering concerns. Notice how she both saves herself and the patient energy and strengthens the image of the other professional while she exhibits at the same time to the patient a certain solidarity among his many helpers and gives him the further opportunity of pursuing any matter in the discussion now admittedly heard by both of them. In a similar vein, she might ask the social worker or minister who was about to visit a patient to carry in the patient's mail; she saves herself steps, makes for the patient one less interruption, and may give the minister or social worker a natural way to begin the conference. And conversely, when this nurse starts the intravenous ordered by the doctor, she may during her same visit to the patient massage his temples or offer some other comfort measure which she dispenses on her own initiative.

Among the nonprofessionals who might theoretically be deemed to be performing activity that realizes a nursing goal are the licensed practical nurses, family visitors, nursing aides, orderlies, dietary aides, volunteers, and housekeeping and maintenance staff. But in what sense can a nonprofessional be an agent of activity realizing a nursing goal? The cheerful, generous, young nurse's aide might be dispatched by the registered nurse to give a backrub to the terminally-ill cancer patient if the aide knows how to give a routine backrub, and the patient has no skin problems or other complicating features. It may be objected that a registered nurse may resort to such a tactic on a busy day; but would it not be better for a fully prepared professional nurse to perform the backrup? Maybe so; but notice

---

[2] This sketchy outline is meant to give a hint of the general scope of content within any section of a survey list; the sketch is surely not wholly clear; nor will the following discussion serve as adequate illumination of the sketch; nonetheless the sketch is included to give both an indication of what might be thought of under any aspect of activity as well as to make again clear that much here suggested needs further amplification and further exploration.

that in some ways the aide may be the preferable agent. She has not the burden of so many other responsibilities and so in discharging her service has not the added difficulty of planning ahead for the disposition of other tasks. Moreover the aide, orderly, or visitor, in being an agent of nursing activity, may be also a *recipient* of the nursing activity of the registered nurse who guides, supports, directs, or encourages another nonprofessional (as she might guide a patient) so that the activity performed by the nonprofessional does *in fact* realize a nursing goal rather than frustrate the goal's achievement.

These considerations of agency are meant to emphasize that activity may perhaps best be regarded as *nursing activity* in virtue of what the activity produces rather than, more narrowly, in virtue only of who is agent (or patient) of that activity. And to admit the theoretic possibility of persons other than registered nurses as agents of nursing activity brings us to the question of how things other than persons could theoretically be agents of activity realizing a nursing goal. Some possible candidates for such agency are things such as computers, instruments, furnishings, equipment, drugs, manuals, or signs, to mention but a few. For example, where two men were once needed to restrain a psychotic patient from self-injury, a drug may now do the restraining.

Theories may vary greatly with respect to who are specified as agents. The practical, and perhaps trivial, examples given here call attention of would-be nurse theorists to this observation: Considering only the registered nurse as agent and considering even here as nursing agent only when she acts *immediately* with or for the patient may be a serious hindrance to arriving at a viable nursing theory. The examples are meant further to illustrate how from practice we could take clues to be exploited in theory.

An agent performing an action may realize a goal whether or not his specific intention is to reach that goal. The point is that someone must entertain the nursing goal and must see that activity is performed which achieves that goal. But that not every agent who contributes activity toward achieving the goal need nec-

essarily entertain that goals as his is an important observation since, for example, economically speaking supply and money may not always permit all agents of nursing activity to be registered nurses. And all economics aside, it may be even highly desirable that at times agents other than nurses, perhaps even the patient himself, perform some of these activities. Still, to emphasize that not every agent need entertain the nursing goal must not be misread as de-emphasizing that *someone* must intend and propel action toward the nursing goal if ever that goal is to be persistently and consistently attained. But the question of just who among the agents to be guided by a theory needs to know that theory in what detail and with what intimacy and depth if the theory is to have impact in practice is a question that warrants careful thought, even at the theoretical level (in considering agents and their preparation), and a question that admits of some empirical test. (For example, among the persons who might need to entertain the theory—both by being aware of it and by adopting it is an acceptable pattern for action— might be medical personnel and hospital administrators.)

Exploring agency along the dimension of internal resources of agent led to the question of the nature of the agent. Within the nursing-theory survey list under the aspect agency there should be specified the kinds of agents expected to contribute to the production of situations bringing the theory's goal content into being, or —in other words—agents to whom the theory provides directives. For each kind of agent the theory should then be explicit as to what internal resources a person or thing must have to function as an agent of that kind. Specifying the relevant internal resources of an agent might involve, say, specifying some or all of these: capacities, skills, education, experience. Nursing theory tends now to offer such descriptions only with respect to the registered nurse. But a nursing theory that can function actually to produce situations realizing its goal content seems likely to require attention to these details of internal resources for all important kinds of agents, and a kind of agent is important if that type of agent has potential for contributing to or frustrating realization of the nursing goal. Again this is an urging to bring to theoretical awareness a demand already somehow "dealt with" in many instances at the practical level; the prompting comes in the hope of theory's contributing to a constructive reckoning with this practical demand of looking to the internal resources of nonregistered nurse nursing agents.

Internal resources of an agent might be taken, then, as those skills, techniques, routines, or policies available to or through the agent; *external* resources of an agent might include those resources other than the agent himself available for maintaining, supporting, developing, protecting, or extending the agent's capacity, power, or flexibility.

Patiency

We have urged as appropriate within nursing theory a broader than usual conception of agency—a view that considers as agent not only registered nurses but also theoretically any other person or thing whose activity contributes to realizing the nursing goal. Such a view of potential agents suggests a correspondingly enlarged theoretical notion of patient or recipient of activity. Under the theoretical notion of patient or recipient of activity are included all those persons or things who receive action from agents under the theory. The notion of patient then embraces not only the sick persons who receive the activity of the registered nurse or even of other recognized agents but includes as well *any* person or *thing* that receives the activity of the registered nurse or of any other agent whose activity contributes to the nursing goal.

Such an enlarged view of patiency emphasizes that perhaps no practical nursing theory can afford to consider as patients only sick persons, since probably much of the activity of persons and things deemed agents by the theory is received or suffered by persons or things other than the ill. And further to regard nurses, other professionals, and nonprofessionals as possible patients of, say, a registered nurse's activity, is to recognize consciously that factors—e.g., how the *patient* views the activity—so carefully taken account of both in current nursing theory and in actual practice might

profitably be extrapolated to the dealings of, say, registered nurses with other professionals and, perhaps especially with nonprofessionals with nursing service—not to speak of generalization to activities of all other agents recognized by the theory. In brief, to regard as patients not simply recipients of a registered nurse's activities but also recipients of all other relevant agents' activities may lead us to give proper theoretical account of some overlooked areas. But even more importantly, this move suggests that findings in areas already recognized as significant—namely, findings in nurse-patient interactions—may be exploited for use in areas more typically overlooked in theory—namely, in nurse-doctor, nurse-nurse, nurse-licensed practical nurse, nurse-aide, nurse-administrator interactions.

To see grouped as "patient" the sick, the non-sick, and even inanimate objects may open the theoretic or practical mind to generalizing—or at least exploring the appropriateness of generalizing—know-how concerning one kind of patient to principles guiding activity directed towards patients of another kind. To suggest that the ill are not the exclusive patients or recipients of nurse activity is not to suggest that we overlook the prime importance of the sick person as a certain focal point in the complex of activity towards a nursing goal. What is being said, however, is that to think the sick person gets that proper focus by being regarded as *the only proper patient* of any activity relevantly considered by nursing practice or nursing theory may be a much oversimplified view. To stress that not only persons but things *too* may be "patients" of a registered nurse's or other agent's activity calls attention to some factors of patiency that may be neglected in theory or looked on in only a stereotyped way unless we see the relevant analogies, on the one hand, between sick and nonsick patients and, on the other hand, between animate and inanimate patients—and, on the third hand, analogies between patients of activities performed by registered nurses and patients of activities performed by agents other than registered nurses but still activities realizing a nursing goal and having perhaps as patient the sick person.

Animate or inanimate, sick or nonsick recipients

of registered nurse activity or recipient of some other agent's activity, whatever kind of patient we consider, two extremes should probably be avoided in any practical conception of patients: (a) the notion that a patient is totally determined in his characteristics and hence not a reactor capable of change, and (b) the notion that a patient can suffer no matter what activity and so is subject to most any change. A patient is perhaps best regarded as having a repertoire of variability such that the characteristics of the patient *qua* patient—that is, of the patient *as receiver of activity*—can perhaps be made to vary so as to produce characteristics more "patient" or receptive to the activity of a certain agent or to activity that has a specified terminus. Moreover, in another sense a patient is not merely passive, for always there will be a reaction, though granted the reaction is not always perceivable or if perceivable not necessarily significant for or against the purposes at hand.

Part of the advantage of enlarging the theoretic notion of patient is that to regard patient as an interaction with agent (among other things) toward activity of a desired kind and as possessed of a repertoire of capacities and limitations (much as is the agent) is to see a great range of latitude as to ways of producing desired outcomes.

Certain quite acceptable practices could be viewed as embodying these enlarged notions of patients. Or alternatively the notion of patient offered here suggests a possible theoretic basis for practices arrived at by routes other than explicit prescription by articulate theory. What is urged here for the realm of nonacademic theory is not unheard of already in the realm of practice. For instance, a human is ordinarily regarded as a conscious being susceptible to pain. But an agent who wants to cut into the stomach wall of that sensitive, conscious human renders the patient at least locally insensate, if not unconscious, before invading his body. Freezing to prevent bleeding is another example. Special diets for building up strength and immunity of feeble patients before surgery is but another illustration. On the other hand, consider how in an interaction of a nurse with, say, an orderly, adding a social dimension to the word-oriented relationship may make the

orderly a more receptive patient of the nurse's activity of order giving, correcting, or instructing and hence enhance the orderly's work directly with the patient (more narrowly conceived).

The fairly bare suggestions given in this discussion of patiency are meant to invite a fuller treatment of the area theoretically and to draw attention to the possible immediate usefulness to practice of a mind consciously aware that change in patient is a factor influencing both agency and outcome of activity. What begins to emerge here too is that exploring any of the six aspects of activity lends inevitably to touching on some of the others of the six.

Framework

And now rather than suggesting factors of patiency or theories relevant to patiency (as might be done in a fuller survey list of a nursing theory), let us move on to consider framework. To view activity from the aspect of framework is to view activity from the aspect of the matrix of that activity. So to view activity is to see it in relation to other things, including persons and other activities, and to see the interrelation of these "other factors" as constituting an organism, unity, or total context of activity. A more startling way to call attention to framework is to remark that "Patient-centered nursing may be a mistake too!" For realizing that we are in the era that has gone beyond task-oriented nursing to develop the ideal of patient-centered nursing, an era when research and study of the nurse-patient dyad is very prevalent—and still nursing problems persist—is to recognize that the admonition toward patient-centered nursing in too literally interpreted may misfire in two ways. First off, the preoccupation with the patient—with emphasis on the patient's being a person and a sick person—may result in the less than adequate respect, concern, or attention for the more "technical" details of interactions with patients. But the second, perhaps more damaging, way the suggestion to center on patient may misfire is that emphasizing the patient as the recipient of the registered nurse's activity may result in the nurse-patient dyad's becoming conceived as a unit flourishing independently in itself. Independently of what? Of other nurse-patient dyads, of dyads of patient with other professionals or nonprofessionals, of dyads or larger groups of nurse with other nurses, professionals, or nonprofessionals, and so on. Independently too not only of other personnel but also of the institution within which the nurse-patient dyad is supported, the climate, policies, location, affiliation, and goals of that institution, its source of funding, staffing, or procuring patients; independently of government support, of insurance coverage for nurse-patient dyads, et cetera, *ad infinitum* if we wished.

In short, though it is an advance in thought not only to consider the task to be accomplished but also to relate it to the patient for whom the task is accomplished and perhaps even to the nurse as agent of the task, still to limit consideration to only these factors restricts us to theoretic analysis that may well be ineffectual for guiding practice toward actual achievement of a nursing goal. We need to take account of the matrix in which the activity takes place. And what is this matrix or framework? To think of framework merely as a setting, a location, the physical structure of ward, hospital, or medical center is not entirely misleading but is much too oversimplified and literal. For taking framework as context of activity implies that not just physical features of time, space, or structure constitute the framework, though surely these are factors within the framework. But consideration tends to suggest that both physical and nonphysical factors demand recognition as parts of framework (and that consideration of one kind illuminates consideration of the other) if framework is to constitute a fruitful aspect from which to regard activity in using, refining, or building a nursing theory.

Perhaps the best way in short scope to give the fullest appreciation of the notion being suggested here is to propose a factorization of framework of activity. This particular factorization grew from a fairly *a priori* invention of initial set of factors; this set was then exposed to criticism, revision, refinement, and extension in a group of nurses, including not just academically oriented persons whose main nursing function is

discharged in education but also persons day-in, day-out involved in substantial and responsible service. (See Figure 46-1.)

Framework Factorization

Granted that framework is complex, and granted too that good sense is needed in knowing the appropriate level of detail for the purpose at hand. For from one point of view, is there anything that could not be thought of as contained within framework, since theoretically at least anything might be potentially relevant as part of the context or framework of activity? But practically speaking what is relevant? Three points that help determine practical relevance (and hence perhaps priority for practice and theory and research) are these:

1. What *can* we take account of if we so wish, which things and how many things, either at one time or given so much time?
2. What things, if we do not take account of them, give us practical difficulties?
3. What things, if we took account of them, would
   a. remove practical difficulties, or
   b. improve the practical situation for the patient, the nurse, the institution, society, et cetera?

Activity is produced within a framework, then, and can be viewed as produced by an agent and received by a patient. But the activity as such can be viewed too from the aspect of its end point, from the aspect of the path to that end point, and finally from the aspect of the power source that enables some agent in a given framework to take the path that leads to this terminus. That is, intimately related to one another— and not unrelated to the aspects of agency, patiency, and framework—are the aspects of terminus, procedure, and dynamics.

Terminus

To treat activity from the aspect of terminus is to view activity from the perspective of the end point or accomplishment of the activity. To regard activity from the aspect of terminus is, then, to consider the activity from the point of view of what is accomplished by the activity. Terminus is relevant whether or not a purpose-

Physical					
Mere Objects	Persons	Structures (Relations of Objects)	Atmosphere	Communiques (Documents: Oral or Written Communication)	Location (Spatial, Temporal

a. Quantity
b. Quality
c. Rights over objects
  1. Right to procure (request, obtain) objects
  2. Right to distribution of objects
  3. Right to use of objects
  4. Right to dispose of objects
  5. Right to restrict the procurement, distribution, use, disposal of objects
	a. Quantity
	b. Quality
	c. Rights over persons
	  1. Right to procure (request, obtain) persons
	  2. Right to distribution of persons
	  3. Right to use of persons
	  4. Right to dispose of persons
	  5. Right to restrict the procurement, distribution, use, disposal of persons
		a. Quantity
		b. Quality
		c. Rights over structures
		  1. Right to procure (request, obtain) structures
		  2. Right to distribution of structures
		  3. Right to use of structures
		  4. Right to dispose of structures
		  5. Right to restrict the procurement, distribution, use, disposal of structures
			a. Quantity
			b. Quality
			c. Rights over atmosphere
			  1. Right to procure (request, obtain) atmosphere
			  2. Right to distribution of atmosphere
			  3. Right to use of atmosphere
			  4. Right to dispose of atmosphere
			  5. Right to restrict the procurement, distribution, use, disposal of atmosphere
				a. Quantity
				b. Quality
				c. Rights over communiques
				  1. Right to procure (request, obtain) communiques
				  2. Right to distribution of communiques
				  3. Right to use of communiques
				  4. Right to dispose of communiques
				  5. Right to restrict the procurement, distribution, use, disposal of communiques
					a. Quantity
					b. Quality
					c. Rights over location
					  1. Right to procure (request, obtain) location
					  2. Right to distribution of location
					  3. Right to use of location
					  4. Right to dispose of location
					  5. Right to restrict the procurement, distribution, use, disposal of location

Figure 46-1   *Factors of Framework*

ful agent is producing the activity in question. Activity characterized in terms of its end point, as opposed, say to its procedure, undoubtedly has greater appeal when recommended for performance to a purposeful agent. But an agent, even a purposeful one, may perform, without explicitly intending to do so, activity realizing the goal as specified in some theory. As an example, consider the person whose highest level goal is to assemble enough funds for a vacation in Bermuda. She may perfectly well be moved by the goal of attaining the money so as to perform actions which (a) procure her those funds as recompense for labor, and (b) happen to or are carefully planned (by some other agent) to realize the nursing goal. But further, a terminus charac-

terization of activity is often necessary simply to record what has been or is to be done or to give a would-be agent enough intellectual grasp of what is to be done to enable him to unify details of activity so as to accomplish the prescribed activity. Tell an aide, "Pick up the sheet, unfold the sheet from edge to center, then from center to end, place on the mattress with sides parallel to the sides of mattress, secure ends under ends of mattress, for each side place the lap over, et cetera. . . ." What aide—or who in the world—could perform when confronted with such directions. An aide might, however, perform the task very ably if told to put on bottom sheet using hospital corner—provided that she knew what constitutes a hospital corner. As

Non-Physical

Potential Energy Domain (Capacity to act)	Other Domains

Potential Energy
Domain
(Capacity to act)

Other
Domains

a. Relationships
   1. Dominion
   2. Direction
   3. Cooperation
   4. Support
   5. Sustenance
   6. Servitude
b. Rights of individuals (or groups of individuals given power to act)
   1. Responsibilities (duties)
       i. Performance of discharging tasks not delegatable
       ii. Performance of discharging tasks delegatable by responsible agent
           A. Delegatable only to capable agent
           B. Delegatable even to noncapable agent
   2. Prerogatives (liberties)
c. Capacities of individuals or groups of individuals
   1. Legal, civil authority
   2. Institutional authority
   3. Physical strength
   4. Mental strength (knowledge, intelligence)
   5. Technical strength (skills)
d. Purpose of individual or groups of individuals
   1. Professional
   2. Personal
e. Other

a. Respect
b. Reward
c. Status
d. Acknowledgment
e. Other

noted under prescription, "judgment" is required to know when to supplement step-wise directions with overall structure of desired terminus and, conversely, to know when to supplement a terminus characterization with step-wise suggestions for arriving at that end point.

Activity can be organized or structured, then, in terms of its terminus. To characterize activity in such a manner gives us an economical and usually graspable language of communication. So to characterize not only unifies activity into graspable units but also presents possibilities for characterizing activity in ways that make the activity either more palatably doable for the agent or more acceptable to the patient. Consider,

for example, what effect the announcement, "I'm going to jab you with a needle," would have on a patient as compared with the proposal, "I'm going to put you to sleep." The second characterization of the activity probably disposes the patient much better to the agent's activity in spite of the patient's having to suffer pain. Visualizing the end product hoped for probably facilitates too a nurse's or doctor's performance of pain-inflicting services on the patient. To hear a practitioner or researcher remonstrate with self about guilt for having to make a patient suffer in a certain way or about guilt when in the interest of research or education she must resist the desire to intervene to alleviate immediate suffering is often to hear a confession of a less than adequate awareness of what she is doing. For example, were the "wet sheet pack" procedure renamed, "somatic induction of psychological rest," a nurse might see the whole "treatment" as less "medieval" compared to the more civilized procedure of just talking with a disturbed patient and even as strikingly modern in its psychosomatic dimension.

Turning attention to activity from the aspect of end point or terminus is to consider how best to describe an activity's end point. To speak in these terms suggests that a given terminus may be described in more than one way. Not only does terminus description make a type of activity graspable or communicable, but the choice of terminus characterization might have further practical implication in making the activity in question more doable for an agent or more acceptable to a patient. To consider the question of acceptability to agent or patient moves us toward the aspect of dynamics; for "acceptability" calls attention to the factor of desire to do or desire to accept as possible power sources for agents and patients. But to consider the question of cognitive grasp of the activity moves us toward the aspect of procedure, for we call attention to the function of knowledge as an enabling factor; and to consider knowledge or grasp not just of terminus but path to terminus is to consider nursing activity from the aspect of procedure.

Procedure

To view nursing activity from the vantage point of the principle, rule, routine, or protocol governing the activity is to treat activity from the aspect of procedure. Considering nursing activity from the aspect of procedure is to stress not the outcome nor the particularizing features of the activity but rather to emphasize the path, steps, rubric, or more generally the pattern according to which activity is performed. "Procedure" in the most obvious sense of the term suggests the steps to be taken towards some accomplishment and may even suggest the proper equipment, arena, or situation for carrying out activity under the procedure's rubric; further a procedure may indicate danger and success signs that occur in the course of following the procedure and

may propose what other activities—follow-up, reporting, or repeating—are appropriate in conjunction with the initiated pattern of activity.

One function of a procedure then is to provide detail sufficient to enable activity to be carried out; but a procedure may function too, as safeguard to agent, recipient, and organization which encompasses the people and the activity. A suggested or prescribed pattern for arriving at some terminus may safeguard the doer by providing knowledge and hence lessening his liability to criticism from recipient or institution. And the recipient and the institution are similarly protected at least against certain aspects or an agent's ignorance. Economy too, as well as safety, may be procured through procedure following. Since an institution is likely to have more than one agent of a given kind (the kind likely to perform the procedure in question), more than one kind of agents (doctors as well as nurses, say) and usually a nontrivial number of recipients of activities of the kind in question, the task of overseeing, maintaining, and securing the institution requires certain regularity of action to insure the proper interplay of many goals and activities without compromising either the existence, good order, good name, or purpose of the institution.

By its very nature a procedure is a general rule rather than a directive to a specified agent at a specified time and place. As an outline of activity, a procedure may specify the typical agent, recipient, and situation for the procedure as well as typical accompaniments of the procedure. So the procedure is not *totally* determinant of activity. Nonetheless, at times it is most important that procedures come as close as possible to specifying such a total determination of path of activity: Where danger to recipient, agent, or institution is great, very determinant procedures may be desirable; and where peripheral knowledge of likely agent is necessarily limited, then again explicit, rote-like procedures may be highly desirable both to enable and to safeguard performance of the procedure.

Probably the greater the potential dangers, especially to the recipient, the more the procedure should be explicitly detailed, whatever the richness of knowledge the anticipated agent possesses. And the danger for the recipient may result either from the character of the interaction or from the state either of the patient or agent at the time of the intervention.

For example, for reasons of economy, custom, or facility, nursing personnel other than registered nurses may be called on to perform activities whose ramifications are beyond the scope of knowledge possessed by the agent and necessary to understand underlying reasons for the activity; properly detailed procedures may both enable and safeguard the performance of that activity. The matter amounts to this: Occasionally an informed agent has the same time and patience to conceptualize a task and its ramifications; then if possessed of the proper communication skill and tenacity, he may be able to translate his conception into followable and safe steps of activity—steps leading to a desired outcome and performable responsibility by an agent who, though he can follow the steps with care, might not, under the circumstances, have conceived the steps and may not see their total ramifications. The translation to activity must somehow or other incorporate the sign posts of which a totally skilled, experienced, and knowledgeable practitioner would be aware when performing the activity even without the guidance of the procedure.

That some procedures should be detailed extensively and that virtually no latitude be given as to how the details be performed is not to say that all procedures should or must be thus minutely specified. For example, as potential danger to recipient, agent, or institution decreases, procedures can safely leave a greater latitude to the agent. And again, the fuller the background knowledge of the likely agent, again the more safely can the degree or detail for the procedure diminish.

Procedures, then, may be more or less detailed but are always general rules or rubrics whose function is to offer guides, safeguards, and economies with respect to activity. The general rule specifies a pattern of activity. In its most usual usage a procedure specifies a pattern in terms of steps to be followed in sequence over time and usually includes at least implicitly reference to a fairly particular and short-range expected terminus. But this recipe or rote-type of procedure does not exhaust procedures in the usage suggested here (or even in current usage). A procedure may specify a rule or protocol for reaching an explicitly specified terminus in terms of the sub-termini to be accomplished—without regard to specific temporal order or minute specifications for reaching the sub-termini. In terms of our discussion, this second kind of procedure tends to leave more latitude for performance of activity under the procedure than does the first kind. And a third type of procedure can be discerned such that some pattern of activity is specified without regard to terminus but solely in regard to the quality of the steps or activity itself. Such procedures are more often termed policies. To see policies as a kind of procedure is to recognize policies of professions and institutions as guides, safeguards, and economy measures for activity. For though policies tend to be nonspecific with respect to typical agent, typical patient, and typical situation and to be unexplicit as to terminus beyond accomplishing the activity itself, in fact policies are perhaps best regarded as procedures to be followed by all agents in all situations to reach a terminus which is so general as to be supplied only as is specified—the goal-content of theory explicitly or implicitly guiding action.

Included then within this broad conception of procedure are the more generalized principles of activity or rules of thumb as well as practice policies or customary patterns of, say, supervision and reporting. Report all known errors immediately to hospital administration and nursing supervisor; visitors are allowed only after 10 A.M., etc.—these might be examples of procedures pretty much at the level of policy. They leave wide latitudes in their being followed but like more detailed procedures function both in a sense to particularize a grander goal and to facilitate and to safeguard agents, recipients, and institutions in the performance of activity towards realization of goal. As procedures are sometimes criticized as restrictive of nursing activity instead of being seen as potential contributions to that activity, so perhaps even more often the more general protocols are attended to only to be criticized as inhibitors and straight jackets. But policies too, at least theoretically, can be deemed to constitute part of the support and safety that can be used to make nursing activity more efficient, palatable, and satisfying.

Dynamics

Finally now to consider activity explicitly from the aspect of dynamics is to emphasize the power sources for that activity. A thorough-going treatment of dynamics would explore all possible power sources—whether chemical, physical, biological, or psychological—for any person or thing functioning as agent, patient, or part of framework for activity realizing a nursing goal. By way of example, however, let us limit ourselves here to considering only psychological power input. Such psychological power input is more familiarly termed motivation, goal-orientedness, drive, or impetus. Such input is relevant, of course, only to persons functioning as agent, patient, or part of framework. So we must pass up for now exploring the analogy of power inputs to inanimate things.

Simply observing whether there are any purposeful creatures involved in a given activity—whether as agent, patient, or other—may be important. For, briefly put, the goals under which people work or live themselves constitute factors which must be taken account of in activity since these goals have ramifications, both positive and negative, for that activity. Entertaining goals can give impetus and direction to performance of the activity, as well as sustenance for that performance; and goals can function too after performance to give a sense of accomplishment for having persisted in creating a reality actually embodying the goal, entertainment of which gave impetus to the activity. Such are some of the positive ramifications. But holding goals that are noble and that excite the desire to fulfill them may have in either of two ways negative potential for activity. The goal may be so beautiful to contemplate that the would-be agent exhausts all his energy extolling to himself and others the goal's nobility so that no energy remains to undertake activity that might realize the goal. Still even such mere "enthusiasm" if it infects more activity-prone people may have

indirectly positive ramifications for activity. The second way a goal may have negative connotations for activity is more nefarious. A would-be agent who is disposed to act to realize the entertained goal often finds he cannot take even the beginning steps; perhaps he does not know what these steps would be; or else, knowing the steps he cannot take them because he is not properly capable, or, though capable, someone else's activity frustrates his attempts. The persistent encountering of difficulties in realizing goals—whether these difficulties come from limitations in the agent's knowledge or capacity to translate the intended goal into doable activity, or else from frustration of his potential by the power of direction of other forces—may eventually make the agent abandon striving for a particular goal and may even tend to make him abandon altogether his purposeful dimension. Even this negative potential of goal-having has a positive correlate. Goal-directed agents require the satisfaction not only of realizing their goals but of being conscious of having realized them. And whereas strong purposeful agents may have no need of commendation from others for having followed and realized worthy goals, still such external praise, recognition, and reward has probably strong force in reinforcing first, feeble, or even developing tendencies to responsible goal-directed activity.

Since here we must necessarily limit ourselves only to illustration, let us further limit the discussion of psychological power input to a discussion of psychological power sources for persons who are registered nurses or other nursing personnel.

Given these restrictions, dynamics can be explored this way. Consider an agent who is knowledgeable, skilled, and adequately strong to function as a nurse and then ask the question, Why should that person function in this way? Or, When will she so function? Or, When will she cease to function in this way? Or even, Under what circumstances will she function to her maximum potential? Why should anyone related by neither blood, marriage, religious, nor even social ties engage in activity that is often emotionally overwhelming, frequently physically repellent, and in any case incredibly onerous with respect to the burden of life, death, and jeopardy for which she is legally liable? Traditionally, service motivation has always been a strong power input for the nursing profession. Other questions of dynamics aside, three main issues are those of:

1. How can service motivation be inculcated, sustained, or increased?
2. How is service motivation decreased, inhibited, or even extinguished?
3. What are reliable sources of motivation other than service motivation? In other terms, what kinds of agents can be expected to have service motivation as an important power source? And what can serve to supplement or support service motivation or even stand in its stead?

To have service motivation might be most simply to desire to serve mankind, say, by working as a nurse. To desire to serve may be to have a warm feeling and lack of repulsion at the idea of supporting and ministering to the ill and disabled. But how stable a power source is such motivation? Doubtless, some individuals possess these feelings to a marked degree; nonetheless, how widespread are they likely to be in a society not predominantly self-sacrificing or independently wealthy that is, in a society where people tend to have cultivated many needs beyond mere subsistence and where few have already in their possessions the means to supply all their wants? But no matter how prevalent service orientation may be, is it realistic to suppose that service orientation ever exists in isolation?

However strong the service impulse, it does have limitations as a reliable power source for the accomplishment of service. The desire alone does not point the way to fulfillment. A generous feeling unaccompanied by an explicit conception of the content toward which the feeling is directed may well result in good intentions coming to less than full fruition—or at the very least, not coming persistently and consistently to fairly full fruition. And such a service desire even accompanied by an explicit conception of terminus may not insure well-directed activity unless there is also some concept of how to fulfill the visualized aim. A strong service orientation may keep an agent functioning despite any conceptual lacks, but doubtlessly such a

person if enlightened with conception would perform even more fruitfully. Knowing what you are doing and how to do it is a very useful complement for service orientation, for such articulate knowledge may allow the agent to succeed or to be frustrated less in the realization of the desire to be of genuine service. For as nothing so kills the spark of "higher motives" as having them frequently misfire, probably nothing more enhances service motivation than satisfactory activity succeeding in its aims of service. And capacity for conceptualization is relevant not only to "know how" but can itself affect "care to," as we noted above in discussing terminus.

The way activity is conceived can make a big difference to performance. But the other side of the coin is that depending on who is to perform the activity, one or another characterization may be more conducive to production of satisfactory activity. A problem that must be faced within nursing practice and hence within nursing theory is that at least some of the agents who must be counted on to carry out activity for the nursing goal may be persons not necessarily capable of conceiving or visualizing a goal, nor of being internally motivated toward that goal, nor of acting imaginatively to realize that goal whether the motivation is external or internal. To take account both of what things can be counted on to motivate people and of what directions people require to perform their tasks safely and responsibly is of no less moment than to say exactly what, say, a professional nurse should allow herself to do.

People may perform, and perform even well, their assigned tasks or roles out of fear of criticism, blame, or even fear of losing the job because of poor performance. They probably fear, too, loss of respect of their co-workers and diminution of status. And what we fear to lose, we value. So, desire for recognition, praise, money, respect, status, and social prestige may all be potential sources of power supply for any kind of activity and hence for nursing activity.

These forces can work perhaps without the company of service motivation, but in any case they doubtless function as strong supports of service motivation. Man's desire to wield power and influence over other things, whether they be sick and disabled humans (patients in the narrow sense) or healthy subordinates and peers might be tapped in the interest of providing nursing service. The pride of membership in a team that performs noble service is another inducement not to be overlooked—and is in fact not overlooked, as witness the pride of wearing pin, cap, or uniform identified with a strong tradition for service. These motivations beyond service motivation are perhaps not ignored in *practice;* still nursing *theory* rarely accords full due to these power sources, either from lack of awareness or perhaps from the inclination to maintain the myth that only pure devotion to duty, especially unpleasant duty, is a worthy and mentionable motive for a person discharging the important task of servicing mankind, especially the sick and disabled.

Two further power sources—both potent because of their relevant independence of the opinions of other people as to an agent's performance—might be tapped. One such source is the desire for the immediate, aesthetic satisfaction available to the true craftsman, the pleasure felt in the very doing, because of the quality of the performance and the agent's awareness and pride in the quality. A second source, that builds on the first, is the desire for self-esteem, a desire resting on a conception of the agent's role as one worthy of fulfilling, a sense of true craftsmanship, and a sense of responsibility in fulfilling the role. Just as for the craftsman's satisfaction there is needed not only the desire to do but also the skill and opportunity to do, so too for self-esteem the capacity to conceptualize both the overall role and the particular activity is of utmost importance. *The more developed is the theory or conception of nursing practice, the more likely will these two power sources be available for producing and sustaining activity realizing a nursing goal.* For example, the more a nurse conceives creatively and proudly as an indispensable part of her nursing function and not as distractions or as invasions of her independent rights her work with, for, or in some cases even under medical supervision, the stronger will be her service motivation for such activities.

We could similarly discuss dynamics as they govern patients or recipients of activity or as dynamics function more broadly within the framework of activity. We could, for instance, consider the dynamics of an institution: What are the power sources that have inputs into a typical health service organization? Some inputs are educational institutions that train personnel, the power potential of the institution's personnel, literally the power lines into the institution—gas, electricity, et cetera—or in a more figurative sense, the endowment, the capacity of the board of directors, and importantly, the reputation and good name of the institution. These are all power sources that tend to supply the motion allowing the institution to create itself, to maintain itself, and to attract to it personnel and patients. A viable nursing theory may have to take up into its theoretical grasp the most pressing practical considerations; e.g., the danger of lawsuits brought against an institution in an era where juries think insurance companies have too much money, the great potential for mishaps in institutions where delicate procedures and vulnerable people must be dealt with even by learners and where the most responsible and competent person would not hope to be omniscient nor omnipotent.

Existing Nursing Theory

Our whole discussion of theory, of situation-producing theory, and particularly of nursing theory as situation-producing theory suggests that a nursing theory *could* exist. But still the question could be asked, "Does nursing theory exist?" We could explore the question from either of two avenues. We could recall what constitutes such a theory and see if anything in the nursing literature has the requisite ingredients developed at the requisite theoretical level. Then probably the answer must be "No." But if we take account of the types of extant nursing literature and consider whether any of them constitute some contribution to or preparation for such a theory, the answer may be less negative.

Inspection shows that within nursing literature embryos of nursing theory do exist. What is also clear is that producers of these fragments have not, for the most part, been aware of the potential theoretical signif icance of the contributions made nor of the relations of some small segment to the total theoretical picture. Doubtless, uncertainty as to what would constitute a nursing theory contributes to this lack of awareness. But also humility as to one's capacity to produce theory and a skepticism as to the worth of theory in a practice discipline tend toward underrating the contributions of self and others. Whatever the source, the results of the confusions are generally unfortunate: on the pessimistic side, nurses are inclined to claim there is no such thing as existing, written nursing wisdom or nursing content. The impression is given that nursing thought started circa 1950 when the federal government first began funding nursing research on any noticeable scale. On the more optimistic side, there is contention as between would-be nurse theorists as to with what nursing theory should concern itself. The contention tends to produce in many contributors a lack of respect for the worth of another's work. We say optimistic side, for perhaps if people began to realize that each may be exploring a different part of a big area, proper attention could be given to integrating results towards an adequate total product. The differences of opinion would be healthy, too, if nurses would be willing to admit that though all nursing theory may be alike in *structure,* still there may perfectly well be *more than one good nursing theory.* For recall that situation-producing theory has as its prime function the enabling of man to create or shape reality in a desired direction. Quite clearly, it is at least thinkable that not everybody conceives the same kind of reality as most desirable. And even given concurrence about goal-content (desirable kind of reality), there may still exist different conceptions as to agent, patient, framework, terminus, procedure, and dynamics and so different concepts of prescription. In other words, a nursing theory may be deemed a good one if by following it activity can be brought about persistently, consistently, and extensively to create the kind of reality conceptually specified by the theory as desirable. And there may be more than one way, even given one job, to get that job done.

Though the most obvious kinds of nursing literature are research studies, historically earlier in appearance—and still appearing—are the inspirational literature of nursing, general or specialized treaties on nursing, and textbooks. These works distinguish themselves from the more recent literature called research studies in a notable way: the older forms for the most part are based on experience gained either in practice or in teaching as opposed to being gotten as an activity planned for the purpose of gathering data on which to make or evaluate theses about nursing. The research studies tend to be restricted to isolated topics. Moreover, the studies in general emphasize the relation of the conclusion to the evidence for that conclusion rather than the relation of the conclusion to practice. And both the treatises and the research studies differ from textbooks in that the textbooks so-called are intended mainly to supply either immediately useful background knowledge or immediately applicable patterns of action rather than serving mainly for the enlargement or deepening of the "body" of nursing knowledge.

But what might these types of nursing literature contain by way of clues for nursing theory? Inspirational literature gives accounts of nursing goals expressed in terms that stir the emotions and fire the desire for service. Treatises, too, tend to contain some considerations relevant to the goal-ingredient of a nursing theory. These treatises, particularly the more general ones but even the more specialized kinds, usually contain some statement of nursing goal. The statement is customarily less grandiloquent than those found in inspirational literature and is often contained in a preface or introductory remarks neatly set aside as the philosophy which, when dispensed with, allows the treatise to move to the more earthy levels of its informations. Though generosity may find in existing nursing literature a contribution to each ingredient of nursing theory, still the treatment is sporadic. The goal ingredient of theory tends to be handled either on an abstract or grand scale without easy potential for relation to action or else in fragmented portions that are easily integrated. Prescription is almost entirely ignored except in inspirational literature (and, of course, implicitly in textbooks at least to the point of specifying agent). And of the six aspects distinguished for the survey list, framework and dynamics are probably those aspects most sparsely touched on, and within the consideration of any of the six aspects there tends to be a considerable absence of any systematic factorizations or of explicit citings of relevant theories with adequate justification for the claimed relevance.

The usually acknowledged parts of nursing literature—treatises, tracts, studies, and textbooks—do not exhaust the written body of nursing content. Other written material exists that might serve as fertile sources of theory. No hospital is without written and rewritten procedure books and policy books. However much or little such works are used, still a great deal of care goes into the writing of them; and, moreover, the writing often tends to be done by people who are in service in at least a supervisory capacity. But what could theory expect to find in, say, the written procedures? As they now stand these procedures incorporate at least implicitly the considered practical judgments of seasoned practitioners or supervisors as to one way of performing a given task. Perhaps more significantly, the procedures contain clues, on the one hand, as to what preventing and promoting theories need to be exploited or developed to provide reasons for nostrums, as opposed merely to presenting nostrums as fiats, and, on the other hand, hints as to what in the framework besides immediate agent and patient impinge directly on planned activity—trivially, equipment and setting are specified and their return to "normalcy" given as part of the procedure so that concern for preserving the institution literally by husbanding its supplies is given written recognition as important. And the return to "normalcy" speaks implicitly to the question of other agents and patients whose activities must not be infringed upon; more directly, noting whose permissions or order must authorize giving the procedure and who must be given knowledge concerning the procedure's performance are implicit mentionings of the unmentionable, namely, the interrelation of professional powers and responsibilities.

To overlook so abundant and fertile a source of nursing content would be wasteful; but it must be acknowledged that "procedures" as they now stand do not have already at an explicit conceptual level their most important potential contributions to theory. Nor insofar as they are at conceptual level do they necessarily constitute theories or parts of theories that have received the critical scrutiny of conscious attempts at validation. Procedures have been subjected, of course, to trial within practice. The amount by which activity nominally following the procedure actually does follow the procedures as written—whether procedure is consulted but not wholly followed or whether in practice no one even bothers to consult the written procedure—gives some indication of the unwitting practical refinement, rejection, or extension of the procedure if regarded as already at the theoretical level. Wittingly to guide research studies on the basis of these clues to theory offers an avenue of research which might before too long have practical output through the improvement of theory.

Procedures provide still another dimension for contributing to nursing theory. A nursing procedure book constitutes in some sense a catalogue, whether or not exhaustive, of typical nursing activities. But the types are not in general named according to terminus or expected outcome of following the procedure but are more often named in terms of some striking feature of process or equipment. A rewarding but difficult enterprise might be to comprehend a procedure well enough to offer a more suggestive name—for example, as mentioned above, to reconceive wet-sheet packs as somatic inducement of psychological peace. Any attempt to implement this suggestion tends to reveal that procedure writers and refiners seem at times to have labored long to conceal the intended end point of the activity for which the procedure is given. This tendency probably reflects a laudable if overly indulged desire to be detailed enough about what specific steps must be taken both to insure safety and to allow performance by less than long-seasoned and highly prepared practitioners.

Policy books are perhaps another kind of non-academic nursing literature. Might not these contain some fruits of nursing observation and experience concerning, at least, framework questions? And yet another source of written material that might offer clues for theory is the day-to-day communications between various levels of nursing service as well as between the nursing service and either institution administration or other branches of service. Such material may provide more fruitful directions for study than, say, patients' comments on hospital treatment or elaborate questionnaires filled out by persons well capable of censorship, intentional or not.

In short, nursing literature, especially if broadly conceived, though admittedly not constituting a total nursing theory or even for the most part any conceptually well-developed part of such a theory, is a rich mine, if we know how to exploit the veins. Nursing theory, insofar as it does exist, surely is an embryonic state having a potential either for extinction or for development. The existence of something concrete which can be critically regarded—written materials and existing practice are two such things—is a necessary stepping stone to any extension, refinement, rejuvenation, or exploitation of the truths or errors thus concretely presented. In other words, even now practice is guided in some incipient way by embryonic theory. What is needed is more explicit guidance by better and more fully articulated and tested theory. To regard this interplay between theory. To regard this interplay between theory and practice as an already-begun and hopefully an ever-increasing development is both intellectually more nearly sound and practically more healthy than to take the stance that no theory exists now, but some day we will have precisely one pat theory in need of no further growth. But if the embryo is to develop, we must be clear not only as to what theory is but also as to exactly what are the sources of the theory.

The Authors Comment

Purpose Preserved and Tested in Complexity
Collaboration With Ernestine Wiedenbach in a Yale Context

Our collaboration with Ernestine Wiedenbach was a natural outgrowth of our interactions with her. She had attended our logic class and subsequent class in concepts, and was an active member of three workgroups we led for faculty and graduate students. One group worked on the problem of measures and attempted to spell out nonverbal indicators as stress measures; a second group attempted to rewrite the ice pack procedure so that the procedure as stated constituted a theory; and the third group, instituted at Wiedenbach's initiative, attempted to formulate a measure that could be used to evaluate a student's nursing activity. The three of us were also participants in the biweekly research seminar of the Yale School of Nursing.

Our recognition of the need to articulate the relatively invisible elements of the complexities of nursing stems in good measure from our collaborative discussions with Wiedenbach. She was always proudly and strongly aware of the accomplishments of nursing, and open to innovations and growth for the discipline.

Ernestine Wiedenbach is a remarkable person—intellectually vigorous, courageous, and compassionate. Her wholehearted commitment to nursing and to educating nurses kept her persistently in touch with the practice setting. Undoubtedly her concern with obstetric nursing and midwifery accounted for her particular sensitivity to the inhibiting and supporting influences to which an individual practitioner is subject from the agency of others.

Ernestine Wiedenbach was visibly excited by the conceptual work of Orlando. And she was venturesome, too. She was more than willing to expose herself to and to work at something ostensibly remote from her immediate interests—for example, symbolic logic. She regarded her study of symbolic logic as an endeavor that *might* further her attempt to know more about nursing and to articulate for others what she had already discovered. Her aim was always the same— to give and to enable others to give the kind of nursing care human dignity warrants. Thus, she was open to new conceptions—to theory and to research for nursing. But her openness was in no sense a quest for status nor an attempt to "elevate" nursing to the status of a profession. Professionalization-talk strikes us as foreign to Wiedenbach's character. To her, nursing was already something special—a calling, one of the highest expressions of the human spirit—although she probably would regard such talk as pretentious and "highfalutin." Of course, nursing could be better. The giving of even better nursing care—that was Wiedenbach's focus. Her watchword was purpose: Know why you are doing what you are doing.

The Friday research seminar at the Yale School of Nursing had as routine participants nursing academics, nursing service personnel, and academics from other disciplines (sociology, psychology, and philosophy). Nursing research at that time (the early 1960s) was still in its swaddling clothes—an avant-garde "thing." Some of the "progressives" who attended the seminar tended to regard Wiedenbach as a "foot-dragger." She often would object when a particular study was being presented: "But that is not nursing." The patronizing reply would be "No, that is nursing research." Her objection was interpreted by some as a rejection of research, the up-and-coming thing. But Wiedenbach was dauntless; she would not be put down. In fact, we could see that she had her finger on a sensitive and delicate point of methodology. What may have appeared on the surface to be a nursing intervention was, Wiedenbach would insist, not a *nursing* intervention: for example, an hour and a half of "deliberative" nursing by a nurse charged with no other responsibilities than the admission of a single patient was not an instance of nursing. The independent nursing variable in the study was actually *not* a *nursing* variable, because no service nurse could realistically be expected to have the leisure to perform such an intervention. (The experimental nurse refreshed herself while waiting for the next subject by an hour or so of novel reading.) It was Wiedenbach's awareness of the conditions of "real nursing" that made her object to the study. She was aware that such a study could be used to damn service nurses. (*They* (service nurses) are not giving good care, they do not know how to give good care; we researchers do, as our research shows.) Wieden-bach's criticism of this viewpoint that bifurcates the knowing researchers from the service nurses was deadly practical; what good is a study if its independent variable cannot feasibly be realized as the activity of a nurse in practice? To go beyond merely condemning ongoing practice—to change practice for the better—requires something more ingenious from research than merely a formally "correct" study whose independent variable bears no relation to what a nurse could feasibly do in a practice setting. In short, "ivory tower" exercises that had no potential payoff in the real world of nursing service were not nursing research as defined by Wiedenbach.

Wiedenbach's experience and mode of thinking had independently brought her to the sense of our proposal concerning the structure of theory for practice-discipline. Our proposal incorporated goals as an ingredient but demanded tests for the goal; it explicated (the survey-list ingredients) the factors and framework dynamics pertinent to the nurse-client interaction without displacing that interaction as a prime concern of the nurse. These features of the proposal probably constitute some of the reasons why Wiedenbach saw promise in the conception and willingly collaborated in pressing particulars of practice forward to help shape the emerging conception.

In our collaboration with Wiedenbach, differences would occasionally arise. Our proposal about the structure of nursing theory had as one of its consequences the broadening of the notion of "nursing activity." We recall a pitched battle we once had with Wiedenbach when we insisted that the thermome-ter, too, was conceptually a patient to the nurse, and in a like fashion so was the doctor. Our point was that in order to give direct care to a client, the thoughtful nurse will do things that do not immediately bear on the client; e.g., will see to it that the thermometer is cleaned and in working order, that the doctor is "positioned" appropriately with respect to the client (the attitudinal positioning in question being determined by the nurse's judgment as to what is appropriate). When Wiedenbach saw the point she, of course, agreed; but in a context where task-oriented nursing was being displaced by patient-centered nursing, the remark that a nurse might appropriately do something that was not immediately and directly concerned with the client was especially difficult to grasp. More generally, we insisted that the concept of agency and the concept of patiency, as we used them in spelling out the structure of nursing theory, did not allow an easy and simple-minded identification of nurse with agency or an identification of client (with patient in the more usual sense) with patiency. In a pre-Orem era, we pressed to suggest that the sick person was a competent agent for some things and—even more scandalously—we pressed for the open admission of the pressures and influences to which any practitioner is patient. Unless the unmentionables become mentionable, there is little hope of improving nursing care. There are factors outside of the client's state and the nurse's knowledge that bear on the quality of care a nurse gives to a client. Our proposal for the structure of nursing theory offered some way to take account of these forces.

Wiedenbach was a person who lived a conception rather than merely voicing it—she "hoofed what she mouthed." A striking illustration of this personality trait emerged from a discussion during our collaboration with her. Wiedenbach was vigorously putting forth the Orlando contention that a nurse should not try to meet an unfelt patient need; a nurse does for a patient only what the patient wants done. We differed equally vigorously with her on this point, and once it became clear to her through discussion that the surveillance routinely practiced by a "good nurse" was a violation of Orlando's conception, she abandoned the Orlando principle as too simple minded. Surveilling for need, presenting herself to a patient to allow a need to be expressed, even instructing to create or provoke needs in a patient—all were routine measures in Wiedenbach's nursing practice. She lived that conception, and once she recognized that she lived it and that experience had validated her living it, her voicing became consistent with her practice.

From Emphasis Merely on Structure and the Verbal to an Emblematic Presentation of a Concept of Nursing

A remark suggesting how our current work contrasts with the Wiedenbach collaboration seems to be called for. Our current work results from a building on, a development, of our earlier thoughts. A theory of theories, we have come to see, is simply an adumbration of a theory of conception and meaning. We now speak of a theory of conception and of concepts as guides to action. Concepts can be regarded as purposeful oversimplifications that can serve as guides to action when they are taken with "procedural bent." (See Dickoff & James, 1984.)

A theory of theories is an instantiation of our more general theory of conception. The notion of a concept as a guide to action has given rise to a new kind of definition, which we call "prospecting definition." Concepts as purposeful oversimplifications, concepts taken with procedural bent, prospecting definitions—these constitute in part what we call a technology for concepts. The most important tool of the practitioner is conception, and the technology of conception provides the practitioner with a habitual agility in using concepts as guides to action.

Words are but one way of presenting a concept. We have devised what we call emblematic presentation of a concept. Such a presentation is other than a merely verbal presentation of a concept and is a powerful way for grasping a multiplicity into the unity of a concept. We have developed an emblematic presentation of the concept of nursing as complexity considerate, thoughtful doing. The emblematic presentation of such a concept constitutes a prospecting definition of nursing. This is not the place to spell out the details of such an emblematic presentation. Suffice it to say, a striking and significant difference between practice theory as offered in our theory of theories and the current emblematic presentation of nursing lies in this: The theory of theories presented situation-producing theory as simply a structure empty of specific content. The emblematic presentation of a concept of nursing is a structure, but the nature of the structure is such that specific "content" is part and parcel of the structure offered.

—JAMES DICKOFF AND PATRICIA JAMES

While I was teaching at the Yale University School of Nursing, Dean Florence Wald invited James Dickoff and Patricia James, members of the Department of Philosophy of Yale University, to give a series of lectures for the nursing faculty on the importance of theory to nursing practice. Coincidentally, I was writing the book *Clinical Nursing: A Helping Art* at the time. I was greatly impressed by their exposition of various levels of theory, and so I asked them to review my manuscript. This they did, and to my surprise they saw in it the elements of a prescriptive theory.

Many hours of valuable discussion followed. As a result of this exchange of ideas, Jim and Pat asked me to co-author their articles, "Theory in a Practice Discipline," which subsequently appeared in *Nursing Research*.

Another outgrowth of my association with Jim and Pat was the format and organization of the material for my book *Meeting the Realities of Clinical Teaching* (New York: Springer, 1969). To paraphrase a paragraph from the book's preface (p. vi):

When developed according to a prescriptive theory, a clinical program gains, I have discovered substance, trenchancy, and stature. It enables the individual (student or practitioner) not only to gain knowledge and skills, but also to apply them in practice and to obtain desired results. The purpose, goals, and objectives of the program are given practical meaning and such commitments as planning, orienting, and evaluating, which often are taken for granted, are recognized as vital to its effectiveness. A program thus developed cannot be lightly undertaken. Its implementation calls for wisdom, perspicacity, and thoughtful review and assessment of actions.

—ERNESTINE WIEDENBACH

REFERENCES

Dickoff, J., & James, P. (1984, January). *Conceptual trends, conceptual needs, prospects for a fit.* Paper presented at the 2nd Annual Meeting of the Society for Research in Nursing Education, San Francisco. (Tapes of this presentation are available from the Society.)

Wiedenbach, E. (1969). *Meeting the realities of clinical teaching.* New York: Springer.

Chapter 47

Theory: The Professional Dimension

Hildegard E. Peplau

One of the most important tasks before the profession of nursing is to establish the nature and uses of theory in professional nursing practice. It is not an easy task. Similarly, to present a paper on an aspect of this task to this group of nurse scientists is not exactly the most comfortable experience. Recently, Merton published an illuminating essay in which is included a description of the climate of scientific communities similarly at work on the task of clarifying and validating scientific theories that are proposed:

> The organization of science operates as a system of institutionalized vigilance, involving competitive cooperation. It affords both commitment and reward for finding where others have erred or have stopped before tracking down the implications of their results or have passed over in their work what is there to be seen by the fresh eye of another. In such a system, scientists are at the ready to pick apart and appraise each new claim to knowledge. This unending exchange of critical judgment, of praise and punishment, is developed in science to a degree that makes the monitoring of children's behavior by their parents seem little more than child's play. Only after the originality and consequence of his work have been attested by significant others can the scientist feel reasonably confident about it. Deeply felt praise for work well done, moreover, exalts donor and recipient alike; it joins them both in symbolizing the common enterprise. That, in part, expresses the character competitive cooperation in science (Merton, 1969, p. 220).

There are many forms of theory. In this paper, the use of established theoretical concepts and processes, and the development of knowledge from observations in nursing situations will be described. These are but two small aspects of the larger task—clarifying the nature and uses of scientific knowledge in nursing.

About the Author

HILDEGARD E. PEPLAU began her nursing career in 1931 as a graduate of the Pottstown Hospital School of Nursing in Pennsylvania. In 1936, she accepted a position at Bennington College, Bennington, Vermont, as executive officer of the College Health Service; she combined this work with study for a B.A. in Interpersonal Psychology, which she received in 1943. She then worked as a staff nurse in the psychiatric department at Bellevue Hospital, New York City. From 1943 to 1945, she was a First Lieutenant in the U.S. Army Nurse Corps, at the School of Military Neuropsychiatry (ETSA). After discharge from the Army, Dr. Peplau continued her education at Teacher's College, Columbia University, receiving a M.A. (1947) and an Ed.D. (1953). While a doctoral student at Teacher's College, she served as director of the Psychiatric Nursing Education program. In 1952, while at Columbia, Dr. Peplau wrote *Interpersonal Relations in Nursing* (New York: Putnam), a text that is still widely read in the original first edition.

In 1954, Dr. Peplau accepted a faculty appointment at Rutgers University in the Psychiatric Nursing Department. She became department chair in 1955 and director of the graduate program in psychiatric nursing in 1958, a position she held until her retirement in 1974. She was made a professor in 1960.

Among Dr. Peplau's numerous professional achievements are publishing more than 50 scholarly journal articles and contributing to at least 10 texts. She has lectured nationally and internationally since 1949; been active on the local, state, and national level in professional nursing organizations; and received various honors and awards from colleges, universities, and nursing associations. In 1983, she received an honorary doctoral degree (her fourth) from her alma mater, Columbia University. In 1984, she was awarded honorary recognition from the American Nurses' Association and, in 1990, received the ANA's Hildegard Peplau Award.

Her long career in nursing has given Dr. Peplau many rewards; when asked about particular satisfactions, she summed it up: "Nursing has provided many opportunities to use and to develop my capacities to meet interesting persons and to enjoy lifelong relationships." About the future, she comments "The full professionalization of nursing depends on scientific research of nursing phenomena, application of theory in nursing practice, and wide dissemination of health knowledge to the public by nurses."

Uses of Established Theoretical Concepts and Processes

Nursing, like other professions, is primarily an applied science. It uses established knowledge for beneficial purposes. One such use is the application of known concepts and processes to observations made in nursing situations. Such application serves the purposes of interpretation of observational data and the derivation of theory-based nursing actions (Peplau, 1968). In nursing practice, the starting point is something observed during a contact with a patient. The name of a particular concept, relevant to that particular observation—or to a selection of the more crucial among diverse phenomena observed at a particular moment— "flips up" in the mind of the professional. Thus naming, categori-

zation, or classification of observed phenomena is a first step in application of theory in nursing practice. It occurs at the point of observation especially for the most effective nursing interventions in instances of crucial observations. Thus, the nurse who observes blood in some amount on the body and sheets of the bed of a patient, "flips up" a concept such as "bleeding" or "hemorrhage"— i.e., choosing this concept— nursing interventions deriving from this concept are likely to follow. It is this point—of using available concepts to name and thus to begin to explain observed phenomena and to derive theory-based nursing actions —which is glaringly omitted in two recent publications on the subject of nursing theory (Dickoff & James, 1968; Sarosi, 1968).

Naming the phenomena observed, however, is

only the first step. The professional goes beyond mere naming (although in some fields, such as psychiatric work, it is not uncommon to note concepts used in a "name-calling," derogating sense). A second step in the application of a selected concept to observation is to use the concept definition as a structured format for obtaining more information, by observation or interviewing[1] (Peplau, 1962).

Such data collection may widen the base of information obtained. Thus, a concept selected initially may be discarded and still other concepts, which arise in the mind of the professional in relation to observations of data being obtained, provide a basis for a new selection of a concept for application. As data being obtained becomes clearer, a particular explanatory concept tends to be selected and its definitional format ultimately serves a third step, which is to consider options for resolution of the difficulty and to judge which option to use.

Known concepts, defined in operational terms—by stating in serial order of emergence those behaviors generally associated with that concept—thus serve several purposes: (a) naming observed phenomena, (b) providing a structure for obtaining more information, and (c) suggesting resolution options relevant to the particular phenomena that were noticed. A professional encounter—whether the nurse-patient contact is for a duration of ten or one-hundred minutes—is a very fluid interaction in which the professional uses observation, then interpretation of observed phenomena, and then responds with theory-based interventions.[2]

Such encounters thus require the professional to have in mind readily available to recall, the definitional components of those concepts crucial to the recurring phenomena pertinent to nursing situations, conscious and well-disciplined use of procedures of theory applications of different types, and critical judgment so as to discriminate and select well from among resolution options that are available.

There are, of course, conceptions—ideas, generalizations—which cannot be used in the manner described, which do not have the specificity, but which are useful in other ways. Whorf's idea that "language influences thought" (and with rare exceptions, not the other way around) can be extended by stating that: (a) language influences thought, (b) thought then influences action, (c) thought and action taken together evoke feelings in relation to a situation or context. The only specificity, then, is in terms of nursing actions—the suggestion that impact upon language behavior of patients is the major point of corrective impact for disturbance of action and feeling. In psychiatric work, that is an important testable hypothesis rather than an explanatory concept at this time.

A concept, as used narrowly in this paper is explanatory of a fairly small amount of behavior. On the other hand, a process represents many concepts which, taken together, provide explanations of a broader range of behavior. The processes of development,[3] socialization, learning, hallucinations (Peplau, 1963), provide instances. A process is, in effect, an organization of concepts into larger components—called phases, stages—each of which includes a series of separate concepts arranged in a serial order showing the emergence of particular behaviors. Thus, the process of development (see appendix II) shows concepts explanatory of some behaviors seen in such phases as infancy, childhood, juvenile era, etc.—both phases and concepts being arranged in the order in which such behaviors ordinarily evolve.

A process provides a somewhat different definitional format for application in professional practice.

---

[1] See Appendix I for two illustrations.

[2] There is also a fourth step in the total process of professional thought at the "bedside" and that is: evaluation of effects of interventions on the phenomena observed and interpreted. Such continuing evaluations, over time, lead to standardization of practices in relation to observation of known phenomena. Such standardized practices can then be developed into manuals for technical nursing practice. Such manuals would point out (a) what to look for—what can be observed under certain circumstances; (b) what to do when such observations are noticed; and (c) a reason or rationale for the action —which, in effect, is a simplified restatement of the theory used by the professional as described above. Thus, technical nursing has to do with known or standardized nursing practices as these have been evolved by professional nurses through repeated use of the four steps described in relation to particular phenomena seen in nursing situations.

[3] See Appendix II, "Tools and Task Outline," for illustration.

Each concept can, of course, be used separately as described previously. The definitional format of the entire process, however, provides a structure for observations of several kinds. The process of personality development provides an instructive instance:

1. The professional can place observed behavior within the established structure. Thus, the behavior of a 30 year old may be recognized as that more compatible with an eight year old, at a given moment of observation.
2. The process definition can be used to anticipate subsequent behavior which should follow observed behavior (as in the case of a healthy child observed *vis-à-vis* the process of development.
3. The process definition can be used to place current behavior *and* to identify "next step" behavior that should be stimulated. Thus, a patient who uses competition recurringly may need help to learn behaviors that tend to evolve subsequently such as compromise and cooperation.

The process definitional structure for development can be used to map out age-related interpersonal competencies that are observable in a patient, those that are lacking, and its serial order of development of such competencies can be followed to design a nursing care plan. Such a plan should help patients to gain interpersonal competencies which are lacking by reason of unfortunate experience, lacks in growth opportunities, or the effects of disease processes upon human functioning.

To this point, this paper has suggested some important uses for established theory in the clinical practice of nursing. It might be useful to keep in mind Stainbrook's noteworthy observation that "some professionals use theory the way a drunk uses a lamppost —for support rather than for illumination." What has been suggested here is the use of known concepts and processes for illumination of clinical observations in nursing, a purpose which requires considerable development of intellectual competencies in professional nurses through collegiate education.

Development of Knowledge From Observations in Nursing Situations

Theory represents a formulation of the meaning of observed phenomena in an order or form which enables the formulation to be used to explain similar phenomena, observed in other situations of like kind, and to guide the professional in choosing interventions relevant to the phenomena observed. Theoretical concepts, therefore, are a shared explanatory language—a shortcut language—of particular use to professionals in the field to which those concepts pertain and from which they were derived. Nursing situations provide a field of observations from which unique nursing concepts can be derived and used for the improvement of the professional's work.

Concepts generally derive first from empirical observations—an astute clinician noting a phenomenon about which there is a question. In another context, Davis (1969) gives a description of this process of "the irrepressible and cyclical gropings of intent minds to *solve a puzzle* that has resisted solution." He says:

> In his description of the quest for a solution, Watson makes us intimate witness to the frailties, opportunities, and unsuspected resources of the creative thinker, be he scientist, artist, or man of affairs; the false starts, the moody setting asides and quirkish picking ups, the imaginative though empirically unsubstantiated leaps forward, the profoundly deflating collapse of an apparently promising line of inquiry, the ego-massaging rehearsals of fantasized future fame, the long-neglected clue thrust suddenly and inexplicably into consciousness and last, though not least, the serendipitous chance remark of a colleague working on seemingly unrelated problems. Instead of some simple-minded cognitive linear progression from problem to solution, Watson gives us a much richer, multi-level, and emergent rendition of the discovery process; a kind of dialectical backing and filling in which concept, data, and empirical focus constantly interact upon each other until some convincing, internally consistent explanation is finally achieved (Davis, 1969, pp.53–56).

And that is pretty much how it will be in delineating concepts relevant to phenomena seen in nursing practice. To name them, as was suggested earlier, is to have at least the name of the concept in mind. As yet, there is not available an organized nomenclature of such phenomena. A second, very important task of the profession of nursing is to develop a nomenclature of nursing problems and to define these concepts in ways that serve to explain the phenomena and to guide nursing actions. In order to do this, the parameters of the field of nursing—in relation to other disciplines—may need to be clarified. Nursing can take as its unique focus *the reactions of the patient or client to the circumstances of his illness or health problem* (Peplau, 1955), thus overlapping medicine only when dealing with disease processes more directly. Assuming that illness provides an opportunity for learning and growth through exposure to professionals, the stress of the event providing the energy, the profession could stake a *claim to a focus on helping patients to gain intellectual and interpersonal competencies beyond that which they have at the point of illness, by gearing nursing practices to evolving such competencies through nurse-patient interactions* (Gregg, 1954).

In order to derive nursing concepts, then, professional nurses would take note of reactions of patients —to illness, hospitalization, effects of these upon life and living—observing those behaviors for which no explanatory concepts are as yet available. Such observations would be sought in other patients, under similar circumstances (Rouslin, 1963). As observations continued, certain regularities would begin to appear—concerning the nature of the data being observed. Thus, a name for the phenomena would occur to the professional. Subsequently, with further observations the concept of the phenomenon would become clear—and thus be defined and tested against still other patients. Eventually, useful interventions would be derived from the explanation of the phenomenon and the effects of those interventions upon it also tested.

Nursing concepts, thus, are the result of a search for recurring phenomena seen in nursing situations. These regularities are then observed in greater detail and their variations and dimensions made more explicit. Initial formulation of the concept then serves as a format for more systematic observations in many similar situations and perhaps even by other observers. Thus a system to record recurring instances of like kind or similar to the phenomenon in question would have to be devised. The initial concept becomes a structured matrix for subsequent observations, and for locating the scope of variations in the particular phenomenon. The initial concept also provides the name (i.e., the concept of) of the phenomenon, while subsequent observations assure identification of all of the behaviors associated with that particular concept.

There are, to be sure, some reactions of patients about which much is already known and concepts are available in the literature (Burd & Marshall, 1963, p.379). Denial of illness is one such reaction. But denial is a concept used by other professions. Consequently, what may be needed at this time is a survey of published nursing literature to locate those concepts, if any, which are solely used by nurses and those shared with other disciplines in the health field. Meanwhile, the search for new concepts derived from nursing situations must and will go on.

Summary

In this paper the use of theoretical concepts and processes already known has been described. An approach to obtaining nursing concepts has been discussed.

References

Burd, S.F., & Marshall, M.A. (1963). *Some clinical approaches to psychiatric nursing.* New York: Macmillan.

Davis, F. (1969). Review of the double helix. *Transaction, 6*(5), 53–56.

Dickoff, J., & James, P. (1968). A theory of theories: A position paper. *Nursing Research, 17,* 197–203.

Gregg, D. (1954). The psychiatric nurse's role. *American Journal of Nursing, 54*(7).

Merton, R.F. (1969). Behavior patterns of scientists. *The American Scholar, 38*(2), 197–225.

Peplau, H.E. (1955). Loneliness. *American Journal of Nursing, 55*(12), 1476–1481.

Peplau, H.E. (1962). Interpersonal techniques: The crux of psychiatric nursing. *American Journal of Nursing, 62*(6), 50–54.

Peplau, H.E. (1963). Interpersonal relations and the process of adaptation. *Nursing Science,* 272–279.

Peplau, H.E. (1968). Operational definitions and nursing practice. In L. Zderad & H.C. Belcher (Eds.), *Developing behavioral concepts in nursing* (pp. 12–15). Atlanta. Southern Regional Education Board.

Rouslin, S. (1963). Chronic helpfulness: Maintenance and intervention. *Perspectives of Psychiatric Care, 1*(1), 25–28.

Sarosi, G.M. (1968). A critical theory: The nurse as a fully human person. *Nursing Forum, 7*(4), 349–363.

Appendix I.

Format for Definition and Application of Theoretical Concepts in Nursing Practice

Serial order of emergence of observable behaviors associated with the concept.	Structure for obtaining more information about a specific problematic situation by further observation or interviewing, inherent in concept definition.	Structure of resolution options inherent in concept definition for choice of theory-based nurse actions based upon professional judgment of which option to use first.
A. Concept of Frustration		
1. A Goal is set.	What Goal? Is it attainable? When set? Was it clearly formulated? Expressed to others?	Identify the Goal. Give up the Goal. Revise the Goal. Discuss Goal with others.
2. There is movement toward the Goal.	What strategies? Were these reasonable? Were these clearly related to Goal?	Change strategies. —Acquire new ones if needed.
3. An obstacle prevents goal achievement.	What obstacle? External or internal? Can it be removed or bypassed?	Remove or bypass the obstacle.
4. Aggression is felt and expressed. —Directly toward the obstacle. —Indirectly away from the obstacle.	Was the relation of Aggression to Goal, movement, and/or obstacle recognized?	Formulate the relation.
B. Anxiety		
1. An expectation (wish, desire, goal, etc.) becomes operative.	What expectations? Is it attainable? Was it communicated to the other(s) in the situation?	Connect the anxiety and expectations —Give up the expectation. —Revise the expectation in relation to what is possible. Communicate the expectation.
2. The expectation is not met.		
3. Extreme discomfort and internal tension is experienced.	Discomfort experienced where—what part of the body?	Name the experience as "anxiety."
4. The energy from the tension is converted, more or less automatically (without thought) into "relief behavior."	What pattern of behavior is used? Is there a series of relief behaviors that are used? Does the series recur in the same order in subsequent anxiety-producing behaviors? The amount of anxiety is also inferred from the relief behaviors.	Connect the anxiety and relief behavior. —Name the relief behavior.
5. Relief is felt and jusitifed or rationalized.		

Appendix II.

The "Tools and Tasks Outline" that is attached was prepared by a group of graduate students in partial fulfillment of requirements for the Master's degree at Teachers College, Columbia University, 1951. The title of the study was: *A Shift in Thinking: Instrument and Manual for Understanding Behavior.* Regrettably, the work was not published. The psychiatric nurses who participated in the preparation of this outline were Mrs. Elrose Daniels, Helen D. Johnson, E. Katherine LeVan (Fountain House, New York City), Claire Mintzer Fagin (Faculty, New York University), Janesy B. Myers (V. A., Northport, Long Island), Naomi Perry, Catherine M. Thilgen, and Gwen Tudor Will.

This instrument was constructed following a review of published literature of 26 authors; 13 of these were selected for study and synthesis and for development of the outline which shows developmental eras and two types of behavior (Tools and Tasks) characteristic of these eras. The outline was then used to classify behavior described in 184 situations—selected according to pre-established criteria. Validation of placement was secured by a panel of experts including Dr. Barbara Biber (Bank Street School), Dr. George Devereaux (Anthropologist), Esther Garrison, R.N. (NIMH), Dr. Arthur Jersild (Educator, Teachers College), Dr. Norman Kelman (Psychoanalyst), Emmy Lanning Schockly, R.N., Dr. Irving Lorge, Jeanette Regensburg (Community Service Society, New York), Dr. Morris Schwartz (Sociologist), Dr. Ellen Simor (Psychoanalyst), and Dr. Otto Will (Psychoanalyst). The results from the placement of 184 situations by graduate students and 29 situations by the jury of experts proved the instrument to be valid and reliable for categorizing presenting behavior according to guides provided in the Tools and Tasks Outline.

The outline was developed as an educational tool to indicate a common frame of reference regarding behavior characteristic of eras of development and constructive capacities that can be released for growth.

The outline has been used in clinical workshops for nurses as a basis for discussion of "tools" and "tasks" that emerge, and can be observed in the behavior of persons, during the process of normal growth and development. Discussion of each tool and task—its definition, its manifestation and variations shown in presenting behavior—leads to understanding of phenomena to be observed. When a variation of a particular tool or task is observed, in the presenting behavior of a patient hospitalized in a psychiatric facility, the outline can then serve to indicate the current "tools and tasks" used by a patient and the next steps in that patient's development which require the help of nursing services if the patient's growth is to be promoted.

—HILDEGARD E. PEPLAU

Definitions

Tool.   The instrument by which learning is effected or accomplished. Each individual has capacities that usually ripen are available to him at each era of development.

Task.   A learning experience which arises at or about a certain period in the life of an individual, as a result of biological maturation, cultural pressures, and level of aspiration. Each task that has been learned becomes a tool for the next era.

Learning.   A process where capacities are actualized in the direction of growth or forward movement. This formulation is particularly oriented toward learning to live with people.*

Era.   A period in time distinguished by certain criteria of a physiological or psychological nature. Each era usually has some characteristics of preceding eras, but is sufficiently different quantitatively and qualitatively to differentiate it from other eras.

Note.   Mastery of task plus movement toward a next task requires the exercise of the capacities of tools available. This leads to development of skill in their use.

---

* Different from conditioning. i.e., adapting behavior to the situation merely in terms of tension reduction.

Tools and Tasks Outline

Infancy.   The period of living that starts with the birth of the individual and proceeds to emergence of the capacity for communication through speech, i.e., when child uses Mama or Dada in the mother-child relationship or father-child relationship. (0–1½ years)

Tools	Tasks
1. *Cry and other prespeech* vocalizations are powerful tools available to the infant to call to the attention of the adults his feelings and/or his needs and, thus, to communicate with them.	1. *Learning to count on others to gratify needs and satisfy wishes.*
2. *Mouth* is the tool for taking in (sucking), cutting off (biting), pushing out (spitting) or holding on to objects (mouthing or sucking) introduced by others in the situation.	a. Struggling to express needs.
	b. Accepting what is given with a feeling of comfort.
	c. Recognizing objects in his immediate environment, i.e. significant people and things.
	d. Directing emotional expression to indicate needs and wishes.
3. *The satisfaction response* occurs when the infant's biological needs are met and when a mutual feeling of comfort and fulfillment is emphasized by both. This is used by the infant as a tool in future relationships. . . . The needs of the infant are for nourishment, care and comfort. . . . The needs of the mother are to give these warmly to her infant.	e. Beginning to see himself as separate from others.
4. *Empathic observation* is a capacity arising in the infant which enables him to perceive the feelings of others as his own immediate feelings in the situation.	
5. *Autistic invention* is a primary unsocialized state of symbol activity which makes the infant feel that he is master of all he surveys. It is a tool with which the infant sees his environment in a highly personal way.	
6. *Experiments, exploration, manipulation* are tools the infant uses to get acquainted with himself and the things about him. These activities are directed toward making his environment more familiar and less threatening by the use of his mouth, eyes, arms and legs in reaching out, holding on, striking, feeling, rooting, playing, etc. Masturbating may start as an exploration of the body. Anxiety and autistic invention may enter in—becomes habit with comfort sought through one's self.	
7. Emergency reactions arise in response to situations perceived as threatening by the infant because they lead to reinforcement of feelings of helplessness and powerlessness. The infant responds by crying, increased motor activity or apathy. Patterns of behavior arise to communicate greater striving for help through increased struggle or greater dependency. The infant responds with	
a. *Fear* that is called out by external events such as a sudden loud noise, sudden movements (falling) or sudden changes in the situation.	
b. *Rage* that is called out by external obstacles that limit his efforts of expression.	
c. *Anxiety* that is the discomfort felt in infancy, which later becomes known as anxiety. It is empathized by the infant experiencing contact with the mother or mother surrogate who is tense or generally uneasy.	

Anxiety is communicated between people in relation to internal events that may lie outside of their awareness, i.e.

(1) One anxious person can make another person feel anxious.

(2) An individual may become anxious by concerning himself with an illusory image who makes him feel anxious.

Childhood.   The period of living which begins with the capacity for communication through speech and ends with a beginner need for association with compeers, i.e. when the child begins to form relationships with people of his own level who share his attitudes toward authority, activities, and the like. (1½–6 years)

Tools	Tasks

1. *Language* is a tool consisting of meaningful sounds used for verbal communication of needs and wishes.
2. *Anus* is a tool of childhood used for giving or withholding a part of himself to control significant people in his environment. It is used to express his feelings (satisfaction-dissatisfaction, comfort-discomfort, power-powerlessness) in response to his present situation.
3. *Self* is a tool made of reflected appraisals. The self-dynamism grows as it functions. The self perceives, organizes and uses experiences in terms of approval and disapproval, and inattends or dissociates experiences not in accord with awareness.
4. *Autistic Invention* in childhood is the tool through which thoughts, feelings and words have a magical power of fulfilling needs, wants and wishes.
5. *Experimentation, exploration and manipulation.* In childhood there is a refinement of these tools. The child's aggressive behavior, his pushing forth into the world, his exhibitionism, imitation, curiosity, increased locomotion (walking), masturbation, and parallel play are his ways of becoming further acquainted with himself and the things about him.
6. *Identification* is a tool which the child uses in an attempt to be like a person who is significant to him.
7. *Emergency reactions* (as defined in infancy) which are used in this era are anger, shame, guilt, and doubt.
8. *Anxiety* is now recognized as anxiety rather than discomfort. It disciplines attention and restricts personal awareness. With the aid of significant adults this energy can be used to focus on learning.
  a. *Anger*—destructive feeling—thoughts which arise in response to a frustrating situation.
  b. *Shame*—feeling of self-consciousness and/or embarrassment that arises because the child feels that there is something unacceptable about his thoughts, feelings, or actions.
  c. *Guilt*—feeling state made up of shame and anger directed against himself.
	1. *Learning to accept interference to his wishes in relative comfort.*
	  a. Identifying and accepting self.
	  b. Seeing to his own wishes in relation to the wishes of others.
	  c. Recognizing that he has the power to stand alone to some degree.
	  d. Beginning to separate from parent and associate with age mates with interest.
	  e. Awareness that postponing or delaying gratification of his own wishes, in deference to others, may bring satisfaction.

d. *Doubt*—makes the child hesitate and/or question what he should or should not do. It helps the child through consistent experiences, to see relationships and lays the groundwork for later consensual validation and critical thinking.

Juvenile.   The period of living which begins with the need for association with compeers and ends with the capacity to love, i.e., "When the satisfaction or the security of another person becomes as significant to one as is one's own satisfaction and security, then the state of love exists." (6–9 years)

Tools	Tasks
1. *Competition* is a tool of the juvenile era used in contesting for affection and/or status with others. It is comprised of all activities that are involved in getting to a desired goal first.	1. *Learning to form satisfying relationships with compeers.*
	a. Loving from family to compeers for gratification.
2. *Compromise* is a tool of the juvenile era which enables the child to give and take in a reciprocal relationship in order to maintain his own position.	b. Testing sharing activities, attitudes, values, and beliefs of the peer group.
	c. Distinguishing his different roles in the various social and authoritative situations.
3. *Cooperation* is a tool of the juvenile era which the child uses in maintaining his own position by adjusting and adapting to the wishes of others.	d. Acting out selected roles in his different situations.
4. *Experimentation, exploration, and manipulation.* In the juvenile era there is further refinement of these tools. The juvenile is experiencing learning as fun through cooperative play, recreation and sexual curiosity. These are his ways of becoming more aware of himself and the world about him.	

Pre-Adolescence.   The period of living which begins with the capacity to love and ends with the first evidence of puberty, i.e., characteristic sexual changes. (9–12 years)

Tools	Tasks
1. *The capacity to love* is a tool in the pre-adolescent era which enables the individual to express himself freely and naturally because he thinks as much of someone else as he thinks of himself. Tolerance, sympathy, generosity, and optimism flow out of this. (The capacity has its beginning in infancy with the satisfaction response.)	1. *Learning to relate to a chum of the same sex.*
	a. Identifying himself with peers of the same sex to the exclusion of peers of opposite sex.
2. *Consensual validation* is a tool in the pre-adolescent era which consists of talking things over, comparing notes with others and coming to a way of action. In this way, the pre-adolescent gets clear about himself and the world and is relieved of guilt feelings and anxiety.	b. Being more loyal to chum than to family members.
	c. Becoming creative through expression of self.
3. *Collaboration* is a tool in the pre-adolescent era which is a step forward from cooperation. Achievement is no longer a personal success in terms of "we." He moves from his desire to maintain his position in the group to derive satisfaction from group accomplishment.	

4. *Experimentation, exploration, and manipulation.* In the pre adolescent era there is still further refinement of these tools. The pre-adolescent is experiencing an interest in learning as a way of implementing future living. He shows signs of rebellion through restlessness, hostility, irritability, taking less responsibility and becoming less obedient. These are his ways of moving from "egocentricity toward a fully social state."

Early Adolescence.
The period of living which begins with the first evidence of puberty and ends with completion of psychological changes, i.e., primary and secondary sex changes. (12–14 years)

Tools	Tasks

1. *Lust* as a tool of early adolescence "is a state of dissatisfaction which orients awareness toward the tendency to integrate situations chiefly affecting the genital zone."
 2. *Experimentation, exploration, and manipulation.* In the early adolescent era there is continued refinement of these tools. The early adolescent is showing an intense interest in becoming an adult by actively rebelling against authority, engaging in fantasies and over-identifying with heroes, cliques, and crowds. This results in a further realization of himself as an individual in relation to other individuals.
 3. *Anxiety* as used by the adolescent is a tool which restricts awareness so that he may function productively despite his feelings of inadequacy and insecurity in his new role (guilt, shame, fears of not measuring up, or achieving full development). This is evidenced by his frequent moods of depression and exaltation.
	1. *Learning to become independent.*
	   a. Evaluating his own limitations and powers.
	   b. Examining and anticipating the consequences of his own decisions.
	   c. Evaluating critically ideals, beliefs, attitudes and values.
	 2. *Learning to establish satisfactory relationships with members of the opposite sex.*
	   a. Accepting himself as a sexual object.
	   b. Finding suitable sexual objects.

Late Adolescence.
The period of living which begins with the completion of the physiological changes and ends with the establishment of durable situations of intimacy, i.e., choice of love objects of opposite sex. (14–21 years)

Tools	Tasks

1. *The genital organs* are tools of the late adolescent era that are used for release of emotional tension through coitus in order that sexual satisfaction and procreation may take place.
 2. *Experimentation, exploration, and manipulation.* In the late adolescent era there is a special use of these tools in the sexual-social situation, i.e., in dating, dancing, sex play, socialized speech (repartee, "lines," jokes, etc). Through these the late adolescent learns to pattern genital and social behavior.
	1. *Learning to become interdependent.*
	   a. Tolerate anxiety and using it constructively.
	   b. Establishing reciprocal relationships with his parents.
	   c. Assuming responsibility for others.
	   d. Making decisions and choices of far reaching importance for his future.
	   e. Becoming economically, intellectually and emotionally self-sufficient.
	 2. *Learning to form a durable sexual relationship with a selected member of the opposite sex.*
	   a. Learning to verbalize consciously and to act out sexual interest.

b. Patterning of genital behavior.
c. Wooing and winning a mate with whom one develops
   (1) Willingness to share a mutual interest
   (2) Mutuality of orgasm
   (3) Willingness to share procreation
   (4) Willingness to regulate cycles of work and recreation.

The Author Comments

The Kansas theory conference was the first of its kind. My paper was written at the invitation of Catherine Norris, who had the vision to see how timely a theory conference would be for the nursing profession. The title of the paper supports my view that theory-directed practice is central to the professionalization of nursing. From 1948 to 1969, I was involved in theory development, with the help of graduate students who studied in programs in psychiatric nursing that I directed. Many concepts were formulated form clinical observations and interview data, tested during varied, supervised practice, and published in various journals and books. The paper summarized some of the major dimensions of what I had learned from that educative process in the previous two decades.

Since 1969, much work has gone forward on theory development in many different universities. In 1986, there are various lines of inquiry toward the formulation of nursing theories. The definition of nursing in the American Nurses' Association's 1980 publication *Nursing: A Social Policy Statement*, and the substantial work on nursing diagnosis since 1973, will give even further impetus to theory development. Theory is needed to explain the phenomena that nurses diagnose and as a guide to nursing treatments.

—HILDEGARD E. PEPLAU

Chapter 48

The Practitioner as Theorist

Rosemary Ellis

When Gulliver traveled to Laputa, land in the clouds, he found rapt theorists wandering about constructing useless ideas. And, generally, that is what we think of theorists. This author, though, says that theorists in nursing are not the ivory-tower thinkers; they are the nurses who work directly with patients. With every patient, she explains, we select an approach, then use, modify, and expand it—whether or not we are conscious of doing so. Because theories in a field have a powerful, long-term influence on the direction that field will take, the author pleads that we struggle to make already-existing, implicit nursing theories— such as TLC, for example—clear and explicit, so that nursing will develop in the direction of more skilled bedside care.

Nursing has been called an applied science. It is, in the sense that it is the application of knowledge from the basic sciences. But nursing care, or nursing practice, is something more. It is not the simple transfer of basic science knowledge. The nurse does not practice chemistry, anthropology, or sociology. She must sort out, select, adapt, and infer from her basic science knowledge. She uses some of the knowledge, orientations, processes of study, or models from these sciences as a guide to understanding patients, their pathology, and therapeutic practices.

This selection, adaptation, and sometimes interpolation from the basic sciences must be done by the practitioner. The physiologist or anthropologist cannot predict what specific knowledge or what concepts the nurse will need. The nurse must identify these, because what is needed depends on the specific purpose intended. The nurse, for nursing, uses some framework for her selection and adaptation. In this action she is a theorist. That is, some theory—often not made explicit—directs her selection of the knowledge or concepts to apply.

By "theory," I mean a coherent hypothesis, or set of hypotheses, or a concept, forming a general framework for undertaking something. Theory means a conceptual structure built for a purpose. For nursing, that purpose is practice.

But the practitioner cannot just select from a rack of ready-to-wear theories, because the knowledges and theories as we find them in the basic sciences are insufficient for practice. Instead, nursing practice requires that she structure converging, and sometimes conflicting, facts from the many fields which produce knowledge about human beings.

The nurse works within the framework of the inseparability and interdependence of one person's human life, so she attempts to relate aspects not yet clearly related in the separate sciences.

That is, we strive to act holistically, though our knowledge does not come for use from any holistic science of humans.

In this, the practitioner differs from the scientist. The scientist, due to reasons of control, feasibility, and measurement in study (due, as well, to the sheer impossibility of mastering all sciences, or even specialties within one science) isolates aspects for study. While the scientist may recognize the interrelationships of, for instance, physiologic and psychologic factors in man, he far less commonly studies these as a whole.

The practitioner of nursing, in contrast, may not have a complete science to nurse the whole man, but nurse the whole man is what she is striving to do. And, she sees the problems that result when one aspect or another is left out.

The practitioner of nursing thus finds herself working from a framework somewhat different from that within which knowledge is typically generated in the sciences. In this translation, the practitioner, of necessity, begins to restructure theory. She—often, at least—must apply the theory or concept in a way its originator may not have foreseen. She cannot simply take concepts from the sciences and directly apply them and hope to have the key to the biologic and psychosocial factors bound together in a patient, because this very interdependence is often a factor in response to and recovery from illness.

Generalities Don't Suffice

Further, because we attempt to nurse the individual, general theories cannot suffice. General theories of human behavior describe the typical or the norm, not the exception or the individual. Or, sometimes, they describe the extremes and not the middle range.

For example, it is a useful notion that self-preservation, both in a physical and psychologic sense, is a major element in human behavior that accounts for or explains much observed behavior. Yet it is not uncommon to see patients who do not act rationally for self-preservation. They appear to have some stronger motive for action. We also see heroic acts of self-sacrifice which are not easily explained by general theories of self-preservation.

As one moves from general theories about human behavior to those relevant to all of the helping professions, and then to those relevant to patient behavior, there is need for an increasing number of conditional statements. What applies is shaped by the context, roles, and, for patients, the physical status that presents. This is yet another reason why the professional is a theorist: she is the person who must identify the conditional factors; she has to make the conditional statements.

Related to this is the fact that the professional can encounter conflicting theories, with each supported by some evidence. If she is to take some action she must choose a theory, either consciously or not, for her action is not independent of history; it stems from some framework.

For example, the concept or theory that guides the common practice of encouraging patients to talk about their problems often is not made explicit. Verbalization is generally conceived to be a good thing. But does this concept support the practice in all circumstances for all patients, or explain clearly the exceptions? Theoretically, indiscriminate practice would seem to involve some risk. Do the reasons behind this concept identify the risks and the benefits? The practitioner who follows a practice based on theory must appraise and criticize the theory if she follows if in nursing patients. She must weigh the risks and benefits in a manner not required of the scholar who theorizes about a phenomenon in the specific or in general, but who does not treat the individual.

The scholar is often concerned with describing and predicting phenomena. He seeks objectivity, so he reduces, to the extent possible, the influence he may have on the variance due to the experimenter. He seeks to eliminate the human, personal element of the investigator.

This is the converse of a practice discipline. As Conant (1967) has highlighted, a practice discipline seeks not only to describe or predict phenomena, but to introduce change. Practice is goal-directed, not to the accumulation of knowledge, but to the prescription and implementation of activity to change natural outcomes to desired outcomes.

Therefore, the clinical testing of a theory is essential if it is used as a guide to practice. It is the professional practitioner who is able to criticize the theory in use, and determine its value for directing actions to achieve defined outcomes. In this she is not only a *user* of theory, but she may be a *modifier* as well. She is also a *chooser* of theory.

Consider a practice of encouraging a patient to verbalize about his operation. Talking about one's operation occurs frequently enough to have become a folk expectation and to have provoked joking. The frequency and persistence of the behavior suggests that there is some potency behind it. One could speculate, too, that there is possibly a folk norm for the time at which such talking is acceptable, excusable, and tolerated by friends and family. There may also be social norms for what content is acceptable. If such norms exist, and the patient exceeds these norms, he runs the risk of being cut off verbally or avoided by others. One hears complaints to suggest this happens.

Can this be avoided through nursing? From one theory it can be argued that if the nurse encourages a patient to talk about his operation, some of the need to continue talking about it can be extinguished, and the risk for the patient of annoying family and friends can be reduced.

But, from another theory, one could argue that if the nurse, an important figure for the patient postopera-

tively, encourages the patient to talk, conveys the expectation that he will talk—and thus, in effect, rewards the behavior—she may prolong or reinforce it, causing the patient to risk violating folk norms.

It is not the originators of alternative theories who can solve a possible dilemma for the nurse. It is the nurse as practitioner and user of theory who must resolve the dilemma—in action, in critique of action, and in further theorizing.

A universal practice of encouraging patients to talk about their feelings may be questioned from another orientation. A medical patient recently talked with one of my faculty colleagues about the graduate student who was caring for him. He could not understand what the student wanted of him. This student, in her clinical course work, had time to talk with patients, and had visited with the patient after she had completed the typical morning care activities of bathing and bed making. Her conversations were patient-focused but were not probing. She did not have any specific goal in mind except to interact with the patient and to get to know him.

This patient, however, told the instructor that he was an orphan, who had learned early that people do not do things for nothing. He interpreted the student's talking with him as evidence that she wanted something from him. This man viewed even conversation as something you get or give only in exchange for something or because you want something. For him, the nurse's attempt to learn more about him by talking with him was seen as a sexual advance. He could not imagine any interaction that did not have an exploitative motive. He was, therefore, made acutely uncomfortable by a very casual attempt by a nurse to encourage him to verbalize. Her motives were significantly misperceived, to the detriment of the patient (though one could argue that perhaps we learned more about the patient because of his discomfort).

There may also be instances where attempting to get a patient to talk about his feelings is contraindicated because it may dissipate the feeling. There may be instances where it is important for someone to experience and to recognize feelings *as feelings*. Talking about them may diminish them, objectify them, and so lose them as feelings. Joy is certainly one emotion that can be diminished by talking about it or attempting to explain it. I can recall an obstetrician father who was so profoundly moved by the birth of his own child that he burst into tears. The intensity of his own feeling totally surprised him, as well as his obstetrician colleagues. It seemed important for him to fully experience the intensity of his feeling and not diminish it until he had really felt it and absorbed it as his own feeling.

Lest I mislead, let me hasten to say that, in general, benefits seem to result from the practice of encouraging verbalization, but what are the exceptions? If benefits accrue, how are they explained? Practice could be more selective, and perhaps more effective, if we knew exactly what patient benefits to expect, and what dynamics would achieve them.

For example, benefits might be due to the patient's recognition, through talking, of the specific content of his feelings.

Benefits could also be due to the sense of companionship which can be achieved by talking with another, without regard for particular content. That is, would talking be effective without a listener? If not, what is supplied by a listener, even a nondirective listener, that is essential?

Is benefit derived from the recapitulation of an event which serves in some sense to produce mastery over, or integration of, the event, as in talking about one's operation? Or are benefits due to some reciprocal system where talking serves in place of some other potentially more detrimental form of discharge, such as acting out or somatization? Choose your theory. It is not likely to hold for all circumstances or cases, nor to support an invariate nursing practice of encouraging verbalization. Thus, the professional practitioner must become not simply a user of given theory, but a developer, tester, and expander of theory. This is not for the purpose of scholarship; it is an essential for intelligent practice.

The Need for Theory

It is essential because of the inadequacies in existing theories for the circumstances of nursing.

It is essential because of the need to synthesize, for practice, knowledge from diverse disciplines not yet fully related in theory.

It also is essential because the basic disciplines often are not pursuing the problems of importance to nurse and patient. For example, there is no extensive study, knowledge, or theory about appetite. As nurses we study nutrition, yet many of our observations and concerns with nutritional problems of patients are not solved by knowledge of nutrition. We need to know more about how to enable a patient to partake of the nutrients he needs, and about patterns of appetite in illness. For nursing, we need theories toward a science of appetite or of taste, and what happens to it in illness.

Conant (1967) gives an example of the complexities of a practice theory for back care: it must encompass maintenance of skin and underlying tissues, nutritional and fluid balance, and physical manipulation of the body. It is unlikely that the theory for back care will be developed from any other discipline than nursing. Existing theories guide the development of a field, because they guide what are seen as the interesting problems for study, the purposes for such study, and the ways in which problems are studied. Ways of defining problems, and of studying them, and what is considered worth pursuing are likely to differ from field to field. What may be significant problems for nursing may not fit with the theories, methods of study, or current focus of any other single field.

It is also unlikely that scientists in other disciplines will rush to collaborate with one another for study of a phenomenon because a nurse finds it important in nursing care. This is perhaps too pessimistic a view of collaboration in view of increasing evidence of interdisciplinary research. There remain, however, significant obstacles in orientation and method which impede cross-disciplinary research.

How Theory Is Built

Of course, we theorize without knowing we do it. A nursing student last fall was relating an experience she had while walking with a young child. The child had to smell every flower in a bush. The student told the child they would all smell alike, but he had to check out every blossom, just the same.

I commented that perhaps the child had made no generalization about flowers. He hadn't yet developed a notion that flowers that are shaped and colored alike, and grown on one bush, have a high probability of smelling alike. One could say the child was operating without any general concept of flower smell, and exploring each bloom was still an adventure.

Over time, the adventure may be lost and the child will conclude—or accept someone else's conclusion—that flowers that look alike, smell alike. And he'll spend time on other adventures.

Now it occurs to me that, not being a flower specialist, I have never really thought about similarities and differences in flower smells in any scientific way. As I think about it, I very much doubt that the visual cues I use to class flowers as the same—such as shape, color, type of petal, and so on—have very much to do with smell. I associate visual similarities with olfactory similarities—probably erroneously as to cause, but not erroneously from an empiric view. But it doesn't matter. I'm not the expert. I don't practice or teach others the practice of flower smelling. Only I suffer from my misconceptions. But if we all acted so confused about nursing matters, we'd be in trouble.

No skillful nurse could efficiently practice like the adventurous little child—testing every detail of every nursing action each time it appeared. Instead, she arrives at some generalizations and begins to accumulate some wisdom over time that allows her to group, to classify, to identify, to focus, and to select what she will spend time pursuing. She will reach at least my level of thinking about flowers and their perfumes—it may be erroneous, but it is at least a concept.

The professional practitioner quickly recognizes differences between patients, or their responses, and accounts for them. She may not do this deliberately or make her theory explicit but, nevertheless, she adjusts her approach, her expectations, and sometimes her activities, accordingly.

She also is theorizing when she *labels* patient behavior. Many nurses have learned to recognize and label behavior as rejection even when the cues the pa-

tient gives do not exactly duplicate any specific definition of rejection. We have in some sense extended this concept or the ideas about it.

Unfortunately, we often stop when we have categorized or labeled the behavior or speculated about its genesis, just as I stopped with color, shape, and odor because I had satisfied one level of understanding. But the skillful practitioner, contrary to me and my flowers, must test out her generalization, her framework. Further, she may have an obligation to change the behavior she has observed and labeled. But too often, when she does attempt to change it, she fails to make explicit the theory which guides her action, though she implicitly is operating from some framework toward some direction. Such framework is at least incipient theory. Recognition of patterns in patient behaviors is also incipient theory.

Everyday Theorizing

We are not sufficiently conscious of the extent to which we use theory in practice, nor of the extent to which we adapt theory in practice. We also rarely recognize when we create or develop theory in practice, yet it does happen.

It is not uncommon for a nurse to sense correctly that a certain patient is not going to be able to follow some prescribed regimen, or for the nurse to predict, correctly, a patient's negative reaction to some element of therapy. Sometimes these perceptions run counter to those of the physician or others. What has happened is that the nurse has related some element of behavior to acceptance of therapy or response to it, that the other persons have not included in their framework, for some reason. And, of course, the converse can be found. Such examples illustrate the differences in the theories that are used pervasively. When the nurse's perception and prediction differ from others, she has developed a different theoretical stance.

The failure to make theory explicit is sometimes from lack of awareness of how one structures something. We do not stop to think, or possibly are not really conscious of our framework. Much of our structuring may be preconscious. Certainly, some failure to make theory explicit is because the practitioner (of necessity, and rightly so) is interested in the goal of nursing care, and not the analysis of the perceptions and processes used to achieve it. Our focus is on action, not on the analysis of it. But if we really have a commitment to the future beyond the personal accumulation of wisdom from patient to patient, and if we wish to communicate this wisdom we must try to analyze our actions and formulate theories from them. We must have practitioners in nursing who are willing to be scholars as well and who have the interest, skill, and time to pursue the analyses and formulations and test them in practice.

A New Look at the Familiar

But there is another reason why theory may not be made explicit. It it because we may overlook the familiar, or perhaps we devalue it.

There is some danger of neglecting, or even rejecting, some of the traditional, familiar components in nursing as we grow in our emphasis on science and research. One such component might be what is termed TLC—"tender loving care." This something or this concept, which someone (it would be fascinating to know who) has tried to capture by a phrase, is non-scientific. We are not likely to do research on it. We do not have tools to measure it. Yet many nurses, as well as non-nurses, recognize it as an essential component in nursing for many patients.

Recently in teaching I used this vague concept, TLC, as a possible example of something that occurs in nursing for which we do not yet have a theory or perhaps, more precisely, that we have not theorized about, yet which we can sense. I felt the idea embarrassed several students. I think this regrettable, but I was not totally surprised. One of my friends has been collecting data from entering, middle, and graduating students from nine schools of nursing, baccalaureate and diploma, religious-affiliated and secular. These data included many, many examples of student dilemmas about expressing their feelings for patients. It would appear that a significant number of students enter with compassion for patients but quickly get the idea they must never convey feelings to patients. Rightly or wrongly, such an attitude will affect one's view of "tender loving care."

My own view is that tenderness and love are essential ingredients in nursing care. We need to theorize about these elements in nursing. Others have valued them as effective components in care, and occasionally TLC is actually prescribed—though I doubt the effectiveness of ordering it.

Whether or not you agree with this view about TLC, it is an example of a concept that exists, that is associated with nursing, that has been felt to be rather specific to nursing, but that we have not yet made explicit, nor yet fully conceptualized. We probably know, at least at a preconscious level, more about it than anybody else, for we can see it in so many diverse actions and situations. It does not seem unreasonable to suggest that theorizing about something as vague and yet as familiar as TLC might be valuable for understanding nursing.

At this stage in theory development I could entertain, even, the use of jargon—in the sense of a special professional language—to express some of the ideas in nursing. For instance, I would endorse the use of this term TLC for the purposes of taking about it until we can more precisely or more elegantly describe what we are talking about.

At this time in theory development it will be profitable to borrow or adapt concepts and theories from whatever source we can, if they will help us to understand and produce nursing. They must, however, be tested for their usefulness in guiding nursing practice in the arena of practice.

Intuitive exploration, speculation, trial and error, introspection, subjective impression—all can be used toward development of theory.

What is needed are attempts to make theory explicit, with tests of theories for nursing *in the practice* of nursing, and with further development or theories emerging *from the practice* of nursing.

Reference

Conant, L.H. (1967). Closing the practice-theory gap. *Nursing Outlook, 15,* 37–39.

The Author Comments

I wrote this article in an attempt to demystify the then-prevalent ideas that theory should be "grand theory" or that what was needed was some "theory" to justify nursing. As was evident from the literature and conferences at national meetings, there was great confusion as to uses of theory and why nurses as practitioners needed theory. With their emphasis on theory and research, nurse scientists often rejected or at least ignored the importance of phenomena of nursing practice.

—ROSEMARY ELLIS

Chapter 49

Nursing Science: The Theory-Practice Linkage

Maeona K. Jacobs
Sue E. Huether

The Status of Science in Nursing

Serious concern about nursing science and its relationship to practice is relatively new in nursing. Although word symbols related to science are familiar to most practitioners, their use evokes many and varied ideas, actions and attitudes. As Schlotfeldt states, "thoughtful nurses are now thoroughly convinced they need, but do not have a body of structured science to guide them in practice" (Schlotfeldt, 1971, p. 140). Perhaps the most certain statement to be made is that there is no consensus among nurses that nursing science exists, is of value to practice or should be pursued. When agreement about the value of nursing science prevails, debate centers around the direction it should take and the method of its derivation. Clearly there are many schools of thought about nursing science which are worthy of pursuit and which will contribute to the advancement of nursing.

The Nursing Tradition

Modern nursing has emerged from a tradition of apprenticeship with a strong image of servitude, humility and humanitarian aims. Good arguments can be made that the tradition still holds—that there has been little change in nursing. Our aims are still humanitarian, and if one reads Nightingale it is evident they have hardly altered. Certainly most of nursing still retains the humble image ascribed to us by professional peers and clients and perpetuated by ourselves. Moreover, most of the changes that have occurred can be argued to have resulted from societal forces such as the knowledge explosion, advances in technology, medical specialization, government policy and wars, rather than from challenges and diversity arising from within the profession.

These external forces will have less influence on nursing when it creates its own internal stimuli for

From Advances in Nursing Science, *October 1978, 1(1), 63–73. Copyright ©1978, Aspen Systems Corporation.*
Reprinted with permission of Aspen Systems Corporation.

About the Author

SUE E. HUETHER was born in Spokane and grew up in Rosalia, Washington, on a wheat farm. She received a B.S.N. in 1963 from the University of Washington, Seattle, then continued her education at New York University, earning an M.A. in 1966. She moved back west in 1966 and accepted a faculty appointment at the University of Colorado, teaching medical-surgical nursing on the graduate level. Before moving to Utah in 1972, she taught at Idaho State University, Pocatello, for 3 years.

At the University of Utah, Dr. Huether has held a number of appointments, including director of the Family Nurse Practitioner Program, research associate professor in the School of Medicine, associate professor in the Physiological Nursing Program, division director, and currently, interim Associate Dean for Academic Affairs in the College of Nursing. Combining her professional work with academic study, she received a Ph.D. from the University of Utah in 1981.

Clinically, Dr. Huether has always been interested in critical care and medical-surgical nursing. She believes that bioinstrumentation and advanced technology can significantly contribute to the progressive development of nursing science and practice. Dr. Huether is also very interested in nursing theory and the issues surrounding the development of theory. When asked about the future, she commented "Developing nursing's theoretical base for practice requires establishing systematic approaches for the incorporation of nursing theory into baccalaureate nursing curricula. There is an apparent failure in either the preparation of teachers to incorporate this content or the expectation that it is a necessary component of basic nursing education."

When asked about satisfactions she has experienced in nursing, Dr. Huether said "One satisfaction is feedback from patients and families that they were truly more 'healthy' and had a better quality of life because of the care they received from knowledgeable nurses. Another is observing students intellectually defend their rationale for a particular nursing act to physicians and other nurses."

change and redefinition based on knowledge and practice generated by nursing science. Unless and until nursing science emerges to define common goals and guide the practice of nursing, our profession can expect to gain very little control over its practice. Without science, 100 years hence we are likely still to be struggling against our traditional image, being directed in our functioning by others and having precious little control over the care provided to clients.

Present attitudes of nurses and others about scientific endeavors in nursing have strong historical roots. Early "nurses" received no formal training and often came from the undesirable element in society. By historical accident, when the Nightingale school was imported to North America, it came under the control of service institutions and did not remain autonomous as Nightingale advocated. The school's superintendent headed the hospital as well as directed the school. Under the pressures of this dual role there was little time to attend to the education of recruits.

During the 19th century, hospital schools proliferated quickly, necessitated by urban growth, industrialization and disease. A period of open recruitment occurred when virtually all who came were admitted for training. The recruits were women, a source of readily available manpower, who conformed to and perpetuated the image of nursing. Early reformers undertook brilliant, farsighted efforts to upgrade the educational preparation of nurses; however, they were not successful in moving this training into the mainstream of higher education.

With the medical school reform which followed the Flexner report of 1910, nurses were needed in even greater numbers to carry out medical tasks delegated to them as physicians became unavailable to staff wards. But the pattern for modern nursing was set. Young women were trained to fill service positions and were locked into a system which demanded obedience, humility and submissiveness. This pattern persisted despite the advent of national organizations in nursing, control by licensing, growth of college-based educational programs and the admonitions of several reports commissioned by governmental and private organizations.

Current Professional Features

Historical influences on professional nursing are evident in present professional characteristics. Nursing is a highly diverse profession. Its practitioners differ widely with regard to level of educational preparation, practice environment or location and area of specialization; they also differ greatly regarding their own role and objectives. Nursing appears, on the surface, to agree on common goals such as those expressed by the concepts of "caring," "health" and "intervention." However, when elements of the concepts are elicited, there proves to be much disagreement both about goals and the means of achieving them.

Multiple suborganizations exist within nursing to support and perpetuate interest group goals. Formally proposed changes which affect large groups of nurses initiate seemingly unending controversy. An example is the 1965 position paper of the American Nurses' Association on educational preparation of nurses which is still under debate today. The unclear goals of nursing are both a result and a cause of lack of clarity and disunity within the profession. Several factors contribute to this state of affairs. Since most nurses are women, they enter and practice nursing with strong and socially sanctioned loyalties to family as well as professional life. This leads to competing demands and conflicts between roles and to a lack of primary commitment to advancing the profession. This in turn works against the development of definite goals.

Without clear goals, nursing has experienced frequent shifts in approaches to care. The profession has seen the eras of team nursing and primary care, problem solving and nursing process, clinical specialization and humanistic nursing as well as technical and professional nurse classifications. Each of these may be viewed as nursing's attempt to come to grips with its purposes and the related educational and socialization processes. Thus today's nursing bears the burden of its heritage—diversity, fragmentation and amorphousness accompanied by confusion and anti-intellectualism.

The accounting appears bleak; however, nursing has always existed in some form and always will. Collectively, nurses are performing needed services and constitute a potentially powerful group of health care providers. Individual practitioners are making contributions which effect positive changes in individuals, families and communities. Moreover, attempts to improve the profession and its functioning are in evidence. Attempts to upgrade the profession's educational level by mandatory continuing education for licensure are underway. Unity is evidenced by groups attempting through legal and legislative processes to implement commonly held goals. There is debate and controversy in nursing, as well as participation in interdisciplinary and intradisciplinary communication and health care services. All this is occurring in the face of encroachment by numerous other groups providing health care services, and represents a collective commitment by nurses to advance the profession.

Advancing Nursing as a Science

Now, more than ever, the nursing profession needs cohesiveness. The concept of cohesiveness implies unity and dedication to certain processes of thought and action which give rise to an evolving and changing, yet known and communicated, goal. Nursing science provides coherence and unity and interrupts processes that fragment and confuse. Assuming cohesiveness to be a desirable goal, fostering the evolution of nursing science will hasten its advent.

What exactly is nursing science? Nursing science is the process, and the result, of ordering and patterning the events and phenomena of concern to nursing. Thus discussions of nursing science can be unclear about what is under consideration—the body of knowledge or the process of deriving that knowledge. This process-product ambiguity of science is discussed by Jacox (1974). In the present context, science refers to the method of inquiry, the process, as well as to the outcomes of that inquiry, the product.

The Nature of Science

Science is morally neutral. When science is equated with technology, one of its many products, the tendency is often to rebel against it, devalue its contributions and espouse humanism as an alternative. Although science is morally neutral, the uses to which it is put are based on values. Thus applications of science can be humanistic or hedonistic, good or bad. The point to be made is that science does not blindly move itself; it is directed toward some purpose.

Science is an attempt to organize experience. To quote Frank (1968):

> science advances through the formulation of a body of postulates and assumptions, a conceptual framework . . . (which) provides a coherent, internally unified way of thinking about the events and processes in each discipline for which it is relevant. This approach fosters the conception of science as a systematic and never ending endeavor . . . (Frank, 1968), p. 45).

Frank's conceptualization suggests that science is a *product* that advances, as well as the *process* by which it evolves. The two aspects are mutually dependent: science is a product created by a process and the process is directly dependent on the product created. Unsatisfactory notions of science are those which assume the existence of an elusive "truth" or which do not help to identify the high order relationships, or theories, that impart coherence.

The Structure and Functions of Science

All sciences function within an area of concern, that is, they deal with delimited events and concepts using specialized techniques. There is nevertheless much blurring of borders and overlap among sciences, especially ones that are interrelated. As scientific knowledge within a discipline advances, branches of the discipline develop and boundaries are extended and redefined. When sufficient differentiation occurs, a new discipline emerges with its own scientific processes. Thus differentiation within anthropology gave rise to the physical and social branches, each concerned with concepts of human beings through time but working with different subconceptualizations of humans consistent with its special interests.

Nursing has not yet achieved the status of a science. The practice of nursing is still directed by medical orders and institutional policy rather than being grounded in the findings of nursing research. However, the science of nursing is indeed evolving as can be seen in the increasing number of research publications, the integration of research content in nursing undergraduate and graduate curricula, the growth of doctoral programs in nursing, the increased federal funds for nursing research, and the development of centers for nursing research.

The major aim of science is to evolve theory. Theory can be variously conceptualized and defined. Herein it means a coherent set of verified relations useful for explanation and prediction, and consequently for control. Classification of facts, description of events and development of instrumentation do not constitute theory but are often required for the theory-building process. Theory, like science, is not static. Theories change as knowledge and concepts evolve. In the empirical sciences, theory depends on the existence of reality-based events and processes. Without nursing practice, nursing theory has no reality to theorize about or impose order on.

If nursing science has the ultimate goal of theory formulation, and if theories formulated are to explain, predict and control the practice of nursing, there must be an intimate and sustaining theory-practice relationship. Theory constructed without a serious consideration of practice will bear a tenuous relationship to practice. Conversely, practice without theory will be carried out intuitively.

Theory Construction in Science

What is the nature of such theory-practice inter-relationships, and how do they bear on nursing science? Answers to such questions require an understanding of how theory derives, that is, how it is constructed. Professional literature in other disciplines offers several approaches to the techniques of theory construction (Hage, 1972; Margenau, 1973; Suppe, 1977). In nursing, Dickoff and James (1968) are well known for their Theory of Theories and their advocacy of situation-producing theory. Strauss and Glaser (1967) espouse Grounded Theory, which derives from the systematic collection and analysis of data. Most nurses writing about theory have dealt with theory-related topics and examples of conceptual approaches to nursing rather than with techniques of theory construction. It is such techniques, however, that determine the theory-practice link.

A scientific system for evolving theory involves an interdependent process of linking concepts in theoretical formulations, such as models and conceptual frameworks, and empirically verifying the linkages in an on-going and evolving manner—a very complex task. According to Piotrowski (1971), there are four essential functions of all scientific theory systems: (a) concept definition, (b) concept representation, (c) formulation of theories and propositions, and (d) propositional validation. In nursing, the manner in which each of these functions is accomplished determines the theory-practice linkage, and hence the state of nursing science.

Choosing and Defining Concepts

Concepts, often called the building blocks of theory, are the most critical elements to be considered when theoretical formulations are undertaken, for they determine the direction of inquiry. Concepts are ideas deriving from perceptual experiences of properties, objects or events. The idea or the concept is different from the empirical referents that represent it. One can have an idea or concept of something without having directly experienced it. Two people do not experience the same event in exactly the same manner; therefore it is assumed that certain characteristics of experientially derived concepts are unique. Conversely, since perceptual experiences do have similar elements, certain attributes of concepts are assumed to be similar. The uniqueness of perceptual experience requires that concepts utilized in theories be carefully explicated.

Concepts change and evolve as empirical events are made known. The formulation and modification of certain concepts have occurred via technological ad-

vances which have made it possible to secure previously unavailable sense data. The concept of the atom has thus changed considerably since first proposed. However, concepts such as consciousness have changed less dramatically since precise and concrete empirical references still do not exist.

If theory and practice are to be directly related, concepts must evolve from or pertain to practice. This is the key to viable theory-practice linkages in nursing, for concepts comprise the theory. Not only must concepts evolve from, and relate to, practice—they must be operationalized in a particular manner.

For example, to formulate a theory useful in nursing practice, the concept of caring would be a likely choice for incorporation into theory. Caring, rather than curing, would be chosen—for curing is often considered to fall within the domain of medicine. The concept chosen, in this case caring, is determined by its fit within an acceptable definition of nursing practice. On the surface, caring seems a reasonable and prudent choice. However, its appropriateness is less clear when the concept is subjected to close scrutiny. Is curing a part of caring, and do physicians therefore also exhibit caring behaviors? Is cure a part of nursing, and if so what is cured? The nature of caring emerges as very complex, and whether or not caring or curing is acceptable behavior for nurses depends on how each concept is defined. Thus the theoretician in making theoretical linkages must choose a concept acceptable to most of nursing and carefully define it in an acceptable manner. This increases the possibility that theories built will be useful, and facilitates the communication within nursing which is needed to implement the results of scientific processes.

Empirical Referents

When concepts acceptable to nursing are defined in reference to practice, it is likely they will be operationalized in a manner ultimately useful to the profession. Unless concepts can be empirically referenced in practice, theories built on them cannot be tested or applied in the practice setting. The requirement that concepts be operationalized in practice tends to limit the breadth of concepts linked in propositional or relational statements. This in turn imposes limitations on the scope of theories derived.

The process of theory building, congruent with the conceptual definition, requires that, once defined, concepts be linked in relational statements; these conceptual links, empirically represented, must then be verified in reality. The nature of concept definition directs this process. For example, assume a theoretical formulation incorporating the global concepts of caring and stress were to be developed. These concepts are of concern to nurses and can be defined in many ways. Suppose the concept of stress were defined to include subcellular changes inaccessible to nurses outside the experimental laboratory. When stress is so defined and operationalized, the theory derived will be of little use to the practicing nurse. If theory which includes the concept of stress is to be useful, then stress must be empirically referenced in terms of behavioral manifestations or clinically available physiological indicators. This does not imply that stress can never be defined as subcellular change. However, it does mean that if finally conceived in these terms, such theory will not be directly useful in practice. The foregoing does not preclude the nurse from developing new means of quantifying important concepts, but the practice area will limit the possible operationalizations of concepts in practice theories.

Many nursing theorists incorporate broad and unfamiliar concepts into their theoretical formulations. These formulations, though useful, do not provide an immediate theory-practice linkage, and often they create an image of separatism between theoretician and practitioner. Broad concepts embody numerous interrelated, diverse and unclear empirical manifestations. They are thus not useful for prediction precise enough to permit control. These "molar" theories, so called because of their broad scope, appear to explain; but for different users, they explain differently since so much can be accommodated under their umbrella. Broad concepts within theories are not inherently bad; however, until they are carefully analyzed, categorized into subconcepts and their empirically verifiable rela-

tionships tested, their utility in guiding practice is limited.

The linking of concepts with their empirical manifestations is part of the scientific process. This operation requires a close relationship between theorist and practitioner. Once concepts are defined and explicated, potential referents for them are evident. Scrutiny of the practice setting for actual referents provides needed input to ensure that possible referents are not excluded and reasonable referents are chosen. The theorist, for example, may wish to reference the concept of stress using a paper and pencil test, along with arterial blood pressure measurements. The practitioner can suggest other references to represent the concept of stress, such as skin temperature or cardiac arrhythmia. The practitioner is also in a position to offer information about the feasibility of testing the theory, and about potential applications for it if it is verified.

Validation

Once formulated, conceptual linkages in the form of empirically referenced, theoretical propositions are validated. Validation in the practice arena is necessary for a viable theory-practice linkage. Practitioners, as well as theorists, are indispensable to the validation process.

To develop usable practice theory, the concepts chosen and the related formulations must be in what may be called the mid-range, that is, their scope must be sufficiently restricted to allow for clear definition, empirical operationalization and testing. These processes are indispensable to validation, and validation is essential for a theory to be confidently used in practice. Thus molar theory must be made mid-range or perhaps even molecular—that is, even more restricted—before it can be validated and implemented in practice without hazard. On the other hand, molecular theories focusing on concrete and narrowly operationalized concepts often do not take into account enough events to be useful in predicting the complex behavior encountered in nursing. Conceptual relationships in molecular theories may thus have to be combined to develop predictive capability.

Mid-range theories might be perfected out of the pain studies completed by Jacox and her associates (Jacox & Stewart, 1973). In these studies the concept of pain was central and a variety of treatment approaches were used in an attempt to alleviate it. For illustrative purposes, pain could be considered a subconcept of stress, while treatment measures employed could be linked with the concept of caring. Mid-range theories formulated from these studies might explain how pain could be relieved in like groups of clients by utilization of differing alleviative methods, method choice being determined in part by factors known to affect the pain sensation and pain-alleviation relationship.

It should be evident that theory can be variously derived. At any point in the theory-building process, the theoretician is concerned with concepts and their relationships. Concepts can be conceived and defined apart from or within the practice environment. Conceptual relationships may also be formulated either by purely cognitive processes or as the result of observation in the clinical laboratory. However, with an empirical verification requirement for theories, concepts must be defined and referenced in a particular manner: neither too narrowly nor too broadly. Empirical referents must be clinically available and feasible. If postulated conceptual relationships are found not to hold, practitioners may offer valuable suggestions for concept redefinition and operationalization, or for control of intervening factors.

Thus the process of nursing science requires that concepts be defined, operationalized, linked into relationships and verified. From verified conceptual linkages accrue the product, which is theory; and the theory explains and predicts nursing phenomena. Predictive power must be used within nursing to control its practice, so the process, among other things, can continue to exist. If the process of science in nursing is to result in a goal-producing product, the current practice of nursing must be linked with theoretical endeavors via the system of science.

In nursing, practice has not been illuminated and ordered by theory; that is, the process of nursing science has not existed in a significant degree, and the product of nursing science has been sparse. There are many reasons for the underdevelopment of nursing science, and they can be classified in many ways, i.e., historical, educational, political, economic and attitudinal. Also, to understand this underdevelopment, the self-fulfilling prophecy associated with the evolution and growth of scientific systems must be comprehended. When a discipline has poorly developed science—both process and product—it becomes difficult to initiate and advance science. Conversely, once initiated and moving, the process of science generates momentum which tends to perpetuate the development and evolution of product.

Attitudes and abilities of nurses are of paramount importance in promoting the evolution of nursing science.

Education for Nursing Science

Differing educational preparation within nursing breeds a multiplicity of aims and means which does not foster science. Nurses who have had limited exposure to theory do not appreciate the importance of developing and using it. Educating nurses to a high uniform level is necessary to the development of nursing science that is usable and used. Uniformly high educational levels will provide a common knowledge and process base. Legislation aimed at requiring the baccalaureate degree for entry-level practice is significant. Consideration should be given to requiring progressively higher degrees for entry-level practice. Today a great need for doctorally prepared persons exists, especially to fill research and clinical practice roles. The evolution of scientific systems requires the design and perfection of multiple tools, methodologies and instruments to validate propositional statements. Since nursing's concepts are extensive, their incorporation into theory requires practitioners with a variety of high-level educational preparation.

The shortage of nurses with doctoral preparation has greatly influenced scientific systems in nursing. The few available individuals uniquely prepared to develop nursing science have tended to work in administrative and teaching positions and have not made the contribution they might have in theory development and research.

Type of doctoral preparation is significant in directing the evolution of scientific systems. Nursing science needs persons with doctoral education in nursing; there is also a need for doctorally prepared persons in all nursing related disciplines. However, the critical requirement for persons educated at this level is not the area of preparation but the commitment to develop science in nursing.

Attention to educational approaches that foster high-level cognitive skills is significant to assuring the future development and use of nursing science. Nursing students must be taught how to think and analyze, and, more importantly, how to synthesize. Coursework that is both related to research, theory and philosophy and offers sound preparation in the content area of nursing is important; it will generate attitudes of inquiry and openness among nurses about values, means and ends, and thereby facilitate the development of science.

Certain attitudes within the nursing profession have formed barriers to the growth of nursing as a science. An important problem has been lack of receptiveness to new and different ideas. Ideas are not deadly, though many people act as if they were. The inability to listen, debate and examine unfamiliar, and perhaps unsympathetic, thought reflects the profession's insecurity. The practitioner must attempt to appreciate the efforts of the theorist, and the theorist must attempt to comprehend the problems of the practitioner—for nursing cannot exist without either. Further, no person can be expected to be the total embodiment of nursing—practitioner and scholar; only collectively can nursing be both.

Why should nursing be concerned with science? The evolution of nursing science will assure the survival of nursing. As theories evolve which allow for control of practice, the power to control that practice increases. Nurses must become the group of persons who know most about caring behaviors in health and illness. If nurses develop theoretical formulations which predict in practice, they will be able to care and they will be allowed to care. The power to care will come only from linking practice with theory, and this link will be made only through implementation of nursing science—the process—to create nursing science—the product.

References

American Nurses' Association (1965). American Nurses' Association first position on education for nursing. *American Journal of Nursing*, 65(12), 106–111.

Dickoff, J., & James, P. (1968). A theory of theories: A position paper. *Nursing Research*,, 17, 197–203.

Frank, L.K. (1968). Science as a communication process. *Main Currents in Modern Thought*, 25(2), 45–50.

Glaser, B.G., & Strauss, A.L. (1967). *The discovery of grounded theory: Strategies for qualitative research*. Chicago: Aldine.

Hage, J. (1972). *Techniques and problems of theory construction*. New York: John Wiley & Sons.

Jacox, A. (1974). Theory construction in nursing—An overview. *Nursing Research*, 23, 4–13.

Jacox, A., & Stewart, M. (1973). *Psychosocial contingencies of the pain experience*. Iowa City: University of Iowa Press.

Margenau, H. (1973). The method of science and the meaning of reality. *Main Currents in Modern Thought*, 29(5), 163–171.

Piotrowski, Z.A. (1971). Basis system of all sciences. In H.J. Vetter & B.D. Smith (Eds.), *Personality theory: A course book*. New York: Appleton-Century-Crofts.

Schlotfeldt, R.M. (1971). The significance of empirical research for nursing. *Nursing Research*, 20(2), 140–142.

Suppe, F. (1977). *The structure of scientific theories* (2nd ed.). Chicago: University of Illinois Press.

The Authors Comment

The thoughts contained in this article had been germinating in our minds for some years before they appeared in print. The immediate stimulus for writing the paper was the availability of a publication outlet in the form of *Advances in Nursing Science.* Before this time, our experiences in attempting to publish articles of this nature had been frustrating, as existing nursing journals did not regard them as consistent with their purposes. Professional trends that related to the nurse practitioner movement and independent practice for nurses, as well as the beginning of a doctoral program at the University of Utah, provided us with the impetus to examine our ideas about the *practice* value of traditional science for nursing. The article was an attempt to express our current thinking about the problem of uniting nursing practice and nursing theory by focusing on the utility of science for practice. In it, we considered how the basic ingredients of theory, and processes for its development, might serve as focal points for linking theory and practice.

Although the thoughts contained in the article are still generally subscribed to for theory as we defined it in this article, some comments about our current thinking seem important. First, we no longer contend that even the narrow brand of scientific theory considered in this article is morally neutral. Second, we no longer view theory as the *major,* or *ultimate* aim of legitimate nursing science. Third, we no longer exclusively subscribe to the definition of theory presented in the article, which reflected the nursing literature at the time the article was written. Since that time, our notion of theory has expanded considerably, and theory as "a coherent set of verified relations useful for explanation and prediction, and . . . control" would only constitute one type of theory. This brand of theory as science, though extremely useful, needs to be augmented with other forms of science, as well as nontheoretical ways of knowing, to significantly influence practice. Other factors affecting practice must also be examined and modified if science, more broadly defined, is to link theory and practice.

—MAEONA K. KRAMER AND SUE E. HUETHER

Chapter 50

The Notion of a Practice Theory and the Relationship of Scientific and Ethical Knowledge to Practice

Jan Beckstrand

By examining the relationship of scientific and ethical knowledge to practice, it can be shown that much of the knowledge required for practice is the knowledge of science and ethics. This brings the notion of the need for a practice theory in nursing into serious question since unique knowledge beyond that of science and ethics must be shown to be required in practice.

In recent years, several authors in different fields have considered the possibility of developing a practice theory that would be different from a pure scientific or ethical theory (Dickoff & James, 1968; Dickoff, James, & Wiedenbach, 1968; Greenwood, 1961; Jacox, 1974; Wooldridge, Skipper, & Leonard, 1968). In almost all these cases, practice theory has been considered to be a prescriptive theory leading to prescriptive directives for carrying out practice. However, for notions of a practice theory to be meaningful, four conditions must be shown to be true. First, practice knowledge must be shown to be different from the knowledge of science and ethics; otherwise practice knowledge would be reducible to these, and no need for a separate practice theory would exist. Second, one must be able to con-

struct a calculus (or a formal system of rules) on which to base a practice theory. Third, practice knowledge must be capable of universalization; i.e., it must be applicable to identical situations over time. Fourth, the application of practice knowledge must be useful in the attainment of the goals of practice.

In this paper, the first requirement is examined in an attempt to show that a practice theory is not useful to the progress of nursing science. Specifically, two primary aspects of practice knowledge, the knowledge of how to make changes and the knowledge of what is morally and nonmorally good, are shown to be identical to scientific and ethical knowledge. As a consequence, the question of whether practice knowledge is reducible to science and ethics is critically raised.

About the Author

JAN BECKSTRAND is a Texan, born and raised in El Paso. She currently holds the joint position of Assistant Dean of Clinical Research, Indiana University School of Nursing, and Director of Clinical Research for Nursing Services, Indiana University Hospital, Indianapolis, Indiana. Dr. Beckstrand received a B.S.N. from the University of Texas-Austin in 1971 and a M.S. from the University of Colorado in 1973. She returned to the University of Texas-Austin and earned a Ph.D. in Nursing in 1978; her dissertation was titled *A Conceptual and Logical Analysis of Selected Health Indicators.* She also holds a M.S. in statistics from Texas A&M University and has completed extensive coursework toward a doctoral degree in statistics.

Dr. Beckstrand has worked in neurology, neurosurgery, and general medical-surgical nursing. She held an assistant professorship at the University of Minnesota in Minneapolis from 1978 to 1981, where she taught graduate-level theory courses and was a thesis advisor to graduate students.

She is a member of the American Nurses' Association, Sigma Theta Tau, Sigma Xi, and the American Statistical Association.

According to Dickoff and James (1968), one may characterize a theory as a conceptual system developed to some purpose that fulfills the goal for which it was developed. Following this guide, one may begin the investigation of whether practice knowledge is reducible to scientific and ethical knowledge by comparing the knowledge used to achieve the purposes of practice with the knowledge of science and ethics. Only if these can be shown to be substantively different, can practice be said to entail knowledge beyond the legitimate boundaries of science and ethics.

It is generally agreed that the purpose of science is to describe, to explain, and to predict natural and social phenomena. The purpose of ethical or normative theory is to describe and to predict what actions and characteristics will lead to the realization of morality and goodness. Finally, the purpose of practice is to bring about changes in entities such that a greater degree of defined good (value) is realized or becomes increasingly capable of being realized.

Science and Practice

The determination of whether practice knowledge is reducible to scientific knowledge depends on whether the knowledge used for accomplishing control in practice is the knowledge of lawlike empirical relationships. This is true because lawlike empirical relationships are the subject of science, and it is the knowledge of these and their empirical implications that constitutes scientific knowledge. An examination of the knowledge of each discipline will show that the knowledge used to control phenomena in practice is the knowledge of lawlike empirical relationships, and hence it is identical to scientific knowledge.

Scientific Knowledge

Science is concerned with identifying lawlike empirical relations, with confirming or corroborating their factual nature, with describing and explaining them, and with determining their interrelationships and their empirical consequences. (Hempel, 1965; Nagel, 1961; Popper, 1968) What causes an apparent lawlike relationship to be elevated to the status of a scientific law is that several different phenomena predicted on the basis of the law have been consistently realized or prevented under specified conditions (Hempel, 1965). The fact that an apparent lawlike relationship may be elevated to a scientific law on the basis of this evidence is a result of the characteristics of the deductive process used in the confirmation of natural laws.

Scientific knowledge is predicated on the notion of predictive certainty that is entailed in valid deductive arguments (Hempel, 1965; Popper, 1968). Predictive certainty, and hence the knowledge of empirical laws, is realized through the valid deduction of specific factual consequences from a set of theoretical definitions, a set of lawlike propositions, and a set of specifiable initial conditions. If the conditions and lawlike relationships are true, logical deduction allows one to expect to bring about the occurrence of the predicted factual event. If the event does not occur, then either the conditions or the proposed law must be considered to be false. In hypothesis testing, scientists use deductive arguments to test the factual nature of proposed scientific laws by predicting and attempting to realize the occurrence of deducible factual consequences.

The potential for controlling a phenomenon is synonymous with lawlike relationships and the potential for prediction that they provide. The knowledge requisite to scientific control rests in the valid deduction of demonstrable factual consequences from confirmed lawlike relationships. To control the phenomenon, "If A, then B," is to initiate the occurrence of the sufficient condition, "A," or to prevent the occurrence of the necessary condition, "B," in a valid logical deduction. This allows the realization of the respective conclusions, "B" or "not A" ("—A"), if the law is true and the initial conditions are met.

A condition or set of conditions are sufficient for the occurrence of an event if and only if whenever the set of conditions is present, the event is also present (Skyrms, 1975). For example, falling from the top of the Empire State Building is a sufficient condition for death. A condition or set of conditions are necessary for the occurrence of an event if and only if whenever the event is present, the conditions are also present (Skyrms, 1975). For example, as far as we know, water and organic matter are necessary conditions for life (Skyrms, 1975). The negation of a necessary condition is sufficient for the negation of the event. For example, if there is no oxygen, one cannot live.

Symbolically, these two valid forms of logical argument can be represented as:

$$\text{"If A, then B" is true}$$
$$\underline{\text{And A is made to occur,}}$$
$$\text{then B must also occur}$$

and

"If A, then B" is true
and B is preventive from occurring,
then A cannot occur.

In words, these would mean that if the lawlike proposition "If loss of blood supply, then gangrene" is true and a loss of blood supply occurs, then gangrene can be expected to follow. In addition, if gangrene is prevented from occurring, it can also be expected that a loss of blood supply will not have occurred.

Speaking more generally, the process of scientific control may be represented as follows:

$$\text{If } L_1, L_2, L_3$$
$$\text{and } C_1, C_2, C_3$$
$$\underline{\text{and A or } -B,}$$
$$\text{then E.}$$

Here L_1, L_2, and L_3 represent scientific laws of the form "If A, then B,"; C_1, C_2, and C_3 represent conditions under which the laws are true; and E represents the result of the laws' operation (Hempel, 1965).

When a law is quantitative, control may be conceptualized in terms of incremental, decremental, or reciprocal relationships. Thus, to control B may mean that one will increase, decrease, or hold A constant. In addition, control may involve altering the conditions for the operation of a law to produce the states under which the law is applicable. Diagrammatically, this can be expressed as follows:

$$\text{If } L_1$$
$$\underline{\text{and } S_1(C_1, C_2, C_3),}$$
$$\text{then } E_1$$

or

$$\text{If } L_1$$
$$\underline{\text{and } S_2(C_4, C_5, C_6),}$$
$$\text{then } E_2.$$

By creating the situation S_1 for the operation of a law, some result of the law's operation, say E_1, can be produced; and by altering the situation to S_2, the former result of the law, E_1, can be changed to E_2, and controlled. Science seeks to establish the knowledge that allows for this kind of control, and this is the knowledge of sufficient and necessary conditions for the occurrence of empirical phenomena.

Control in Practice

To accomplish change one must be able to exercise some control over the relevant variables operating in a situation. Therefore, practice requires the knowledge of scientific laws and logically valid relationships, but in practice attempts to control phenomena may be made on the basis of the invalid forms of deductive arguments, on functional arguments, and on empirical generalizations. All these methods are based on the knowledge of scientific laws and logical relationships, but they lead to uncertain conclusions because the reasoning processes being used are not deductively valid. It is this fact that may account for the belief that practice requires some special knowledge beyond the knowledge of science and ethics.

The invalid argument forms are the reverse of valid arguments in logic. These are called (a) the negation of the antecedent and (b) the assertion of the consequent (Salmon, 1973). In contrast to valid deductive argument forms, the truth of the premises in invalid deductive arguments does not ensure the truth of the conclusion. The reason that these invalid forms do not lead to true conclusions, given true premises or scientific laws, is that one is asserting or implementing necessary rather than sufficient conditions for the occurrence of the conclusion of the logical argument.

For example, in practice one might wish to argue that "if ventricular tachycardia (VT) exists, then ventricular fibrillation (VF) is soon to follow," and "if one can alleviate the tachycardia, then fibrillation can be prevented." Diagrammatically this can be represented as follows:

If VT, then VF
and if the condition "not VT" can be realized,
then the condition "not VF" will follow.

This is the opposite of the valid forms of logical argument. Instead of an argument of the form

"If A, then B"
and A occurs,
then B occurs;

we have an argument of the form

"If A, then B"
and A does not occur,
then B does not occur.

On reflection, one can easily see why the first argument form leads to a certain conclusion and the second does not. The absence of an antecedent condition like ventricular tachycardia in the lawlike proposition "If VT, then VF" cannot ensure with certainty that ventricular fibrillation will not occur. Ventricular fibrillation may result even though ventricular tachycardia is not present. Alleviating the tachycardia will prevent fibrillation ensuing from tachycardia, but it will not prevent fibrillation which may result from many other factors that may exist in the situation.

In using invalid logical forms like this to control situations, one cannot predict with certainty that the desired conclusion will result because only a necessary and not a sufficient condition for the occurrence of the result has been realized. These logical forms do not afford predictive certainty, but they are frequently utilized in practice.

Closely related to invalid deductions from scientific premises are a class of relationships called "functional relationships." These are being used when a series of necessary conditions for an occurrence is brought about as a means of controlling the situation. An example of how this kind of argument is used in practice is as follows: water, oxygen, nutrients, respiration, and so forth are necessary for life; therefore to maintain life, provide these. The fallacy is similar to those encountered in invalid deductions since providing any number of necessary conditions will not maintain life even though it is certain that life cannot be maintained without them.

Finally, control in practice is often facilitated by the use of empirical generalizations and other forms of inductive arguments. Empirical generalizations are based on regularities known in experience for which no scientific explanation has yet been given. In fact, it is these kinds of regularities that science seeks to explain and to validate as scientific laws. An example of this type of control formulation is the use of aspirin for fever and headache. It is used because it is known from experience that it works, but no scientific explanation exists for explaining why it works. The logic of this situation is inductive; and there is no scientific reason like that afforded by a scientific explanation that allows us to expect that the empirical generalization will work in any given situation.

In addition to the use of reasoning methods that do not logically afford predictive certainty, practice differs from science in the amount of predictive certainty that is realizable even when control methods are validly derived from scientific laws. The control afforded by valid deductions and scientific explanations depends on how closely conditions in practice reflect the initial conditions necessary for the working of a given scientific proposition. For example, a popliteal bypass may restore circulation in the extremity, but it will only do so if circulation above and below the bypass is reasonably patent. This leads to three additional possibilities: one in which control is certain because it is based on scientific laws and on the replication of conditions specified as necessary for the operation of scientific premises in valid arguments; and two in which conditions vary from the ideal.

In these latter two cases, it can be said that even though control methods are based on valid deductions from scientific laws, they are still uncertain. This is due to the fact that conditions for valid deductions from laws can vary in practice in two ways. The conclusion of valid scientific arguments will be true if and only if (a) certain auxiliary conditions exist in the situation and (b) no other intervening sufficient conditions are operable. Neither of these assumptions can be supported consistently in practice. Even though practice methodology proceeds by valid deduction from scientific laws, the outcome may be uncertain if the initial conditions for the laws' operations are not met and intervening conditions are uncontrolled and operating in the situation.

Therefore, practice utilizes scientific knowledge in attempting to control phenomena, but allows the use of reasoning processes that do not provide predictive certainty. These reasoning processes describe the methodology of control in practice. As a consequence, it may be concluded that even though the methods used for control in practice are different from those used in science, the knowledge on which these methods are based is the same. This is the knowledge of lawlike empirical relationships and logical reasoning. Science uses the knowledge of logical relationships and apparent empirical relationships to establish scientific laws and to predict empirical events; practice uses the knowledge of science and logical relationships in attempts to alter undesired empirical events.

Ethics and Practice

The field of philosophy known as ethics is concerned with the knowledge of what is right, good, or obligatory. The branch of philosophy dealing with these questions is called normative ethics. In normative ethics, one is primarily concerned with determining a set of acceptable standards for appraising moral obligation, moral value, and secondarily, nonmoral value (Frankena, 1973; Taylor, 1972). Another area of concern within the field of ethics is known as metaethics. Metaethics is concerned with such problems as the logical, the epistemological, and semantical meanings of ethical terms; the justification of ethical judgments and value judgments; the distinction between moral and nonmoral; and the meaning of the notions of freedom and responsibility. Both normative ethics and metaethics have relevance to practice and to the discussion of whether practice knowledge can be reduced to the knowledge of science and ethics. An examination of the knowledge of ethics and the knowledge of practice will show that the knowledge used for determining the moral conduct of practice and for determining the goals of practice is the knowledge of moral obligation and moral and nonmoral value.

Moral Obligation

One of the problems considered in normative ethics is the question of moral obligation. Theories of moral obligation are concerned with developing standards for deciding what a person ought to do in a given situation. Therefore, they provide a basis for determining what actions are morally right. In examining the relationship existing between ethical theories of moral obligation and practice knowledge, one can see, first, that general theories of moral obligation are equally relevant to people regardless of any special role they might play in society.

However, it is usually the case that practitioners in different fields are bound, in addition, by a special set of moral obligations, which are specifically applicable to their roles as practitioners. For example, physicians are considered to be bound by a special theory of moral obligation which is reflected in the Hippocratic Oath and in codes of professional conduct. Still, theories of the special moral obligations of practitioners are identical in form to other theories of moral obligation. The only difference is that in ethical theories specific to practitioners, the agent is defined not as all reasonable people, but as a certain group with capacities for certain actions not held by others. As a result, the special moral obligation is limited to members of this group. Nevertheless, a theory of moral obligation in practice is an ethical theory.

Moral Value

A second topic of normative ethics is the theory of moral value. Theories of moral value are concerned with standards for evaluating the moral goodness or badness of people and their attributes. As with moral obligation, ethical theories of moral value may arise in practice because of the extraordinary skills of practitioners in certain situations. However, like theories about moral obligation, theories of moral value in practice do not represent unique forms of theory. Rather, these are merely ethical theories which assume that the agent holds special capacities for action not held by others.

This means that if one were to construct a theory of the moral obligations for practitioners or a theory of the moral virtues of practitioners, in both cases one would have an ethical theory and not a practice theory. Therefore, the moral knowledge used in practice derives solely from ethical knowledge and not from some special form of knowledge in practice.

Nonmoral Value

We are left, then, with the theory of nonmoral value. Here, one is concerned with the ascription of the qualities of goodness and badness on nonmoral grounds to things like cars, hospital care, and movies; to the outcomes or results of actions like nursing interventions; and to people and their traits. These are known as value judgments. Value judgments imply that a thing is good in particular or in general with reference to some standard. For example, a thing may be regarded as good because it is good in itself or because it is useful for some purpose.

If a thing is considered good because it is useful for some purpose, it may be called a utility value. Other things may be considered good either because they are means to a good end or because the experience of them is good. These are called, respectively, extrinsic values and inherent values. Two other types of nonmoral values are intrinsic values and contributory values. Intrinsic values are things that are considered good in themselves as ends. Contributory values are things that contribute to or add to good experience. A thing may be good in more than one of these senses, or a thing may be considered to be good in one sense and not to be good in another.

Instrumental Values

In addition, one may also observe that some of these values can be classified together as instrumental values. These are values that lead to the achievement of an end or goal (Hempel, 1965). Instrumental values would include utility values, extrinsic values, inherent values, and contributory values.

The fact that several different kinds of values can be viewed as instrumental values is relevant to the relationship between science, ethics, and practice. Instrumental value judgments are reducible to empirical assertions that are amenable to scientific testing and explanation. According to Hempel, an instrumental judgment of value asserts either that [a course of action] M is a (definitely or probably) sufficient means for attaining the end or goal G, or that is a (definitely or probably) necessary means for attaining it (Hempel, 1965, p. 85).

This means that the knowledge of instrumental value is scientific knowledge, and it can be used in practice in the same way.

However, the practitioner often needs to know more than that a particular course of action will lead to a certain result or goal. Most practitioners must frequently determine which course of action among several alternatives is the best in a particular situation, and it is this question that one seeks to answer through normative theories of the intrinsic value of a thing, an event, an act, or a person.

Intrinsic Values

Intrinsic values are those things considered to be good in themselves. An ethical theory of intrinsic value is concerned with determining what is good in itself as an end and what standards or norms one might use to determine what is good in a nonmoral way. Like questions of moral obligation and moral value, the knowledge of what is intrinsically good in practice does not differ in form from the knowledge of what is good as an end in ethical philosophy. Again, the theory of value in practice is simply the ethical theory of value applied to a special case or set of unusual circumstances.

The goals of practice must be either intrinsic values considered good in themselves as ends or derivative values considered to be instrumental for achieving intrinsic values. Derivative values in practice can be justified because they are instrumental to the realization of intrinsic values, but the intrinsic values ultimately used to define the goals of practice must be justifiable as intrinsic values within an ethical theory of nonmoral value. For example, for the promotion of a healthful life, the cure of disease, and the education of the gen-

eral public to be considered valuable as ends in practice, they must be considered valuable in relation to intrinsic values held within some ethical theory of value.

Conclusion

In this paper, the question of whether practice knowledge is different from scientific and ethical knowledge has been addressed. It has been shown that (a) the knowledge used to make changes and to control phenomena in practice is the knowledge of science and logic, (b) the knowledge used to direct the moral conduct of practice is the knowledge of moral obligation and moral value, and (c) the knowledge used to define and to justify the goals of practice is the knowledge of nonmoral value.

Dickoff and James (1968) characterized theory as a conceptual system developed for some purpose that fulfills the goal for which it was intended. The purpose of practice is to bring about changes in entities such that a greater degree of defined good (value) is realized or becomes increasingly capable of being realized. Considering the findings of this paper, it appears that science and ethics are conceptual systems that may completely fulfill the purpose of practice when used in conjunction with the activity of the practitioner and client.

Therefore, it would appear that there is no need for a practice theory distinct from scientific or ethical theory. As a consequence, one might revise the definition of the purpose of practice to say that the goal of modern "scientific" practice is to bring about changes in entities through scientific and moral means so that a good that is acknowledged and defined within the ethical theory of value is realized or becomes increasingly capable of being realized. The knowledge of moral obligation, moral value, and nonmoral value is required in practice, and it is identical in form to the knowledge of these questions in ethics. The goals defined in practice are nonmoral values which may be determined by the methods of ethical philosophy and no others. In addition, the knowledge used in practice for achieving these goals is the knowledge derivable from science, logic, and theories of moral obligation.

References

Dickoff, J., & James, P. (1968). A theory of theories: A position paper. *Nursing Research, 17,* 197–203.

Dickoff, J., James, P., & Wiedenbach, E. (1968). Theory in a practice discipline: Part I, Practice oriented theory. *Nursing Research, 17,* 415–435.

Frankena, W.K. (1973). *Ethics* (2nd ed.). Englewood Cliffs, NJ: Prentice-Hall.

Greenwood, E. (1961). The practice of science and the science of practice. In W. Bennis, K.D. Benne, & R. Chin (Eds.), *The planning of change.* New York: Holt, Rinehart and Winston.

Hempel, C.G. (1965). *Aspects of scientific explanation.* New York: Free Press.

Jacox, A. (1974). Theory construction in nursing. An overview. *Nursing Research, 23,* 4–13.

Nagel, E. (1961). *The structure of science: Problems in the logic of scientific explanation.* New York: Harcourt, Brace, and World.

Popper, K.R. (1968). *The logic of scientific discovery* (2nd ed.). New York: Harper and Row.

Salmon, W.C. (1973). *Logic* (2nd ed.). Englewood Cliffs, NJ: Prentice-Hall.

Skyrms, B. (1975). *Choice and chance: An introduction to inductive logic* (2nd ed.). Encino, CA: Dickenson.

Taylor, P.W. (Ed.). (1972). *Problems of moral philosophy.* Encino, CA: Dickenson.

Wooldridge, P.J., Skipper, J., & Leonard, R.C. (1968). *Behavioral science, social practice, and the nursing profession.* Cleveland: Case Western Reserve University Press.

The Author Comments

My two 1978 papers and my 1980 paper on practice theory were originally one paper that I wrote as a doctoral student at the University of Texas-Austin. Prior to entering the doctoral program, I had studied philosophy of science on my own, reading Popper's *Conjectures and Refutations* (New York: Harper Torchbooks, 1968) and other works. This allowed me to take a series of colloquia on philosophy of science and metaethics outside of the nursing department in the fall and spring of 1975 to 1976. I had trouble deciding on a final paper tonic for metaethics and still had not completed a paper for the course when I took Dr. Lorraine Walker's course on the philosophy of nursing theory. We studied Dickoff and James *again*, along with many of their predecessors and critics. I decided to try to use what I had learned in each of these courses to evaluate the notion of a prescriptive practice theory and to submit the paper as a final paper in both nursing and metaethics. The topic interested me very much and the result was a 75-page paper for which I happily received the course credit I desired. In addition, Dr. Walker gave me excellent criticisms and suggestions.

I decided to rework the paper for publication when I began job interviews and found that several schools were planning to base doctoral course work in theory development exclusively on various (and often ambiguous) notions of practice theory. I thought this trend was a serious mistake for nursing.

I believed that the brevity enforced in many nursing articles made what would have been valid arguments appear as mere statements of opinion. I thought the logical development of my paper was important and I submitted it whole, mainly hoping that it would be good enough to be published as a monograph or in several parts. I sent the entire paper with some explanation to *Nursing Research*, but the editor sent it back without reading it, saying it was obviously too long. I then contacted *Research in Nursing and Health* by phone. Dr. Harriet Werley, who is extremely patient and always polite, suggested I divide the paper into shorter parts before the review. I rewrote the paper in three parts, making substantial changes, and Dr. Werley sent the three for review sequentially (to save work, I suppose, in case the first had been rejected).

Because the papers were reviewed sequentially, much time elapsed before I received the reviews—especially for the second and third papers. This allowed me some distance from which I could evaluate my work, and again I rewrote substantial portions of the second and especially the third papers. At least some of the continuity of the argument was lost in the process. I regret deleting some of the arguments in my second paper because I thought it would be too long. Other aspects of the papers were very much improved. In all cases, the comments on the reviewers were very helpful to me in developing this series of articles.

—JAN BECKSTRAND

The Need for a Practice Theory as Indicated by the Knowledge Used in the Conduct of Practice

Jan Beckstrand

By examining the knowledge used in the conduct of practice, the knowledge required for practice can be shown to be completely reducible to science, ethics, and logic. Consequently, all notions of a practice theory in nursing are likely to represent some combination of these kinds of knowledge. As a result, no need for a practice theory exists.

In a recent article (Beckstrand, 1978), four requisites for evaluating the meaningfulness of a practice theory were outlined. First, the conduct of practice must require theoretical knowledge beyond that supplied by existing knowledge systems such as science and ethics. Second, a calculus of practice must be constructable. Third, practice knowledge must be capable of universalization. Fourth, practice knowledge must be useful in attaining the goals of practice. From an examination of relationships of science and ethics to practice, Beckstrand (1978) concluded that the aims of practice can be achieved using the knowledge of science and ethics alone. However, the discussion did not demonstrate conclusively that practice knowledge was completely defined by the knowledge of science and ethics since some other heretofore unformalized theoretical knowledge might still be required in the conduct of practice.

One way to test whether practice requires a knowledge system other than science and ethics is to examine the knowledge used in the conduct of practice. Through this process, the knowledge used in thinking and making decisions becomes apparent. By examining this knowledge in relationship to science, logic, and ethics one can determine whether practice requires something more. In this article, the knowledge required in the conduct of practice is examined in an

From Research in Nursing and Health, *1978, 1(4), 175–179. Copyright © 1978, John Wiley & Sons, Inc. Reproduced by permission of John Wiley & Sons, Inc.*

effort to assess whether the theoretical knowledge used in practice is completely defined by science, ethics, and logic.

Change and Action

One may begin to determine what knowledges are used in the conduct of practice by analyzing the knowledges implied in the definition of the purpose of practice. Practice attempts to *change* an entity or phenomenon in such a way that a *greater good is realized*. Therefore, practice requires knowledge of change. Accomplishing change in practice necessitates action, so practice requires the knowledge of both change and action.

As has been shown (Beckstrand, 1978), the knowledge of what is needed to make a change is scientific and empirical. In addition, the knowledge of the actions required to make changes is scientific, ethical, and psychomotor. However, there may be a knowledge of change and of action that is distinct from the usual kind of scientific knowledge and from the usual kind of propositional logic related to events. This is the knowledge of change and of action in themselves. While this knowledge is empirical and logical, it may be different from the knowledge of necessary and sufficient conditions for events.

For example, one way change can be represented is suggested by von Wright's (1963) expressions of the forms "pTp, pT-p, -pTp, and -pT-p." In these expressions, "T" stands for "transpose or change," and "p" or "-p" stands for events. To say "-pTp" is to say that an event capable of change is being transformed. For example, if "-p" stands for the event "a closed window," and "p" stands for "an open window," the expression "-pTp" stands for the act of opening the window.

Similarly, action is susceptible to logical and empirical analysis as a phenomenon in itself. Among the many authors who have addressed the question of the logic of action are Chisholm (1966), Davidson (1967), and von Wright (1963, 1967). The logic of action entails the logic of change, but it is more complex. Nevertheless, the determination of the empirical process of change and action lies within the legitimate boundaries of science, and the logic of both action and change rests within the domain of logic in general. In this regard, the knowledge of change and action required in practice is describable within the knowledge of science and logic, while the morality and value of action and change is the concern of ethical philosophy

A Description of Practice

The conduct of practice requires the knowledge of science, ethics, and logic in general (Beckstrand, 1978), as well as specific scientific and ethical knowledge of change and action. Can these knowledge systems, however, be used to answer *all* the questions that arise in the conduct of practice?

In determining what changes to bring about in a particular situation, the practitioner is required to answer several questions: (a) What conditions exist in the situation? (b) Which conditions need to be changed? (c) What outcomes are scientifically and practically possible to achieve within the situation? (d) What is the relative value of changes and their outcomes in terms of the desired ends? and (e) Which of the possible outcomes represents the greatest good that can be achieved in the situation?

Conditions

To be able to practice, a practitioner must first identify the conditions that exist in a situation. How this is accomplished can be understood by examining the structure of practice situations. In general, a practice situation results from two distinct sets of conditions. These sets depend on the source in the situation from which they derive. The first set consists of the conditions defining the client's situation, and the second is composed of the conditions defining the circumstances of practice.

The client's situation refers to all the empirical conditions—both deductive and inductive implications—that characterize the client. For example, the conditions in the client's situation would include the totality of the person's life experience as well as the meaning the individual assigns to the current situation. In addition, the client's situation would include the client's abilities, limitations, and expectations. In contrast, the circumstances of practice refer to all the empirical conditions and their logical implications, as they relate to the practitioner. Examples of these conditions are the totality of the practitioner's life experience and the person's knowledge and skills. In addition, the circumstances of practice include conditions in the environment in which the practitioner operates.

The client's situation may be represented as a set, called A. This set is composed of single conditions in the client's situation and of subsets of single conditions interacting with each other to create new conditions. An interaction between two single conditions, a_1 and a_2, may be represented in the set A by the figure "a_1a_2." This representation does not take into consideration the order of occurrence of the two events. One should notice, however, that the interaction "a_1a_2" may produce completely different results depending on whether a_1 precedes a_2, a_2 precedes a_1, or a_1 and a_2 occur simultaneously. Similarly, the circumstances under which practice takes place may be represented as a set, called B. Like A, this set is composed of single conditions (b_1, b_2, and so forth) and the interactions of single conditions.

Sets A and B interact to create the conditions existing in a practice situation. For example, suppose that set A is composed of only three single conditions and their possible combinations, and that set B is composed of only three single conditions and their possible combinations. When these two sets merge in a practice situation, a whole new group of conditions is created. These conditions are the interaction conditions of the two sets, and they are describable by the Cartesian Product of the elements in sets A and B.

The interaction of sets A and B form the conditions of practice. Only when meaningful interactions occur between the conditions existing in the client's situation and the circumstances of practice can practice take place. To say that an interaction is meaningful is to say that the interaction has logical implications in relation to existing scientific or ethical knowledge. When only three single conditions and their possible interactions exist in the client's situation and in the circumstances of practice, respectively, a total of 49 unique and potentially meaningful conditions may result in a practice situation.

Based on this result, one might reasonably say that the totality of relevant conditions in a practice situation is never actually identifiable since it is potentially infinite. However, the human potential to perceive the environment, and the personal knowledge of the practitioner are limited in the situation. Consequently, only a limited number of conditions in the situation are ever attended to and identified at a given time. Because of limitations in knowledge, the conditions that seem to be meaningful in the situation are likely to always be fewer than those that are actually meaningful. Thus, what the practitioner identifies as the relevant conditions for practice is most dependent on the practitioner's scientific and ethical knowledge.

Values and Goals

Once conditions in the practice situation are identified, the practitioner must determine what changes are necessary. The goal of practice is to make changes in the client's situation so that a greater good is realized. The practitioner determines what changes are necessary by comparing the empirical conditions that exist in the client's situation with the values of the practice discipline. When existing conditions contradict these values, the conditions are considered candidates for change. The values of the discipline reflect normative ethical theories. The realization of conditions reflecting these values are the desired ends of practice. Accordingly, only changes which will lead to outcomes reflecting the intrinsic values of the profession, values derivative from these intrinsic values, or values instrumental to their attainment are considered appropriate as ends in practice.

This process is not as simple as it first appears, however, since any given condition or event may simultaneously reflect one value and contradict another. To help solve this problem, a hierarchy of values is often established. In general, only higher order derivative values and intrinsic values are really applied in determining whether conditions existing in the client's situation contradict the values of the practice discipline. For example, the preservation of the vital signs of respiration, pulse, blood pressure, and body temperature may be considered appropriate in practice as an instance of the value, "preserving life." Here, other consequences and other questions of value that could be raised may be initially ignored.

Often, a practitioner has a pre-established hierarchy of values for given situations. This procedure facilitates the speed in the decision-making process that is required in practice. A practitioner sometimes accepts a hierarchy implicitly and uncritically, but these hierarchies and their implementation represent ethical decisions. In addition, a hierarchy of value can not always provide a solution when values conflict. As a consequence, what actually leads one to consider a change to be necessary in practice is a complex and often situationally dependent process. The process involves ethical theories and difficult ethical decisions, as well as various strategies, such as maximizing the gain, minimizing the losses, or other optimization procedures that require the simultaneous minimizing of losses and maximizing of gains. Even the choice of a given strategy, however, represents an ethical decision, so the question of what changes are necessary in the client's situation is ultimately an ethical question. As a consequence, assessment of the need for change in practice depends on the ethical knowledge of the practitioner.

Outcomes

Once the conditions requiring changes in the client's situation are determined, a practitioner examines the situation to identify the possibility of making the changes desired. First, a practitioner uses scientific knowledge of necessary and sufficient conditions to determine if desired changes are realizable. Next, a practitioner examines the situation to determine whether conditions for achieving the desired changes exist. In practice, the requisites for making changes may not be present in either the client's situation or the practice circumstances. As a result, values initially highly regarded in the assessment of need may be completely abandoned on the basis of exigency. As a result,

the set of realizable outcomes in practice is determined by what is scientifically possible within the exigencies of the practice situation.

The Greatest Good

From this narrowed set, a practitioner must select the changes to be brought about. Selecting changes to be implemented requires a practitioner to determine which set of realizable outcomes represents the greatest good in terms of the intrinsic values previously identified. Here, the value of the possible changes in relation to the realization of the intrinsic values lacking in the practice situation must be considered and compared. The determination of the value of a particular change entails consideration of its consequences. These consequences include the realization of the outcomes of the changes as well as the methods used to realize that change.

As a result, there are two ways the value of a change can be assessed. First, the intrinsic value of either an outcome or a method can be considered and, second, either an outcome or a method may have instrumental value in the achievement of intrinsic values.

With respect to the possible outcomes of changes, the scientific relationship existing between an outcome and a value will determine whether the outcome is intrinsically or instrumentally valuable. For an outcome to be considered intrinsically valuable, the outcome must be an empirical instance of an intrinsic value. On the other hand, an outcome may be instrumentally valuable in relation to other intrinsic values. In this second case, the outcome must be regarded as an aspect of a method and must be subjected to the same valuation criterion as other methods.

With respect to alternative methods of achieving change, again the scientific relationship existing between a method and a value determines the value of the method. A method is intrinsically valuable when the method represents an empirical instance of an intrinsic value.

For example, the use of recreational therapy for certain persons with minor depression and withdrawal may be considered intrinsically valuable regardless of whether it is an effective method of alleviating depression. Similarly, the provision of emotional support and acceptance may be regarded as intrinsically valuable.

More frequently, however, alternative methods are evaluated in terms of their instrumental value in achieving a desired outcome. In this respect, the value of a method depends on whether (a) the method is sufficient for realizing the outcome under the conditions existing in the practice situation, (b) the method is sufficient for realizing the outcome under certain conditions that are not completely realized in the practice situation, (c) the method is sufficient for realizing the outcome under the conditions in the situation, but other conditions also exist that are sufficient for its negation, (d) the method is empirically related to the outcome by empirical generalization, (e) the method is necessary for the outcome, or (f) the method is considered functionally related to the desired outcome. In general, the value ascribed to each of these ways of realizing an outcome is related to the degree of predictability associated with it. Thus, realizing a sufficient condition for a desired outcome is the most valued of these methods.

From the values assigned to the possible outcomes and from the methods of achieving them, a practitioner must determine which changes will realize the greatest good. To identify the greatest good, one must determine what is the best of all the possible combinations of outcomes (ends) and methods (means) that can be realized in a practice situation. The criterion for determining what is best is the hierarchy of values held within the profession as amended by the practitioner. This process entails questions of both moral and nonmoral value as well as scientific and logical questions. The process can be characterized as a rational betting game under conditions of uncertainty. Here, one does what seems most likely to lead to the realization of the intrinsic values of the profession within the limits of ethical propriety. Because the processes require prediction of empirical and ethical consequences, the quality of the bet depends on the practitioner's scientific and ethical knowledge. This knowledge allows one to increase the likelihood of successful betting by allowing a greater number of options and increased knowledge of the odds. i.e., the likelihood of gains and losses. The

outcome depends on this knowledge and on the skills of the player in implementing the requisites for the desired changes in the situation.

Summary and Conclusion

From this description of practice, it appears that the knowledge required to answer the question of what changes to make in practice is only the knowledge entailed by science, ethics, and logic. The conditions identified as being relevant in practice depend on the scientific and ethical knowledge of the practitioner. The values used to determine needs for change and desired outcomes in particular situations are determined by the knowledge of ethics. The knowledge of the changes that will realize these outcomes is scientific, and the value ascribed to outcomes of the changes depends again on the ethical theory of value and scientific relationships. Finally, the question of the greatest good is related to the knowledge of moral right, nonmoral value, and scientific possibility under conditions of uncertainty. This is the concern of the discipline of mathematical and statistical decision theory, and is primarily a scientific and logical discipline. This means that practice knowledge is entailed within the disciplines of science, ethics, and logic, and that any given notion of a practice theory is likely to be reducible to the simple conjunction of these kinds of knowledge. Thus, the knowledge of practice depends not on some special aspects of practice but on science and ethics alone.

References

Beckstrand, J. (1978). The notion of a practice theory and the relationship of scientific and ethical knowledge to practice. *Research in Nursing and Health, 1*, 131–136.

Chisholm, R.M. (1966). Freedom in action. In K. Lehrer (Ed.), *Freedom and determinism*. New York: Random House.

Davidson, D. (1967). The logical form of action sentences. In N. Rescher (Ed.), *The logic of decision and action*. Pittsburgh: The University of Pittsburgh Press.

von Wright, G.H. (1963). *Norm and action*. New York: Humanities Press.

von Wright, G.H. (1967). The logic of action: A sketch. In N. Rescher (Ed.), *The logic of decision and action*. Pittsburgh: The University of Pittsburgh Press.

A Critique of Several Conceptions of Practice Theory in Nursing

Jan Beckstrand

The thesis of this article is that the Dickoff, James, and Wiedenbach (1968a, 1968b) conception of a practice theory is roughly equivalent to a plan of action. This idea is contrasted with other conceptions of a prescriptive practice theory, especially the set-of-rules conception described by Jacox (1974). The set-of-rules conception is shown to be untenable, and other conceptions of practice theory are shown to be nothing more than examples of established forms of knowledge.

Practice theory is considered a form of prescriptive theory, distinguishable from scientific theory, which is predictive (Dickoff, James, & Wiedenbach, 1968a, 1968b) or descriptive (Greenwood, 1961). The purpose of this article is to examine the notion of practice theory and determine the usefulness of the ideas proposed by Dickoff et al., as well as the other conceptions of practice theory.

The Notion of Dickoff et al.

Dickoff et al. (1968a) argued that practice theories consist of a well-described goal, a prescribed set of actions to realize the goal, and a survey list. Although the earlier ideas of Dickoff et al. (1968a, 1968b) were often imprecise and vague, two later publications by Dickoff and James (1970, 1975) provided some clarification. From these publications it seems that what Dickoff and James intended to denote by practice theory was the articulation of the conceptual frameworks (i.e., the systematized ideas, both explicit and implicit) practitioners actually use to direct their own actions in carrying out practice. Such a conceptual framework includes all the scientific and ethical reasoning and personal motives that account for a nurse's behavior. According to Dickoff and James (1970), in order to guide action these ideas must be crystallized and exhibited in the mind as directives for action along with a survey list

From Research in Nursing and Health, *1980, 3, 69–79. Copyright © 1980, John Wiley & Sons, Inc. Reproduced by permission of John Wiley & Sons, Inc.*

used to attend to relevant details when implementing actions to achieve a well-described goal. Thus the components of a given practice theory are a goal, directives for action, and a survey list.

A practice theory so constituted actually and primarily serves to enable "man to create or shape reality in a desired direction." (Dickoff et at., 1968a, p. 433). Therefore, whenever anyone claims knowledge of how to achieve a goal in action and tries to alter reality through action in a specific way, as for example in changing a flat tire, a "practice theory" is being employed in the performance of the task.

According to Dickoff and James (1970), one reason to making practice theories explicit is that discrepancies may exist between what a practitioner actually thinks, says, and does. This lack of consistency may interfere with a practitioner's ability to bring about a desired situation and may even prohibit the practitioner from knowing what is wanted as a result of a given activity. Other reasons for making practice theories explicit are to allow for examination and criticism of a nurse's preconceptions and assumptions and to allow for creative freedom to invent new and constructive alternatives. In addition, this process helps other practitioners adopt well-conceived plans. (Dickoff et al., 1968a).

Apparently (see, for example, the implied questions concerning engineering in Dickoff & James, 1975) some people have suggested that practice theory can be reduced to at least one connotation of the term "technology," i.e., the science of achieving a desired aim in action. Here the meaning of technology is broadened from its narrower denotation of instrumentation, techniques, or skills to mean the totality of a plan of action used to bring about a goal that is presumed desirable. Indeed, the criteria suggested by Dickoff et al. (1968b) for evaluation of practice theories reflect the identity between practice theory and this notion of technology. According to these authors, practice theory is evaluated in terms of the ability of the specified activity to achieve a goal (coherence), the desirability of the goal actually achieved (palatability), and the potential for cost-efficient implementation given the actual factors in a situation (feasibility). That coherence and feasibility are essential criteria for the evaluation of a plan of action is easily seen, but that palatability is also an essential criterion for the evaluation of a plan is often obscured in modern society by the tendency toward what Habermas (1974) called the "scientification" of life.

To state Habermas's insight simply, in modern society scientific control is valued so much that the desirability of the end is often ignored. Consequently, the question of the palatability of the result of a plan of action is frequently deemed irrelevant or less relevant that the achievement of control. This situation often reflects the state of affairs nurses encounter, especially (but not exclusively) in the performance of delegated medical tasks.

Therefore, in reminding nurses of the question of palatability, and in showing nurses how action is cognitively based. Dickoff et al. (1968a, 1968b) rendered nursing a great service. Dickoff et al. began the description of the last step in the cognitive translation of thought into action. However, Dickoff et al. (1968a) did not fully explicate or formalize their theory so that their work on practice theory in nursing presents only an undeveloped idea.

As a result, in response to the query. "What does it mean to talk about a nursing theory?" Dickoff et al. (1968a, 1968b) answered only fairly well with respect to the act of practice and not well enough with respect to science, ethics, logic, and philosophy. Thus many nurses are still confused about the place of these four types of theory and of practice theory in nursing. Dickoff et al. (1968a, 1968b) have been misinterpreted, and other conceptions of practice theory have developed (Jacox, 1974). It is the purpose of this article to show how these other conceptions of practice theory are erroneous in themselves and as interpretations of Dickoff, James, and Wiedenbach's (1968a, 1968b) original conception.

Prescriptive Rules for Practice

Perhaps the most common understanding of the notion of practice theory of Dickoff et al. is as a set of rules for practice. This conception of practice theory is reported by Jacox and is exemplified by the following statement: "A practice theory of pain alleviation would prescribe when a sympathetic, supportive approach by the nurse, combined with administration of an analgesic might be most effective" (Jacox, 1974, p. 10). Here, the Dickoff et al. notion of practice theory is viewed as prescribing when certain methods are to be used to achieve specific goals. However, the prescriptions or directives in the Dickoff et al. conception do not specify when nurses should achieve a certain goal in a certain way. Instead, the directives merely indicate what actions individual practitioners are committed to and thus regard as necessary and compelling in given situations when a well-defined goal is to be achieved.

This distinction is subtle, but very important, and it might be clarified by observing the differences in the following constructions. In using the Dickoff et al. (1968a, 1968b) and the Dickoff and James (1970) conceptions, a given practice theory might appear as follows: When a nurse desires to bring about a well-defined goal (G) in a situation (S), considering certain factors (F) in the survey list, then B is a useful belief set with respect to the goal, when B is articulated as directives for action. Here usefulness refers to the fact that the intended purpose is served: i.e., B is both coherent and feasible, and G is palatable. The belief set B is a set of directives derived from the scientific theories and facts and the ethical ideas to which a given practitioner is committed in action and, therefore, compelled to perform. Another practitioner may hold a different but equally valid practice theory in the same situation (Dickoff & James, 1970).

In contrast, the set-of-rules conception of a practice theory can be characterized as follows: When confronted with a specific situation (S), defined by certain relevant conditions (C_s), the nurse ought to perform a given set of actions (A_s) and achieve a specific goal (G_s). To understand why the example reported by Jacox (1974) can be represented in this way, the question of what it means to talk about the best or most effective course of action must be considered.

Contrary to popular belief, the question of the most effective course of action is not just a question of the relative usefulness of different methods. To illustrate this, suppose that two different courses of action M_1 and M_2 are both known to be instrumentally valuable in achieving a desired goal G. Suppose also that M_1 accomplishes G in time T_1, with additional effects E_1. M_2 is different from M_1 and accomplishes G in time T_2, with additional effects E_2. Given that both methods are sufficient to achieve the goal G, the question of which of the methods is most effective or useful is reducible to the question of which consequences (E_1 or E_2) are the most desirable (intrinsically valuable) as additional ends. When neither method fully achieves G, a similar situation results. Therefore, to prescribe a method is tantamount to prescribing the goal to be achieved.

Since the prescription in practice theory, as described by Jacox (1974), prescribes the action used to achieve a goal, it necessarily prescribes the goal. Consequently, this conception is different from that of Dickoff et al. (1968a, 1968b). Dickoff and James were committed to self-determined practice, as was clearly stated:

> A guide to action is a principle or pattern that describes either the process or end point of the action in question. A belief is a guide that is or can be articulated by the agent. Two features of belief so construed interest us here: (1) that the principle is or can be articulated and is not merely a dumbly followed rule, and (2) that the articulator is the agent himself, not some outside force or spectator describing or controlling an action (Dickoff & James, 1970, p. 418).

Nurses using the former conception of practice theory are compelled to conform not to their own belief sets in carrying out practice activity but to a set of rules imposed by an external authority. In contrast, nurses using the Dickoff et al. (1968a, 1968b) conception are merely following the dictates of their own knowledge, conscience, and circumstances in deciding goals and in establishing and implementing actions.

An essential difference between the notion of practice theory that we attribute to Dickoff et al. (1968a, 1968b) and that described by Jacox (1974) is the nature of the prescriptions in the two types of theory. In the Dickoff et al. (1968a, 1968b) conception of practice theory, the norm-giver and norm-authority is the practitioner acting to achieve a goal. The prescriptions or directives for action derive from the practitioner, even though the practitioner may accept as legitimate and adopt into a belief system ideas that were originally proposed by an external authority. Consequently, sanctions imposed on actions are both created and self-imposed by the practitioner. On the other hand, in the conception described by Jacox (1974), the norm-giver and norm-authority are not necessarily individual practitioners, and are not likely to be. Thus, when practitioners fail to adopt a behavior specified by a prescription, they are liable to externally imposed sanctions. This result obtains even though the prescription is considered illegitimate by a practitioner. In essence, prescriptive practice theory becomes a set of universally prescribed rules for practice, and it is with the set-of-rules notion of a practice theory that we here take issue.

Problems With the Set-of-Rules Conception

When practice theory is viewed as consisting of sets of rules, several problems arise. First, in order to legitimatize the compulsion inherent in the prescription, some justification for requiring a behavior must be given. But how do we know that nurses ought to perform a set of actions or achieve a certain goal in a situation? Maybe nurses ought not to perform those actions or achieve that goal, or maybe they ought to take another set of actions instead.

Problems in Justification
Instrumental Value

According to Dickoff et al. (1968a, 1968b), one way to justify a prescriptive theory is to check the theory to see if it fulfills its purpose. This formulation works well when practice theory refers to the cognitive workings of a practitioner that lead to action in a given situation. Either the theory actualized in practice achieves the goal or it does not. But when practice theory is conceived as sets of prescribed rules for behavior, the fact that the behavior realizes the goal no longer serves to justify the prescription. The goal is actually prescribed, and the fact that a set of behaviors achieves a goal cannot justify the prescription of the goal. In prescribing the goal, intrinsic values are being prescribed, and the only way to justify the prescription of intrinsic value is through ethical arguments.

Ethics

Therefore, a second way in which a set-of-rules type of practice theory might be justified is by appealing to ethics. What is asserted by the set-of-rules conception of practice theory is as follows: Of all the possible actions (A_p) and all the possible goals (G_p) available to the practitioner in given situations (S_p), the good and right goals are G_s, and the good and right actions to use in achieving them are A_s. To justify this statement, a theorist need only justify that the prescribed goals and actions are good and right. But justification of what is good and right is no small task, as the history of ethics shows. One method popularly used is consensual agreement of rational and morally minded people, and either a decisionist or a nondecisionist perspective can be adopted.

When a decisionist perspective is used, the method holds great potential for disagreement. For example, Hempel pointed out that no one set of criteria for rationality exists. Rather, these criteria may depend on the "inductive attitudes of the decision maker and in some cases . . . [on] different degree of optimism or pessimism as to what to expect of the world" (Hempel, 1965, p. 468). Hence the decisionist will conclude that because of conflicting criteria for rationality, only a few sets of rules are likely to gain consensus. Certainly the numbers of consensually accepted goals and actions in specific situations will be far fewer than what is required if practice is to be directed by prescriptive theories of the specifically necessitated in the set-of-rules conception.

In contrast to the decisionist, the nondecisionist maintains that normative questions can be consensually decided in practice through the use of dialogue focused on the critique of attitudes leading to differing viewpoints (Habermas, 1974). However, in spite of the fact that consensus can be achieved, the nondecisionist's perspective cannot be used to justify the prescription of goals. In using this system, the prescription of the consensual goal will suppress the requisites for further dialogue and will contradict the aim of achieving consensus in the first place, i.e., freedom, autonomy, and knowledge. Thus the prescription of the goal will be irrational within this system. Therefore one must conclude that some question exists as to how practice theory of the set-of-rules type can be justified.

Problems in Use

Practice

In addition, problems also arise in the use of prescriptive sets of rules for practice. First, the complete set of relevant conditions defining a situation in which a given set of rules is to be applied cannot be specified. Practice theories of the set-of-rules type can therefore never be truly prescriptive. Second, if anything less than a complete prescriptive system is instituted, it logically follows that depending on how conditions are selected in a situation, two equally applicable and perhaps contradictory prescriptive theories may be appropriate. In this case, the practitioner must arbitrarily choose between the two, and practice will no longer be prescribed.

If other criticisms are not sufficient to conclude that a prescriptive set of rules will not be useful in practice, certainly the two preceding criticisms should be. The construction of a completely prescriptive theoretical system for practice is impossible, but to prescribe anything less incapacitates the system because its application may lead to contradictions about what is prescribed.

Finally, even if the conditions defining different situations were completely specifiable, it is questionable that a practitioner could ever actually identify which set of rules fits a situation. For example, if a practice situation were defined by only 10 relevant conditions, a separate practice theory would have to exist for each situation definable by the possible subsets of the 10 conditions. Looking only at subsets containing 2 conditions, 45 different practice theories would be needed. The potentially huge numbers of possible combinations that could occur, each requiring a distinct practice theory, would serve to make the system completely untenable.

In using such a system, the practitioner would have to identify not only all of the conditions existing in a given situation but also all of the prescriptive theories relevant to each condition to select appropriate actions and goals. As a result, practice would be reduced to matching the potentially huge sets of conditions in a situation with the conditions specified for the application of each prescriptive theory. This procedure would lead to a rapidly expanding system. These results show that a truly prescriptive set of rules for practice is untenable. One can easily imagine the real-life complexity, if not impossibility, of this procedure.

Still, one might argue that if a prescriptive practice theory of the set-of-rules type cannot be justified, then no decision can be made about what to do in practice. For, after all, this theory is just an attempt to codify this process. In addition, it might be said that practice theory of the set-of-rules type would be useful because each practitioner would know exactly what to do in a given situation, and this would guarantee a standardized quality of care. Here, the use of practice theory of the set-of-rules type could be viewed as a way of mitigating the problems currently arising in practice based on scientific and ethical judgment and the personal discretion of each practitioner. However, there are several problems with these arguments.

First, there are many differences in what may be considered an adequate justification of an action and an adequate justification of a prescription. Second, even if a system of prescriptive theories could be justified and developed, scientific and ethical judgment would still be required in practice. Thus the existence of practice theory of the set-of-rules type would not lessen the need for judgment nor the problems of incomplete knowledge or erroneous assessment of factual and ethical conditions in given situations. Moreover, misapplication of prescriptive theories is as likely as misapplication of any other knowledge; so the problem of erroneous diagnosis and treatment would still exist. Finally, the existence of prescriptive practice theory would not reduce the problem of incomplete and imperfect knowledge, even of prescriptive theory. The practitioner might still suffer from knowledge lags and the vagaries of erroneous recall and interpretation.

Inevitably, the problems currently arising from erroneous scientific and ethical judgment and incomplete scientific and ethical knowledge would not be reduced by the existence of prescriptive practice theory. Therefore, prescriptive practice theory of the set-of-rules type cannot be considered more useful than the application of scientific and ethical knowledge in practice.

Education

Since practice theory of the set-of-rules type is not particularly useful in practice, it cannot be very useful in the education of practitioners. However, what appear to be prescriptive systems have frequently been used in teaching. In fact, it may be these normative systems that have led to the idea that prescriptive sets of rules for practice are needed. These systems are the principles of practice and the standards of current practice.

The principles of practice are shorthand ways of referring to fundamental truths to be considered and general customs to be followed. Most principles of practice reflect a factual relationship between a situation and valued goals. Examples of these principles are the following: "When a client has gallbladder surgery, keep him placed in a low Fowler's position." "Relieve high anxiety before attempting to teach." Each of these statements reflects the knowledge of a factual relationship and the knowledge that certain outcomes are considered desirable or undesirable.

For example, it is known that if people with high abdominal surgery are allowed to remain in a reclining position, impingement of traumatized tissue on the diaphragm leads to a reduction of movement of the lungs. As a consequence, pulmonary function is likely to be impaired, and the impairment of pulmonary function has potentially severe implications for recovery. The "low Fowler's position" principle reminds us of this danger and of the situation considered to be its cause, and it instructs us to negate the antecedent in a scientific relationship.

The principle also implies that a position considered instrumentally valuable in this regard is the low Fowler's position. Since we know that impaired pulmonary function can lead to situations contradicting values in several professions, we will want to place the client in a low Fowler's position and closely monitor pulmonary function. In so doing, the principles of practice correspond to technical norms or directives as defined by von Writh (1963) and perhaps to some therapeutic, logistic, and prudential rules as defined by Walker (1971).

Other principles of practice represent nothing more than statements of common practice or customs. For example, in nursing schools, students are frequently admonished to reinforce dressings in the early postoperative period rather than change them. This is the common method for keeping accurate accounts of the amount of wound drainage and for lessening the possibility of infection. Although this method has been a good one, there is no scientific reason to prevent the attainment of an equally good result using some other procedure. The principle merely reminds the practitioner of a commonly used practice.

A second kind of normative system encountered in the education of practitioners is based on the standards of current practice. These standards reflect the value consensually accorded to the practice techniques available within a profession. Standards of practice differ from customs in that they are not based on habits, but on scientific relationships. Thus the standards of practice, like some principles of practice, may imply technical directives. In addition, the standards of practice indirectly recommend a hierarchy of values to be used in a given situation.

An example of a standard in medical practice is given in the following statements: "External cardiac massage, prompt ventilation, and electrical defibrillation is the treatment of choice" (Krupp & Chatton,

1973, p. 198) for ventricular fibrillation. In addition, these authors suggested that a coronary bypass procedure not be done unless the patient has difficulty in controlling angina pectoris and at least 50% to 70% occlusion of the proximal segment of the artery is involved. In nursing, McCarthy's (1972) attempt to construct a practice theory is a good example of a set of standards for practice. As can be seen, most standards are expressible as empirical statements about what most practitioners think ought to be done in certain situations. Implicit in standards are ideas about the values thought to take precedence in each situation. Additionally, standards often provide general empirical and ethical criteria for instituting a change in treatment or a change in values in scientifically related situations. Finally, a great deal of empirical evidence is provided to support these contentions.

Therefore, standards for practice are attempts to specify what most practitioners in a field think is the best choice for action in a situation, given the values of the profession and the current state of scientific knowledge. Although it is true that practitioners who frequently violate these standards are called into question, the standards of practice reflect less the prescriptive rules for practice than the results of applying what von Wright called "the rules of the game" (von Wright, 1963, p. 6). The standards of practice reflect what practitioners consensually view as the best move within the almost always unstated rules of the game of applying existing scientific and ethical knowledge to the problem of achieving a desired end in an uncertain situation.

Practitioners who consistently draw unpopular conclusions are examined to determine whether they are applying the rules incorrectly or whether they perhaps know a better choice. But conclusions drawn appropriateness of practice will depend on empirical consequences of practitioner's actions and the rationale for making them, not on the standards themselves. As a result, standards are not prescriptive, since the ultimate assessment of the appropriateness of practice does not depend solely on violation of the standard itself. The same may also be said of the principles of practice.

Therefore norms currently used in teaching and in practice are not really prescriptive in nature, since they are not imperatives carrying sanctions for their adoption or violation.

Research

Thus far, three things have been shown: first, practice theories of the set-of-rules type are not justifiable on empirical or ethical grounds; second, it is impossible to develop completely prescriptive theories of this type for practice; third, anything less may lead to contradictory prescriptions in given situations. Moreover, it has been shown that the set-of-rules types of prescriptive theory will not lessen the problems currently existing in practice. Thus it has been found that prescriptive practice theory of the set-of-rules type cannot be useful in practice or education.

In addition, sets of rules for practice cannot be useful in scientific research. One way to look at the research process is as a means of establishing the usefulness of a hypothesis in predicting logically derivable consequences. The use value of the hypothesis is established if it provides for empirically accurate predictions when logically combined with other established or hypothetical empirical relationships. In this process, evidence for the truth of the hypothesis is considered to be obtained by the existence of the predicted occurrence. If predictions are found faulty, at least one hypothesis in the logical system is considered false. The value of the hypothesis is thereby established by empirical testing for truth and falsity. However, prescriptive theories of the set-of-rules type are not amenable to empirical testing because as prescriptions they imply no deductively derivable empirically true or false consequences (predictions). Accordingly, it follows that prescriptive practice theories cannot be useful in scientific research.

Other Notions of Practice Theory

Although the set-of-rules interpretation of practice theory is probably the most common, several other conceptions of practice theory are also possible. Among these is the notion that practice theory is a conceptual framework of (or for) nursing practice. This conception may derive from the idea espoused by Dickoff and James that "a theory is a conceptual system or framework invented to some purpose" (Dickoff & James, 1968, p. 198). This statement is obviously true, but it is often not realized that a conceptual framework is merely a system of well-related ideas. As a result, any system of ideas, such as a legal code or a political perspective, may qualify as a conceptual framework (Gale, 1979). Therefore, although it is true that theories of differing kinds are all conceptual frameworks, not all conceptual frameworks are theories. Moreover, even when several conceptual frameworks are theories, they are not necessarily theories of the same kind. Especially, conceptual frameworks of nursing, such as Roy's (1970) or Jones's (1978), are not scientific theories but ideologies, and in this sense they may be considered a kind of prescriptive practice theory, albeit different from the Dickoff et al. (1968a, 1968b) conception. These frameworks attempt to define and therefore to prescribe what nursing is in terms of its goal, its orientation to care, and its methods. Conceptual frameworks of nursing can be derived from either idealizations or descriptions of current practice. But regardless of how they are invented, conceptual frameworks of nursing are not scientific theories, because these frameworks are legitimately alterable on the sole basis of personal or public discretion. Like the Dickoff et al. notion of practice theory, conceptual frameworks of nursing are not amenable to testing for truth or falsity. As normative theories, conceptual frameworks of nursing are roughly analogous to delineating rules for playing a game such as baseball.

Two misconceptions have arisen from the equation of conceptual frameworks of nursing with scientific theories, especially in regard to the role conceptual frameworks of nursing can play in the development of scientific theory. The first is exhibited in Peterson's statement that "a discipline comes to have a body of scientific knowledge by first clearly defining its relevant concepts" (Peterson, 1977, p. 24). Here the use of the pronoun "its" implies that the identification of concepts relevant to nursing as an ideological discipline

will lead to scientific theory development in nursing. (Other arguments made in Peterson's article support to this interpretation.) However, a conceptual framework of nursing cannot lead to scientific theory development as proposed.

Concepts useful in scientific theories are invented as a way to understand empirical events and phenomena. For example, to understand the nature of water, concepts might be invented to describe its properties (like wetness and fluidity) and its structure (like hydrogen, oxygen, and ionic bonding). Similarly, the practice of nursing can be scientifically studied as an empirical phenomenon, and concepts may be invented to characterize it. However, concepts relevant to nursing as a phenomenon can only be used to explain and describe the properties and structure of nursing, not the problematic client-related phenomena encountered by nurses.

For example, one might hypothesize that nursing behavior can be understood as the beneficent implementation of medical regimen and as attempts to reduce suffering from problems outside of medicine or poorly understood by medicine. One may even hypothesize more specifically that one way nurses seek to reduce suffering caused by grief is by empathizing. Whether or not nurses are aware of the hypothesis relating empathy to grief implicit in the action and whether or not the action is successful may even be investigated. However, none of these observations provides understanding of the grieving process or of the means of facilitating grieving to a good end. Yet the scientific body of knowledge needed in nursing is precisely knowledge, like the knowledge of the grieving process, that is relevant to bringing about changes in a client's condition. This knowledge is largely that of client-related phenomena encountered in practice, not knowledge of the properties of nursing or how nursing is constituted. Thus, identifying the concepts relevant to nursing as an activity will not help nursing develop comprehensive scientific knowledge of its clients' problems and how to deal with them.

Moreover, even if Peterson (1977) meant that scientific knowledge will be developed by first literally defining the concepts relevant to the achievement of nursing goals, the position espoused is still untenable. The phenomena (concepts) relevant to achieving the goals of nursing or those of any other discipline cannot be known a priori. Otherwise, all scientific problems (such as how to cure cancer) could be easily solved. Instead, as the history of medicine shows, the most relevant discoveries in medicine are often made researchers and theorists working in unrelated fields or working on what seem at the time to be unrelated problems. For example, Leeuwenhoek (a lens grinder) did not set out to discover microorganisms; neither did Semmelweis (a physician) nor Pasteur (a chemist and physicist) intend to discover that putrid matter and Leeuwenhoek's microorganisms could be linked to the occurrence of disease (Kutumbiah, 1971).

Related to Peterson's (1977) ideas is a second misconception propounded chiefly by Dorothy Johnson, who argued that nursing theory development has been hindered because of "the failure of nursing . . . to explicate a common ideal goal in patient care" (Johnson, 1978, p. 2). In this view, a model of nursing, especially with respect to its goal, is considered essential for scientific theory development. According to Johnson, such a model would provide both direction for determining relevant areas of research and a means of integrating diverse research findings. Johnson cited the history of medicine as evidence for the validity of her claim. But in relation to these points, the history of medicine shows again that the mere knowledge of a goal gives neither direction as to relevant areas of research nor any real basis for "integrating diverse research findings." The reason is the same as before: The knowledge of what constitutes a relevant area for research and the knowledge of how diverse areas are related cannot be known a priori on the basis of an aim. Rather, this knowledge is generated through scientific theorizing and testing.

However, a conceptual framework of nursing may lead to scientific theory development in nursing in one way. When a conceptual framework of nursing entails scientific assumptions explaining the operation of a group of empirical phenomena and how intervention

can be accomplished with respect to these, then these assumptions may form a basis for scientific investigation. For example, implicit in Roy's (1970, 1971) conceptual framework is the suggestion that specific nursing activities can influence stimuli affecting the adaptive state and adaptive response of an individual.

In essence, Roy (1970, 1971) argued that the effectiveness of at least some nursing actions (interventions) depends on the ability of the intervention to produce adaptation. If this is indeed the case (which is scientifically verifiable), then perhaps some problematic phenomena encountered in nursing can be controlled and improved from a similar basis. As a result, the process of adaptation may provide a scientific theoretical model for explaining some problematic phenomena encountered in nursing and for devising a means of intervening. To the extent that conceptual frameworks of nursing promote creation and clear articulation of these kinds of assumptions, they may be useful developing nursing science.

Another kind of theory that might legitimately be regarded as a practice theory is metatheory. Metatheory is a type of philosophical theory that attempts to describe the logical and methodological foundations of a discipline or body of knowledge (Carnap, 1966). Two familiar areas where metatheories are encountered are metascience (i.e., the study of the nature of science) and metaethics (i.e., the study of the nature of normative statements and their justification). Metatheories arise when an attempt is made to characterize the knowledge of a discipline and to describe how it is developed and appropriately used. These are theories about the nature of certain kinds of knowledge, and they belong in the realm of epistemology.

In this respect, it is perfectly correct to attempt to construct a theory of practice. For example, one might wish to characterize and evaluate the methodology of practice. In this effort, and attempt might be made to describe and logically analyze the rules and procedures used by practitioners in gaining knowledge of a client and in making decisions. In addition, one might wish to examine how science and ethics are used in practice and to define the logic of intervention. All of these are possible, and some may require the study of practice as an empirical phenomenon. The Dickoff et al. (1968a, 1968b) conception of a practice theory, as well as the Orlando (1961) and Yura and Walsh (1973) nursing process theories, might be considered beginning metatheories of nursing practice.

In addition, as previously stated, practice and aspects of practice may be studied as empirical phenomena in themselves. For example, Hammond and Adelman (1976) recently spoke of the need for empirical study of human judgment and provided an example of empirical research of this kind. In studying practice as an empirical phenomenon, one might attempt to describe and account for the conduct of practice under different conditions, such as in different organizational circumstances. Alternatively, one might be more interested in the use value of certain theories, methods, and procedures under differing conditions. Here the survey list developed by Dickoff et al. (1968a, 1968b) might be used to help identify potentially relevant experimental variables in the practice situation.

Still other notions of practice theory are actually incorporated in pure science. According to Popper (1968), science is concerned with certain kinds of problems. Some examples of the problems that science might be concerned with are the following: "Why are trees green?" "What does the red blood cell do, and how does it work?" "How can polio be prevented?" "Does preoperative teaching affect postoperative recovery?" But with respect to the place of what is often regarded as "pure science" in nursing, many nurses have experienced confusion.

First, some nurses have thought that they needed to define what scientific study in nursing was before any scientific study was begun. This idea ignores the fact that the existing scientific disciplines arose not from definitions or conceptual frameworks but from purely scientific attempts to answer previously unanswered empirical or practical questions. Second, although myriad unanswered questions open to scientific investigation are encountered daily in nursing practice, nurses and others have wanted to restrict the questions investigated by nurses to ensure that these do not belong to some other discipline like sociology and physiology.

However, in attempts to circumscribe nursing's unique area of knowledge, what constitutes the legitimate knowledge of certain disciplines is frequently misidentified. Particularly, the scientific investigation of a realm of phenomena is often confused with the character of knowledge used to explain the phenomena under study. It is as if psychologists were to say, "We cannot study the physiology of learning because that's physiology, not psychology." Statements like these reflect confusion over the relationship between the character of a phenomenon under study and the character of the knowledge used to describe and explain it. This kind of confusion has led many nurses to consider nursing a discipline where scientific knowledge is merely applied, not discovered.

What is overlooked is that science is a unitary system. For example, at certain levels of theory development and scientific investigation, physics and chemistry are interrelated; i.e., physics is used to explain chemical phenomena, and chemistry is used to explain physical phenomena. The same is true for other social and natural sciences, and many new questions often cannot be answered without reference to previously established knowledge systems. In nursing, the fact that a problem or question may have a sociological explanation does not mean that the knowledge derived in discerning a cause is sociological knowledge. It is nursing knowledge.

In addition, any scientific knowledge is at least potentially applicable to answering questions arising in nursing practice. Therefore, for the time being, any questions or problems encountered by curious nurses are legitimate questions for nursing science. Whether the information gained becomes the science of nursing or the science of something else must await the test of history.

In addition to the types of theory previously mentioned, the notion of a practice theory may even refer to ethical theory for practice or to philosophy in nursing. Ethical theories for practice are theories about right and obligation, moral value and responsibility, and nonmoral value that are used in practice disciplines. Although ethical theories are not necessarily empirical, they may, depending on how they are defined, have empirically researchable implications. For example, one might wish to investigate the value accorded to practice decisions and their consequences using a moral criterion that defines relief from pain as the ultimate good.

Finally, practice theory may refer to philosophy in nursing. Philosophy is concerned with ethics and metaethics as well as other kinds of knowledge, such as the nature of beliefs, experience, and the universe. Many aspects of philosophy are entailed in the knowledge used in nursing. For example, philosophy is the basis for one's view of man and the nature of his experience. As Dickoff and James (1970) pointed out, philosophic knowledge requires the same rigor and precision as any other form of knowledge. And since philosophy underlies all forms of knowledge, rigorous thought in this area is very important. The work of Paterson and Zderad (1976) is an example of philosophy in nursing, and it illustrates several aspects of philosophic investigation and theorizing.

However, none of these ways of theorizing is unique to practice. Rather, these are methods available to all who would comprehend some aspect of the world. As a consequence, it does not seem useful to call an ideology, a metatheory, a scientific theory, an ethical theory, or a philosophical theory related to practice a practice theory. Rather, when these theories arise within the purview of a particular discipline, they can be called the scientific and philosophical knowledge of the discipline.

Conclusions

Often, exactly what is meant by "practice theory" is vague, and the implications of any one conception are not carefully described. However, two distinct conceptions are prominent in the literature. In analyzing these, several conclusions can be drawn. First, the Dickoff et al. (1968a, 1968b) conception refers not to any kind of scientific theory but to the fact that

thoughts must be formulated in a certain way before they can be used and evaluated as guides to action. Second, a set-of-rules conception of practice theory, reported in Jacox's (1974) examination of theory in nursing, is difficult to justify and to use. Consequently, the set-of-rules conception is not useful in achieving the goals of nursing practice, education, or research. In addition, it has been suggested that all theoretical knowledge relevant to practice can be discovered within existing systems of knowledge such as metatheory, philosophy, science, and ethics.

However, this does not mean that a specialized body of knowledge for nursing is impossible to achieve. Although this knowledge is frequently not well articulated or recorded, the knowledge already exists and can be furthered by the rigorous application of the methods of science, ethics, and philosophy to the problems encountered in the professional experience of nurses.

References

Carnap, R. (1966). In M. Gardner (Ed.), *An introduction to the philosophy of science.* New York: Basic Books.

Dickoff, J., & James, P. (1968). A theory of theories: A position paper. *Nursing Research, 17,* 197–203.

Dickoff, J., & James, P. (1970). Beliefs and values: Basis for curriculum design. *Nursing Research, 19,* 415–426.

Dickoff, J., & James P. (1975). Theory development in nursing. In P. J. Verhonick (Ed.), *Nursing research I.* Boston: Little, Brown.

Dickoff, J., James P., & Wiedenbach, E. (1968a). Theory in a practice discipline: Part I, Practice oriented theory. *Nursing Research, 17,* 415–435.

Dickoff, J., James, P., & Wiedenbach, E. (1968b). Theory in a practice discipline: Part II, Practice oriented research. *Nursing Research, 17,* 545–554.

Gale, G. (1979). *Theory in science: An introduction to the history, logic, and philosophy of science.* New York: McGraw-Hill.

Greenwood, E. (1961). The practice of science and the science of practice: In W. Bennis, K.D. Benne, & R. Chin (Eds.), *The planning of change.* New York: Holt, Rinehart, and Winston.

Habermas, J. (1974). *Theory and practice.* Boston: Beacon Press.

Hammond, K., & Adelman, L. (1976). Science, values, and human judgment. *Science, 194,* 389–396.

Hempel, C.G. (1965). *Aspects of scientific explanation.* New York: Free Press.

Jacox, A. (1974). Theory construction in nursing: An overview. *Nursing Research, 23,* 4–13.

Johnson, D.E. (1978). State of the art of theory development in nursing. In *Theory development: What, why, and how?* (Publication No. 15–1708). New York: National League for Nursing.

Jones, P.S. (1978). An adaptation model for nursing practice. *American Journal of Nursing, 78,* 1900–1906.

Krupp, M., & Chatton, M. (1973). *Current diagnosis and treatment.* Los Altos: Lange Medical Publications.

Kutumbiah, P. (1971). *The evolution of medicine.* Madras, India: Orient Longman.

McCarthy, R.T. (1972). A practice theory of nursing care. *Nursing Research, 21,* 406–410.

Orlando, I.J. (1961). *The dynamic nurse-patient relationship.* New York: Putnam.

Paterson, J.G., & Zderad, L.T. (1976). *Humanistic nursing.* New York: John Wiley & Sons.

Peterson, C.J. (1977). Questions frequently asked about the development of a conceptual framework. *Journal of Nursing Education, 16*(4), 22–32.

Popper, K.R. (1968). *Conjectures and refutations: The growth of scientific knowledge.* New York: Harper Torchbooks.

Roy, C. (1970). Adaptation: A conceptual framework for nursing. *Nursing Outlook, 18,* 42–45.

Roy, C. (1971). Adaptation: A conceptual framework for nursing. *Nursing Outlook, 19,* 254–257.

von Wright, G.H. (1963). *Norm and action.* New York: Humanities Press.

Walker, L.O. (1971). Toward a clearer understanding of the concept of nursing theory. *Nursing Research, 20,* 428–435.

Yura, H., & Walsh, M.B. (1973). *The nursing process: Assessing, planning, implementing, evaluating* (2nd ed.). New York: Meredith.

Beckstrand's Concept of Practice Theory: A Critique

Rosemarie Marrocco Collins

John H. Fielder

This article sets forth objections to Beckstrand's (1978a, 1978b, 1980) claim that the knowledge required for nursing practice is reducible to the knowledge of science, ethics, and logic. Her view overlooks the role of knowledge of individuals and of moral ideals in nursing, neither of which fits her conceptions of science and ethics. We conclude there are questions unique to nursing that a practice theory must address.

One of the contemporary debates in nursing concerns the status of a practice theory. Using Stevens's definition of theory as "a statement that purports to account for or characterize some phenomenon" (Stevens, 1979, p. 1), there are important questions concerning the characterization of nursing practice. Does nursing require a unique practice theory, or can nursing be fully articulated in terms of other disciplines? Should nurses seek to develop their own theoretical framework for their work and research, or should they acknowledge that nursing borrows its conceptual apparatus from various other kinds of established inquiry? Most of the literature on this subject simply advocates one view or another. Very little writing is directed to a critical assessment of the opposing point of view (Stevens, 1979).

We believe that if the nursing profession is to come to grips with this important issue there must be critical argumentation concerning the merits of each position, so that the strengths and weaknesses of each way of looking at nursing practice can be exhibited and duly considered.

Our contribution toward this goal consists of a critical assessment of a point of view advocated by Jan Beckstrand. In two articles concerning the need for a practice theory in nursing, Beckstrand (1978a, 1978b) argued that practice knowledge is composed of knowledge of science, ethics, and logic. The essence of her view is that nursing applies scientific knowledge and logical reasoning to meet ethical goals. Consequently, there is no need for a separate practice theory, because

About the Authors

ROSEMARIE MARROCCO COLLINS grew up in the Pennsylvania-Maryland area and has continued to work and study in the same geographic region. An American Nurses' Foundation Scholar, she currently is in private practice as an individual, couples, and family therapist in Wallingford, Pennsylvania. She is also the administrative director of the Pastoral Counseling Service of the Marianist Center in Folsom, Pennsylvania. Previously, she taught nursing at Widener University and Villanova University.

She is a graduate of Bon Secours Hospital School of Nursing in Baltimore, Maryland, receiving a diploma in 1960. Dr. Collins continued her education at Neumann College (Aston, Pennsylvania), receiving a B.S.N. in 1976. She also studied at the University of Pennsylvania, receiving a M.S.N. (1977), a M.A. in Social Gerontology (1983), and a Ph.D. in Nursing (1985).

Dr. Collins is active in the areas of ethical decision making, aging, and mental health. Her current research-in-progress is a study of the relationship between depression and attributional style in the elderly. She has spoken to various professional audiences on topics such as child custody decisions, spiritual and emotional health, and intergenerational issues. She comments that clarification and refinement of theoretical issues and positions is a source of great challenge and satisfaction in nursing.

JOHN H. FIELDER is an associate professor of Philosophy at Villanova University, Villanova, Pennsylvania, where he has held a faculty appointment since 1969. Dr. Fielder is a graduate of Tulane University, receiving a B.S. in Mathematics. He continued his education at the University of Texas-Austin, receiving a Ph.D. in Philosophy in 1970.

Dr. Fielder's principal area of teaching is professional ethics. He stresses the analysis of actual cases of ethical problems using the techniques of decision making. He teaches on both the undergraduate and graduate levels. He directed a project funded by EXXON to develop a course stressing the connections between engineering and the humanities.

Dr. Fielder has published over 15 articles in professional journals dealing with topics in Ancient Greek philosophy, ethical issues in engineering, health care, and the professions generally, and problems in teaching and the curriculum in professional education. His book on the DC-10 case is in press. About his work with nursing professionals, Dr. Fielder comments, "I enjoy using my skills and knowledge in philosophy to help clarify and solve interesting problems in nursing."

all of the theoretical concepts in nursing can be found in science, ethics, or the logical relationships connecting these branches of knowledge. A similar argument is used in her recent article criticizing certain conceptions of a practice theory in nursing (1980).

If true, this conclusion has important implications for our perception of nursing for it means that on a conceptual level nursing has no claim to uniqueness: Unlike the specialized disciplines it draws upon, nursing raises no special set of questions, employs no special methods, or creates no special knowledge through research. All of these will be "borrowed," to use Dorothy Johnson's (1968, 1974) term, rather than unique.

This is not to say that nursing is not unique in other ways. Even if Beckstrand is correct, nursing

would still be a unique field. No one else has responsibility for the particular set of activities assigned to nurses, nor does anyone else face the unique collection of ethical and technical questions present in nursing. Beckstrand's thesis does not alter the fact that nursing has special tasks, problems, and rewards, but the rewards would not include having to deal with technical, philosophical, and ethical problems that spring from a unique conceptual framework that is necessary to describe nursing practice.

Beckstrand's views are therefore of more than semantic interest. If she is right, it is a mistake for nurses to think of themselves in the way suggested by Dickoff and James (1968), as members of a profession requiring a practice theory of even greater sophistication than those of physics or biochemistry. Instead of the challenge to invent practice theories and test them against empirical reality, nurses would be left with a conception of their work that guarantees them a kind of intellectual second-class citizenship, forever dependent upon other disciplines for their theoretical substance.

The implications for nursing research are even more important. With no unique concepts, methods, or goals, nursing research would simply involve the usual kinds of scientific investigation applied to problems in nursing situations. Nurses would borrow the methods and theories of the biomedical and social sciences and use them for their own research projects without redefining and synthesizing them according to nursing's unique perspective. Instead of focusing on the development of special research procedures, nurses would be advised to concentrate on acquiring and applying standard research techniques from the established sciences. Time and ink spent on trying to develop a unique nursing paradigm would be better employed in standard research.

Because of its important implications, Beckstrand's view needs to be given a careful critical examination, one that is responsive both to the adequacy of her account of nursing and to the philosophical issues she raises. We believe there are a number of serious difficulties with her account that must be addressed before her conclusion can be accepted. Fortunately, the clarity and directness with which her thesis is argued makes it possible to address the issues she raises regarding a practice theory more clearly and fruitfully than much of the other writing in this area.

Beckstrand's Argument

Beckstrand's (1978a, 1978b) argument begins with a distinction between two primary aspects of practice knowledge: (a) knowledge of how to make changes, and (b) knowledge of what is morally and nonmorally good. Nurses must know how to initiate and control changes in the reality they face in their work and how to make these changes with the aim of bringing about goals that are good and worth seeking. Caring for an ill person, teaching health practices, diagnosing, counseling, and executing various nursing procedures and regimens, require that the nurse understand what outcomes are to be sought and what changes will bring about those outcomes. The former knowledge is found in ethics, the latter in science. An ethical theory will supply the knowledge of the obligations of the nurse to her clients, as well as the nonmoral goods to be sought. Once this knowledge is acquired, knowledge of how to make the changes that will enable the nurse to reach these goals is all that is required. This knowledge, in Beckstrand's view, is scientific knowledge. It is the knowledge of law-like empirical relationships and the conditions under which they hold. Using this knowledge involves manipulating and controlling the conditions so that the desired outcome is obtained. Of course, our knowledge of such relationships is incomplete, but the important point is that nursing is a matter of borrowing existing scientific and ethical knowledge and applying it to nursing situations. This being the case, there is no need to seek a special practice theory for nursing.

Nursing does draw much of its content from other disciplines, but we believe there are important features of the knowledge used in nursing practice that are left out in Beckstrand's analysis and that these features require a unique practice theory for their incorporation into nursing. Further, Beckstrand makes a significant mistake in her treatment of the ethical aspects of nursing practice; and this mistake serves to invalidate her argument that a practice theory in nursing is reducible to knowledge of science, ethics, and logic. Our critique will focus first on the view that the knowledge of how to make changes in nursing practice consists of scientific knowledge. We will then turn to her claim that the ethical knowledge in nursing is borrowed from ethical theory. Finally, we will discuss two major problems for a practice theory that this critical analysis of Beckstrand's position reveals.

Scientific Knowledge

Beckstrand claims that the knowledge nurses need to effect changes is scientific knowledge, which she views as consisting of statements of law-like empirical relationships. Certainly much of the knowledge that nurses use in their work does consist of empirical patterns that can be stated as general laws. But it is a mistake to characterize the knowledge nurses draw upon as exclusively scientific. In an article on clinical judgment and understanding, Stephen Toulmin pointed out that in a clinical situation *"our task is to recognize the plurality of different types of medical knowledge"* (Toulmin, 1976, p. 41). The same point has been made by a number of nursing investigators regarding nursing knowledge (Carper, 1978; Donaldson & Crowley, 1978; Haller, Reynolds, & Horsely, 1979). Toulmin showed that in a clinical situation the clinician employs many different kids of knowledge. While the most obvious is that of general theoretical knowledge—roughly what Beckstrand calls scientific knowledge—it is not the only kind, nor is it always the most important. In addition to knowledge of general theoretical relationships, clinicians also must have knowledge of particulars—that is, of specific persons and events. It is one thing to know a variety of theoretical relationships that apply to some feature of a client's situation, but it is quite another thing to know that client as a particular human being with a unique history. Frequently this latter knowledge is of primary importance in health care, both for understanding the impact of health problems on clients, and for their ability to recover.

With respect to knowledge of individuals, the role of the nurse and the biographer are similar; both must turn their attention to knowing individuals in all of their uniqueness and particularity. The biographer must know scientific laws that are relevant to the subject—for example, how opium addiction affected Coleridge's health. But one cannot help but be struck with the need to get beyond this kind of knowledge to present subjects in their individuality as human beings. No collection of law-like empirical generalizations can make the subject come alive as a real person, although empirical generalizations are important in our understanding of the person. Knowing persons as individuals requires that we see the world from the individual's unique point of view, that we take the particular facts of a life and construct a sense of the personal coherence of that life.

The search for law-like empirical relationships focuses on the similarities shared by different individuals; knowing a person as a person emphasizes what is unique and different about that individual. The biographer approaches this task as a detached examiner of facts, seeking to create a judicious portrait of the subject. The role of the nurse is similar, in that the nurse seeks to understand clients as individuals and help them deal with their health problems within the framework of their individual ways of being. But the nurse's role is perhaps closer to that of the priest, intimate friend, or therapist—seeking not only knowledge of the individual but also the person's well-being. Understanding is not the primary goal, but a way of becoming an effective advisor and advocate for the person's interests.

Knowing persons as individuals requires sensitivity to their subjective, inner life. To know this aspect of an individual it is necessary to see the world from the individual's standpoint and have a sense of how that world is experienced and felt. It demands empathy toward their subjectivity, to the unique constellation of feelings, thoughts, attitudes, fears and hopes that persons bear within themselves. Here, too, the stress is on moving away from the strictly "objective" knowledge embodied in scientific laws, toward the no-less-real understanding of the subjective individual. The philosophical mistake of regarding only general, theoretical knowledge as genuine is an ancient and persistent one that can be traced back to Plato. The best cure for this type of mistake, as Wittgenstein (1971) pointed out, is to avoid sweeping generalizations about knowledge and undertake a detailed examination of the actual types of knowledge being used—as Carper (1978) has done.

Clearly, both of these modes of knowing are essential to nursing practice. A person can, for some purposes, be regarded as simply a complex set of ongoing chemical reactions governed by empirical laws. To control the balance of electrolytes in the blood, for example, it is necessary to know these laws and how to use them for the client's benefit. But the person seeking health care must respond to health-threatening conditions and to treatment. An individual responds as a unique person, bringing a particular collection of strengths, weaknesses, and needs that must be understood and dealt with by those who care for that person. Beckstrand's conception of nursing knowledge includes only the former. Caring for the client as a particular individual, however, also requires knowledge of particulars, a humanistic knowledge not based solely on law-like empirical generalizations (Silva, 1977).

It might be objected that individuals are unique but their uniqueness is the product of factors which, if fully understood, would provide a scientific knowledge of the person. Thus, if we knew all the laws governing all the factors in a person's life, we would need only scientific knowledge in nursing. This is an important philosophical issue that cannot be treated fully here. For our purposes it is sufficient to point out that the claim that there is a knowledge of particulars distinct from the knowledge of theoretical generalizations has been forcefully argued in a recent article dealing with clinical judgment (Gorovitz & MacIntyre, 1976). Even if Gorovitz and MacIntyre are wrong, it is true that at the present time and for the foreseeable future nurses must rely on a type of knowledge that does not spring from theoretical structures but from a grasp of the unique facts constituting an individual life. This knowledge is not derived from empirical generalizations.

If science is not the only kind of knowledge nurses use in their work, then nursing knowledge is not reducible to scientific knowledge. The task of articulating the kinds of knowledge nurses must call upon is one part of a practice theory in nursing. Because nursing is concerned with caring for the whole person and not just curing illnesses, it must draw on a number of different disciplines and types of knowledge. This means that a practice theory must show how these partial views of man (e.g., chemical reactions) can be adapted for nursing without contradicting the basic, humanistic orientation of nursing. Whether or not there is an area of knowledge unique to nursing, it is clear that nursing seeks to employ knowledge shared with other disciplines in its own way, incorporating this knowledge into the special perspective of nursing (Andreoli & Thompson, 1977; Donaldson & Crowley, 1978; Jacox, 1974). Thus nursing theorists are rightly concerned with examining the assumptions inherent in other forms of knowledge (Stevens, 1979) and their compatibility with nursing's ideals.

Ethical Knowledge

We believe Beckstrand's treatment of the role of ethics in nursing is also mistaken. She holds that any ethical aspect of nursing practice, whether it be professional obligations, a concept of moral good, or an account of nonmoral goods, must be part of an ethical theory. Hence any ethical features of nursing practice will be borrowed from an ethical theory and not unique to nursing. Nursing may provide a unique setting in which the moral theory must be put into practice, but it is only the conditions that are unique, not the ethical conceptions.

As with the treatment of knowledge of how to make changes, there is much that is valuable in this account. It is true that any claim that a practice is ethically obligatory or prohibited must be justified by appealing to some ethical theory, for that is exactly what an ethical theory does. It provides an account of what makes right actions right and wrong actions wrong. Similarly, the claim that certain things are nonmorally good (ascribing goodness to things on grounds other than moral obligation; e.g., health, pleasure, freedom, etc.) will also be justified by some appeal to an ethical theory. Thus Beckstrand is right to point out that these features of nursing practice must be justified by an ethical theory. But it does not follow from this observation that the entire ethical content of nursing is borrowed from or reducible to ethical theory. Although every ethical claim must be justified by an ethical theory, that theory will not answer all of our questions about the ethical dimensions of nursing because not all the questions about ethics in nursing have to do with justifying ethical claims.

There are many goals, activities, and practices that

are not morally obligatory but which are morally praise-worthy. Their performance is not morally required but is morally applauded. These are what Bernard Gert (1973) called "moral ideals." For example, if we take it upon ourselves to plant flowers in vacant lots so that the appearance of the neighborhood is improved and benefits everyone, this would be regarded as a worthy practice and we would be praised for doing it. But others would not be seen as morally remiss if they did not do likewise, going forth armed with Burpee seeds to brighten drab corners. Duty does not require one to engage in such an activity, but it is morally praisewor-thy to do so.

The question of which, if any, moral ideals an individual pursues is not answered by an ethical theory. The theory may be used to justify an ideal as a moral ideal, but the choice of which ones to pursue must flow from an individual's concept of what kind of life the person wishes to lead.

In the same way, the determination of what ethical ideals a profession stands for cannot be answered by an ethical theory. Nursing, like all bona fide professions, pursues goals that provide something valuable to the public it serves. But what are the goals of nursing? What moral ideals should it pursue? The profession of nursing has only recently emerged from the role of being the physician's handmaiden and is now in the process of defining itself as a profession in its own right embodying certain moral ideals. Just what those ideals should be is one of the major elements of a practice theory. While it is clear those ideals are associated with the idea of caring for the whole person, it is necessary to provide more systematic and specific content to this conception in light of the particular set of moral ideals nursing serves. The activity of developing such an ac-count of nursing and how it is related to and differen-tiated from other professions serving moral ideals (e.g., medicine) is a central part of a practice theory in nurs-ing. The fact that any moral ideal must be justified as a moral ideal by appealing to an ethical theory does not eliminate that task. Nor does this fact establish that the content of the ethical dimension of the practice theory is borrowed from ethical theory. The particular constel-lation of moral ideals of nursing, how they fit together, and how they are related to other concepts of nursing practice will not be supplied by an ethical theory. The question of which moral ideals are to be sought and how they are related to other aspects of nursing is a nursing question, and the answer must be provided by a theory of nursing practice.

Practice Theory

The above considerations show that the need for a practice theory in nursing is not easily dismissed. Im-portant issues remain despite the fact that much of the content of nursing is borrowed from other disciplines. We have stressed the need for a nursing theory that will set out the kinds of knowledge utilized in nursing prac-tice and the particular set of moral ideals that nursing practice seeks to bring about. In both cases there is the need to redefine and synthesize the elements found in other areas of knowledge (Stevens, 1979). They are not items to be simply listed in a theory of nursing practice; they must be given new meaning, within a conceptual framework appropriate to nursing.

It is somewhat ironic that an illuminating example of this comes from the role of theory in science. Scien-tific laws are not simply generalizations drawn from collections of observations; on the contrary, they ex-press these observations with a new conceptual appara-tus (Hanson, 1965; Toulmin, 1965, 1977). Indeed, the-ories contribute to our conception of what is to count as a fact. Major scientific changes thus result in a new way of looking at the worlds, not simply the discovery of new regularities (Kuhn, 1971). Nursing is in a similar situation, seeking a conceptual framework in which the items borrowed from other disciplines will be ex-pressed with the theoretical concepts of nursing. New-ton's genius was not in gathering additional observa-tional data, but in developing a scientific vocabulary (concepts of force, mass, etc.) in which observations could be interpreted. In a similar way, nursing theorists are seeking an appropriate conceptual vocabulary for the interpretation of that which has been borrowed from other fields.

Our investigation has not examined the question of whether nursing is unique because of a separate body of knowledge. What our critique has attempted to make clear is that where knowledge is borrowed, whether from science or ethics, significant questions arise concerning the status of those borrowings within nursing. These questions are unique to nursing, and a nursing practice theory is required to answer them in a systematic and coherent way. We plan to address some of these questions in another paper.

References

Andreoli, K., & Thompson, C. (1977). The nature of science in nursing. *Image, 9*, 32–37.

Beckstrand, J. (1978a). The notion of a practice theory and the relationship of scientific and ethical knowledge to practice. *Research in Nursing and Health, 1*, 131–136.

Beckstrand, J. (1978b). The need for a practice theory as indicated by the knowledge used in the conduct of practice. *Research in Nursing and Health, 1*, 175–179.

Beckstrand, J. (1980). A critique of several conceptions of practice theory in nursing. *Research in Nursing and Health, 3*, 69–79.

Carper, B. (1978). Fundamental patterns of knowing in nursing. *Advances in Nursing Science, 1*(1), 13–23.

Dickoff, J., & James, P. (1968). A theory of theories: A position paper. *Nursing Research, 17*, 197–203.

Donaldson, S., & Crowley, D. (1978). The discipline of nursing. *Nursing Outlook, 26*, 113–120.

Gert, B. (1973). *The moral rules.* New York: Harper and Row.

Gorovitz, S., & MacIntyre, A. (1976). Toward a theory of medical fallibility. *The Journal of Medicine and Philosophy, 1*, 51–71.

Haller, K., Reynolds, M., & Horsley, J. (1979). Developing research-based innovation protocols: Process, criteria, and issues. *Research in Nursing and Health, 2*, 45–51.

Hanson, N. (1965). *Patterns of discovery.* Cambridge: Cambridge University Press.

Jacox, A. (1974). Theory construction in nursing: An overview. *Nursing Research, 23*, 4–13.

Johnson, D.E. (1968). Theory in nursing: Borrowed and unique. *Nursing Research, 17*, 206—210.

Johnson, D.E. (1974). Development of theory: A requisite for nursing as a primary health profession. *Nursing Research, 23*, 372–377.

Kuhn, T. (1971). *The structure of scientific revolutions.* (2nd ed.). Chicago: University of Chicago Press.

Silva, M. (1979). Philosophy, science, theory: Interrelationships and implications for nursing research. *Image, 9*, 59–63.

Stevens, B. (1979). *Nursing theory.* Boston: Little, Brown.

Toulmin, S. (1965). *The philosophy of science: An introduction.* New York: Harper and Row.

Toulmin, S. (1976). On the nature of the physician's understanding. *The Journal of Medicine and Philosophy, 1*, 32–50.

Toulmin, S. (1977). From form to function: Philosophy and history of science in the 1950s and now. *Daedalus, 106*(3), 143–163.

Wittgenstein, L. (1971). *Philosophical investigations.* New York: Macmillan.

The Authors Comment

We had done a number of workshops on ethical problems in nursing and had discussed problems concerning ethical theories and the role of theory in nursing generally. The Beckstrand articles raised these questions, once again, in a clear and forceful way for us.

The series of articles by Beckstrand also proposed to reduce a complex professional practice to a few basic features, something that is familiar in the history of philosophy. We were aware of work in philosophy and nursing that stressed the diversity of types of knowledge and concepts in medicine, science, ethics, and nursing. Unless that diversity was acknowledged, the main task of nursing theory as we saw it—showing how all the borrowed elements were placed within a nursing perspective—would be overlooked.

Finally, we wanted to encourage more critical analysis of points of view in nursing theory. If there is to be some sort of consensus about nursing theory it will have to emerge from an ongoing debate about the strengths and weaknesses of different conceptions.

—ROSEMARIE MARROCCO COLLINS AND JOHN H. FIELDER

A Reply to Collins and Fielder:
The Concept of Theory

Jan Beckstrand

The purpose of this article is to show that Collins and Fielder (1981) misinterpreted Beckstrand's (1978a, 1978b, 1980) thesis, and to criticize their argument against the idea that theory in nursing can be borrowed from the existing body of scientific and ethical knowledge. Collins and Fielder employed a question-begging definition of theory and distorted Beckstrand's claim in a way that made it easier to attack. In addition, emotional language and appeals to authority were frequently substituted for careful analysis of the issues. I agree that much of the theory needed in nursing cannot be borrowed even though it is likely to be scientific and ethical in form. As a result, I have tried to give some better reasons for believing that theory needed in nursing cannot be borrowed. In addition, many issues concerning the conception of theory in nursing are addressed in this article.

In a recent article Collins and Fielder (1981) critiqued several papers on practice theory (Beckstrand, 1978a, 1978b, 1980). Collins' and Fielder's paper is important because the potential for a serious misunderstanding of Beckstrand's work was pointed out. There also is much of value in Collins' and Fielder's account of the need for moral ideals in nursing. Certainly, deciding what moral ideals nursing should pursue is important in developing a conceptual framework, or more correctly, a professional ideology for nursing. In addition, because of their insight, the appropriate concerns of metapractice theory will need to include an understanding of how the moral ideals of a practice profession are decided, as well as given specific content, how these may be justified.

Collins and Fielder were right to inquire whether the need for ethical and scientific forms of theory implies that these may be borrowed. But Collins' and Fielder's evidence that practice necessitates knowledge or individuals, other particulars, and moral ideals will not refute the proposition that the theoretical knowledge required in practice can be borrowed. The prob-

From Research in Nursing and Health, *1984, 7, 189–196. Copyright © 1984, John Wiley & Sons, Inc. Reproduced by permission of John Wiley & Sons, Inc.*

lems with their reasoning on this issue exemplify several important fallacies in the discussion of theory in nursing.

To adequately understand the mistakes in Collins' and Fielder's argument, several disparate topics need examination. The first section of this article identifies potential sources of misunderstanding in Beckstrand's papers and attempts to clarify them. The second section provides a critique of Collins' and Fielder's (1981) paper. Since Collins and Fielder failed to adequately defend their position that much theory needed in nursing cannot be borrowed from the existing body of science and ethical philosophy, the third section of this article offers an argument in favor of this position.

Sources of Misunderstanding

Although Collins and Fielder credited Beckstrand's papers with clarity and directness, the work apparently was not clear enough to prevent a serious misunderstanding. They interpreted the papers as saying that the knowledge needed in nursing practice consists solely of theories and methods borrowed from the existing branches of science and ethical philosophy. The intent of the papers, however, was not that the substantive scientific and ethical knowledge needed in practice must be borrowed from, or developed within, the existing branches of science and ethical philosophy. The point was that the theoretical knowledge required in any kind of practice activity was scientific and ethical in form, and that practice could not be helped by a proposed new form of theoretical knowledge known as prescriptive practice theory.

A major source of misunderstanding in Beckstrand's papers is likely to be the cursory presentation of the criteria used to examine the need for a new epistemological class of theoretical knowledge, particularly practice theory. When Beckstrand (1978a) specified the minimum requisites for the notion of practice theory to be meaningful, she incorrectly assumed that the relationship of these criteria to her subsequent discussions was apparent. The two most important criteria were that some example of knowledge needed in prac-

tice be capable of universalization, and different from the concerns of science and ethics as epistemological classes. The capacity for universalization is a generally accepted criterion for considering an instance of knowledge to imply the need for theory, to be part of a theory, or to embody theory (Carnap, 1966; Dubin, 1978; Popper, 1968; Toulmin, 1960).

For example, the empirical law "all crows are black" and the moral imperative "killing is wrong" are instances of knowledge capable of universalization; these imply the need for theory as explanations or justifications. The scientific law "to every action there is an equal and opposite reaction" is knowledge capable of universalization contained in a theory. Because theories are concerned with and contain knowledge capable of universalization, they are also capable of universalization.

Theories are dependent on instances of knowledge that are capable of universalization. As a result, Beckstrand allowed that the need for a new form of theory in nursing can be shown by finding any instance of knowledge needed in practice that is capable of universalization, but outside the concerns of science and ethics as epistemological classes. She sought such an example, first, by investigating possible differences between scientific or ethical forms of knowledge and the knowledge capable of universalization needed to achieve the goals of practice (Beckstrand, 1978a) and second, by examining the knowledge forms capable of universalization and needed to answer the questions that arise in practice (Beckstrand, 1978b).

Beckstrand reasoned that not all knowledge capable of universalization constitutes theory, so that even if an example of this type of knowledge was found, some additional criteria must be met to show that practice theory is possible. Beckstrand's (1978a) other criteria addressed this problem. Systems of ideas accorded the status of theory must rest on a thought process that can be constructed and evaluated for consistency (Braithwaite, 1968). Such a thought process represented in symbols is called a calculus and is a precise way of requiring that theories ultimately be comprised of pieces of knowledge whose relationships can be spec-fied and used to make valid inferences. In addition, a theory must be useful. This means that inferences from theory cannot be contradictory or ambiguous. This last requirement abrogates the set-of-rules conception of practice theory (Beckstrand, 1980). The criteria for the meaningfulness of the notion of practice theory given by Beckstrand referred to these requirements.

As the evidence given by Collins and Fielder to refute Beckstrand's position showed, Collins and Fielder misunderstood that the practice knowledge sought in Beckstrand's papers must be capable of universalization. In addition, Collins and Fielder were confused about the dual meanings of terms like scientific and ethical knowledge, science, ethics, ethical theory, moral theory, normative theory, and the theory of nonmoral value. Each term may refer either to an epistemological form of knowledge characterized by the kinds of questions each attempts to answer, or to instances or existing bodies of knowledge of a particular form.

In Beckstrand's papers, terms were used for the most part in the epistemological sense. The term scientific knowledge was used to refer to a form of theoretical knowledge concerned with observable occurrences. Such knowledge is capable of universalization and is gained from systematic investigation of empirical phenomena accomplished in concert with potentially testable speculations about their workings. The term ethical knowledge was used to refer to another form of theoretical knowledge also capable of universalization, but gained by systematic investigation of what actions are right or nonmorally good and of how these judgments may be justified. Both types of theory employ other kinds of philosophical theories as assumptions and rely on various kinds of logic for reasoning. In Beckstrand's papers, the term practice knowledge usually referred to theoretical knowledge needed in practice and the word knowledge often was intended to denote theoretical knowledge according to the context of the discussion. In addition, the words knowledge systems or systems were used to indicate epistemological forms of knowledge.

However, in other literature, the dual meanings of terms such as scientific and ethical knowledge often are

distinguished by referring to the accrued knowledge of science and ethics as systematized knowledge. Therefore, the similarity of the terms knowledge systems and systematized knowledge may have been confusing.

The problem of the dual meanings of these terms was perhaps complicated by the use of the words derives and applied. For example, Beckstrand stated that "the moral knowledge used in practice derives solely from ethical knowledge and not from some special form of knowledge. . ." (Beckstrand, 1978a, p. 135), and that the knowledge used for achieving the goals of practice "is knowledge derivable from schemes, logic, and theories of moral obligation" (Beckstrand, 1978a, p. 136). Beckstrand also stated that "the theory of value in practice is simply the ethical theory of value applied to a special case or set of unusual circumstances" (Beckstrand, 1978a, p. 135).

In the first two examples, the word knowledge was used initially to refer to existing or potential substantive knowledge, and later to epistemological forms of knowledge. Thus, the first sentence should be understood as follows: Because moral questions require theory of ethical form, the real or potential substantive knowledge of moral standards used in practice must derive solely from theoretical knowledge which can be classified as ethical in form and not from some special form of knowledge, i.e., practice theory. The second example should be interpreted similarly. In the third example, an attempt was made to emphasize the prior argument that special theories of ethical form needed in practice will have characteristics similar to other theories of ethical form. The difference required is that the concern of the theory not be the right action of all people but only of those with extraordinary skills and capacities to act. Each of these sentences was a summary statement concluding longer arguments intended to convey their intent more adequately.

Finally, use of the term disciplines to refer to science, ethics, and practice, and comments on particular bodies of knowledge such as mathematical and statistical decision theory and the theory of change and action, (Beckstrand, 1978b) may have been confusing. The word discipline usually refers to an existing field of study or to a subject which is taught. The meaning was stretched when the term was used to describe science and ethics as epistemological classes of investigation.

The discussion of the existing theory of change and action and of decision theory was included in anticipation of criticism that these are required in practice and might be considered forms of theoretical knowledge distinct from science and ethics (or philosophy). Evidence was given to support the premise that such knowledge is scientific, ethical, or logical in form, by examining the form of the knowledge accrued thus far about these topics (Beckstrand, 1978b).

In addition to Collins' and Fielder's misinterpretation, another misunderstanding of the papers has been communicated privately. Some readers thought that the last paper (Beckstrand, 1980) attributed authorship of the set-of-rules conception of practice theory to Jacox (1974) who reported the conception but did not originate it. Jacox's fine article stated clearly that she was merely reporting the set-of-rules conception and not propounding it. The words reported and described were used literally by Beckstrand (1980) in referring used literally by Beckstrand (1980) in referring to her article. There was no intent to attribute authorship of this view of practice theory to her.

The intent of the Beckstrand papers should have been clear from their context which was a response to those who thought that practice required a new epistemological category of theoretical knowledge, especially the set-of-rules conception of prescriptive theory. I have shown that the set-of-rules conception of prescriptive practice theory is not useful in practice (Beckstrand, 1980). I would not claim, however, that other forms of theory may not exist or be useful. I think that none has been adequately formulated, and I have been unable to find a confirming example of the need for such theory in nursing (Beckstrand, 1978a, 1978b).

As a consequence, I think that the theoretical knowledge needed to practice is likely to be both scientific and ethical in form, and that the reasoning necessary is common to all human endeavors. Yet, I completely agree with Collins and Fielder that much of the theoretical knowledge needed in nursing practice can-

not be borrowed from existing bodies of knowledge or developed within the existing arenas of scientific or ethical investigation. The errors Collins and Fielder made in attempting to substantiate this claim often are not a product of confusion over terminology. Instead, many of the mistakes are pitfalls in reasoning that arise within the discussion of theory in nursing. As a result, the next section of this paper is devoted to a critique of their argument.

A Critique

Collins and Fielder wanted to refute the claim spuriously attributed to Beckstrand that the theoretical knowledge needed in practice can be borrowed from the existing body of scientific and ethical knowledge. They argued that if some part of the knowledge needed in practice cannot be borrowed from science and ethics, then nursing requires a unique practice theory. Knowledge of particulars is needed in practice and is not scientific (or ethical or theoretical) knowledge, and knowledge of moral ideals is needed in practice and is not the subject matter of theories of moral obligation. Therefore, a unique practice theory is required.

The argument follows a standard deductive form. The first sentence of the summary provides the premise that is supposed to be true. Next evidence is given that the antecedent—or "if" part of the premise—obtains. By deductive logic when the entire premise is true and the antecedent described in the premise is true, the consequent—or "then" part of the premise—can be inferred as a conclusion. Since Collins and Fielder believed their premise was true and gave evidence that the situation in the antecedent part of the premise is fulfilled, they felt warranted in concluding that nursing requires a unique practice theory.

However, Collins and Fielder made three serious mistakes in their argument. First, Beckstrand's claim was misinterpreted in a way that made it easier to attack. Second, specious assertions and appeals to emotion and authority were substituted for careful analysis of the issues; and finally the conclusion of the argument was guaranteed by an all-encompassing definition of practice theory.

Distorting the Claim

Instead of arguing against Beckstrand's claim that the theoretical knowledge needed in practice is likely to be scientific and ethical in form, Collins and Fielder attacked the claim that all knowledge needed in practice can be borrowed from science and ethics. Beckstrand's claim requires that some example of nonscientific or nonethical universalizable knowledge needed in practice be found for a refutation, but the interpreted claim is refutable on the basis of the need for any nonscientific or nonethical knowledge at all. As a result, the interpreted claim is easily refuted since it is plainly false. Beckstrand (1978b) pointed out refuting evidence when she referred to the need in practice both for psychomotor knowledge and knowledge of particulars. Beckstrand (1978a) also argued that practitioners' extraordinary capacities to act seem to necessitate a new and special moral theory beyond that already existing in ethical philosophy. Collins and Fielder thus committed a well known mistake of not giving the author the benefit of the doubt (Scriven, 1977) by supposing that Beckstrand would identify, explicate, and then ignore such obvious evidence against a claim.

Specious Assertions

In addition, Collins and Fielder ignored many other cardinal rules of argument (Damer, 1980; Scriven, 1977). Their argument rested on specious assertions and appeals to emotion and authority rather than on a careful analysis of the issues. Certainly, several of Collins' and Fielder's assertions reflected a misunderstanding of the meta-theory of science. For example, they used Stevens' (1979) definition of theory and the terms conceptual framework and paradigm in a way that indicates they do not know that these ideas fail to distinguish theory from other large and diverse categories of knowledge (Kuhn, 1974). Collins' and Fielder's explanation of Beckstrand's view of scientific knowledge indicates they do not understand the technical distinction between scientific and empirical laws. In addition, their

supposition that borrowed theories applied to nursing problems will abrogate the need to develop new research methods reflects a lack of knowledge of the history of science and the requisites of the research process.

Collins and Fielder also drew a faulty analogy between the scientific vocabulary, developed by the famous physicist Isaac Newton for interpreting and predicting empirical laws of motion, and the conceptual vocabulary that a conceptual framework of nursing might provide. The analogy rested solely on the similarity of the jargon used for vague ideas about the functions of a conceptual framework in interpreting borrowed knowledge, and the jargon produced by a technical explanation of Newton's accomplishments used out of context. Newton's theory explains and amplifies scientific theories existing in other fields, as many good scientific theories do. However, in no sense does Newton's theory interpret theories borrowed from other fields in the ways envisioned by Collin's and Fielder's conception of a practice theory.

Even more damaging to their argument was Collins' and Fielder's reliance on emotional claims and appeals to authority. For example, their paper began with a series of false dilemmas that evoke popular sentiment and threaten the self-interests of nurses. Next, they adopted a confident manner assuring us of their good intentions and of the value of the contribution provided by their paper. Then, even more threats to nurses' self-interests were made, for example, the assertion that accepting the idea that nursing theory can be borrowed means relegating nursing to a second class status. These assertions were accompanied by more appeals to popular sentiment—that nursing requires theory of even greater sophistication than physics or biochemistry. This demagoguery was crowned with an emotional epithet reflecting another false dilemma and a challenge to nursing's interests: "Time and ink spent . . . would be better employed" (Collins & Fielder, 1981, p. 318).

Even more detrimental was Collins' and Fielder's use of appeals to emotion and authority in the section on scientific knowledge. The significance of the fact that nurses require knowledge of the particular person is argued entirely by emotion, comparing nurses to priests, biographers, intimate friends, and therapists needing "to present subjects in their individuality as human beings," and "in all their uniqueness and particularity" (Collins & Fielder, 1981, p. 319). Employing more jargon, Collins and Fielder justified the importance of this goal by claiming that nurses seek to help individuals "within the framework of their individual ways of being" (Collins & Fielder, 1981, p. 319). General approval of these goals was assumed, and they contrasted this view with the opinion spuriously imputed to Beckstrand, that all that really matters is the machine.

In the process, Collins and Fielder succeeded in referring to the irrelevant authority of Coleridge and Plato, in paraphrasing Wittgenstein, in approving Carper, and in deferring to Silva, Gorovitz, and MacIntyre. All this name-dropping and posturing gave the illusion of weight to an insubstantial argument.

To Collins' and Fielder's credit, the position concerning ethical knowledge was better developed. The major flaw in this part of their paper rests on the use of a question-begging definition of theory to be discussed in detail in the next section. The result of using a question-begging definition is that nursing's need to define its moral ideals does not imply the need for a unique practice theory as Collins and Fielder supposed. In addition, one may take issue with Collins' and Fielder's assumption that the choice of moral ideals in nursing, as with individuals, does not require the use of an ethical theory. Instead, the pursuit of a moral ideal by professions may be justifiable less by the moral praise worthiness of the ideal and more by its nonmoral goodness.

Begging-the-Question

The most serious error Collins and Fielder (1981) made in their argument was using a question-begging definition of theory. Question-begging refers to the mistake of invoking ideas that assume a question or thesis already is proved as part of the premises or evidence given to prove it. Begging-the-question often occurs at the starting point of an argument and renders the whole argument invalid.

In Collins' and Fielder's argument, what they meant by practice theory was described by its functions. But the functions of practice theory, and hence its definition, already assumed the conclusion they wanted to prove. Thus, the definition of practice theory used by Collins and Fielder begs-the-question and renders their argument invalid in its inception.

Collins and Fielder viewed a nursing practice theory as a unique conceptual framework that is needed to describe nursing; for example, see page 319 or 321. According to them, a practice theory functions to determine and specify nursing's moral ideals, relating these to each other and to other conceptions used in the discipline. This kind of theory would provide systematic and specific content to nursing's conception of caring in relationship to these ideals, and would relate and differentiate nursing from other professions also serving moral ideals.

In addition, a practice theory would articulate the kinds of knowledge used in practice and provide a conceptual vocabulary for interpreting and incorporating borrowed knowledge in nursing, redefining and synthesizing it according to nursing's unique perspective. As a result, a practice theory would establish the status of borrowed knowledge in nursing. The problem with the view of practice theory is that the conclusion Collins and Fielder wanted to prove, that nursing requires a unique practice theory, was already assumed in their definition. There are several ways to understand exactly how this happened.

One way is to note that practice theory is just nursing conceptualized. This is apparent both where Collins and Fielder equated the idea of practice theory to a unique conceptual framework needed to describe nursing (pp. 318 & 321), and where they described the functions of practice theory.

The question of whether nursing needs to be conceptualized is not in dispute. As a result, when Collins and Fielder equated practice theory with a conceptual framework of nursing, the conclusion they wanted to defend, that nursing needs a unique practice theory, was assumed in their definition of practice theory.

A more rigorous way to explain how Collins' and Fielder's definition begs-the-question is to show that the definition makes empirical evidence irrelevant to evaluating the truth of the premise used in their argument. Their argument depended on the allegedly empirical premise that if knowledge needed in practice cannot be borrowed from science and ethics, then nursing requires a unique practice theory. The premise can be considered empirical only if it is conceivable that some observational evidence may be given to refute it. The observation needed for a refutation is an example of knowledge needed in nursing that cannot be borrowed and that does not require a practice theory. But, Collins' and Fielder's definition of practice theory makes this kind of observation inconceivable.

Practicing nurses use all the kinds of knowledge needed in practice, and since a function of practice theory is to articulate these kinds of knowledge every example of knowledge needed in practice implies the need for a practice theory by Collins' and Fielder's definition. As a result, the Collins and Fielder definition of practice theory precludes the possibility of finding any evidence that might refute the premise of the argument; thus, the premise is not empirical. Instead the premise is true by virtue of the definition of practice theory alone. This means that Collins and Fielder used a question-begging definition of theory because the allegedly empirical question of what theory is needed in practice is completely settled on the basis of the definition. The empirical problem is simply defined away.

The Concept of Theory

A problem that contributed to the mistake of begging-the-question is that the definition of theory Collins and Fielder used is too broad to restrict the class of what may count as theory. Using Stevens' (1979) definition, Collins and Fielder viewed theory as a statement or system of ideas that fulfills the purpose of accounting for or characterizing some phenomenon, namely nursing. Collins and Fielder ignored the fact that categorizing the profession of nursing as a phenomenon is sub-ject to debate, and their view conforms more to Dickoff's and James' (1968) notion that theory is any conceptual system that fulfills the purpose for which it was developed. (Note, however, that the views of practice theory in the Collins' and Fielder's and in Dickoff's and James' papers are very dissimilar.)

The Dickoff and James (1968) conception of theory, and to a lesser extent the Stevens (1979) definition, imposed only the restrictions of systematization and usefulness on the class of ideas that may count as theory, so almost any conceptual system may be awarded the status of theory. For example, a given individual's description of another particular person's perceptions and motivations is both systematic and useful and so is a city's fire code. Yet, the first example is simply a description of a fact and the second a set of technical requirements.

Thus, any conception of theory and that requires only that knowledge accorded the status of theory be speculative, useful, and systematic cannot be used to distinguish theory from many other merely speculative and useful systems of thought. A similar mistake is made in equating theories to paradigms, conceptual frameworks, solutions of problems, or ideologies. All instances of the latter are not examples of theories, but theories are subclasses of these larger sets. Such conceptions lack an additional and essential requirement that theories be ideas capable of universalization. The importance of this criterion can be seen in the fact that it is unsatisfactory to claim that nursing is a theory-based practice because each nurse constructs a systematic conception of the personhood of each client.

Collins and Fielder dropped the requirement that theory be knowledge capable of universalization, and as a result their concept of practice theory does not possess the minimal characteristics of theory. Nursing practice is a volitional activity, i.e., it is what the actors make it. The requirement of a capacity for universalization dictates that theoretical knowledge claim to be independent of time or historical perspective. However, an adequate conceptual framework, or any conceptual entity, that accounts for the totality of nursing practice must change as the activity responds to circumstances that develop in the world. As a result, an adequate conceptual framework of nursing cannot claim to be universally true. Instead, what Collins and Fielder called a nursing practice theory or a conceptual framework accounting for nursing is more likely to be some other (no less worthy) conceptual entity such as a professional ideology.

A serious consequence of equating the theory needed in practice to a conceptual framework for nursing is that no satisfactory conception of theory independent of practice is provided to serve as a criterion for evaluating exactly what theory is needed in practice. In addition, by equating theory needed in practice with a conceptual framework that can account for the totality of what nurses do, the notion of theory is reduced from a generally accepted generic conception used by Beckstrand to an eccentric conception used in nursing.

Better Reasons

When knowledge implying theory is required to be capable of universalization, the evidence given by Collins and Fielder will not support the premise that the theory needed in nursing cannot be borrowed. Knowledge of particulars and the specification of the profession's moral ideals are not examples of knowledge capable of universalization. As a result, Collins and Fielder did not show that theory needed in nursing cannot be borrowed.

The question of whether the theory needed in nursing can be borrowed is an empirical one that can only be answered by experience. However, some good reasons exist for supposing that much of the knowledge capable of universalization and needed in nursing cannot be borrowed from the existing branches and knowledge of science and ethics. The question will be addressed first in relationship to ethical theory.

As argued previously, (Beckstrand, 1978a, 1978b) one reason is that existing ethical theory usually has been constructed to apply to the public in general. As a result, such theory cannot provide a sufficient basis for deciding action when people, such as practitioners, possess extraordinary abilities to act. In becoming a practitioner, a person acquires capacities for action different from those of the general population. Thus, the acceptance of professional status in the pursuit of moral ideals necessarily obligates the practitioner to take action which for others is not obligatory. For example, one can conceive of some circumstances where one would certainly agree that a capable physician, given the opportunity, who does not attempt to relieve pain or prevent death is morally censurable but the average and, therefore, relatively incapable person is not.

In addition, the practitioner has a moral obligation to acquire and implement a sound knowledge of how to achieve a professed moral ideal; an obligation that is not shared by non-professionals. For example, a practitioner is bound morally to attempt to provide tangible help in instances where the church guild pursuing the same moral ideal is not. Therefore, a moral theory useful in practice must address both the special skills and obligations of practitioners in a way that is not likely to be a simple extension of a moral theory applicable to all rational people.

With respect to the question of the theory of nonmoral good, practitioners do not only pursue the good, they decide what constitutes its particular manifestations. Moreover, practitioners develop and control powerful means for achieving what they have defined. Consequently, practitioners must be concerned with theories of the good and with how these might be interpreted.

Certainly, practitioners need a theoretical justification for assigning hierarchies to various kinds of good that might be achieved. Such a justification constitutes a theory of the good itself because it addresses the question of a good way of deciding the ascendant good among competing potentials. Such knowledge is capable of universalization and might be considered a part of either ethical theory or metapractice theory in nursing. Although I am not adequately acquainted with the theory of nonmoral value to know whether this kind of theory can be borrowed, I suspect that it cannot be.

However, even if such theory might be borrowed, there are other possibilities. For example, nurses must provide substantive interpretations of theories of the good, since nurses need to know what constitutes health or what makes sets of coping mechanisms good in certain situations. Given that the conditions of applications are well defined, these kinds of knowledge are capable of universalization and thus imply the need for theory. However, these are not likely to be borrowed from existing theories of the good.

The need to determine the nonmoral good in nursing points out an additional need for moral theory in practice. Questions of morality are involved in the acts of defining and implementing the good so that moral theories concerning the use of power and sanctions in promoting the good are especially needed in practice. Existing ethical theory approaches this problem mostly from the perspective of social control and this does not encompass the full range of the question in practice.

To answer fully the question of whether scientific theories needed in nursing can be borrowed, the question of what it means to borrow scientific theory needs analysis. While many nurses express confusion on this point, several things are clear.

First, the categories of scientific knowledge needed to explain nursing's phenomena cannot be known *a priori*. This means that nurses cannot be sure that educating themselves in an existing basic science discipline will help them understand the phenomena of nursing. Fortunately, this is not an unusual occurrence in science where many discoveries are made by people educated in the "wrong area" for the phenomena they are investigating. Like other scientists, nurse scientists must be ready to seek the information that will help them to understand phenomena of the discipline as hints about their character are revealed in the process of an investigation. What is important is an understanding of scientific method and experience with the phenomena of interest.

Second, the fact that some phenomena investigated by nurses may be explainable using forms of knowledge characteristic of an existing discipline does not signify that the knowledge is borrowed. Knowledge from one discipline is often useful as a tool in many others, and nurses should expect to use and contribute to the development of existing arenas of knowledge. What is important is that the explanations are made,

or, the problems are brought by people concerned with nursing. The understanding of the phenomena that is gained is not borrowed, but created, and can be considered original nursing theory.

What will establish nursing as a scientific practice is not only the discovery of new realms for scientific investigation, but the investigation of any empirical phenomena of interest to nurses producing results that eventually help nurses achieve particular objectives with clients in practice. All phenomena that may be of interest to nurses are not currently identifiable, but whether an investigation of nursing's phenomena will reveal them to be completely new phenomena or new manifestations of what was previously known is unimportant to the development of nursing science or to the ultimate acquisition of scientific status for nursing.

In spite of this, the question of whether the ethical and scientific knowledge needed in nursing must be produced by nurses alone still remains. Again, one cannot tell a priori. However, one can assert that with respect to ethical theory, those who do not completely comprehend the range of a practitioner's capacity to act, while able to judge isolated constellations of action, are not able to provide comprehensive moral theories for practice. Therefore, the participation of practitioners in the development of ethical theories for practice is essential.

With respect to scientific theories, investigators must have some experiential knowledge of a phenomenon to formulate questions for scientific investigation. Nurses have experiential knowledge of the phenomena they encounter, and they are currently the sole possessors of the skills, knowledge, and interest which allow them to gain access to these experiences. Therefore, given sufficient scientific training, nurses should be the persons best suited to initiate scientific investigation of the phenomena of interest in nursing practice. To the extent that others do not possess the skills or the desire to encounter the phenomena experienced in nursing, nurses must be involved.

The process of analyzing and describing this unique experiential knowledge for the purpose of scientific investigation requires interaction with other nurses. (This fact constitutes a good argument for educating nurse scientists in schools and departments of nursing.) In fact, until nurses develop sufficient scientific information to document the existence of nursing phenomena and begin to publicize and describe them, scientists outside of nursing are likely to have little interest in them.

Therefore, it seems likely that a large part of the scientific and ethical knowledge needed in nursing cannot be borrowed and requires research by nurses for its development.

References

Beckstrand, J. (1978a). The notion of a practice theory and the relationship of scientific and ethical knowledge to practice. *Research in Nursing and Health, 1,* 131–136.

Beckstrand, J. (1978b). The need for a practice theory as indicated by the knowledge used in the conduct of practice. *Research in Nursing and Health, 1,* 175–179.

Beckstrand, J. (1980). A critique of several conceptions of practice theory in nursing. *Research in Nursing and Health, 3,* 69–79.

Braithwaite, R. (1968). *Scientific explanation.* New York: Cambridge University Press.

Carnap, R. (1966). *An introduction to the philosophy of science.* New York: Basic Books.

Collins, R., & Fielder, J. (1981). Beckstrand's concept of practice theory: A critique. *Research in Nursing and Health, 4,* 317–321.

Damer, T. (1980). *Attacking faulty reasoning.* Belmont, CA: Wadsworth.

Dickoff, J., & James, P. (1968). A theory of theories: A position paper. *Nursing Research, 17,* 197–203.

Dubin, R. (1978). *Theory building.* New York: Free Press.

Jacox, A. (1974). Theory construction in nursing: An overview. *Nursing Research, 23,* 4–13.

Kuhn, T. (1974). *The structure of scientific revolutions* (2nd ed., enlarged). Chicago: University of Chicago Press.

Popper, K. (1968). *Conjectures and refutations: The growth of scientific knowledge.* New York: Harper Torchbooks.

Scriven, M. (1977). *On reasoning.* New York: McGraw-Hill.

Stevens, B. (1979). *Nursing theory.* Boston: Little, Brown.

Toulmin, S. (1960). *The philosophy of science: An introduction.* New York: Harper Torchbooks.

The Author Comments

I had just started working on a degree in statistics when Collins and Fielder's criticism appeared. Due to the demands of course work and teaching responsibilities, I was delayed in responding to their article for several months.

After submitting my reply, I had the opportunity to meet Rosemary Ellis. She acknowledged my work and encapsulated the problem with my work and Collins and Fielder's work in less than 2 minutes. I thought to myself "it took me a month and a half to figure it out."

My purpose in writing the reply to Collins and Fielder is summarized in the abstract.

—JAN BECKSTRAND

Chapter 51

Highly Technical But Yet Not Impure: Varieties of Basic Knowledge

James Dickoff
Patricia James

A practice discipline may be disesteemed by others—or even itself, because the discipline deals only in "applied" areas, not basic research or knowledge. Basic knowledge is often taken as synonymous with pure knowledge, and pure knowledge is distinguished from applied knowledge. We have tried to begin a constructive assault on the imperious distinction of pure from applied knowledge.[1] Here we go on to propose a notion of basic knowledge that seems more salutary than what is often the "received" or unquestioned or dogmatically recited notion of basic knowledge. Then we propose also a distinction of highly technical concepts from merely technical concepts, and suggest a parallel distinction of kinds of action. We suggest that professionalism is highly compatible with the development and use of highly technical concepts. Moreover, we note that nursing might find that among those concepts it could develop for export[2] would be some of these highly technical concepts.

Basic Knowledge and Use

To prize, parrot-like, pure above applied knowledge is a habit of the academy that action-oriented professions

---

[1] Except for slight modifications, mainly change of examples, the paper reprinted here was published in the January 1988 *Dental Hygiene*, *62*(1), pp. 41–42, after presentation at the University of Iowa at the Second National Conference on Dental Hygiene Research. Three related papers by us found in the same journal issue: "Organization and Expansion of Knowledge: Toward a Constructive Assault on the Imperious Distinction of Pure from Applied Knowledge, of Knowledge from Technique" (ibid., pp. 15–20); "New Calls for Knowledge Development in the Practice Discipline of Dental Hygiene", (ibid, pp. 25–29); and "Taking Concepts as Guides to Action: Exploring Kinds of Know-How" (ibid., pp. 38–41, and reprinted in this volume as Chapter 52). These four papers respond, in part, to Carol Lindeman's proposal of knowledge worker as a conception for researchers within the practice discipline of dental hygiene.

[2] (See J. Dickoff and P. James, "New Calls for Knowledge Development in the Practice Discipline of Dental Hygiene," *Dental Hygiene*, *62*(1), pp. 27–28.)

would do well to resist. To counter the unhealthy influence of the imperious distinction[3] of pure from applied knowledge we wish specially to resist, and invite others to do so too, the tendency to think that pure knowledge is knowledge with no prospect for use, knowledge unrelated to any interest in use; knowledge not sought or developed for a use; knowledge carefully sought by keeping the mind free of the "bias" of any special care or concern or alert. Our suggestion is that a more salutary conception of knowledge is that some knowledge, some tested concepts, may have uses and users beyond those and other than only those for which the concept was developed. Other concepts have a more narrow use, fewer possible users, and may be tailored for specific uses. Use and usefulness is not a source of impurity.

To think of "applied knowledge as concepts (or knowledge that might possibly be of more restricted initial use than other knowledges) is a more salutary stance for practice disciplines toward the knowledge question—given that the *raison d'etre* of practice disciplines is not merely to describe the world but to bring into the world existence of situations of a described kind. To view "applied knowledge" as concepts of a more restricted initial use is more helpful than to be misled into thinking that there is something conceptual

(call it knowledge) that is pure of relation to action, that is, pure in virtue of having no relation to action, and that this pure knowledge must then in the course of an action be "applied" without further conceptual guidance.

Still some concepts or knowledge might be regarded as more basic than others in having more uses and users than those others. We might call *basic* those knowledges (concepts) that have uses beyond those for which the concepts are initially developed; or that have uses outside the use of those who developed the concepts.

Highly and Merely Technical Knowledge

Another parrot-like downgrading that wants resistance is the denigrating of technique, technology, technicians, and the technical—as such. To counter the unhealthy influence of the imperious distinction of knowledge vs. technique, we contrast what we call here the *merely technical* with the *highly technical*.

To flee technique and technology—and so inadvertently to flee the highly competent, technically demanding action that might be at least some part of professional domain—may be done to seek freedom from inappropriate subservience or from inappropriate denial of occasions for using one's own guidance powers. To flee thus may be to flee also—unsuitably, we think—from development and use of concepts that can guide action where the concepts leave few degrees of discretion but where, nonetheless, action in absence of such conceptual, constraining guides would be impossible or irresponsible.

Consider the relatively resentful, robot-like doing of something deemed relatively insignificant and done according to a plan imposed upon the doer. Now compare this first doing with another. This second doing involves considerable detail where no degrees of freedom are left open either because knowledge is limited and the risk is great or because the person carrying out the action is depending importantly on the itemized guidance of another conceiver. The first way might

---

[3] For a discussion of imperious distinction, see J. Dickoff and P. James, "Organization and Expansion of Knowledge: Toward a Construct Assault on the Imperious Distinction of Pure from Applied Knowledge, of Knowledge from Technique," *Dental Hygiene*, 62(1), pp. 15–20. For some detail here, note from page 16:

"In an imperious distinction, the things distinguished are joined at least implicitly by a 'versus' or by an 'or' of conflict. The 'or' of conflict tends to "exclude" any middle ground between the two alternatives—excludes overlap, excludes options. For example, knowledge-worker or technician; A or B; A vs. B. The two, A, B (knowledge-worker, technician) come to be thought of as mutually exclusive of one another; so, as never found together; hence, as in conflict. The two tend also to be thought of as jointly exhaustive of the possibilities; thus, no alternatives to the two are thought to exist. An imperious distinction, then, passes—and often legislates—without question even though questioning might propel thought to a more fruitful and flexible perspective.

. . .To distinguish knowledge-worker and technician imperiously may bring two presumptions: Thinking that to become a knowledge worker it is necessary to avoid techniques and technical doing; thinking that to become as knowledge worker it is sufficient simply to avoid techniques and technical doing. We would quarrel with both presumptions.")

describe someone doing the merely technical. The second way might describe a responsible professional involved in something that is highly technical. To concentrate on the way a concept is used rather than only the content of the concept might be important in helping to remove inappropriate "merely technical" activity without inappropriately discarding or failing to develop both concepts that are highly technical and the capacity to use non-robotically even concepts that are "highly technical".

Another way to put the point here is this: The second kind of doing, unlike the first, is compatible with real conceptual agency and with professional doing once we realize that not only are some things to be done which ask for careful, precise, detailed capacity, information, and reaction, but also that:

- Not all is known by anyone.
- Not all of what is known is at the ready command of every doer who depends in some ways on or takes advantage of that information in the doing.
- Human doing calls for using the best guide possible and using it with alert rather than waiting endlessly for a perfect antecedent guidance.[4]

A distinction we would like to propose for use, then, to counter what we see as an imperious distinction[3] of knowledge from technique is the distinction of the *merely technical* from the *highly technical*. Though we might also speak of actions, procedures, or persons as merely or highly technical, we propose our distinction here in terms of two kinds of *concepts:*

A concept that is merely technical is one specified for use by someone who knows so little or will attend to so

little that the steps, items, explicit procedures, mechanisms, instrumentation, etc., are the only things to be specified in the concept and the only things to be noted in the doing.

A concept that is highly technical is one specified with elaborate detail, precision, complexity, with elaborated details on variance and the differences variance makes. Such a concept is specified for use by someone with:

- Strong and suitable background knowledge, experience, schooling, instruction, practice placement
- Command of the notation or other economies of presentation used to exhibit the highly technical concept
- Access and capacity of assess propriety of use of the concept in specific places and to assess where the use of the concept is counter- indicated as a guide to activity
- Time, energy, and capacity for invention and initiative in following up on the immediate and later consequences of using the concept as guide to activity in the instances chosen
- Status and credentials enough to have the right to put the client in harm's way to take advantage of the concepts at hand to use for enhancement, cure, or staving off or slowing down degeneration, etc.

Moreover, the highly technical concept may be a concept that would be proposed and developed as knowledge by a person with the five specifications just noted.

There may be some temptation, as nursing continues its expansion into psycho-social-economic-political dimensions, to think that poorer guides to action are purer, are more valuable knowledge; that acting in areas where there are few constraints (because there is more complexity, less risk, more adequate options) is always freer or more professional acting than is acting where there is highly technical knowledge available to function as part of the guide to activity. To bear in mind our proposal for distinguishing the *highly technical* activity from the *merely technical* activity on the basis of whether the activity is or is not guided by a *highly technical* concept may be helpful in the next stages of nursing development.

---

[4] Quoting ibid., p. 17:

"Generally, it seems to us that doing with thought (including physical doing)— activity that is guided by thoughtfully used conception—may be the highest human enterprise. In the academy—and probably more broadly—the customary talk of "pure" knowledge, "disinterested" knowledge quietly suggests application as impure, interested, less worthy, and so insidiously suggests that the activity that applies this knowledge is somehow less valued than is the knowledge applied."

See also, for a link to ethical value, Dickoff, J., & James, P. (1990). Humanizing health care practice through a more humane technology of concepts. In G.L. Ormiston & R. Sassower (Eds.), *Prescriptions: The dissemination of medical authority* (pp. 41-79). Greenwood Press.

Similarly, to bear in mind our suggestion that knowledge be considered as more or less *basic* depending on its usefulness beyond the area for which it is first discovered or developed —often for use—instead of on some fiction that some knowledge is "pure" of all use may be helpful in the next stages of nursing development. Realizing this conception of basic knowledge might encourage nurses to take responsibility for export as basic some of those tested concepts that nursing itself has originated or developed, either because of nursing's special need, special access, or special capacity, but such that nursing is far from the only discipline that could benefit from this knowledge.

To have knowledge for use well beyond only the occasion or setting that called for the development of that knowledge is a mark of reciprocal responsiveness for a growing discipline that has worth beyond only just its service worth. Still the allegiance to service would seem to be the condition for developing such knowledge, for nursing use and for export beyond only nursing.

Putting together these two suggestions on basic knowledge and highly technical knowledge might lead nursing to realize that among the richnesses nursing might have for export as a basic knowledge—useful well beyond only the restricted area for which the knowledge was first developed—would be some of its highly technical knowledge. Allegiance to the clinical dimension, suitably conceived, of nursing may need to be well cultivated to make possible the call for, development, nursing use. Nursing export of such concepts— along with whatever else nursing might develop.

Chapter 52

Taking Concepts as Guides to Action: Exploring Kinds of Know-How

James Dickoff

Patricia James

In this paper[1] we focus on a pair of notions—"knowing-that" vs. "knowing-how"—to illuminate some aspects of the knowledge question for a practice discipline such as nursing.[2]

Setting aside the detailed articulation of "knowing-that's" that can be differentiated, we can list three sorts of "knowing-that" which seem pretty clearly to be important on their bearing on know-how:

- Knowing that the world is x (some descriptive or representational statement such as: the antiseptic of choice for surgical wounds is. . .).
- Knowing that these (x, y, z, . . . [—say, heat, color, odor, . . .]) alerts and points of reference need to be taken into account in the doing.
- Knowing that someone of a given kind has to do something in a given way for a person in a given situation if there is to be effective, safe, satisfying service or practice.

The distinction of "knowing how" from "knowing-that" is a fairly going distinction used to differen-

[1] Except for slight modifications—mainly change of examples and update of references—the paper reprinted here is the same as that published in *Dental Hygiene*, *62*(1), pp. 38–41, after presentation at the University of Iowa at the Second National Conference on Dental Hygiene Research. Three related papers by the authors are included in the same journal issue: "Organization and Expansion of Knowledge: Toward a Constructive Assault on the Imperious Distinction of Pure from Applied Knowledge, of Knowledge from Technique" (pp. 15–20), "New Calls for Knowledge Development in the Practice Discipline of Dental Hygiene" (pp. 25–29), and "Highly Technical But Not Yet Impure: Varieties of Basic Knowledge" (pp. 41–42, and reprinted in this volume as Chapter 51). These four papers respond, in part, to Carol Lindeman's proposal of knowledge worker as conception for researchers within practice disciplines, whether nursing or, say, dental hygiene.

[2] See Dickoff, J. & James, P. (1968). A theory of theories: A position paper. *Nursing Research*, *17*(3), pp. 197–203; Dickoff, J., James, P., & Wiedenbach, E. (1968). Theory in a practice discipline: Part I, Practice oriented theory. *Nursing Research*, *17*(5), pp. 415–435; Dickoff, J., James, P., & Wiedenbach, E. (1968). Theory in a practice discipline: Part II, Practice oriented research. *Nursing Research*, *17*(6), 545–554. These articles are reprinted in this volume as Chapters 8, 46, and 53, respectively. See also Dickoff, J., & James, P. (1984). Towards a cultivated but decisive pluralism for nursing. In M. McGee (Ed.), *Theoretical pluralism in nursing science* (pp. 7–83). Ottowa: University of Ottowa Press. This piece contains a good set of references to other earlier Dickoff and James pieces.

tiate, usually, being able *to do* something from conceiving or being able *to conceive*, articulate, thematize, or be "thetic" about something. The "something" could be a piece of information (say, copper is a good conductor of electricity) or a doing, an activity (the activity, say, of changing a dressing or comforting a patient).

In common speech we say, "We know that copper conducts electricity." The piece of information, the "fact," is conceptualized as something known. Knowing that copper conducts electricity is a case of "knowing-that," is a "knowing-that." A "knowing-that" is a case of conceptualizing.

On the other hand, when a nurse changes a dressing or comforts a patient, the activity involves a "knowing how," a capacity to do that often does not involve conceptualizing how to do what one is said nonetheless to know how to do. That is, the distinction of knowing-that from knowing-how, as it was originally and still is used, assumes that knowing-that is a conceptual matter but that knowing-how is a doing and is not on a conceptual level.

It is often said that know how is a "disposition" of an agent: A nurse just comforts the patient or changes the dressing; she does not explicitly conceive the activity; she just does it. Being soluble in water is a disposition of a cube of sugar. Dropped in water, a cube of sugar does dissolve (engages in the activity of dissolving) without thinking about the matter at all. In a like fashion, if a nurse has the disposition of comforting or of changing dressings, she just engages in that activity without thinking about it in any but a trivial way when placed professionally before a client wanting or needing comforting or a dressing change.

The distinction of knowing-that from knowing-how was originally elaborated in a context of the discussion of rule following, and examples employed were following rules of games. Before being able to give an account of the rules, or without ever being able to give an account of the rules by listing them, reciting them, appealing directly to them a person could be said to "know how" to play the game whose very essence is granted to be given by the rules governing the play of the game.

As originally set up the distinction of "knowing-that" from "knowing-how" reflects or can be interpreted as reflecting the bias that pure knowledge is something distinct from applied knowledge. The original distinction of "knowing-that" from "knowing-how" can be extrapolated to support or reflect the view that once we have been "trained" or "educated" to do something, then we just do it without any further recourse to thought (or to concepts) in the doing. [3] In fact, some philosophers or other analysts of practice (or praxis) go so far as to suggest that conceiving can hinder the efficient, "expert" doing of an activity. Some thinkers would hold that "knowing-that" destroys "knowing-how." Others go so far as to claim that some things are in principle not susceptible to becoming articulate.[4] The emphasis on socialization to a practice in some ways embraces this latter view.

Benner's work offers empirical evidence to support the notion that the Dreyfus model is a "fit" for expert nursing practice.[4] If it be granted that there is good support from the evidence for the claim, still for starters two questions of interest arise: 1) Are there other notions that are as good or better a fit? 2) Are

---

[3] There is sometimes explicit statement of hierarchy of values among kinds of knowledge. For instance, Polyani (the chemist who wrote *Personal Knowledge* and *The Tacit Dimension*, among other works), discussing the integration managed by what he calls tacit thought, states that "the highest forms of integration loom largest now. These are manifested in the tacit power of scientific and artistic genius. The art of the expert diagnostician may be listed next, as a somewhat impoverished form of discovery, and we may put in the same class the performance of skills, whether artistic, athletic, or technical" (*The Tacit Dimension*. New York: Doubleday Anchorbooks, 1967, p. 6).

We take this quote to reflect a customary tendency, to which we take exception, to regard the "purer" kinds of knowing to be "higher." Higher on what grounds? More general? Less polluted in terms of use? It is hard not to think the second is what ends up being the case. This case worries us particularly since nursing has come to "receive" Carper, who depends relatively uncritically on Polyani, perhaps without adequately considering whether the dependence is suitable for a practice discipline that values highly—maybe most highly—its practice capacity. (See Carper's "Fundamental Patterns of Knowing in Nursing," originally from *Advances in Nursing Science* and reprinted in this volume as Chapter 19.) Not for here is a discussion of what constitutes "scientific" in this matter.

[4] For instance, Patricia Benner, who follows what is called "the Dreyfus model" in her *From Novice to Expert: Excellence and Power in Clinical Nursing Practice* (Menlo Park, CA: Addison-Wesley, 1984).

there notions or models for practice that, were they followed, would give a higher quality practice, a higher quality life than exists in the following of the Dreyfus model? These notions are more fully discussed in a paper given at a conference at Oregon Health Sciences University School of Nursing in June 1987.[5]

The Dreyfus model itself has some sympathy with the philosophic notion from some phenomenological positions, to the effect that man cannot render thetic, bring to concept, all that guides his action; that man "lives" in a world in part not subject to critical rejection or conceptual reflection and enhancement. We tend to refer to such notions as notions that "empeasant" mankind. Empeasanting know-how is one (1) kind of know-how; but we suggest there are also other kinds. We name three other kinds: (2) psittisitic (following Piaget's term for parrot-like) know-how; (3) pedantic (or schooled) know-how; and (4) a more humane, humanizing, know-how that we call complexly considerate thoughtful know-how. This last know-how is a thinking doing where the thought (the concept or conceiving) of the thinker stays perpetually open, including especially an opening to the phenomena in the scene and circumstances of action, including an opening to the special perspectives of the patient or client.[6]

The imperious distinction of knowing-that from knowing-how reflects or embodies or at least fails to challenge the bias that pure knowledge is something noble, more elevated than that "applied" knowledge that guides action.[7] Notice, then, the implications for a practice discipline of the original distinction of "know-

ing-how" from "knowing-that." First, there is the expectation that once "trained" or "educated" to perform a certain activity, a practitioner requires no further thought in any very significant way to engage in the activity. Secondly, the novice, after being instructed in selected concepts, theories, generalities, is put in a clinical environment on the assumption that education will be completed with heavy dependence on role models and other "socializations to practice."

These views play down the role of thought and conception in learning and enhancing capacity for practice. By contrast, we conceive a practitioner (whether functioning in education, research, theory development, administration, or direct practice) as importantly also a thinker, a conceiver (as part of being an inquirer). We propose that "knowing-that" can be a part of at least some kinds of "knowing-how" and that a genuine practitioner, a professional practitioner, an ethical practitioner, a practitioner who aspires to be a knowledge worker and not a "mere technician," is well conceived as a thinking doer. Let us sketch out briefly what we have in mind.

Surely, sometimes there can be "know-how" without "knowing-that" for some or all the relevant "knowing-that's." Without explicit and conscious conception either of what you are doing or any information relevant to the doing, the doing occurs. Empirically speaking, this is probably at best a limiting case of know-how, since in fact it can be said at some level of awareness is the realization that, a client or patient is there and that, say, a sterile pad, etc., is being used. So it could be said that these "knowing-that's" are present in the doing that is a dressing change. Such awareness is customarily called, though, "non-thetic," since in many relevant senses there is not thought used in the doing just portrayed. The practitioner is not guiding the practice activity by concepts. Hence, this gives us a case of "knowing-how" virtually without "knowing-that."

Conceding the possibility of acting virtually without guidance by concept, our contention is that this is not the only possibility open to a practitioner, that is, to an agent who must act. We would hold that there is a great variety of "know- how's," that "know-how" as

---

[5] The conference, titled "International Perspectives and Implications for Doctoral Education in Nursing," took place at Portland and Lincoln City, Oregon, from June 22–26, 1987. The proceedings are published and available from Oregon Health Sciences University School of Nursing. The relevant paper, titled "Thinking, Doing, Differences and Nursing Doctorates: A Prepared but Prospecting Survey," appears in those proceedings, pp. 107-148.

[6] For some further details on complexly considerate thoughtful doing as ethical doing, see, by the same authors, "Humanizing Health Care Practice Through a More Humane Technology of Concepts," in G.L. Ormison & R. Sassower (Eds.), *Prescriptions: The dissemination of medical authority* (pp. 41–79). Greenwood Press.

[7] See "Highly Technical But Not Yet Impure: Varieties of Basic Knowledge," reprinted in this volume as Chapter 51.

originally distinguished from "knowing-that" is but one of the many "know-how's" that can be distinguished. More, these various kinds of "know-how" can be ranked with respect to the degree that "knowing that's" are invoked in the doing. We suggest that responsible practitioners know or "know- how" in virtue of (a) resorting to concepts as guides to action the practitioner is doing and (b) exercising judgment in a given situation about both the appropriate concepts to use and the appropriate explicitness of use (if any) of those concepts (if any) to use as guides to action in the particular situation.

For a slightly more particular sense of what we are trying to bring to special notice here, consider these various kinds of "knowing-how" say, knowing-how to comfort or to change a dressing.

1. Knowing-how, just barely managing to do what could be recognized as comforting or changing a dressing.

2. Knowing-how, taking into account a specified range of factors in the course of adjusting the comforting or the dressing change to the particular situation.

3. Knowing-how, doing while surveilling the activity for the plus and minus features of this particular act today or comforting or dressing change in relation to the specified range of factors noted in (2).

4. Knowing-how, doing while surveilling and taking responsibility for deviations conscious of these "deviations," rather than mindlessly letting them happen and leaving them untouchable for repetition, correction, or report for special attention.

5. Knowing-how, doing while surveilling and taking responsibility for deviation (as noted in (4)) but taking into account a broad rather than a narrow scope of factors, maybe including some previously unnoted surveillance factors as avenues of possible towardness or untowardness of comforting or dressing change.

6. Knowing-how, doing while surveilling for the plus (toward), minus (untoward) features of the action, bearing in mind an explicitly held and retrievable goal and maybe also a protocol or prescription for the comforting or dressing change, and assessing in the doing even the goodness of the goal and protocol as guides.

7. Knowing-how, doing, guided by conception of goal, prescription or protocol, while surveilling for things indicated by a well developed survey list that points up factors and theories that bear or might bear on the doing of the dressing change or giving comfort, even though exactly how

each of the factors or theories bears on the activity is not spelled out antecedently—yet.

This list makes apparent that there are many sorts of "know-how." (Patently, the kinds of know-how distinguished call for considerable further exemplification and elaboration.) To characterize "know-how" as a doing unguided by concepts is at best misleading. To maintain that any "know-how" must be a doing unguided by concepts is dogmatic. Hence our proposal: "Knowing-how" is compatible both with "knowing-that" and with not "knowing-that" for some relevant "that"—say, for example, the antiseptic of choice for a wound of given origin.

What difference does it make whether or not we recognize the existence of various kinds of "know-how"? It could make enormous differences to a practice discipline attempting to "professionalize" itself. Grasping the variety of "know-hows," such a discipline would no longer speak of "pure knowledge" and the "application of pure knowledge" in the accustomed way. The accustomed way cultivates the view that knowledge is "just applied," unthinkingly, the way a band-aid is applied to a scratch. In short, the application (doing) does not call for new conception beyond the "pure" concepts. In this "use" of the "pure," this view of application does not explicitly call for any further conceiving in the very activity (moment) of doing. Application, on this view, is not an activity requiring thought, is not as valuable or worthwhile as the seeking of pure knowledge, and those who "apply" are persons of lesser capacity, giftedness, and social worth than are those who develop "pure" knowledge. This view of pure and applied knowledge, in our eyes, denigrates or underesteems practitioners inappropriately and renders practice less excellent than it could be.

Our proposed conception of the various kinds of know-how has ramifications for those interested in further developing knowledge for nursing. Recognizing that "know-how" can be guided by concepts and so involves thought (before, after, and during doing) makes it possible to use thought to improve practice by developing better conceptual guides. Practice, on the proposed view, is no mute thing that happens fortuitously or unfortuitously by chance, no matter how much circumstances are, admittedly, not under control of the practitioner. Practice is activity guided by concepts and is better or worse at least in part depending on the quality of the concepts guiding the practitioner's activity and in part depending on the capacity of the practitioner to use concepts as guides to action.

More specifically, then, one difference it might make to recognize that know-how can be guided by concepts is a heightened sense of the urgency for devoting energy and resources to develop and test concepts that would guide activities of suitable kinds, with know-how of suitable kinds; suitable to give safe, effective, well received services; suitable also to make the giving of the services gratifying to the giver; suitable to make the teaching of future practitioners an excitement to students and instructors alike. The inquiry attitude would need to be cultivated to see which concepts, used in what manner, helped how, hindered how, in the learning, delivering, and sustaining safe awareness for delivering or teaching of the various elements of practice.

Further, suppose knowledge is thought of as whatever can be expressed conceptually (or in some other articulation) and submitted to a suitable test. Beyond descriptive or more generally representational concepts, there need to be developed concepts that function as guides to action but which do not reduce simply to these representational types. Without elaborating detail, we can suggest that for us a non-representing concept presenting itself as a guide to action is a tested concept, is knowledge, when it has been ascertained to (a) who, (b) using the concept how, (c) when, (d) for what, (e) performs what purposeful activity, (f) accompanied by (1) what towardness, (2) what untowardness, and (g) with what (1) coherence, (2) feasibility, and (3) palatability for agents, recipients, and other surrounding persons, institutions, and other environing elements.[8]

Summary

We have focussed on the various kinds of know-how to suggest some of the expansions, organizations, detailings that might be of particular importance to nursing in its organization and expansion of knowledge. These organizations and expansions of knowledge might be overlooked were overly narrow notions of knowledge, its organization and expansion, to blind the minds of would-be knowledge developers. But there is one further point. Practice, conceived as activity guided by thought, can help make doing, practice, activity, recognized as an important empirical encounter. Doing may be a privileged occasion for expanding knowledge, both in the sense of getting "starters" of awareness not hitherto articulated, but awareness that comes to a doer in repeated careful doings; and in the sense of giving a suitably varied and complex empirical setting for the testing in every use of any concept taken as guide to action, whether not the use is in a formally labelled research context.[9]

Further, in the course of doing that is guided by concepts one may be in a privileged position to realize what "knowing-that's," known with what level of recall and command, are most essential in the "knowing-how" question (clues to the factors and theories for the survey list referred to in 7 above in the list of the kinds of know-how). Elsewhere[2] we have described the conceptual guide informing the "know-how" characterized as the seventh kind in that list as practice theory. For such concepts contribute to the developing of theory for a practice discipline, a theory that incorporates but is not limited to that "knowing-that" some would call either "pure" or "applied." So the resources as well as the persons developing such knowledge for a practice discipline are not to be limited to only those persons who are not (mere) practitioners in the most common sense of that term.

---

[8] Compare note 2, especially Dickoff, James, and Wiedenbach, Part II.

[9] See, again, note 2. Also see, relative to conceptual-empirical interplay, by the same authors, "Theoretical Pluralism for Nursing Diagnosis," in R.M. Carroll-Johnson (Ed.), *Classification of nursing diagnoses: Proceedings of the eighth conference, North American Nursing Diagnosis Association.* (pp. 98–125). Philadelphia: J.B. Lippincott.

Unit Six

Nursing Theory and Nursing Research

Unit Six, Nursing Theory and Nursing Research, continues to investigate the need for theory in the reality of nursing experience. While Unit Five explored the nature of theory in clinical practice, Unit Six presents ten articles that examine the role of theory in research.

Research has been accepted widely as one very useful method for generating, testing, and validating nursing knowledge. Although it is not the only method, research is a readily identifiable process that can be applied to a variety of situations to aid in understanding and to provide some degree of meaning. Gortner has stated that research is the tool of science; properly conducted research should contribute to the scientific body of knowledge in nursing.

However, in perusing journals that publish nursing research, it is easy to find examples of studies that are not, in actuality, nursing research. One might reasonably ask why this occurs.

Part of the answer comes from the fact that many people have a difficult time defining nursing, and in turn, lack a clear understanding of the nature of nursing inquiry. Also, research conducted by a nurse is not automatically nursing research. This may seem obvious, but in the literature, some examples of "nursing research" seem to have no direct connection to nursing other than the author's affiliations.

The authors of the ten chapters in Unit Six point out that theory can be used to help resolve this dilemma. Theory provides a structure to define nursing and from that structure, to identify those questions that are nursing questions. Nursing research can and will be done if the researcher starts by asking a nursing question.

This preceding discussion should not be seen as an argument for only experimental, reductionistic research. Rather, it is an acknowledgment of the need for research methods that are effective in answering nursing questions. It is apparent that due to the nature and complexity of phenomena and concepts of interest to nurses, traditional research methods may not always be appropriate for their investigation.

The ten chapters in Unit Six examine these issues and posit some solutions. As with so many of the other chapters in this book, the evolution in thinking is clear. Earlier articles argue the need to use research for testing and verification of nursing actions. More recent articles consider what types of research methods are appropriate for investigating nursing questions.

In Chapter 53, "Theory in a Practice Discipline Part II: Practice Oriented Research." Dickoff, James, and Wiedenbach continue the discussion initiated in Unit Five, emphasizing the importance of research in the practice of nursing. Schlotfeldt, in Chapter 54, "The Significance of Empirical Research for Nursing," also argues for the role that research can play in developing a body of nursing knowledge.

Chapter 55, "Conceptualizing the Research Process" by Marjorie V. Batey, outlines a scheme that can be used in relating research to conceptual structures. The impetus for this article came from Batey's dissatisfaction with texts that emphasized how-to-do research and did not stress the theoretical structure that must accompany the process.

In Chapter 56, "Research for a Practice Profession," Susan Gortner provides a brief overview of the status of nursing research at the time, 1975. When this article was written, Gortner was Chief of the Nursing Research Branch of the Division of Nursing. The examples used to illustrate the points in the article come from research that was funded by the Division at that time. Chapter 57, "The Interaction Between Theory and Research" by Jeanne Quint Benoliel, continues to stress the need for research grounded in a theoretically based structure. This theme is strongly re-emphasized in Chapter 59, "The Relationship Between Theory and Research: A Double Helix," by Jacqueline Fawcett. Fawcett states that theory and research are interdependent and one without the other is meaningless.

Chapter 58, "Philosophy, Science, Theory: Interrelationships and Implications for Nursing Research" by Mary Cipriano Silva, and Chapter 60, "Nursing Philosophy and Nursing Research: In Apposition or Opposition?" by Patricia L. Munhall, both question which research methods are appropriate for nursing. They stress that the method must come from the nature of the research question asked; it is inappropriate for the method to dictate the question.

Chapter 61, "Toward a New View of Science: Implications for Nursing Research" by Mindy B. Tinkle and Janet L. Beaton, addresses the nature of science in nursing. This is a point that has been made repeatedly in articles throughout this volume, but Tinkle and Beaton's approach presents a slightly different conceptualization of many of the issues involved in the debate.

Finally, Chapter 62, "Scientific Inquiry in Nursing: A Model for a New Age" by Holly A. DeGroot presents an optimistic view of the future of nursing research and nursing science. I find this a particularly positive note on which to end this book.

The articles in Unit Six are discussions of the nature of theory and research; none of these articles is a research report. Gortner discusses some research that was being done, but her discussion is limited and brief. However, issues raised in Unit Six have an impact on much of the research that is being done and reported in the literature. A probable step after reading these ten chapters would be to read and critique research reports, keeping questions such as these in mind: Is this a nursing research question, and why? Is the method appropriate to investigate the question? What is the theoretical structure of the research that is presented? If a goal for the discipline is to establish a tested and conceptually verified body of knowledge, then the nursing research being done must address and attempt to answer these questions.

Chapter 53

Theory in a Practice Discipline Part II: Practice Oriented Research

James Dickoff
Patricia James
Ernestine Wiedenbach

The following article is Part II of a two-part article on "Theory in a Practice Discipline." Part I, entitled "Practice Oriented Theory," appeared in the September-October 1968 issue of Nursing Research *and dealt with the relation of theory to practice and with the appropriate structure of any practice theory and, more appropriately, of nursing theory.*

To have a nursing theory what sources must be tapped? At least these three: awareness of status of practice theory; interest in developing practice theory; and openness to relevant empirical reality. If you do not know what you are looking for, you will not recognize it even if you were to find it; if you know what something is but do not see it as worth your trouble, you will spend no energy getting it; and if you are not willing to stimulate and risk your inventions in the fire of reality, your conceptions, however magnificent, have no claims beyond the academic.

The first two of these sources have been touched on in part one of this two-part article. Of the three mentioned sources of nursing theory, perhaps the most easily overlooked is this first-cited one, namely, the need for an awareness of what constitutes theory of the kind needed for nursing. A main purpose of the previous article was to make available for criticism and refinement initial thoughts consciously directed to bringing appropriate attention to this area. Hence we discussed in considerable detail the questions, What is theory? What is practice theory? and what is nursing theory? Awareness of the status of theory involves knowledge of what constitutes theory, of what the various levels of theory are and of their interrelation; how to go about developing a theory; and the possible uses of a theory. Knowing the state of existing theory in any specific area of interest is another helpful awareness, for conceptualization is always a bootstrap operation. Happily, theory can build on conceptualization that occurs before there is an explicit desire for or even a knowledge of exactly what theory is. So a first step in theory-building is clever exploitation of the conceptualization existing more or less precritically in the area for which a theory is sought; hence, our interest in pointing up fertile regions of extant conceptualization, ripe now for further development into explicit nursing theory.

Interest as a second essential source for theory is related to our earlier analysis of nursing situations, where we suggest that critical reaction even at the merely conversational level bespeaks three valuable commodities. First, criticism at the verbal level demands conceptualization; secondly, a beginning awareness of goal or at least of a better state is implicit in any criticism. But particularly relevant at the moment is the further ingredient of criticism—the interest betokened in the subject matter criticized.

A problem-oriented criticizer's interest in the subject matter incorporating the problem areas criticized is one sort of interest needed as a source of nursing theory. A call for this interest is not to be taken as a pronouncement that only nursing practitioners could be interested in producing nursing theory. Instead, what is meant to be emphasized is that theory is *never* produced in any discipline unless there is interest in or expectation from the theory—whether the hope be for clarity, status, reappointment, or a real desire to reshape and structure reality to a better dimension. But interest not only in the problems of nursing but also in practice theory as such is required for production of a nursing theory. What is needed is persons who both care about the problems of nursing *and* see vividly practice theory's potential as a help towards the resolution of these problems. No sane person, however much his interest in nursing, would invest the extensive energies requisite to move further in the development of nursing theory were he not convinced of the potential worth of that theory. But what too often exists is either persons really disturbed about the problems of practice and characterized by researchers as mere "problem solvers" or else researchers who fear their commitments to practice as biases against a true research orientation. Given the sophistication and complexity involved in helping any development, it is somewhat dubious whether motives of achieving academic status or desire for freedom from less fastidious areas of nursing would ever be sufficient to provide persistently untiring and nondespairing energy for what is admittedly a difficult, exacerbating, and not-soon-to-be-finished enterprise.

The third source needed for theory is *openness to relevant empirical reality.* But if the theory to be produced is to be a nonacademic theory for a practice discipline, what kind of "openness" is appropriate and what kind of reality is relevant?

Openness to Relevant Empirical Reality

Research is purely a part of the required openness. But practice, too, present and past, constitutes an important and not always recognized part of this third source of nursing theory.

The Features Requisite for Openness

To function as a source of theory, openness to empirical reality must have two important features. First of all, this openness must be founded on an appreciation of the worth—in fact, the indispensableness—of consulting or contemplating empirical reality if the theory to be produced is to have not only proper form but also "relevant" content. Secondly, this openness must be constituted by both the opportunity to look at and the capacity to see relevant things. That is, does the researcher as such always have a better opportunity to view empirical reality relevant for nursing theory than does, say, a full-time practitioner? Are there some aspects of reality to which only the keen senses of an experienced practitioner would be sensitive? And would a nonnurse rather than a nurse be more likely to spot certain aspects of, say, administration or power lines within a health complex?

But *what* empirical reality is going to be relevant or is going to merit the contemplation of someone whoever it be? Probably as with survey-lists within theories, so with openness to reality in research: nothing can be *a priori* excluded as irrelevant. But, on the other hand, certain kinds of reality would seem *prima facie* to demand early consideration; and for nursing theory, perhaps nursing practice as now carried on makes such a first demand. At times there is some doubt as to whether current nursing researchers are really alive to such reality both in the sense of thinking this reality worth looking at and at the same time having the opportunity and capacity to see this reality. And might it be too narrow-minded to conceive a one-to-one patient interaction as *the* nursing reality or to think that only a participating nurse can see nursing reality?

And now a second remark in the same vein. Whatever is taken as relevant, care must be exercised that the empirical reality gazed upon is of the kind the viewer claims to be inspecting. For example, is the interplay between patients and a nurse with no service responsibilities beyond those accidentally accrued as a participant observer collecting data about nurse-patient interaction really an instance of nursing? Or is the interplay a laboratory situation of some kind despite its location on a clinical floor? And if so, what ramifications has this fact for conclusions drawn about nursing on the basis of the data so gathered?

Research and Practice—Distinctive Kinds of Openness to Empirical Reality

The claim here is that practice and research are alike in being types of openness to empirical reality. But there are important differences. Research, like practice, is an openness to the present but, unlike practice, an openness that has as essential ingredients, a remembered past and a future planned beyond whatever accomplishment occurs in that present. More fully, though practice is activity that may have fruits beyond its own accomplishment and though a practitioner may be reflective and self-critical in the performance of practice, the essential output and virtue of practice as opposed to mere research lies in the accomplishment of something in the here and now. Research, on the other hand, is activity that has planned goals beyond the immediate accomplishments. That is, research is an activity whose main function is inquiry and what is accomplished in addition to inquiry is *as research* gratuitous. Conversely, inquiry accomplished through practice is accidental to the activity *as practice*. In a sense practice is for itself; research, for something other than itself. Research is an *instrument* or *tool* whose activity is inquiry and whose end product is early vintage theory, theory that has undergone some test of reality; in short, research is not an end in itself.

Research is conscious of the past and so is well named as a kind of reflection back to or a planned re-encounter with a certain sort of reality. Research is activity which occurs, at least in part, as a confrontation of an empirical reality deemed relevant to something which in a sense brought about the research. Narrowly conceived, the "past" may be the hypothesis guiding the inquiry. More broadly conceived, this past can be seen as the practical problem or conceptual unclarity producing the initial discomfort. From that discontent may have arisen the energy as well as the inspiration, hunch, or perhaps guess about a hypothesis but more generally also about what kind of empirical reality might be fruitfully encountered in an inquiring mood.

Though similar to practice in being a planned activity taking place in the present, research is inclined to be more formal than is practice. Research tends to be vitiated when not done according to preconceived plan, whereas practice—activity having as its main goal the accomplishment of a task in the present—can alter its planned routine in the interest of achieving that immediate purpose. Formality is both a virtue and a drawback of that kind of openness called research. (In terms of our earlier discussion, practice is terminus oriented; research, procedure oriented.)

Also in orientation to the future, research tends to differ from practice. Research has a planned future beyond its own accomplishments, in the sense of a planned increase in knowledge. Practice, too, may be said to have a planned future; but the main aspect of that future expectation is not an increase in knowledge. Providing a basis for future good practice, for well-being of the patient of the practice—or even for increase in funds or goods for the practitioner, thanks to accomplishment of practice—these are more likely future expectations of practice.

Research—Objectives as Related to Methods

Research, then, differs from practice in that research has as its essential goal input to knowledge beyond the immediate particular. To have knowledge is to have conceptual frameworks or grasps which have genuine capacity to structure reality. And research is useful both in arriving initially at a conception and in testing that conception for adequacy. Three avenues are available to man both for arriving at initial conceptions and for assaying the conception in its relation to reality. These three modes are first man's conceptualizing power, secondly his senses, and finally his capacity to interact with reality—whether in plain daily living, in professional practice, or in research. Research properly conceived in its relation to theory—a conceptual framework—and to reality (the reality of practice where the theory is a practice theory) is man's systematic way of exploiting in conjunction all three avenues towards inventing, testing, or readjusting a conceptual framework.

Possible Research Objectives

Research is perhaps unfortunately described as an "abstracting" of theory from reality. For as we noted in the nursing episodes characterized earlier, no amount of interaction with reality—even if the encounter is planned—dictates a conceptualization that fits that reality. But though interaction cannot dictate, still, planned or unplanned interaction with reality may supply impetus as well as direction for some initial invention of concepts; and certainly planned interaction can help establish the knowledge warranty of some proffered conceptualization. In other words, research is an activity that may have either of two objectives—both of which are related to knowledge-getting. First, research may function to stimulate conception and then is engaged in as heuristic towards theory. Openness to empirical reality presents the observer with a manifold or multiplicity that tend to demand a unification in terms of a concept; the manifold's content directs in some fashion the concept that will be invented for the unity. At the very least, proper openness to empirical reality eliminates as obviously unfitting an incredibly large number of the infinity of possible concepts that might be invented. This quick elimination of inadequate concepts we often tend to take for insight towards the relevant. But perhaps more fruitful methods for inviting invention result if we view the situation thus: Every concept is equally relevant unless we have indication of nonrelevance.

The second objective of research is to test, assay, or validate a conception already made. And we test the concept's fit to reality—or more properly the adequacy to purpose—by giving the conceptualization every chance to be discounted as a good fit. Our warrant increases in proportion to the number of opportunities the conceptualization has had to fail to fit and yet has not failed.

But theories are big, research studies small in scope. So how could research stimulate or validate a theory any more elaborate than a set of a few factors or more extensive than one or two statements of prediction? This very query emphasizes the importance of knowing just what theory is as a whole and what is a theory's part. For in inventing, testing, or readjusting a theory the work must progress on a part only. This need for fragmentation sometimes makes us forget that the fragments require putting together—and makes us overlook too that work on a part may be vitiated if during the progress of that work no proper account is taken concerning the relation of that part to the whole.

We can say that research has two objectives or that research has theory as its immediate objective but in two different ways. Research may be aimed at helping towards a statement of theory where none exists or where the existent one is thought to be inadequate; or research may be aimed at testing the adequacy of some already stated theory or of some part of that theory. For simplicity's sake let us say research can function as a tester of theory or a stimulator of theory.

Method as It Varies with Theory Level and Research Objective

Research or openness to empirical reality has as objective, then, either the stimulating of conception or the testing of a conception. Research methodology might be viewed as the rules, rubrics, or procedures governing research. Research methodology, in other words, should be a stipulation of those rules that allow research to fulfill its function. These rules may vary accordingly as research is done to stimulate or to test theory. Moreover, methodology needs to vary also accordingly to the level of theory being stimulated or tested.

To stimulate a given level of theory is to dispose the mind to conceptualize factors, relations of factors, relations of situations, or goal-contents, prescriptions, and survey lists accordingly as the level of theory being stimulated is factor-isolating, factor relating, situation-relating, or situation-producing theory. To test a given level of theory requires realizing that a theory is a conceptual framework invented to some purpose and then assessing whether or not the theory serves the purpose for which the conceptual framework is invented. The aim of theory changes with the level of theory. To propose a theory as valid is to claim that it has met its aim, and to test a proposed theory is to assay this claim.

To stimulate the proposal of a theory, then, is to encourage the invention of a conceptual framework that could meet the specified aim. Two explicitly planned ways to stimulate theory at whatever level can be discerned. In the first way a researcher, after having immersed his mind in all existing "relevant" theory, however embryonic or developed, which the newly sought theory might supplant or extend, encounters again and again, and with as many variations as possible, empirical reality of kinds deemed relevant. Such planned "staring" might stimulate theory invention at any level. The second planned way to stimulate theory at a given level is to test theory at the just-preceding level. Such testing provides a structured context and a properly set mind for taking advantages of "insight" generated by interaction with reality. This mode of stimulating theory reflects that theory at any given level exists as significant for theory at the next level. But what then stimulates theory at the first level? Practice. For practice can give a set of relevance; and reflective practice can constitute a mode of research. In a sense, the two kinds of openness to empirical reality tend to reduce to one when the objective of research is stimulus of theory and the level of theory is the most basic. (Actually, such reflective practice can constitute stimulus-research for higher levels of theory, too.)

But let us move to the much more recognized kind of research—where the objective is testing theory. To test a theory is to ascertain whether or not the proposed theory fulfills its claim. For example, a factor-isolating theory claims to give a complete set of significant factors (or names for these factors) for relevant kinds of real situations. Research that tests this claim must first translate into terms of a setting the characterization of relevant real situations as specified by the theory. For each factor there must be specified what empirical indicators are taken as signalling the factor's presence in the real situation. Then confronting realities as specified by the setting for each such situation, a researcher should note whether or not that factor is present. He should note also whether any "significant" factor falls to be nameable from the set of terms specified by the theory. After the encounters, analysis of data recorded should include noting: (a) which factors were never noted, (b) which were most frequently noted, and (c) which factors were present and deemed significant and yet not noted by the theory. The claim of the theory is warranted by the research-activity findings if no significant factors are unprovided for by the theory. In some ways testing a level-one theory is most difficult of all testing-research, since there is a demand that the researcher follow, as an important aspect of the test, his judgment without the guide of formal rules. Only a researcher with a sense of significance could carry on such research. Perhaps only a practitioner can perform this testing; as noted with respect to nursing, in an unplanned way the conduct of practice itself helps both to produce a first-level theory and as we see now, perhaps also to test as well as revise that theory. In other words, relevant situations—that is, states of affair—are initially the set situations in which we find ourselves; the initial clue to significance is found in both the aim we have in those situations and the difficulties experienced in fulfilling that aim. As we observed elsewhere—particularly in discussing embryonic nursing theory—theory emerges initially from practice and the first movements are not self-consciously theoretical.

To realize that to test a theory is to see whether it fulfills its aim enables us to be suggestive as to what constitutes testing of a situation-producing theory. That factor-relating theories and especially predictive theories can be tested is fairly well accepted and hence not particularly discussed here, except to remark that to test such theories is exactly to ask if they fulfill their own claims. In fact, methods of testing factor-relating or situation-relating theories are almost the only kinds of methodology that routinely have their due—or at least have characteristic procedures specified, however much lack of clarity exists as to what following such procedures amounts to or has significant terminus. We are more familiar with the procedure by which we make these tests than we are with seeing at what these tests aim. One advantage of looking at the extreme levels of theory is to make necessary the articulation of the larger context of theory-testing.

As for any level of theory, to test a situation-producing theory is to assay whether or not the theory meets its aim. The purpose of situation-producing theory is proposed as threefold: (a) that the activity called for by the theory if done by the specified agents will achieve the theory's goal; (b) that guiding activity by this theory will produce desirable results; and (c) that guiding action by this theory is feasible when considered in relation to the worth of the goal achieved and the costs of achieving that goal in a way set forth by the theory, where the computed costs include the opportunity costs of those goals sacrificed or subordinated to the production of activities toward the goal as specified by the theory.

To test the theory requires testing all three dimensions of the theory's claim. To test the first claim is to

test the theory's coherency; in a sense goal-incorporating theory or situation-producing theory specifies one of its own measuring rods. For the theory claims that doing what it says in the way it says will produce what it says. To test this claim, theory-specified agents must perform according to the theory and then measure must be taken of whether the resultant activity produces or moves toward the theory-specified goal. The theory's coherency claim fails to be rejected by a research study if the produced activity is not predominantly or even in significant amounts destructive of reality as pictured by the goal. Notice that among the many tasks of setting up appropriate research methodology for assessing coherency would be the task of agreeing on a procedure for discerning effectively whether theory-specified agents are acting as specified by the theory. The procedure needed may be distinctively different from those now provided to test lower levels of theory.

To test the claim that action in accordance with the theory not only produces activity toward the theory's goal but that such activity when produced turns out in fact to be desirable as an achievement is to test the theory's "palatability." Despite the frequent attempts to call such questions policy matters or matters of taste, still ways to test such palatability claims against empirical reality suggest themselves if we distinguish between professional judgment of practitioners —judgment based on knowledge, experience, and professional aims—and mere subjective whim of a person who happens to be a practitioner and allow that professionals may be, practically speaking, capable of making decisions of preference on the basis of such distinction. Very often a goal as conceived is found repugnant when realized, or some factor necessary to the realization is found repugnant. Putting a theory into practice and observing the outcome, once there is some warrant that the theory is coherent and hence that the produced activity does move to the achievement of the theory's goal, is sometimes the only way man has to ascertain what he does desire or deem worthwhile. He must produce the something and watch for his reaction of repulsion from or attraction to the results. Such a test is no less empirical for involving reactions beyond the level of "single sensation"; and where provision is made for assessing not only one man's idiosyncratic reaction but for canvassing a significant number of relevantly sensitive individuals, perhaps an adequate kind of testing might result, adequate particularly if we recall what the purpose of the theory is with respect to practice. Theory in its highest reaches is tested in situations that come closer and closer to being practice itself. And the cost of testing such a theory becomes in itself a very important question—and not simply from the viewpoint of the commodities spent in the testing. Far more significant is the cost as computed in terms of the value or disvalue of the reality produced in the course of the test. This question of cost applies just as readily to the testing of any level of theory; we are simply less aware of the issue at the other levels because there the absolute costs involved tend to be less. (What, for example, in terms of nurse-discomfort, ward peace, and patient's privacy is the cost of a study performed to test whether a nurse's open-ended or closed-ended questions produce more satisfaction within the patient? Not to speak of the cost to the researcher herself.)

Testing not the coherency or palatability claims but now the feasibility claim of a situation-producing theory has two important dimensions: (a) the assessment of whether there exist agents not only who could but who could in fact be induced to produce activity in accordance with the theory; and (b) the assessment of whether the cost of supplying the inducement and so using the agents is worthwhile in view of what is sacrificed—including other goals left unachieved—to move such agents to act.

No question about it—testing practice theory is a wide-ranging business. But unless within his limits man makes such an attempt he is forever compelled to act without the light of theory and so to remain at the level of inarticulate art—a position having grave consequences for educating an adequate number of able practitioners, as well as for the quality of practice. Or else he must dumbly follow a theory of dubious validity. Is there any sense to excluding conceptualization from a realm where reason has high potential for significant contribution not only to man's clarity but to his well being?

Method as Essentially Nonabsolute

Research methodology, then, can be expected to vary accordingly as theory is being stimulated or tested as well as with the level of theory in question. When the task to be accomplished shifts, the clever way of doing the task may shift also. Yet another way of putting the point is to observe that research methodology is not an absolute entity. Talking about methodology without specifying that for which the methodology is a methodology makes as incomplete sense as to call something simply *equipment for or tool for*. Because method as such can constitute a study, the term "methodology" is quite fittingly used to denote the science of method. But notice that in common research parlance, methodology has come to mean the way a study is done—not reflection about how the study is done or is to be done.

Even if we regard research methodology not merely as reflection about method but as the articulation or stipulation of what rules shall govern method, again we see that research method is not an absolute standard. Research-methodology in this guise is happily regarded as a code of rules set down before conduct of research, and meant to hold not for a single researcher but for the total community of researchers. The existence of such a code permits a given researcher to structure his activity explicitly in accordance with these rules; he thereby knows pretty clearly what he has done and how to repeat it, hopefully without essential variation, as often as he desires. And if we take into account more than one researcher, the code of rules sets a common standard that can be referred to when one researcher reports his work to others in the community. A two fold advantage results: When the initial researcher makes available his results together with explicit indication of the method used in reaching those results, he can hope for collaboration from his fellow-researchers. They can now supply checks and corrections to idiosyncratic directions his search may have taken—whether he inadvertently slipped from his stipulated method or whether, though method was explicitly followed, not all sources of variation were covered by the provisions of the method used. But further, other researchers may place confidence in work done according to a method known and accepted as appropriate for the study reported and so stand on the shoulders of the first researcher. Even if fault is found with the initial research, its very evaluation in terms of the common standards may let the next researcher profit from the limitations of the first one or from his suggestive half-starts. In short, for consistency within the research of one individual and for community among researchers, codes for method are essential.

But if research-method is regarded as a preset and common code governing certain aspects of research-activity, why call research methodology nonabsolute? Because the code is not natural law but convention. Confidence is placed in studies guided by the code not because the community of researchers has some absolute guarantee that studies guided by the code can confirm theories in any *absolute* sense or has even any *absolute* proof that such guidance moves us any closer to theories capable of structuring reality. Man's reason tells him what would be required for absolute proof or absolute guarantee of the right-headedness of a method; but reason tells man also that he cannot achieve such guarantee. Yet faced with his desire and the recognition of his inability to fulfill that desire, he does not despair. Reason is moved to invent clever ways to take account both of man's limitations and of his aims for knowledge. "Methodology" in its most honorific sense could be used to label reason's inventions for allowing man, despite his limits and in the light of awareness of those very limits, to come ever closer to reaching his aims. These aims are to understand, control, and shape reality to man's own safety, pleasure, and satisfaction. And he has contrived to use these very aims to extend his limited capacity for knowing—and hence to come closer to those aims. For research is that kind of inquiring activity which uses reason, senses, *and* interplay with reality in activity—at the very least in eye activity—to get an answer for reason's inquiry. Research is an activity to which man resorts, not one to which he aspires.

A good way to see the nonabsoluteness of methodology for research methodology designed, say, to test theory, is to look, for example, at each level of theory and ask what would reason unqualifiedly demand for the verification of the claim of theory at that level. Consider next wherein it is impossible to fulfill those demands; view research-methodology as the compromise formation invented by reason in the light of its aims and the realization of its limits and agreed upon by a community of researchers who acknowledge the same limitations, espouse the same aims, and have enough confidence (or faith) in the agreed-on method to spend time, energy, and sometimes a life in following the method's dictates.

More particularly, we would have to ask these three questions:

1. In order to allow a given experience to serve as a warrant that the reality so confronted can be structured in terms of given conceptualization whether that conceptualization is a set of factors, one or a collection of statements of relation among factors or relations, or is a total practice theory, what does absolute reason require by way of (a) conditions obtaining in the reality to be confronted and (b) information from the senses.
2. What of these demands does reason itself see as unmeetable without omniscience or as unmeetable given man's access to empirical reality or his limited supplies of energy and commodities?
3. What are the *formalities* men can invent and agree upon as adequate if followed (a) to serve as a substitute for an absolute guarantee that preconditions are met and (b) to supplement or make more economical the limited access to empirical reality?

Methodology is nonabsolute in yet another way. Since a methodology as a code governing research activity has status as a code in virtue of being accepted as such by a community of researchers who acknowledge the same limitations, espouse the same aims, and have enough confidence in the agreed-on methods to spend precious commodities following its dictates, any difference with respect to limitations, aims, or commodities at one's disposal may have ramifications for the kind of code or methodology adopted. In other words, it is conceivable that there would be more than one research community—provided researchers were consciously aware of their own limits and aims. And even given no difference with respect to limits, aims, or energies, when we see methodology as reason's invention for complementing and exploiting reason's limitations then it is fairly clear that methodology is nonabsolute in still another sense—namely, reason may be capable of (and perhaps should be stimulated to) more than one way around its difficulties.

We particularly emphasize the conditional nature of methodology to prepare our minds for the task of asking creatively what kind of research is needed or possible to test or to stimulate practice theory for nursing. Rather than take over uncritically a preformed code, note should be taken not only of what must be accomplished to produce or test a nursing theory but also of what are the striking features of the aims, capacities (the converse of limitations) and privileged access available to potential researchers for nursing theory. And especial attention needs to be directed to the distinctive potential of those persons who are skilled practitioners in the discipline for which "confirmed" theory—that is, useful theory—is sought.

Conclusions: Situation-Producing Theory—A Common Denominator of Practice and Research

In considering nurse as theorist, we have emphasized:

1. Practice-oriented theory (Part I)
2. Practice-oriented research (Part II)

Considering theory in a practice discipline requires considering not only theory in itself but requires discussing also the question of such theory's relation, on the one hand, to practice and, on the other hand, to research. And to render explicit the interrelations as among practice, theorizing, and research requires a prior distinguishing of the characteristic features of each of these three activities. Of the triad—theory, practice, and research—most elaboration has been given to the theory component. The presentation offers

probably a novel viewpoint on theory—or, in other words, constitutes a certain contribution to the theory itself. So why not discuss only theory or at least make theory the first and focal point of the discussion? Because equally essential with pointing out what must be characteristic of theory for a practice discipline is the pointing out of such theory's place in the context of the recognized activities of practice and research—even if the indication, as here, is somewhat sketchy, with promise of and need for elaboration elsewhere by us and by others. Without such indication the proffered theory of theories for practice disciplines risks remaining merely academic.

In this paper the treatment of theory here is prefaced by practice considerations and followed by remarks on research. Why this order? Partly to trace out what would seem to be a natural interest pattern for a person professionally engaged in practice: If practice be the professions why go to theory if there is not an awareness of theory's link to practice or a demand from practice for theory? And since theory—to have any ramification for practice—must take disciplined account of empirical reality, any practical consideration of theory must envisage theory's intimate interplay with research. But in addition to tracing out a fairly natural interest pattern, the placing of theory between practice and research literally "pictures" two points fundamental to this presentation.

1. Theory is an economic and appropriate mediation, go-between, or common ground as between the two empirical activities of research and practice; and perhaps even more important, research is done not for its own sake but to produce knowledge or, more elaborately, to produce theory.
2. Theory for a practice discipline is not an end in itself but is produced for the sake of practice; in a practice discipline practice is the thing that is done for its own sake.

Research is for theory, theory for practice, so that practice fittingly has first place and theory the mediating role.

Suggesting the ranking that puts practice in first place seems properly to mirror what are instrumental goods or values and what are ultimate goods for a person who has professional interest as a nurse. Pointing up this ranking is meant also to call attention to the difference between the ranking suggested here and the hierarchy that might be offered were we to consider the scales of status and monies accorded as external rewards to the three types of activity—especially in situations where questions of academic status are involved.

However we resolve the questions of relative worth of the three activities of practice, theorizing, and research, still the question of their interdependence arises. The upsurge in nursing energies devoted over the past one or two decades to research suggests an awareness that practice could be contributed to by research. And researchers in and out of nursing tend to be aware that research eventually contributes to theory and aware too that usually research is done in the context of or is guided by existing theory. But that practice, therefore, must depend on theory is realized much less explicitly. And even among professionals willing to see what research can give to practice, there is often a reticence to acknowledge any similar potential for theory. The paper tries to render explicit this dependency of practice on theory; but the paper calls attention to further dependencies often overlooked: the dependence of theory on practice and the dependence of research on practice. Diagrammatically:

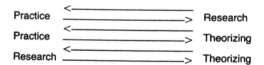

There is a thorough-going mutual interdependence as among the three activities of practice, theorizing, and research. But though the dependence is circular, the activities can or must be ranked linearly, not only when we consider comparative worth or questions of final significance but also when we consider these questions: In what order are these activities to be engaged in by some one individual? Or, in what order should instruction be given in the various activities? What competence is presupposed in the other two areas by any agent titling himself expert in any of the three areas?

What competence is presupposed in any person deemed capable of directing or *administering* activities in any or all of the three areas?[1]

In summing up the presentation's findings or contributions about nursing theory, it may be helpful to emphasize first of all what the presentation does *not* purport to do. The presentation does not offer a nursing theory; rather what is proposed is a theory of theories in general and a thesis is offered as to what sort of entity a nursing theory is or should be, both *qua* theory and *qua* nursing theory. But the offered theory of theories is not a full-scale investigation in minute detail either about theory in general or even about the various levels of theory. Rather the presentation tries to give a map of theory so as to allow the location of nursing theory in relation to other theories and other levels of theory (thereby showing how other theories are ingredient in or presupposed by nursing theory), as well as to sketch the relation of nursing theory to nursing practice and to nursing research. Finally, granted the findings offered are novel in certain aspects, still they are not radically new and, moreover, are a generalization beyond rather than a refutation of some current—perhaps more orthodox—views on theory. The presentation points out how some views of theory may be overly restrictive and perhaps even stultifying, especially for practice disciplines, and suggests a higher perspective from which to view theory *qua* theory. This new perspective gives a notion of theory broader than but not incompatible with fairly accepted notions of theory.

In other terms, this presentation comments on nursing theories in general, rather than supplying some one nursing theory and so is a so-called "meta-level" discussion, at least as regards nursing theory. The tech-

---

[1] Pointing up the interrelation of the three types of activity with the claimed interdependence between the most abstract—theory—and the most concrete—practice—recalls the age-old Platonic theory of the interdependence of our various ways of "knowing" (see Plato's *Republic*, especially, particularly Book VI), and brings to mind also the more contemporary discussions on the interrelation of "knowing how" and "knowing that," as, for example, in Gilbert Ryle's *The Concept of Mind* (London: Hutchinson House, 1949), especially Chapter II.

nique used in arriving at the broadened notion of theory was to scrutinize carefully the ordinary doctrine of predictive theory to lay bare the implicit presuppositions of such doctrine and to draw attention to the not-often-explored extensions of such doctrine. (Brief indication is given also to this same generalizing move with respect to research methodology which must parallel the more sophisticated view of theory).

More particularly, once existence of predictive theory is acknowledged, analysis discloses that predictive theory presupposes capacity to conceptualize the components necessary to conceptualize a prediction. Claim is made, that is, that two kinds or levels of theory are presupposed by predictive theory—a first level that in a sense contributes factors, units, or concepts; and a second level that contributes theoretical descriptions of situations in terms of these factors so that at the third level predictive theory can supply relations between these situations. Seeing predictive theory as giving relations between situations allows seeing the general point that at a similar level we might be interested in relations more elaborate or more subtle than mere casual relations as between situations. Moreover, seeing the stages or levels of theory preceding the predictive level helps render plausible the existence of a level of theory more elaborate than situation-relating theory (of which predictive theory is the predominant example)—namely, situation-producing theory, in which are conceptualized not only the kinds of situations deemed worthy to be produced but also the means for producing such situations as well as the areas to be given attention in so-producing such situations.

To be theoretical is to deal at the conceptual level.[2] One sign of being at the conceptual level is articulate verbalization. That is, while emphasizing the possible existence of theory at higher reaches than mere prediction, further claim is made that theoretical activity starts long before the stage of prediction. Capacity to name factors and to describe situations through relating factors are theory-using capacities.[3] Advancing this claim makes clear that theory may be used non-self-consciously and brings up the question of, so to speak: How many concepts make a theory? Or, when is a theory fully explicit? Rather than elaborating answers to these questions, the suggestion is made as to the importance of realizing that always many things may be left implicit but that explicit attention at times needs to be given to the examination, refinement, or perhaps reconstruction of theories presupposed at whatever level.

In addition to holding that all theory is conceptualizing, the thesis is offered that a theory is fruitfully regarded as *a conceptual invention to some purpose*. Theory at whatever level is a conceptual invention; the purpose of the invention varies according to the level of theory. And an invention is deemed validated or good insofar as known to fulfill its claimed purpose. This analysis of the general features of theory needs to guide the detailed search for methodologies appropriate to building and testing theory at each of the levels.

Seeing theory in this broader light makes clear that theory for practice discipline is not theoretically an impossibility. Nor is such theory—and this awareness is of paramount significance—merely the trial and error, intuitive "application" of predictive theory. What is required as theory for a practice discipline is situation-producing theory. Such theory constitutes conceptualization of the *relations* that must exist between, on the one hand, whatever predictive theories are required and, on the other hand, other things and theories necessary to produce situations of the kind deemed professionally good by the practice discipline in question.

But if there are four levels of theory, why not five? Because theory begins and ends in practice. Situation-producing theory has as its purpose the production of situations of a given kind—that is, has its ultimate reason for being not to provide conceptual basis for a more sophisticated theory but to provide a basis for action. And—looking at matters from the other end of the

---

[2] For a contrast with the theoretical in the sense used here, consider the function of the non-thetic in, for example, Maurice Merleau-Ponty's *Phenomenology of Perception* (New York: Humanities Press, 1962), especially Part III, Section 1.

[3] For an example of a contrary view that seems unfruitful and restrictive for theory, see, for example, Gilbert Ryle's *Dilemmas* (New York: Cambridge University Press, 1964), especially the first section.

scale—realizing that self-conscious conceptual activity presupposes non-self-conscious conceptual activity, such as grows out of disciplined activity, focuses on the birth of theory in practice or action.

The remarks about theory for nursing practice are not relevant only to nursing practice. The "First Vintage"[4] structure of situation-producing theory in terms of goal-content, prescriptions, and survey list, though only sketched, is relevant for the structure not only of a nursing theory but for a theory for *any* practice discipline—whether it be medicine, law, teaching, engineering, or city-planning. Moreover, the six-fold analysis of activity suggested as structuring the survey-list ingredient—agency, patiency, framework, terminus, procedure, dynamics—might, quite beyond nursing practice as such or even its theory as such, serve as a stimulus or heuristic device for thinking through problematic situations in nursing research, education, or administration, or, even outside of nursing, in any realm where activity is in question.

Moreover, even the treatment here given practice itself could be suggestive beyond the confines of practice. The practical considerations in part one of this article were presented through a series of problematic situations. The situations were analyzed and re-analyzed in a movement toward both articulate awareness of the "problem's" nature and articulate presentation of possible solutions to the practical problem. This movement could constitute a depiction in miniature of the thesis that nonacademic nursing theory must begin and end in practice and that practice itself and its demands can contribute criteria of significance and priority as to what areas want theory and hence research. The practice situations were seen upon analysis to present problems that could be grouped in three not unrelated areas: conflicts of interest, practice stereotypes, and questioned nursing image. Focus on these same areas reveals significant problems in nursing *research,* too.

A nurse-researcher is very likely to be aware of conflicts of interest which she has with other re-

searchers as to prerogatives, priorities, and jurisdiction over populations for use as research subjects. And these jurisdictional and priority conflicts the nurse-researcher experiences arise not only in her relations with other researchers but arise perhaps even more tellingly in her relations with nursing or medical service, hospital administration, and educational programs. What's more, the nurse-researcher probably feels certain conflicts *even as among her own interests:* How can she reconcile her practice and teaching commitments with the research demands? And even within the research interests themselves, should she devote herself to basic research or to more problem-oriented research? Will the values of clinical research offset the advantages of neatly controllable laboratory studies? And should she lean more towards the biological sciences or the psychosocial sciences in choice of both methodology and background theory for the research? Should she try for broad explorations with fairly obvious nursing significance or discipline herself to narrow topics and more precise controls with "significant" results but with less obvious nursing significance?

Awareness of these conflicts may be a sign of progress toward their resolution, provided the conflicts are not regarded as so severe that research activity ceases or becomes radically unsatisfying to engage in, or seriously distracted from its proper purpose. What seems to be the case is that some of these conflicts are submerged or are resolved by explicit or implicit appeal to certain nursing-research stereotypes:

1. Don't invent methodology but rely on methodology from some "established" science; experimentation is the most reputable research.
2. Give priority to basic research so as to avoid mere problem-solving or other bias from your own profession; no usable research measure is profession dependent; as researcher, a nurse must forget she is a nurse.
3. Policy questions are not researchable; research can supply predictive theory but that theory then needs to be applied by the practitioner.

Two more overarching guiding protocols are often these—again implicitly if not explicitly:

4. Fundable research is the only research worth doing.
5. Significant results are publishable results, and conversely.

---

[4] In the sense of Francis Bacon, *New Organon*, Book II, Aphorism XX.

And finally the general research climate gives rise to the policy that there can be no legitimate body of nursing knowledge except what is produced through research.

Nursing researchers may well operate under these stereotypes. Should they? Should they what—operate under stereotypes? Or, operate under *these* stereotypes? Wittingly or only implicitly? As was noted both in terms of practice and in the discussion under theory of procedure as an aspect of activity, stereotypes or protocols or policies make real contribution to economy and stability they are consciously proposed, followed, and are habitually re-assessed in terms of the purpose of the activity they are supposed to render economic and stable. So the questions become—How can a nurse-researcher resolve inevitable conflicts? And under what rubrics or protocols ought she to carry on her research activity? Answering these questions requires taking account of the purpose or image of nursing. The danger is, however—partly because, as noted concerning practice, the image of nursing is not totally unambiguous—that the easiest or least painful resolution of conflicts will be accepted and that any available procedures for research will be adopted provided only they are already established and reasonably simple and explicit. For as Nietzsche in particular pointed out,[5] not only the nurse-researcher but any human finds it unsupportable to be without explicit standards of activity. And further, the human will take over for his activity standards that may totally defeat his own purpose rather than work with no standards or with standards having no one else's stamp of approval. And though all humans, claims Nietzsche, have this demand for "security," the tendency is found in marked degree where there is self-awareness of any weakness. So here and now in nursing research it would be surprising were such a tendency not apparent; for here is the profession of nursing, largely made up of women, engaging in activities somewhat new to it and often in academic institutions where other disciplines have had consider-

able head start in research activity. But, as with Nietzsche, the reason for our pointing out this tendency is to warn the nursing profession against being victimized by this desire for certainty, a desire often stronger than the desire to persist on the path that secures self-preservation of a profession's own aim. Practically speaking, what is needed is for a nurse-researcher to develop both her self-surveillance and her self-esteem so as to be able to take advantage of the help and securities of established disciplines without thereby sacrificing her nursing impetus or nursing identity.

What is the nursing image in terms of which to legislate on conflicts and discern genuinely helpful stereotypes? Or, how can we discover this image if it is not already known? There is the rub! And now we come to another aspect of the point Nietzsche urged, a point signalled also by John Dewey, for example, in entitling a book *The Quest for Certainty*.[6] Intellectually we humans tend to think of a realm somehow outside and above work a day reality, a realm wherein all knowledge is present; and we see our task as that of laying bare or discovering what was put there somehow by an agency beyond our own. But just as Nietzsche would emphasize the importance of learning to live with self-imposed standards, so Dewey translates this emphasis into a method of inquiry that urges capacity to live with the tentative. The function of intelligence is, as Dewey urges, one of rising invention rather than of making pre-patterned discoveries. So what is required to supply nursing research with the wanted criterion is an invention as to what the most fruitful and yet feasible image of nursing should be. But the invention, though risky, need not, therefore, be baseless: past experience and thought, present research, as well as foresight, can guide the invention. Nor, once offered, need the invention be accepted either forever after or without test. The courage to risk an invention, the capacity to operate in terms of that invention as guide, while not losing

[5] See, in particular, Nietzsche's *Genealogy of Morals*, especially Essay III.

[6] See also John Dewey's *Reconstruction in Philosophy* (Boston: Beacon Press, 1957) and especially *Human Nature and Conduct* (New York: Modern Library, 1930).

the capacity to subject the guide itself to further assessment, and the stamina to risk yet another invention if the present one proves unsatisfactory—these are needed.

In short, *to supply a nursing image is to venture a nursing theory.* Theory at any level requires invention. Theory for a practice discipline requires theory at the highest level—situation-producing theory. Theorizing at such a level involves in a double sense the risks of novelty. Such theories are creative not merely because knowledge must be invented rather than simply discovered but because they have as purpose not merely an awareness of the world as it is but rather the bringing into being segments of reality according to the pattern of the theory's conception.

As coda be it remarked that a theory of theories too is an invention. The theory offered here should be assessed not only in terms of its variants from certain "approved" standards but rather in terms of its fruitfulness and feasibility as a guide to theoretical activity—especially for theorizing for a practice discipline.

Chapter 54

The Significance of Empirical Research for Nursing

Rozella M. Schlotfeldt

Thoughtful nurses are now thoroughly convinced that they need but do not yet have a body of structured science to guide them in nursing practice. The clamor is thus growing to convince investigators that they should engage in deep thinking in order to produce theoretical formulations that are worthy of testing and that hold promise of contributing to the development and structure of nursing science.

With acceptance of the need for promising theories and verified science to guide practice two questions must be addressed:

1. With what phenomena should nursing theories be concerned?
2. What is the most promising approach to the development of theories significant for nursing?

The first question can be answered by delineating the foremost objective of nursing—that which provides the central focus for practice, education, and research.

An answer to the second question involves a choice of approach to the generation of new knowledge.

One of the first requirements of theorists is to identify the essential nature of the particular knowledge system about which they inquire. Recognition of the interrelationships between and among disciplines does not relieve theorists of this requirement. Thus for nursing, as for any practice discipline, investigators must identify the central focus of practice and delineate the phenomena about which theories need to be developed.

Nursing is a service to Man. The central focus of nurse practitioners is care of people who need help in coping with problems along the continuum of health-illness. Although nursing encompasses a variety of intervention modalities, all are designed to enhance each individual's health-seeking behavior, to stimulate his avoidance of disease and disability, and to promote productive use of his own inherent capacities to be re-

About the Author

ROZELLA M. SCHLOTFELDT was born and raised in DeWitt, Iowa, and is a magna cum laude graduate of the University of Iowa, receiving a B.S. with a major in Nursing in 1935. After graduation, she worked in various clinical positions at the University of Iowa Hospitals and the U.S. Veterans Administration Hospital in Des Moines. During World War II, she served as a Lieutenant in the U.S. Army Nurse Corps, Domestic and Foreign Service (ETO). After discharge from the Army in 1946, she returned to school for graduate study at the University of Chicago, receiving a S.M. (1947) in Nursing Education/Administration and a Ph.D. (1956) in Education and Curriculum Development.

Dr. Schlotfeldt has worked as a nursing educator for more than 50 years. She has held faculty appointments at the University of Iowa, University of Colorado, and Wayne State University. In 1960, she joined the faculty at Western Reserve University (now Case Western Reserve University) as Dean and Professor of the Frances Payne Bolton School of Nursing. She served as Dean for 12 years and returned to teaching as a Professor of Nursing in 1972. Since July 1, 1982, Dr. Schlotfeldt has been officially retired, but is still active. She comments "My interests and concerns include theory development and the identification, discovery, selection, and structure of nursing's corpus of knowledge."

Among Dr. Schlotfeldt's numerous professional achievements are more than 120 scholarly works that have appeared in books and journals. She has received more than 35 honorary awards, including an endowed lectureship at Case Western Reserve University and seven honorary degrees. Dr. Schlotfeldt has spoken widely, both nationally and internationally, on a multitude of subjects since beginning her professional career. About her success in nursing, she comments "I have, throughout my long and sustained career, considered nursing to be an exciting and personally fulfilling profession." When asked about the future of nursing, she responded "Nursing leaders have the option of promoting nursing as a learned profession and a scholarly discipline through emphasis on scholarly practice, high-quality professional education, and systematic inquiry."

stored to health and maximum capability in circumstances of genetic inadequacy, trauma, disease, or deprivation of several kinds. Nursing practice encompasses compensating for man's inadequacies and sustaining and supporting him throughout periods of temporary or permanent dependence caused by infirmity, disease, or dysfunction. Since the object of nursing intervention is man himself, the professional must have command of knowledge about man as a rational, sentient, valuing, reacting, and dynamically interacting, producing, and reproducing being. A holistic conception of man is appropriate for practitioners whose interventions are designed to alter and improve man's function as a total being (Spring, 1969).

Conceptualizing the nature of nursing points up that nurses' proper study of mankind should be his behavior as it relates to attaining, retaining, or regaining health and maximum function. The focus of inquiry designed to generate useful theories for nursing includes man's behavior relative to his motivation to seek

health as well as his behavior in coping with crises encountered throughout the life process—birth, genetic failure, infirmity, deprivation, disfigurement, changes in life style, disease, disability, and periods of development and decline. The focus of inquiry must also include man's behavior as he copes with a wide variety of diagnostic and therapeutic modalities. The feature that distinguishes nursing science from other science is the type of knowledge about man that nurses need and use in practice. Inquiry to advance nursing science, quite obviously, must be concerned with man's behavior in response to circumstances that require nursing action and his behavior in response to that action as well.

There are two reasons why delay has been encountered in the development and structure of nursing science. Within the nursing profession there has been uneasy and tenuous harmony with regard to the nature of research that the profession has supported and valued. To date there has been a paucity of research concerned with man's coping behavior on the health-illness continuum. This circumstance has resulted because nursing practice has not been highly regarded by many nurses in positions of leadership and power, and also because nurses in large numbers have abdicated the role nurse *qua* nurse. Certainly if knowledgeable nurses do not routinely deal with problems of nursing practice, they can hardly be expected to think deeply about them, to inquire about them, and to seek new insights into their resolution.

A second reason for delay in structuring nursing science can be attributed to the approach followed by investigators. Within the nursing profession there has been undue reliance upon theoretical constructs borrowed from other disciplines and uncritical acceptance of them—both with regard to their inherent validity and to their usefulness in explaining and making reliable predictions about the complex phenomena encountered in nursing practice. The observation does not deny the usefulness of knowledge from the "basic" disciplines to nursing practice; rather it points up the need for conscious, critical analysis of the validity of theoretical formulations from the several fields of knowledge and the need to assess their significance for nursing practice. Only as knowledgeable, observant nurse-investigators systematically study problems of nursing practice will they be able to test the validity and relevance for nursing of theories set forth by other scientists; only as they ideate about their observations will they be able to develop theoretical constructs that hold promise for advancing and structuring nursing science.

The title of this paper conveys confidence in empiricism and in inductive thinking. This orientation leads to reliance on empirical inquiry for generation of new nursing knowledge rather than acceptance *a priori* of knowledge vouchsafed from "outside" sources. It should be noted that commitment to the advancement of knowledge through empirical inquiry assumes commitment to the use of knowledge to gain more of it. Immediately the observation must be made that justifiable inductions are based upon antecedent knowledge. The question that logically follows relates to the justification of *initial* inductions; and therefore, the question concerning the validity of all knowledge gained

through inductive inquiry must be posed. The answer to that query is that new insights must always be confirmed or rejected by empirical evidence viewed in the context of logic and relevancy to all other existing beliefs within any knowledge system at any one time. Making it explicit that propositions and beliefs generated through empirical inquiry must bear logical relationships to one another points up that both refinement and advancement of knowledge are inherent in the process of empirical research. Elements of any knowledge system are reformulated and rearranged as logic dictates at any point in time, and are revised and corrected through repeated tests of hypotheses in several ways over time. This represents the process of advancement of knowledge and the structure of science through empirical inquiry (Hawkens, 1964).

The history of progress in any knowledge system attests to the fact that observation and ideation are two crucial aspects of theory development. A third essential ingredient is the capacity of the one who observes and ideates to conceptualize creatively and to think systematically. These two types of thought processes might seem to be antithetical, for creativity connotes lack of restraint, whereas systematic thinking imposes pattern and rigor in intellectual processes. However paradoxical these requirements may seem to be, it is important to note that in the process of systematic inquiry there are two time periods when ideation should be quite unrestrained. They are prior to decisions about the purposes and design of an investigation and after data reduction and analyses have been completed. Rigorous and systematic adherence to procedures should prevail in the intervening period. It is creative thinking about empirical data that leads to hypotheses worthy of test and to the generation of promising theories as well. How then will empirical research contribute to theories useful for nursing?

Firstly, empirical research is essential to establish the existence of order in human phenomena of concern to the investigator. Repeated, systematic observations can be expected to distinguish facts from pseudo facts. The order assumed to be inherent in nature generally can be assumed to extend to human beings. Making explicit those phenomena that persist over numerous observations permits extension of knowledge about the behavior of man as it relates to his seeking of health and coping with threats to health, with disease, and with disability. Such behavior must be broadly conceived to encompass that which is physiologic, psychologic, social, voluntary, and involuntary. Facts deriving from such observations are ingredients needed for generation of theories having relevance for nursing.

Secondly, empirical research reveals inadequacies in currently held explanations of human phenomena as they are pertinent to man's attaining, retaining and regaining health and to his restoration of function. Even though attempts to develop grand theories of the life process of man are ongoing, there is as yet no verified science that leads to the understanding of all behavior of human beings (Mathwig, 1969; Rogers, 1970). Findings from empirical inquiry do illustrate the interrelationships between man's physical and emotional responses as he attempts to cope with problems inimical to health and with his therapeutic regimen (Chapman, 1969). Findings suggest hypotheses that, when tested, may lead to the synthesis of knowledge from several disciplines useful in the explanation of human phenomena and for making reliable predictions as well. For nursing and other practice disciplines, empirical inquiry leads to knowledge that can be used to explain and predict. It must also contribute to the structure of verified science relevant for practitioners.

Thirdly, and most importantly, empirical research leads investigators to develop theoretical formulations that are useful for the continuous improvement of practice. Such formulations serve as guides *for* practice and when tested *in* practice, provide data that are self-correcting with regard to the validity and usefulness of the theories generated. Empirical inquiry thus becomes the instrumentality through which theories are generated and systematically tested, refined, and restructured; it is also the means through which practices are improved when they are guided by verified knowledge.

Scientists have long accepted the need for investigators to inquire into phenomena relevant to their fields as the means for advancing knowledge. The chemist deals with chemical phenomena and by so do-

ing, searches for the logical relationships between theories and observable facts. His quest for developing new chemical knowledge thus has hope of fulfillment. The advancement and structure of knowledge for its own sake, however, is insufficient for the theorist in a practice discipline. The nurse-investigator-theorist must be in a position to contribute to building theories concerned with antecedents to and consequences of nursing action as they are revealed in responses made by those they serve (Ellis, 1969). Intelligent nursing action will result only to the extent that practices can be guided by theoretical constructs about man's health-seeking and coping behavior—tentatively held until they are repeatedly subjected to test.

Summary

Acceptance of the assumption that there is need for theories to serve as guides for nursing practice makes empirical inquiry mandatory. The focus of that research must be on man's behavior as it relates to his seeking health and coping with disease and dysfunction. Since nursing action should be designed to assist the persons nurses serve, it becomes essential to determine through empirical investigation the several mechanisms that are and can be productively utilized by man in his coping with threats to health, life crises, infirmities, disabilities, and dysfunctions. Concomitantly, nurse theorists must concern themselves with determining the nursing interventions that have predictable chances of augmenting the health-seeking behavior of individuals and groups and of enhancing their successfully coping when their health and productivity are in jeopardy. Empirical research is thus significant for generating theories and equally significant for improving nursing practice. It is as crucial to the structure of nursing science as knowledgeable nursing practice is to the well-being of mankind.

References

Chapman, J.S. (1969). *Effects of different nursing approaches upon psychological and physiological responses of patients.* Cleveland: Case Western Reserve University.

Ellis, R. (1969). Practitioner as theorist. *American Journal of Nursing, 69*, 1434–1438.

Hawkens, D. (1964). *The language of nature*. San Francisco: Freeman.

Mathwig, G.M. (1969). Nursing science. *Image, 3*(1), 9–14.

Rogers, M.E. (1970). *An introduction to the theoretical basis of nursing*. Philadelphia: F.A. Davis.

Spring, F.E. (1969). *Man: A holistic conception for nursing*. Cleveland: Case Western Reserve University.

The Author Comments

In this paper, I sought to acquaint a listening audience (thoughtful nursing clinicians and clinical investigators) and also readers of *Nursing Research* with values to be derived from empirical inquiry. Although I could have addressed the significance of other kinds of research as well, it seemed appropriate then (and now, too!) to pose two questions—namely, which phenomena nursing scholars should generate theoretical statements about and which approaches were most promising for the development of theories *for* nursing. Now, I would broaden the second question—the emphasis then was *primarily* on searching for *scientific* knowledge useful to nursing practitioners and on seeking to close the gaps in knowledge that practitioners recognize.

Although I believe that the paper accomplished its goal, it contains a term I no longer use and believe is not helpful. The idea of a health-illness continuum is not productive for nursing scholars (my bias). Nursing's intellectual focus should be on enhancing (through research) knowledge concerning the health-seeking mechanisms and behaviors of all human beings. Nurses should study human beings, not only those who have problems. Nursing's *main* concern (intellectual) can be conceptualized as a health continuum (surely physicians are primarily concerned with human pathologies and the *mechanisms* of disease processes). Both continua can be conceived as existing simultaneously. Gradients of health can be conceived as health status and also as health potentials to be fulfilled. Health-seeking mechanisms and behaviors can be viewed as health assets. Knowledgeable nurses can render these assets most effective by promoting (enhancing) human beings' *use* of their health assets and *achievement* of their health potentials through deliberately selected nursing strategies. Of course, nurses must know about the myriad factors that affect the health of humans, too; only some of them can be influenced by legitimate nursing action.

I am also now critical of the term "nursing theory." I believe that nursing scholars should propound theories about human phenomena of concern to nurses; some of the theories may be useful to scholars and practitioners in other disciplines and professions. I would like to have nursing scholars' names attached to those theories they propound that prove to be productive of valid science. Nursing does not *own* theories. When nurses become known by the theories they propound, their membership in the scientific community is enhanced and, more importantly, nursing will become known as a scholarly discipline.

—ROZELLA M. SCHLOTFELDT

Chapter 55

Conceptualizing the Research Process

Marjorie V. Batey

In a general way the purposes of a nursing research colloquium are to provide a forum for research concerned with health, illness, and delivery of health care and to stimulate research ideas among the colleagues who are present. Yet these can only be means toward a broader purpose—the quest for an expanding body of knowledge made up of ordered facts and generalizations which are both reliable and valid. Such an expanding body of knowledge forms the basis for health care delivery, for the instructional programs for new recruits to the health care professions, and for the continuing search for new insights. There is no other rationale appropriate to all of the work and expense of the research enterprise. Basically, research is a tool of science. For it to serve well as a tool of science, each component of the total research process must be clearly and rationally conceived, to the extent possible, a priori to the action elements (data assembly and analysis) of research.[1]

The Nature of Science

If research is a tool of science, then what is science? Following the work of Rose (1965), there are four essential characteristics. First, "science is objective and unbiased" (p. 9). It seeks truths; that is, facts which are relevant to that being studied and which are valid. Guided by the objective and unbiased criterion, the

---

[1] Few specific references are cited in this paper. Through the years the sources of the ideas have become blurred as I have attempted to form meaning. To the extent that there is clarity of meaning. I wish to acknowledge former teachers and colleagures—the graduate students, faculty, and other work associates—who have caused me to think through what I do mean by the research process.

About the Author

MARJORIE V. BATEY was born in Hamburg, Iowa, but considers herself a "westerner." She received her professional education in Washington State—a diploma from the Sacred Heart Hospital School of Nursing in Spokane and a B.S.N. from the University of Washington—and at the University of Colorado (M.S. and Ph.D). Since 1956, she has been a member of the faculty at the University of Washington; thus, Seattle is home.

Dr. Batey's clinical preparation was in psychiatric nursing; in the early 1960s, she was director of those programs at UW. Following her doctoral studies, she organized and directed the UW School of Nursing's Office for Nursing Research Facilitation, a unit devoted to strengthening the research component of faculty role. She also has served as a consultant to schools of nursing on the topic of faculty research development. Currently she holds a professorship in the School of Nursing's Department of Community Health Care Systems. Her teaching activities include undergraduate- and graduate-level research methodology and units of the graduate nursing administration program.

Dr. Batey's research interests have been consistent throughout the years: structural and process conditions that impact on goal attainment. Her past research has examined organizational structure as it relates to faculty research productivity; autonomy as both structural and perceived conditions relative to administrative and clinical practice; and structural autonomy, as manifested by law, for its bearing on nurse practitioner prescribing practices. Current inquiry attends to organizational culture in the contexts of clinical and administrative nursing environments.

In her leisure time, Dr. Batey is an avid gardener.

---

scientist's wishes, personal motives, or personal prejudices may not guide the research enterprise which serves science. (It is not posed that science is value free!)

Second, science "is interested in arriving at generalizations" (Rose, 1965, p. 10); those are ultimately of a cause-and-effect type. Generalization is used here to emphasize the search for that which is common and general, not simply accidental and different. In this sense, science is not concerned that a child with a physical handicap is teased by an age mate, nor is it concerned that a patient whose eyes are bandaged following surgery feels lonely. Science would be concerned with such tentative generalizations as children with handicaps receive forms of harassment from age mates or that the sensory deprivation fostered by bandaging the eyes is associated with increased alienation manifested as loneliness.

Within this second characteristic, science seeks at least two types of generalizations: theoretical and empirical (Rose, 1965). The empirical generalization is a summary statement about facts derived by systematic methods. For example, "children in residential treatment centers for mental retardation are older than are those in community-based treatment centers." This is simply a general statement about ordered facts. In many areas of health care research, it is necessary first to assemble such ordered facts before it is possible to move to more refinement of meanings.

The theoretical generalization is a "statement about what takes place *if* certain conditions occur" (Rose, 1965, p. 11). The theoretical generalization is derived from two sources—often from an interaction of the two. It is a guess derived from "logical and abstract thinking (reflecting) about observed phenomena and from previously discovered empirical and theoretical generalizations" (Rose, 1965, p. 11). The aim and characteristic of science is to seek generalizations; the two forms which these generalizations may take have particular relevance for the comments to be made later in this paper on the conceptual phase of the research process—the interrelation among the research problem, conceptual framework, and purpose.

The third characteristic of science is that it constantly strives to develop "better methods for securing the facts deemed necessary to arrive at the generalizations which it seeks" (Rose, 1965, p. 11). The facts which science seeks are embedded in the real world of ongoing reality. These facts are not readily accessible, they are not sitting and waiting for the easy grabbing. "The facts, to have relevance for science, must be observed within a specified frame-of-reference, must be measured with precision, must . . . be related to other relevant facts" (Rose, 1965, p. 11). In summary, ferreting out these facts may require methods not immediately accessible; may require methods which need refinement in their precision; or may call for methods not yet devised. Science seeks such improvement and refinement, plus appropriate use of these methods. The ingenuity of this effort is what can lead to truly creative studies.

The fourth characteristic of science as posed by Rose is that it provides "a coherent body of theoretical generalizations into which all new research is integrated" (Rose, 1965, p. 12). The various disciplines and professions meet this criterion with different degrees of completeness. Yet if our values are congruent with the values of science, our endeavors can lead us in this direction.

The Research Process

Since research is seen as a tool of science, and not as an end unto itself, the characteristics of science have been presented first in order that the remainder of this paper may be placed in that context. The research process has three phases: (a) the conceptual phase, (b) the empirical phase, and (c) the interpretative phase. Most of this paper will be addressed to the conceptual phase: the interrelation among the research problem, the conceptual framework, and the purpose. The empirical phase is the conduct of the activities necessary to obtain the information and to order (analyze) the facts needed to satisfy the purpose. The interpretative phase is the determination of the meaning of the facts (findings) once they are obtained and in relation to the purpose and the

conceptual framework. Less emphasis will be placed on these two phases in this paper.

The word research, for many of us, conjures up images about answering questionnaires, doing observations, looking in microscopes, or handling statistical manipulations. Research uses these empirical procedures, but it is more than these procedures. Prior to doing observations, for example, the investigator had to have made a variety of decisions. What was he going to observe, what would he look for, why look for these points and not others, to name but a few. Whether aware of it or not (and hopefully he is) one does not simply look at facts, classify them, and run t tests. The investigator's "way of selecting certain facts and searching for order among them is guided by some prior notion or theories about the nature of the phenomena under study" (Riley, 1963, p. 5). For example, two investigators may have observed in emergency room that patients receive differential treatment. One investigator might be guided by concepts such as social class and social distance as he attempts to discover the nature of the observed differential treatment. The second investigator might be guided by concepts such as incongruence between self and other role expectations to address the same problem. While the two investigators might have been stimulated by the same real world phenomenon, their notions of why it occurs, their conceptual organization about the problem, the knowledge base they select for studying that problem, may differ. But while they may approach the presenting problem with differing knowledge bases, it is important that they make overt the knowledge base which will guide each of their research decisions.

Following the writings of Riley, the research process requires an "organizing image of the phenomena to be investigated. It starts with a set of ideas—whether vague hunches or clearly formulated propositions— about the nature of these phenomena" (Riley, 1963, p. 6). This organizing image, this set of ideas, is the knowledge base or conceptual framework of the research. "It is this conceptual framework (model) that determines what questions are to be addressed by the research," and hoped to be answered by the research, "and how the research procedures are to be used as tools in finding answers to these questions" (Riley, 1963, p. 6). But the investigator, before he arrives at this stage of developing his study, must have already accomplished important steps in the research process.

The Research Problem

If the conceptual framework is the organizing image of the phenomena, what is the phenomenon to be investigated? This is the research problem. It derives from observations of real world phenomena and/or the orga-

nized body of knowledge. On Figure 55-1, "Paradigm of Research Process" (as adapted from Riley,) these two areas are depicted with broken lines. This is intended to reflect that our perception of the real world of events is always selective and incomplete and that the existing body of knowledge is incomplete and is selectively used. The problem is that unanswered question which started the investigator thinking in the first place. One might observe that certain events occur and wonder why, or observe events which seem to occur with certain regularity and wonder if that regularity would hold

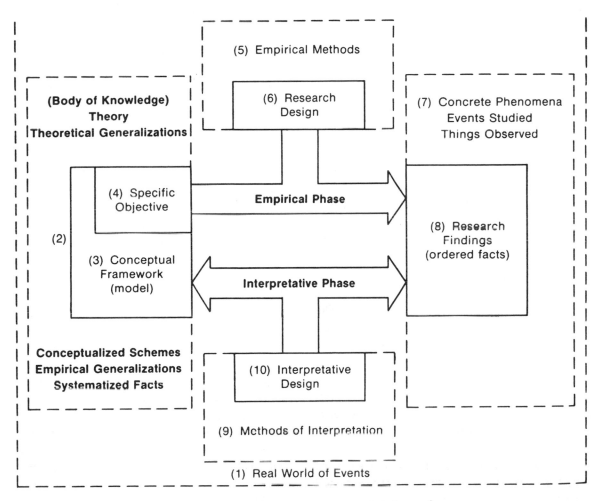

Figure 55-1 *Paradigm of the Research Process*[1]

[1] Adapted from M. Riley (1963), *Sociological research*, p. 4.

with systematic study. One might read certain state-ments and question their validity or might be provoked to examine an untested proposition. The problem may be generated by an unexpected insight during reading, observation, or conversation, or it might be field-in-duced, that is, generated by a need to take some action in some sector of social life. As Hoffman has stated, the problem is "the extended statement of the area where answers are needed". (Hoffman, 1969, p. 6) The initial statement of problem is often rather crude, but the words or concepts it contains can give some direction to the type of literature to be searched for ideas which will give further elaboration and clarification.

The Conceptual Framework

The state of existing knowledge about that which the researcher elects to study strongly influences how he will proceed to develop his conceptual model for the research. To the extent there is some accumulated body of knowledge about or related to the phenomena, the researcher will build his conceptual framework within the context of such knowledge. While there may be glaring gaps in the body of knowledge, the investigator builds his framework such as to use accumulated facts which have been classified, organized, and analyzed. The researcher rounds out his framework with any first-hand knowledge he may have of the particular phenomena to be studied, or any hunches of his own that seem to merit further investigation. But he builds his conceptual framework, insofar as possible, not sim-ply from such *ad hoc* fragments, but also from the available general theories that seem germane and from appropriate portions of the larger body of knowledge. It is in this process of building a conceptual model that one finds the interaction between the real world of events and the systematically accumulated body of knowledge (Riley, 1963).

At this stage of nursing research, it would seem important to call attention to the fact that a conceptual framework is not a review of literature. The review of literature conducted by the investigator is but one tool for the development of the conceptual framework. The

conceptual framework represents a product derived through creative appraisal and use of literature, the source of the accumulated body of knowledge. One does not simply accept a published statement; it must first be examined for its relevance to the image one is attempting to develop. As Helen MacInnes stated in one of her spy sagas, "If we demand an honest state-ment of the ingredients of every package of food we buy, it seems odd that we should treat our minds more carelessly than we do our stomachs" (MacInnes, 1941, p. 7). We can not carelessly accept published research findings into our emerging conceptual framework until they have stood the test of critical appraisal using rele-vant criteria.

Earlier conceptual framework is described as the researcher's organizing image of the phenomena to be studied. It is the researcher's image of how the phenom-ena he wants to study exist in the real world. The researcher may want to study certain aspects of behav-ior, characteristics of human beings in given circum-stances, or the relevance of a given concept in interac-tive process. His framework will generally consist of ideas—more or less clearly formulated—about (a) these human beings (his conceptual cases), (b) these aspects of behavior or characteristics (the conceptual properties of the cases), and (c) the ways these aspects fit together and/or affect each other (the relationships among properties of the cases). In this way, one set of ideas in the framework describes that portion of human beings he will use as the case or point of reference for his investigation—the case may be groups, individuals, cells, et cetera. A second set of ideas in the framework refers to certain properties of the case, for example, role expectations held, attitudes of one specified case (mother) toward another specified case (child), age, edu-cational attainment, levels of integration within groups (cases). The third set of ideas within the framework, if the state of existing knowledge warrants such expres-sions, postulates certain relationships among these properties. For example, the greater receptivity of pa-rental behavior toward the nurse, the more readily will the child move into active play groups in the treatment center.

The extent to which the existing body of knowledge and the investigator's creative use of first-hand knowledge can interact to permit specification of the case, its properties, and the relation among properties, will determine the research objective and ultimate research design characteristics which are possible. We have all heard the expression "It's just a descriptive study" expressed in a tone of bare tolerance and conveying mediocrity. In like manner, we have heard the expression "It's an hypothesis-testing study" or an "experimental design" expressed in a tone conveying superiority and high-level achievement. Neither is acceptable; neither is justifiable! The conceptual framework of a study, when conscientiously and purposefully developed, dictates the type of research design which is appropriate. If we know very little about the properties of the cases we wish to study, it would certainly be foolhardy to predict relations between these properties. On the other hand, if we have available to us an accumulation of well-documented facts (empirical generalizations) about these properties, nothing will be gained to set out to acquire more of the same kinds of descriptions.

The Research Purpose

The research objective or purpose is dictated by the conceptual framework. It is plotted as cell 4 in Figure 55-1. It states which elements in the model are to be investigated—which levels of which kinds of cases, which properties, and which connections between properties. Therefore, the research objective can be no more clearly formulated than the set of ideas from which it is drawn, and the clarity of the relevant portion of the framework will affect the main emphasis of the objective. In this manner, the research objective may be to describe certain patterns of behavior of mentally retarded children in crisis situations; it may be to explore differing patterns of behavior in crisis situations in relation to extent of retardation; or it may be to test a specific hypothesis predicting patterns of behavior evoked by specified types of crisis situations when degrees of retardation are held constant. The purpose (objective) thus may be stated in several forms, to de-

scribe, to explore, or to explain. The latter two forms will likely be presented as hypotheses, while the first will likely be a setting forth of what one will describe. The conceptual framework would identify which of these research objectives would be the logical outcome of the framework. In a research program, rather than in a specific research study, all three objectives might be undertaken—that is, to the extent that findings derived from the first frame of the program led to the natural consequence of the next study. These comments are intended to illustrate how several studies can derive from one conceptual framework. Further comments about a research program as contrasted with one study will be made below.

The Research Design

The research process starts with the conceptual framework. Not only does it start there, the entire process is dependent upon the conceptual framework. What has been described thus far, somewhat briefly, is how the conceptual framework serves the investigator in selecting significant problems when gaps in the theory make exploration necessary, or when theoretical propositions require further testing. Essentially it is through the content of the conceptual framework that we have the rational basis for selection of the specific research purpose(s) of the specific study.

The second critical use of the conceptual framework is to guide the selection of appropriate methods for the empirical phase of the process. The reservoir of empirical methods and the specific design selected for a study are depicted as cells 5 and 6 of Figure 55-1. Again, the broken lines depict the incompleteness and, at times, the inadequacy of empirical methods. Methodological research, an area not dealt with in this paper, is needed before many important studies can be initiated. The research design is the investigator's selection—from all available methods—of a particular set of methods that he will follow in obtaining his research findings, hence, in approaching his research objective.

Prior to selection of what we ordinarily think of as methods—interview, observation, et cetera—the investigator must first translate his conceptual framework into empirical terms. In his framework, the investigator has presented his conception of the case, his conception of the property, and has postulated, possibly, something about a relation among properties. He must now translate his conception of cases into what will be the concrete case(s) of his study. Will the case be the individual, will it be a dyad (for example, mother-child, nurse-child), will it be units of behavior? Next, he must translate his conception of properties into empirical indicants of the properties of his cases. Throughout, the term property is used in this paper in much the same sense we usually use the term variable. It is preferred in the context of this paper because it seems closer to our ordinary conversational language. It is intended to denote something which the case has; it's his property. Across cases the property varies, and hence the property is a variable. For example, one property may be expected functions to be served by an emergency service. An empirical indicant of that property may be the stated reasons by a case (a patient) for seeking emergency room care. The variable aspect of the property is that it can differ across cases.

In addition to the above components, the research design will specify the setting in which the study is to take place, the method for selecting the cases to serve the study, the specific instrument to be used as the empirical indicant of the conceptual property, the specific methods and steps which will be used for analysis of the obtained information in relation to the objective, and a time-phasing of the remainder of the study period through completion of the written report. Such a time-phasing plan permits the investigator to reexamine each step he projects throughout the empirical phase of the research process to insure that all relevant steps are included in his plan.

Data Analysis

The empirical phase of the process continues through the actual data assembly process and the analysis of the obtained information. Cell 7 of Figure 55-1 depicts the environment of the data assembly process and the concrete phenomena studied. Conceptually, this is what the investigator has chosen to extract from the real world of events for studies which occur in natural settings and it is his construction of events in laboratory settings. The results or findings of the study are depicted in cell 8. The methods of analysis to be used to derive the ordered facts reflected by that cell will be dictated by the form of the research objective.

Interpretation

As to all other components of the process, the conceptual framework is also essential to the interpretative phase of research. Once the research findings are known, the investigator has not completed his work. The conceptual framework was the investigator's a priori image of his research problem. Was this image supported empirically? Were the findings contrary to the image? Did the conceptual framework as developed lead the investigator to study properties or to use empirical indicants of them which, on post hoc examination (also called 20-20 hindsight!), were not those which best illustrated what was to be studied? Do the findings lead the investigator to develop an alternate explanation for his findings? The interpretative phase requires the investigator to examine his findings for their meaning in relation to the provoking problem, the conceptual framework, the purpose, and all research decisions made in developing and implementing the empirical phase of the study. It is in this phase that reconceptualization occurs; this in turn leads the investigator to the next step in his research program.

The Research Program

Earlier it was suggested that several studies might derive from a single conceptual framework. The investigator might consider his research problem in such a way that it has a number of diverse facets, each of which he wishes to study. Depending upon his resources, these studies might be undertaken simultaneously or in sequence. The sequence of studies may be considered as a research program. As the first study is completed, the reconceptualization of the guiding knowledge framework is likely to lead to a new organization of a priori baselines for decisions in the empirical phase of the next study. If the first study were descriptive in design, the second study in the sequence may call for additional description. On the other hand, the second study may now have a sufficient knowledge base to permit hypothesizing relationships among properties and call for an exploratory design.

Figure 55-2 depicts one conception of the research program. Each component of the research process as described for the single study is shown, though in different form, on the overlay of the paradigm. The intent of the paradigm is to convey how the reconceptualization of the initiating research problem and the derived conceptual framework in relation to the research design, as accomplished in the interpretative phase of a study, lead to the next stage of investigation. The type of study pursued, whether it be descriptive, exploratory, or explanatory, will depend upon the state of the body of knowledge upon which the study is based. Whether considering the single research process or the more encompassing research program, the critical ingredient is consistently the investigator's imaginative use of the body of knowledge available to him. Through careful conceptualization of the research process, the total study design, each study will move closer to the ideal of serving as a tool of science.

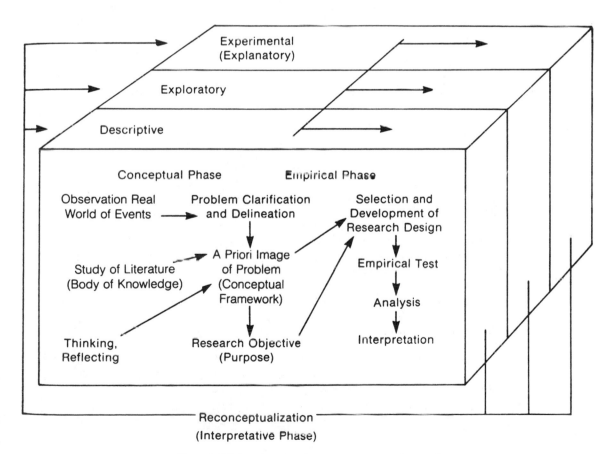

Figure 55-2 *Paradigm of the Research Program*[1]

[1] Adapted from paradigm developed in conference with Barbara Bates, Melvin Sachs, and Donald Yett, May, 1970.

Summary

Prepared for presentation at a nursing research colloquium, this paper covers a discussion of the nature of science and the place of the conceptual framework in research with respect to the research problem, the purpose, the research design, the analysis of data, and the interpretation of findings. It is suggested that several studies may derive from a single conceptual framework, that is, a research program, and a model of a research program is presented.

References

Hoffman, K.J. (1969). Problem identification and the research design. In *Communicating nursing research: Vol. 2, problem identification and the research design.* Boulder, CO: Western Interstate Commission on Higher Education.

MacInnes, H. (1941). *Above suspicion.* New York: Dell.

Riley, M.W. (Ed.). (1963). *Sociological research: Vol. 1* New York: Harcourt, Brace, and World.

Rose, A.M. (1965). *Sociology: The study of human relations* (2nd ed.). New York: Knopf.

The Author Comments

The ideas underlying this paper were drafted initially as teaching notes for a graduate-level research methodology course in the late 1960s. At that time, the nursing research texts and related teaching resources were in my view unduly focused on how to do research, emphasizing specific procedural operations in data production and analysis. In reality, if the purposes of the graduate-level research preparation were to be realized, the inquiry process needed to be understood for its potential richness as a means for building a knowledge base that, in turn, would contribute to the science and practice dimensions of nursing. Procedural operations were needed, of course, but they required a reference point to provide criteria for making decisions about them. That reference point is developed in the paper as the conceptual phase of research.

While my ideas in the paper were taking shape, I was serving on a research review committee for the U.S. Department of Health, Education, and Welfare, Division of Nursing, and on a planning committee for the Communicating Nursing Research conference series sponsored by the Western Council for Higher Education in Nursing (WCHEN). These experiences exposed me to a large number of research proposals and completed studies and helped me to sort out characteristics of the inquiry process that contributed to greater or lesser strengths of studies. I am indebted to colleagues on those committees as interchange with them enriched my thoughts immeasurably.

The culmination of the paper occurred when the faculty of the University of Washington School of Nursing renewed its commitment to research as a vital component of the faculty role. This was symbolized with the opening of the school's Office for Nursing Research Facilitation. This paper, presented at the first of a series of research colloquia designed to implement that commitment, was intended to set a context for examining the research process for both a single project and more extensive research programs.

My thinking about the inquiry process has not changed markedly since I wrote this paper. The inquiry process is a set of interactive components, each with a vital function toward achieving validity of the whole, and, thus, toward the total process serving nursing's knowledge base. Although the level of inquiry (e.g., descriptive, exploratory, explanatory) or the mode of inquiry (e.g., scientific, philosophic) may vary across studies and among investigators, I view the process *per se* as having underlying regularities.

—MARJORIE V. BATEY

Chapter 56

Research for a Practice Profession

Susan R. Gortner

Research for any practice profession necessarily deals with professional arts and skills, with the base of knowledge underlying the practice field, and with the initial and continuing education of the professional. Recent developments and activities in the above areas are discussed, including growth in the investigator pool and studies that deal with the process and outcomes of nursing care.

Why research for nursing? Why indeed research for any service or practice profession? Closely linked with this initial query is another: What is nursing research? Nursing research, in brief, is a systematic inquiry into the problems encountered in nursing practice and into the modalities of patient care, such as support and comfort, prevention of trauma, promotion of recovery, health education, health appraisal, and coordination of health care.

As nurses, we ought to be able to accomplish research in our practice concomitantly with the evolution and verification of nursing theory as a science of practice[1] and concomitantly with research into the educa-

tional system that is charged with the responsibility of preparing practitioners. We must move on all fronts vigorously and not allow one to fall behind the other. This is the particularly heavy charge of all service-oriented professions. Freidson (1971) commented that autonomy of technique is at the core of what is unique about a profession; mastery of the technique together with professional and lay belief in the value and efficacy of the professed knowledge and skill serve as reinforcement.

The value placed on nursing knowledge and skills is a reflection of the capacity nursing has to bring about

---

[1] I am indebted to my colleague, Doris Bloch, for the naming of nursing theory as a "science of practice"; others have written to the

appropriateness of practice-oriented theories (see Dickoff and James, Folta, Ellis, and Jacox in particular); I am not aware that the term, "science of practice," has been used before as employed here.

Copyright © 1975, American Journal of Nursing Company. Reproduced with permission from Nursing Research, May-June 1975, 24(3), 193–197.

positive or "good" results in the health status of its clientele. So research takes on an aspect of social relevance when conducted in and for a service occupation such as ours. Although perhaps little understood by the layman and by the bulk of practitioners, it is nonetheless perceived as necessary to document effectiveness or the lack thereof. Hence, the Resolution on Priorities in Nursing Research passed in 1974 by the House of Delegates of the American Nurses' Association (ANA), submitted by the ANA Commission on Nursing Research, is a significant development in our professional awareness and sense of responsibility for our practice:

> WHEREAS, nursing is a discipline in need of further developing and testing its body of knowledge, and
> WHEREAS, the communication of nursing knowledge would be enhanced by the existence of tested concepts and constructs, and
> WHEREAS, research is one of the primary means of documenting efficiency and the effectiveness of nursing practice, and
> WHEREAS, nursing lacks significant influence, power, and prestige because of its inability to specify its contribution to health care; therefore, be it
> RESOLVED, that the American Nurses' Association make a concerted effort to build a public image of nursing research as an essential contributor to knowledge in the health care field, and, be it further
> RESOLVED, that during the next decade the principal thrust of nursing research be a threefold one, namely,
> a. the development of systematically derived information relevant to the practice of nursing,
> b. the development and testing of theories in practice,
> c. the identification of criterion measures, tools, and instruments to document the outcomes and effectiveness of nursing practice. (ANA, 1974, p. 5)

Nursing Research Defined

Some writers have attempted to distinguish between nursing research and research in nursing. The first has as its subject the care process and the problems that are encountered in the practice of nursing: maintenance of hygiene, rest, sleep, nutrition, relief from pain or discomfort, counseling, health education, and rehabilita-

tion. The second has as its subject the profession itself —its practitioners and the characteristics of their practices: utilization, costs, administration, career patterns, educational levels of nurses and nurse students (Folta, 1968; Notter, 1968). The semantics are of less concern than the relative values attached to each major subject area by theorists, educators, practitioners, and scientists in nursing and in related health fields. For values are what influence human behavior, and the relative worth attached to nursing research or to research in nursing education or nursing practice or nursing administration is going to have an effect upon the amount of research activity ongoing, upon the extent to which it is supported, and upon how quickly application can be made to the practice field.

Considerable value is being attached today to practice research, and particularly to the antecedents to, correlates of, and outcomes of effective practice. There are several reasons for this valuation. First, the health professions can no longer assume infallibility with regard to their pronouncements and ministrations, because of the high costs of services and heightened consumer interest and awareness. There is activity now under way to examine health care practices with regard to both costs and benefits, as public concern and governmental interest in the judicious use of the tax dollar for social security beneficiaries prompted legislation for quality assurance (see, for example, Orme & Lindbeck, 1974). Second, the theorists in the health fields have rather consistently maintained that practice research can be particularly fruitful with regard to the production of practice theories. There appears to be no question of need for such research to evaluate the efficacy of practice; of concern here is the development of praxiologic theories, through such research, that will contribute to a body of nursing science. The research literature in nursing recently has reflected increasing attention to this problem. Examples are to be found in proceedings of conferences on science and theory development in nursing held under the auspices of the Nurse Scientist Program at Case Western Reserve University and the University of Colorado in 1967 and 1968 and to the theory conferences in 1969–1970 held at the University of Kansas—in particular, the conference on the nature of science and nursing, 1968; Norris, 1970; and the symposium on theory development in nursing, 1968. The participants at these conferences were and remain concerned with the nature of nursing theory, its origins, possibilities for development, and potential for impact. Considerable debate continues over the most fruitful sources of nursing theory, as well as the most promising sites for theory testing. There is agreement, however, that the field of practice must figure prominently as the empirical source of many theoretical models, and as the setting for their subsequent verification. Folta summarized the situation well:

> Nursing is at a new stage of development. While recognizing clinical practice as its stated reason for being, nursing has generally accepted research as an integral aspect of its professional development. This acceptance, while not without its own problem, has led the profession to a new degree of sophistication and prestige. Most research has been of the theory testing nature with little concern from whence came the theories. Now nursing appears ready to move to the stage of developing its own theories, and, consequently the issue of nursing theory is of increasing importance in today's scene. Perhaps a degree of security within the profession in its ability to conduct its own research is a factor moving nursing in the direction of positing the development of nursing theory as a value which is seen as both necessary and desirable. The pinnacle of scientific disciplines is the development of theory, and nursing is moving towards this pinnacle (Folta, 1971, p. 496).

The Interrelatedness of Research on Theory and Practice

Hence, the symbiosis between theory and practice, and the artificiality of any distinction between theoretic (that is, abstract, nonutilitarian) knowledge and practical knowledge; such a distinction, says the philosopher team of Dickoff and James, "leads to a kind of theorizing that will never make a difference in nursing practice. . . . Have nurses any business indulging themselves in the luxury of theory unless theory can make a difference? Our view is that they do not" (Dickoff & James, 1971, p. 502). A provocative final point, and one with which I only partially agree, because the relationship of theory to practice is a complementary one but one that to date has not been well balanced. The stretching of the mind, the rationalism, reflection, and the abstraction that is a necessary part of theory development in and of nursing is welcome! We have seen too little rather than too much of erudition in nursing; hopefully, others besides nursing theories will become concerned with the theoretic as well as the utilitarian outcomes of the nursing process. When that occurs, we will have achieved some major revolution in the way we see ourselves as a professional group.

An Increase in the Pool of Nurse Investigators

A third reason why practice research is gaining momentum across the health fields, and particularly in nursing, is that there is increased professional endorsement for it, and that practice research has interested a growing number of capable nurse scientists. To sort out which factor has been more influential is difficult, but I would bank heavily on the nurse scientist factor, for through this program the number of nurses with research preparation has increased dramatically in recent years, and the number of well-designed studies that deal with the practice field has increased proportionately. Although incapable of proof, I believe there is direct relationship between these two variables—the size of the investigator pool and the extent of research activity ongoing.

Actual counts of nurses who complete the doctorate annually are difficult to obtain, but Division of Nursing fellowship records alone indicate that 50 new nurse doctorates were added in 1973–1974, and that the total prepared (N = 120) in the 3-year period 1970–1973 alone is greater than the total prepared (N = 109) during the 5-year period 1964–1969 (Bourgeois, 1975, p. 185). Since early 1973, the Division of Nursing has responded to over 900 inquiries from nurses interested in fellowship support at pre- and post-doctoral levels. The number of active fellows that we were supporting as of August 1974 was 80, down considerably from the 183 we supported at midyear in 1971. Were we able to solicit and review new fellowship applications, an activity that ceased early in 1973, we would see a young, extremely bright clinician or faculty member presenting for review. It is a telling, promising situation that Bourgeois documents (Bourgeois, 1975, pp. 184–188).

Graduate students did continue to enroll, frequently part time, despite the unavailability of research training support for predoctorals until the passage on July 12, 1974, of Public Law 93–348, the National Research Service Act. Under this new legislation, individual awards for up to three years are available upon competitive review to students at the post- and predoctoral levels for research training in the biomedical and behavioral sciences. While clarification is being sought on the applicability of this legislation to other programs than those administered by the Alcohol, Drug Abuse, and Mental Health Administration and the National Institutes of Health, we are following with interest the review of applications by nurses to the participating institutes.

Increased Knowledge Base for Practice

Some time ago I had a conversation with a research program administrator in the Heart and Lung Institute who commented that the field of cardiac physiology was open to all investigators of ability, irrespective of background or experience. I agreed. He then went on to describe what he thought nursing research was. What more, beyond the examination of techniques, such as how to make an impeccable-looking bed? It dealt, he felt, with the care aspects of patient management: custodial, supportive, educative, restorative, and rehabilitative, (i.e., patient care research), which is of considerable social and practical relevance. We agreed, and then I cited some of the more recent work we were supporting: the energy cost of certain bedmaking procedures for cardiac patients, the effect of an upper extremity positioning protocol for stroke patients, the effect of extratactile stimulation of premature infants, the

effect on subsequent welfare of structuring expectations of patients toward potentially unpleasant diagnostic or surgical procedures, and patient-nurse perceptions of pain and suffering. Note the key words: patient and effect. This is the critical nucleus of patient care research, of nursing research, of research for any practice profession. For the final determination of effective medicine or nursing will occur ultimately through deliberative processes yielding significant outcomes. We are at a stage of sophistication in some areas where nursing process can be well defined and controlled in order to concentrate on outcomes. Several of the above studies are at this level (e.g., positioning, bedmaking, preoperative or prediagnostic preparation). Hence, I become particularly excited when years of work on one or more of the above problem areas yields consistent enough data to be widely applied and when the development of outcome criteria for specific patient populations, such as those described in the June 1974 issue of *Nursing Clinics of North America,* (Zimmer, 1974) can be used for prospective investigators to determine goodness of fit of the criteria. Prospective (i.e., longitudinal) studies will greatly increase the knowledge base for practice, as they allow for cause and effect inferences and for confirmation of prediction. They will yield what Dickoff, James, and Wiedenbach (1968a, 1968b) have called situation-producing theory. Retrospective work is extremely helpful in specifying antecedent conditions to the phenomenon under study; we have a few such ongoing, especially one dealing with dying and death patterns in teaching hospitals.

Current Research on the Process of Care

Some of our work deals with investigation of current practice, not because care is thought to be exemplary, but because little is known about a phenomenon. Primary care as practiced within hospitals is an example; appraisal of the activities of nurse practitioners is another. Both examples represent rather recent developments that as yet do not have substantial bases of information so that we are documenting nursing activity, nursing process, if you will.

One study that deals with nurse practitioners in an ambulatory care setting presents excellent quantitative data on patient-nurse encounters, but we are missing, for lack of adequate measurement devices, the qualitative data on nursing process.[2] How does the clinician go about her planned visit? how does she review progress? formulate priorities for management? examine, question, and counsel the patient? reevaluate outcomes? how does one measure process unobtrusively to obtain its full dimensions, its artistry so that it can be captured intact for reproduction (replication) and teaching? It can be done, through process recordings (such as those we filled out as students), through diaries, and through witnesses such as human observers and television. It is difficult to quantify the process of care. Yet, two investigations in particular focused on process and methods for its recording and subsequent analyses. Communications, verbal and nonverbal, between patients and staff have been intensively studied by Daubenmire at The Ohio State University, using continuous videotaping, and sophisticated techniques for analyzing interactions have been developed.[3] Butts at the University of Kansas Medical Center is concerned with the totality of medical patient-staff interaction during usual hospitalization; he has used process recordings and analytic techniques developed in the field of ecological psychology.[4]

Under contract with Rush-Presbyterian-St. Luke's Medical Center and the Medicus Corporation we have developed a computer-based methodology for monitoring the process of inpatient nursing care in medical, surgical, pediatric, obstetric, and intensive care units. A patient-oriented approach has been taken through development of a general classification of patient needs for care, based on intensity of illness, to which the general components of nursing process, namely, assessment, planning, implementation, and evaluation, are adapted for measurement of specific objectives of direct nursing care and supporting unit services and management. Procedures call for noncontinuous monitoring of the quality of services through random selection of units to be observed, as well as times of observation, random selection of patients to be observed by trained observers on the units, and computer generation of observational work sheets by patient type and unitwide criteria. The development of items contained in the total instrument set was a long and exhaustive activity; the research team reviewed all existing instruments for assessing nursing care, and with the assistance of a scientific advisory committee, developed a master list that was then examined logically and statistically for applicability (i.e., validity), redundancy, and reliability. Sources of information for use of the criteria include review of patient records, interviews with patients and staff; and direct observation of patients, staff, unit environment and management. Preliminary trials of the total instrument were carried out in two major medical centers; based on the promising preliminary findings, the instrument has been used in 19 test hospitals across the nation. The goodness of fit of the instrument, and its now several hundred individual items, to the process of nursing care appears reasonable; unknown at present is whether favorable responses on the instrument (i.e., a high quality reading) represent a measure of favorable change in patient state. Hence, in a limited number of the test hospitals, patient outcomes are being examined concurrently with the use of the process criteria and with simultaneous examination of structural correlates of quality; namely, characteristics (educational, experiential) of the nurses who provide care, mixes of nursing staff, organizational climate, availability of expert clinical leadership on the unit, et cetera. Recognition that the environment or setting in which health care is rendered may have a potent influence on the quality of that care has been widely assumed in the health field. The data, when analyzed, should allow inferences regarding those factors in the structure or

[2] "Nurse Practitioners in a VA Clinic: Definition of Their Scope of Practice." Inter-agency agreement with the Veterans Administration, Therese K. Cheyovich project director, concluded in December 1974.

[3] Daubenmire, Jean, "A Study of the Interactive Communicative Process" (ongoing Research Grant NU 00401).

[4] Butts, Stanley. "A Descriptive Study of the Patient Hospital Interface" (ongoing Research Grant NU 00405).

environment that have particular influence (Jelinek et al., 1974).

Trends in the Development of Research

The search for the correlates and antecedents of effective practice continues both through careful investigation of specific practices; that is, validation and revalidation of existing and new techniques, and through the accumulation of evidence that is not spurious and that will stand the tests of reproducibility of findings under like circumstances or conditions.

Nationally, at least two major trends appear to reflect the current interest in practice research. One is that nurse clinicians and nurse administrators are increasingly looking to completed research for information on and means to resolve persistent problems of organization, delivery, and evaluation of care. It is becoming hearteningly more common to read of a major innovation in practice or education that does acknowledge the state of the art to date and that does allow for some evaluation of the innovation. Second, there is increasing interest in consortia or multiple-site investigations of a common problem; the base of knowledge will grow considerably with such cooperative and collaborative efforts. Although prominent in education for some time, consortia are only recently apparent in some clinical areas. For example, the problems associated with the management of trauma, with the management of burns, with respiration and alimentation are at once specific to the several health professions because of specific responsibilities for management, yet have dimensions that are of common interest to all professions. Research and research training can be the common meeting ground for health professionals in providing a concerted attack on these and other problem areas.

Implications for Education

Recently, a second interdisciplinary graduate training program in the clinical management of the thermally injured was launched, again involving the cooperative efforts of departments of surgery and of medical-surgical nursing. The common features of both training sites, one at Dallas and one at Cincinnati, are the prior existence of federally supported trauma research centers and ongoing clinical and laboratory research on burns, and the recognition by the health professionals involved that (a) nursing management must be as expert as surgical management, (b) research specific to the nursing care process could be beneficial and major research problems in thermal injury lie in wait of well-qualified clinically oriented investigators of different professional backgrounds, and (c) there were no current graduate programs in nursing (i.e., at the masters level) that had as their focus the thermally injured.[5]

Again, the complementary nature of research, practice, and education for service professions is noted. Aspects of these educational programs have been built on advances through research in the underlying pathophysiology, clinical symptomatology, and treatment of the burned. Again, we are curious about some of the major questions that have long interested educational researchers in the health field: what are the characteristics of students who present for specialty choice? on what criteria should suitability for admission be based? how should student progression be assessed? what is the order, nature, and sequencing of didactic and clinical instruction? what research opportunities should be provided and when? what is the particular impact of the teaching faculty on preceptors and role models? what are the components of effective environments for learning in the specialty areas?

As momentum is gained through research in practice, so must the structure and characteristics of nursing's educational programs, basic, graduate, and con-

[5] "Nurse Clinician and Researcher in Burns Program" Contract NO1-NU44135, between the Bureau of Health Resources Development, Health Resources Administration, Department of Health, Education, and Welfare, and the University of Cincinnati College of Nursing and Health. "Contract for the Development of Clinical Specialists in the Nursing of Burns." Contract NO1-NU34014, between the Bureau of Health Resources Development, Health Resources Administration, Department of Health, Education, and Welfare, and the University of Texas, Southwestern Medical School in conjunction with the School of Nursing, Texas Woman's University, Dallas, Texas.

tinuing, reflect both research advances in the practice field and continual reappraisal of the efficacy of education itself. The student is a key determinant of educational outcomes. For those who select a health professional career, and to whom we will entrust the best of our skills, the totality of our current and evolving knowledge state, and the ethic of concern for human welfare, we have two aspirations: one is that students learn early the joy of discovery that can come with early exposure to research. Ellis said:

> Nursing is essentially a special type of human caring. Some perceive human caring and science to be antithetical. Science, for some, conjures up images of test tubes, laboratories and increasing remoteness from the real world. This is not the whole story. Science is also the careful measurement of strain in the pinned hip joint as a patient goes through various movements attendant to selected nursing activities. Measurement of the strain on a hip union during the movement of the patient by means of a draw sheet, or other nursing maneuvers, is for the ultimate purpose of selection or development of nursing maneuvers that produce the least strain on the healing, reconstructed bone. It is a means of achieving the kind of caring that is not simple sentiment, but a kind of caring that includes deliberate, scientifically selected action. Science can be an effective tool of the humanist. It is not his enemy (Ellis, 1970, p. 444).

The second aspiration is that those whom we prepare will far exceed us in their achievements in practice, education, and research. So does advancement in any discipline, any profession occur.

References

Bourgeois, M.J. (1975). The special nurse research fellow: Characteristics and recent trends. *Nursing Research, 24,* 184–188.

Conference on the nature of science and nursing. (1968). *Nursing Research, 17,* 484–512.

Dickoff, J., & James, P. (1971). Clarity to what end? (Commentary on Walker's "Toward a clearer understanding of the concept of nursing theory"). *Nursing Research, 20,* 499–502.

Dickoff, J., James P., & Wiedenbach, E. (1968a). Theory in a practice discipline: Part 1. Practice oriented theory. *Nursing Research, 17,* 415–435.

Dickoff, J., James, P., & Wiedenbach, E. (1968b). Theory in a practice discipline: Part 2. Practice oriented research. *Nursing Research, 17,* 545–554.

Ellis, R. (1970). Values and vicissitudes of the scientist nurse. *Nursing Research, 19,* 440–455.

Folta, J.R. (1968). Perspectives of an applied scientist. *Nursing Research, 17,* 502–505.

Folta, J.R. (1971). Obfuscation or clarification: A reaction to Walker's concept of nursing theory. *Nursing Research, 20,* 496–499.

Freidson, E. (1971). *Profession of medicine: A study of the sociology of applied knowledge.* New York: Dodd, Mead.

Jelinek, R.C., et al. (1974). *A methodology for monitoring quality of nursing care.* (Report of Phase 1 of Contract NIH 72-4299). Bethesda, MD: Nursing Research Branch, Division of Nursing, Bureau of Health Resources Development, Health Resources Administration.

Norris, C.M. (Ed.). (1970). *Nursing Theory Conference: 1st, 2nd, and 3rd Proceedings.* Held at University of Kansas Medical Center, Department of Nursing Education, March 20–21, 1969; Oct. 9–10, 1969; Jan. 29–30, 1970. Kansas City, KS: University of Kansas.

Notter, L.E. (1968). The nature of science and nursing. (Editorial). *Nursing Research, 17,* 483.

Orme, J.Y., & Lindbeck, R.S. (1974). Nurse participation in medical peer review. *Nursing Outlook, 22,* 27–30.

American Nurses' Association Commission on Nursing Research (1974). Resolution on priorities in nursing research. *American Nurse, 6,* 5.

Symposium on theory development in nursing. (1968). *Nursing Research, 17,* 196–227.

Zimmer, M.J. (1974). Quality assurance (Guest editorial). *Nursing Clinics of North America, 9,* 303–386.

The Author Comments

This article grew from a request for me to speak on research for a practice profession as part of the University of Rochester School of Nursing's series of invitational addresses on behalf of the school's new direction under Dean Loretta Ford. I attempted in this article to distinguish research in nursing from nursing research. The characteristics of a research based profession were drawn briefly, and a number of current studies, then supported by the Division of Nursing, were described. I have retained much of my original thinking over the years about nursing research, but have increasingly wondered about the importance of basic research in nursing, as contrasted with applied or clinical research.

—SUSAN R. GORTNER

Chapter 57

The Interaction Between Theory and Research

Jeanne Quint Benoliel

In any discussion of the cyclical nature of philosophy, theory development, and research in nursing it is also necessary to explore some relationships between theory and research as reciprocal elements in an ongoing process through which scientific knowledge relevant to nursing and health care is created, expanded, tested, and refined. Before turning to these considerations, however, let me clarify my beliefs about the relationship of knowledge to nursing practice, because practice itself can serve as a stimulus to research and thus form part of the cyclic process.

Sources of Knowledge

As an applied field, nursing occupies a middle position in the health care system—a position located in the interface between the lay world of the consumer and the technical world of medical specialization. Regardless of the details of their work, most nurses have what can be termed a generalist orientation toward their practice. Whether they are explicitly aware of it or not, they depend on and use knowledge drawn from various sources, including law, ethics, religion, medicine, intuition, technology, and science. Clearly, only some of the knowledge underlying sound nursing practice is derived from scientific investigation. Yet one sometimes gets the impression from the nursing literature that research is a magical process capable of providing solutions to almost all the profession's problems.

One of nursing's critical needs today, for instance, may be for a clear explication of the moral-ethical knowledge requisite to decision-making in nursing practice. In my opinion, this is one subject that research *per se* cannot clarify, although certainly systematic inquiry into values, goals, and approaches to practice will make a contribution to that explication. Indeed, I would agree with Schlotfeldt (1975) that, given the nature of nursing work, the profession has given scant

About the Author

JEANNE QUINT BENOLIEL currently is a Professor in the College of Nursing, Rutgers University at Newark. She was appointed to the faculty of the University of Washington, Seattle in 1970 and retired from that appointment in December 1989. Previously, she held faculty appointments at the University of California, San Francisco and at UCLA.

After graduating from St. Luke's Hospital School of Nursing, San Francisco, she continued her education at Oregon State University, earning a B.S. in Nursing Education in 1948. During World War II, she served for 3 years in the Army Nurse Corps. In 1955, she received a M.S. from UCLA and continued on at UCLA for postmaster's study in physiology and statistics. In 1969, she received a D.N.Sc. from the University of California, San Francisco, in Nursing and Sociology. Clinically, she has worked in various medical-surgical positions at hospitals throughout California.

Dr. Benoliel's interest in the humanities—art, music, and literature—has contributed to her thinking about the human condition and the continuing dialectic between separation and connection. This interest is reflected in her research and professional activities. Recent research projects have focused on patterns of care for dying patients, oncology transition services, and psychosocial analysis of patients' responses to cancer. She has written about and spoken widely to national and international audiences on similar topics.

When asked about the past and the future of nursing, Dr. Benoliel commented "I have enjoyed sharing my ideas with nurses and other health professionals and knowing that I have played a part in the growth of the profession. The future of nursing, to me, is directly tied to the emergence of women as equal partners in the world. A major problem is that so many nurses seem to suffer from low self-esteem and a lack of commitment to themselves and their work. But the times are changing—and it is exciting to see the appearance of women willing to tackle the central issue of being human—becoming a person."

attention to the relationship of philosophy both to practice and to science. As an applied field, nursing cannot be responsive only to the search for knowledge in a purely academic sense, but must also be responsive to public interest and public demand.

In my view, science is only one of several sources for nursing knowledge. The art of nursing practice rests in a judicious and thoughtful application of insights and inferences drawn from many fields of human endeavor, including the arts, the humanities and the physical, biological, and behavioral sciences. The overshadowing importance attached to knowledge acquired from science and technology is not unique to nursing but can be seen in other fields as well, reflecting no doubt the strong influence of empiricism and mathematics on the development of modern thought in Western societies (Burtt, 1954; Pearson, 1957). The importance that nurses attach to the word "research" may also reflect nursing's relatively recent emergence into research ac-

tivity and training (Schlotfeldt, 1975). The problems of establishing a science of nursing with an intellectual identity accepted by others as a bounded scientific discipline are not unlike those of ecologists, who are also newcomers to the community of scientists (Nelkin, 1976).

In an interesting way, the eclectic nature of nursing has produced scientific investigators representing a range of disciplines, including education, educational psychology, educational administration, public health, epidemiology, human growth and development, and statistics, as well as the natural and behavioral sciences (Bourgeois, 1975). As a result, the scientific work being done by nurse-investigators extends from the traditional laboratory experiment exemplified by Koltoff's (1969) and Parson's (1972) studies of physiological phenomena to anthropological field investigations such as Ford's (1973) study of cultural criteria and determinants for acceptance of modern medicine among the

Teton Dakota on the Rosebud Indian Reservation. Yet regardless of their discipline, it is probably fair to say that the problems chosen for study by many of these nurse-investigators had their origins in observations made while they were nurses in practice. They cycle for them began when nursing practice served as a stimulus for research.

Practice: Stimulus for Research

In my own case, entry into a serious career in research was directly influenced by some observations of the behavior of patients whose bodies were literally changed by having undergone disfiguring surgeries. Questions began to emerge in my mind as to whether nurses really knew very much about the emotional needs of people who had to live with the aftermath of these procedures; yet the nursing rhetoric of the time was glibly full of commentary about "meeting the emotional needs" of patients.

The opportunity for post-master's study soon presented itself, and after two years of concentrated graduate work, those questions about surgical disfigurement evolved into a research problem. Eventually they were formalized into a funded project to study the processes of adjustment following one instance of surgical disfigurement, radical mastectomy. Details about that study have been reported elsewhere and are not pertinent to this discussion (Quint, 1963, 1964, 1965). Two aspects of my experience during and after that study, however, speak directly to the cyclic interactions of theory, research, and peer contacts among investigators.

Although the mastectomy study was designed to investigate the dual impact of breast loss and cancer diagnosis, the extent to which death and fear of dying became integral parts of the lives of these women was not anticipated nor were the difficulties they encountered in attempting to adjust to the uncertainties of their futures. Furthermore, I was not prepared for the amount of time, effort, and energy required to provide a support system so that the research associate on the project could cope with her own reactions of distress

and then return to the process of data collection. As a result of immersion in death data, however, I eventually joined Anselm Strauss and Barney Glaser on a study of dying patients and hospital personnel, thereby becoming one of the pioneers in the emerging field of thanatology.

As these examples show, one piece of research leads to another in ways that often cannot be predicted at the outset. One idea leads to another idea. Contacts with other investigators open new horizons. Sharing research findings can bring unexpected opportunities for new directions, collaboration with other scientists, and information helpful for completion of work in progress.

The contacts with Anselm Strauss were important to my research activity in a second way. They introduced me to a theoretical orientation—symbolic interaction theory—that subsequently provided the organizing framework of "status passage" to guide the analysis of the mastectomy data (Denzin, 1970; Glaser & Strauss, 1971). The lack of a clear conceptual framework for the original mastectomy proposal was a direct result of the ad hoc way in which I had been introduced to research. Since I had not been socialized into an established scientific discipline characterized by a systematic body of knowledge and an orderly set of rules and procedures governing research activities, my work until then had not been guided by a clearly understood paradigm and set of theories and propositions (Kuhn, 1970). The identification of a theoretical perspective within which the mastectomy data made logical sense was therefore a major step in my development as a social scientist.

This roundabout rather than direct route to a research career can best be understood within the context of the period. Nursing had not yet begun to emerge as a discipline with a systematically organized body of theoretical knowledge (Benoliel, 1973). My movement into a research career took place by atypical means that did not include a sound introduction to theoretically based knowledge and a clear understanding of the differences between theoretical and operational concepts and the relationship of these differences to the research enterprise (Blalock, 1968).

Relationship of Theory to Research

Whether the research aims toward the development of theory grounded in empirical data or the testing of theory through the control and manipulation of variables under experimental or quasi-experimental conditions, the investigator's work is based on a theoretical orientation toward knowledge (Glaser & Strauss, 1967; Johnson & Rice, 1974). In other words, the creation of new knowledge rests on some assumptions accepted *a priori* as truths about that portion of nature selected for investigation. Thus, new knowledge is built upon accepted and tested theories about a particular substantive field, and these concepts and theories are accepted as given constraints on how the research can be done and how its results can be interpreted.

For instance, the building blocks for physiologic research are concepts and theories developed in the physical sciences of physics, chemistry, and mathematics (Donaldson, 1976). These theories set limits on how the researcher in physiology can state a hypothesis, set up an experiment, and interpret the outcomes. For example, the historic series of experiments performed to test the hypothesis that calcium ion release was the intracellular trigger for muscle contraction was based on knowledge about the physical structure of the specialized muscle proteins and the effects of changes in ionic environment on proteins (Ashley & Ridgway, 1970; Heilbrunn & Wiercinski, 1947; Jobsis & O'Connor, 1966). These experiments also illustrate a fundamental characteristic of the scientific enterprise—namely, that indirect evidence and a time-sequencing argument are basic elements used to make inferences about a given phenomenon.

Investigators in the social sciences are somewhat handicapped in their research efforts, because their underlying theories do not have universally recognized paradigms such that model problems and solutions are commonly accepted among them. Nevertheless, the organization and implementation of social research are guided by particular theoretical perspectives and, as Denzin (1970) has noted, the choice of approach and methodology ultimately rests on the scientist's "conceptions of the empirical world" (p. 96). In the study of dying patients and hospital personnel, the theoretical base was that of symbolic interactionism—a theoretical perspective that makes a good fit with the use of participant observation as a methodology. The goal of that research was the collection of empirical data for use in the development of grounded social theory and, eventually, two grounded paradigms were created—one a paradigm for the awareness context in which dying takes place, and the other a model for describing the dying trajectory (Glaser & Strauss, 1965, 1968). Both paradigms have contributed to an understanding of social reality that is useful for nurses in both practice and research.

Both the theory of symbolic interactionism and the inductive approach to the collection of qualitative data hold considerable promise, in my judgment, for the creation of nursing knowledge. The symbolic interactionist perspective sees human beings as creatures who define and classify situations, including themselves, and who choose ways of acting toward and within them (Rose, 1962). This theoretical orientation is centrally concerned with understanding people as social beings. In my case, it provided a perspective on human behavior that made a good fit with my interests in the effects of social interactions on the development of a new identity, such as being a diabetic (Benoliel, 1970).

One of the most exciting aspects of the scientific enterprise is the opportunity it affords for creative thinkers to combine theoretical perspectives from more than one discipline into elegant research operations out of which new understandings can emerge. In recent years, for instance, nursing is among the disciplines making important contributions to the growing body of knowledge about the growth and development of premature infants. Investigations such as Neal's (1971) and Barnard's (1973) are not only elegant in design and research procedure'; they also provide information that has a great deal of promise for practicing nurses.

This kind of elegant pulling together of theory, research design, and knowledge drawn from the world of direct patient care can also be seen in the work of nurse investigators in other fields. For example, drawing on observations from nursing practice, Johnson and her colleagues have combined a perceptive knowledge of psychological theories pertaining to cognitive processes and distress reactions to threatening events with soundly developed laboratory and clinical experiments. They have used their experiments to test hypotheses about the effects of accurate and inaccurate expectations concerning forthcoming threatening events on various measurements of distress. Thus, the finest sense of the word, Johnson's work (Johnson, 1972; Johnson et al., 1975; Johnson & Rice, 1974) illustrates the ongoing cyclical interaction of theory, research, and practice in a person whose contributions to the literature are increasing not only in numbers but also in depth of focus and breadth of application. The ongoing interplay between psychological theory and the real experiences of people living through such frightening events as orthopedic cast removal are beautifully conveyed in her experiments and her writings.

Signal for Change

The process of research for the individual investigator means active involvement with change in the form of new ideas, new investigations, and new contacts with other researchers. Similarly, the process of research can also be a trigger for social change, usually when research findings find their way into the common marketplace. Over the past ten years, for example, a good deal of research and writing has been focused on death and dying as significant human phenomena worthy of serious consideration. One of the interesting by products of this increase in death-focused research may be that it provides public reinforcement to the idea that open talk about the subject of death is legitimate and need no longer be avoided. Furthermore, the paradigms of awareness context and dying trajectory certainly offer professional practitioners two conceptual frameworks that can serve as reference points for understanding practical social situations in which patients are dying.

Another way by which research has been instrumental in introducing change is through joint activities engaged in by university-based investigators and practitioners in service agencies in order to examine problems of mutual interest. An example of such a collaborative endeavor is Walike's study of patient problems related to tube feeding (Walike et al., 1975).

Perhaps the primary way by which research activity serves as a signal for change is through the ongoing influence of one set of research findings on the emergence of new methodologies and new fields for study. Nursing, for example, has shifted from its earlier focus on studies about nurses to an increasing concern with problems of practice (Gortner et al., 1976). In a recent analysis of funded studies in nursing research, Gortner and her colleagues found them to be concerned with the emergence of knowledge in five major fields of study: (a) systematic study of health problems and health needs of patients as well as aspects of relationships between nurses and patients (studies related to a science of practice); (b) laboratory and field studies to evaluate nursing procedures, methods, and techniques (studies related to the artistry of practice, clinical therapeutics); (c) descriptive, analytical, and experimental studies of the physical and social environments in which nurses and consumers interact with each other, including structures that relate to service costs and relative efficiency; (d) studies to develop methodology and measurement tools for clinical as well as nonclinical problems of concern to nursing; and (e) studies that apply the findings of research through demonstrations or replications of original investigations. This latter type of study, the article notes, (Gortner, 1975) has so far been relatively scarce compared to the others. In my judgment, this limitation needs to be viewed simply as an indicator of the current stage of development of nursing research.

Another interesting way in which interactions among theory, research, and practice are bringing about changes in knowledge basic to nursing is through studies of clinical problems by investigators with widely different perspectives. Pain, for instance, has been studied from the vantage point of social psychology by Johnson and Rice (1974), as a biopsychosocial phenomenon by Jacox and Stewart (1973), and as a social phenomenon with organizational and interactional consequences by Strauss and his associates (1974). As new theories about pain emerge from these studies they will create new opportunities for combining theoretical perspectives into a new cycle of research activity that eventually may contribute new ideas for the management of pain in clinical settings.

The theoretical formulations invented by Glaser and Strauss for describing the process of dying and the context in which death occurs have already stimulated additional research. My present research, which involves examination of empirical data from hospital records to describe the characteristics of patterns of dying as these can be identified from these records was designed with the dying trajectory as its theoretical framework. Using the grounded theory approach to data collection, Degner and Glass are using participant observation in a variety of health care settings toward the goal of developing a grounded theory of decision-making about prolongation and nonprolongation of life. At a conference in Canada in 1975, they presented an interesting analysis of some findings describing the calculations of risk versus benefit in health care decision-making (Degner & Glass, 1975). The work of Degner, a former student of mine, amply demonstrates the cyclic nature of the process of research in human-to-human form—an extension of what was done in the past into the present and on into the future.

The Continuing Cycle

These three pieces of research (the study of dying patients and hospital personnel, the study of dying trajectories based on retrospective analysis of records, and the inductive study of decision-making in life-threatening situations) very effectively serve to illustrate the flowing nature of the process of scientific inquiry and the application of different philosophical approaches to the study of a particular human phenomenon—in this case, the social situation of dying.

First, Glaser and Strauss created a substantively grounded theory of dying, based on an inductive analysis of empirical social data obtained through participant observation in a number of different hospitals. Several years later, my present investigation (Benoliel, 1975) was formulated using a deductive approach to test whether or not the types of dying trajectory proposed by the theory could be identified in another set of empirical data, patient hospital records.

Moving another step forward, Degner and Glass have now identified a delimited area for study within the broad field of social thanatology. Using these previous studies as foundations, they have identified a more refined problem for study—the process of decision-making in life-threatening situations. As a new investigator, Degner brings to this important scientific enterprise the sensitive awareness of a nurse who knows from pragmatic experience the complexities of patient care and the rigorous self-discipline of the able participant observer (Benoliel, 1975).

In summary, then, I believe that knowledge production in the fields of health care and nursing depends on a flowing kind of interaction—a movement back and forth between the concrete realities and pragmatic domains of nursing work and the abstract world of those interrelated propositions known as theories. The value of theories is that they can serve to explain and interpret at a variety of levels the world of nature, including human behaviors in health and illness. They also provide the basis from which definitions of reality emerge.

Thus, nursing has a great deal to gain from the work of its growing body of scientific investigators. Ultimately, the future of nursing knowledge will rest less with the particular philosophies, theories, and methodologies that are used and more with the imagination and creativity of nursing's investigators and their willingness to experiment with new ways of examining the complex social world in which we live.

References

Ashley, C.C., & Ridgway, E.B. (1970). On the relationship between membrane potential, calcium transient and tension in single barnacle muscle fibers. *Journal of Physiology, 209,* 105–130.

Barnard, K. (1973). The effect of stimulation on the sleep behavior of the premature infant. In M.V. Batey (Ed.), *Communicating nursing research: Collaboration and competition* (pp. 12–33). Boulder, CO: Western Interstate Commission for Higher Education.

Benoliel, J.Q. (1970). The developing diabetic identity: A study of family influence. In M.V. Batey (Ed.), *Communicating nursing research: Methodological issues* (pp. 14–32). Boulder, CO: Western Interstate Commission for Higher Education.

Benoliel, J.Q. (1973). Collaboration and competition in nursing research. In M.V. Batey (Ed.), *Communicating nursing research: Collaboration and competition* (pp. 1–11). Boulder, CO: Western Interstate Commission for Higher Education.

Benoliel, J.Q. (1975a). Research related to death and the dying patient. In P.J. Verhonick (Ed.), *Nursing Research* (pp. 189–227). Boston: Little, Brown.

Benoliel, J.Q. (1975b). Social characteristics of death as a recorded hospital event. In M.V. Batey (Ed.), *Communicating nursing research, Volume 8.* Boulder, CO: Western Intestate Commission for Higher Education.

Blalock, H.M., Jr. (1968). The measurement problem: A gap between the languages of theory and research. In H.M. Blalock & A. Blalock (Eds.), *Methodology in social research* (pp. 5–27). New York: McGraw-Hill.

Bourgeois, M.J. (1975). The special nurse research fellow: Characteristics and recent trends. *Nursing Research, 24,* 184–188.

Burtt, E.A. (1954). *The metaphysical foundations of modern physical science* (rev. ed.). Garden City, NY: Doubleday.

Degner, L.F., & Glass, H.P. (1975). Calculations of risk versus benefit; indicators in health care decision making. In *Development and use of indicators in nursing research* (pp. 141–147). Proceedings of the 1975 National Conference on Nursing Research, held in Edmonton, Canada, November 3–5.

Denzin, N.K. (1970). *The research act.* Chicago: Aldine.

Donaldson, S. (1976). *Personal communication.* Seattle: University of Washington.

Fagerhaugh, S.Y. (1974). Pain expression and control on a burn care unit. *Nursing Outlook, 22,* 645–650.

Ford, V. (1973). Cultural criteria and determinants for acceptance of modern medicine among the Teton Dakota, Rosebud Indian Reservation, South Dakota. In M.V. Batey (Ed.), *Communicating nursing research: Collaboration and competition* (pp. 41–62). Boulder, CO: Western Interstate Commission for Higher Education.

Glaser, B.G., & Strauss, A.L. (1965). *Awareness of dying.* Chicago: Aldine.

Glaser, B.G., & Strauss, A.L. (1967). *The discovery of grounded theory: Strategies for qualitative research.* Chicago: Aldine.

Glaser, B.G., & Strauss, A.L. (1968). *Time for dying.* Chicago: Aldine.

Glaser, B.G., & Strauss, A.L. (1971). *Status passage.* Chicago: Aldine.

Gortner, S.R. (1975). Research for a practice profession. *Nursing Research, 24,* 193–197.

Gortner, S.R., et al. (1976). Contributions of nursing research to patient care. *Journal of Nursing Administration, 6,* 22–28.

Heilbrunn, L.V., & Wiercinski, F.G. (1947). The action of various cations on muscle protoplasm. *Journal of Cellular and Comparative Physiology, 25,* 15–32.

Jacox, A., & Stewart, M. (1973). *Psychosocial contingencies of the pain experience.* Iowa City, IA: The University of Iowa.

Jobsis, F.F., & O'Connor, M.J. (1966). Calcium release and reabsorption in the sartorius muscle of the toad. *Biochemical and Biophysical Research Communications, 25,* 246–252.

Johnson, J.E. (1972). Effects of structuring patients expectations on their reactions to threatening events. *Nursing Research, 21,* 499–504.

Johnson, J.E., et al. (1975). Altering children's distress behavior during orthopedic cast removal. *Nursing Research, 24,* 404–410.

Johnson, J.E., & Rice, V.H. (1974) Sensory and distress components of pain. *Nursing Research, 23,* 203–209.

Kolthoff, N.J. (1969). Relationship of neurohormones to vascular characteristics of and regenerated adrenal tissue in the rat during stress. In *American Nurses' Association Fifth Nursing Research Conference* (pp. 1–15). New York: American Nurses' Association.

Kuhn, T.S. (1970). *The structure of scientific revolutions* (2nd ed.). Chicago: University of Chicago Press.

Neal, M.V. (1969). Relationship between a regimen of vestibular stimulation and developmental behavior of the small premature infant. In *American Nurses' Association Fifth Nursing Research Conference* (pp. 43–57). New York: American Nurses' Association.

Nelkin, D. (1976). Ecologists and the public interest. *Hastings Center Report, 6,* 38–44.

Parsons, L.C. (1972). The effect of stimulation of the "nonspecific region of the thalamus" upon the intracellular activity of neurons in the motor cortex made epileptic with strychnine. In *American Nurses' Association Eighth Nursing Research Conference* (pp. 101–112). New York: American Nurses' Association.

Pearson, K. (1937). *The grammar of science.* Folcroft, PA: Folcroft Library Editions.

Quint, J.C. (1963). The impact of mastectomy. *American Journal of Nursing, 63,* 88–91.

Quint, J.C. (1964). Mastectomy—symbol of cure or warning sign? *GP, 29,* 119–124.

Quint, J.C. (1965). Institutionalized practices of information control. *Psychiatry, 28,* 119–132.

Rose, A.M. (Ed.). (1962). *Human behavior and social processes.* Boston: Houghton-Mifflin.

Schlotfeldt, R.M. (1975). Research in nursing and research training for nurses. *Nursing Research, 24,* 177–183.

Strauss, A., et al. (1974). Pain: An organization-work-interactional perspective. *Nursing Outlook*, *22*, 560–566.

Walike, B.C., et al. (1975). Patient problems related to tube feeding. In M.V. Batey (Ed.), *Nursing research, Vol. 7* (pp. 89–112). Boulder, Co: Western Interstate Commission for Higher Education.

The Author Comments

This article was the result of an invitation by Joanne Sobol Stevenson to give the keynote address at a research symposium held at the Ohio State University School of Nursing in 1976. The title came from the focus of the symposium, but I took the opportunity to broaden the topic by incorporating my ideas about the influence of both practice and theory on nursing research. Preparation of the article offered me the opportunity to clarify my thoughts about the nature of knowledge in nursing and to consider some of the people and events that had influenced my personal development as a nurse scientist.

At the time, I was distressed that academic nursing appeared to be preoccupied with science as the only means for generating nursing knowledge, and I used the article to argue that nursing knowledge comes from various sources. Being something of a frustrated historian, I also used the article to offer an autobiographical statement on the complex process of being socialized into the world of science.

When I reread the article, I think it is as relevant today as it was when first published. It is a personal statement of beliefs about the nature of scientific knowledge in a practice discipline and the interacting factors that contribute to its development and accumulation.

—JEANNE QUINT BENOLIEL

Chapter 58

Philosophy, Science, Theory: Interrelationships and Implications for Nursing Research

Mary Cipriano Silva

If nurse researchers are to study the structure of nursing knowledge, they must first understand the relationships among philosophy, science, and theory. Although many articles have spoken to the nature of theory or science in nursing (Andreoli & Thompson, 1977; Hardy, 1974; Jacox, 1974; Leininger, 1968; Walker, 1971), few have examined the links between them and fewer yet have examined the role of philosophy in the deriving of nursing knowledge. To bridge this gap, I would like to present an overview of the relationships among philosophy, science, and theory, and then describe some implications for the conduct of nursing research.

Relationships Between Philosophy and Science

Although in western civilization the precise origin of what we call pure knowledge is difficult to trace, most scholars agree that significant advancements occurred during the great Age of Greece (500 B.C. to 300 B.C.). During this time those ideals commonly associated with western civilization—freedom, optimism, secularism, rationalism, and high regard for the dignity and worth of the individual—were developed (Burns, 1955).

Greek learning formed a single entity called philosophy and, even into the nineteenth century, this term was used to designate man's total knowledge. To designate all knowledge as philosophy was possible because our body of knowledge was relatively small and no real distinctions were made between different kinds of knowledge.

The industrial Revolution, however, dramatically altered man's perception about the structuring of knowledge. The Darwinian hypothesis of natural selection, cell and germ theories, revolutionary discoveries about energy and matter, and the advent of psychoanalysis were but a few contributors to the knowledge explosion. No longer was philosophy considered adequate to answer questions about natural phenomena, and science divorced itself from it. New disciplines were formed—embryology, cytology, immunology, anesthesiology, to name a few—each asking their own questions and seeking their own answers.

This specialization, however, created a new problem: Although each discipline revealed unique and enlightening aspects of man, the ultimate questions about his nature and purpose went unanswered. Science had taken man apart but had not put him back together. Once again philosophy was sought out—this time to unify scientific findings so that man as a holistic being might emerge. This is in keeping with Kneller's (1971) view of the philosopher as one whose work begins before and after the scientist has done his job.

The philosopher is concerned with such matters as the purpose of human life, the nature of being and reality, and the theory and limits of knowledge. Questions the philosopher might ask are "Is man inherently good or evil?", "Is truth absolute or relative?", "What does 'knowing' mean?". His approach to understanding reality is characterized by formulating sets of assumptions and beliefs derived from his own personal experience and his contemplation of it in relation to the studied experiences of others (Association for Supervision and Curriculum Development [ASCD] Commission on Instructional Theory, 1968). Intuition, introspection, and reasoning are some of his methodologies.

The scientist, on the other hand, is primarily concerned with causality. Cause and effect, in one way or another, are central to his goal of deriving scientific laws (Labovitz and Hagedorn, 1976). Questions the scientist might ask are "Does treatment X, and only treatment X, cause Y?", or "What is the relationship between X and Y?" His approach to understanding reality is characterized by tentativeness, verifiability, observation, and experience. Reality becomes interpretable to him through such mechanisms as hypothesis-testing, operational definitions, and experiments. The scientist's position is summarized by Kerlinger (1973): "If an explanation cannot be formulated in the form of a test-able hypothesis, then it can be considered to be a metaphysical explanation and thus not amenable to scientific investigation. As such, it is dismissed by the scientist as being of no interest" (p. 25).

However, despite different focuses and methodologies, the philosopher and scientist share the common goal of increasing mankind's knowledge.

Relationships Between Science and Theory

Before analyzing the relationships between science and theory, let us first briefly review some characteristics of science as a system, based on principles of Van Laer (1963, pp. 8–19):

1. **Science must show a certain coherence.** Science must constitute a coherent whole of interrelated facts, principles, laws, and theories which are appropriately ordered. An explication of unrelated data, no matter how valuable, does not constitute a science.
2. **Science is concerned with definite fields of knowledge.** Man is no longer able to know all things. Consequently, he must specialize so that he might know one field, or an aspect of it, well.
3. **Science is preferably expressed in universal statements.** Science ultimately is concerned with commonalities of properties that transcend the specific; science seeks to discover the universal characteristics of phenomena under investigation. Its goal is to reduce data to their most fundamental common denominator.
4. **The statements of science must be true or probably true.** What constitutes truth is a vexing epistemological question. One may suggest, however, that scientific statements are true if they express the nature of things as they are. But man, being finite, frequently does not know the true nature of things. And so it is to the scientist we often turn to help us find reality in a systematic, scholarly, and trustworthy way. His job, according to Scheffler, is "not to judge the truth infallibly, but to estimate the truth responsibly" (Scheffler, 1965, p. 54).
5. **The statements of science must be logically ordered.** One does not draw conclusions before stating hypotheses. Science is usually best served through careful observance of scientific methods such as the deductive-inductive or analytic-synthetic method.
6. **Science must explain its investigations and arguments.** Scientists have a responsibility not only to report

their research findings, but as importantly, to explain the arguments and demonstrations which led them to their conclusions.

The above six principles certainly are not the exclusive domain of science. Many of them apply equally as well to philosophy or theory, once again underscoring the ebb and flow of relationships among philosophy, science, and theory.

We again see these relationships when we ask the question, "What is the aim of science? " Typical responses are that science aims to describe, understand, predict, control, or explain phenomena. But Kerlinger offers a different perspective: "The basic aim of science is theory" (Kerlinger, 1973, p. 8).

But what are the components of theory and how do they relate to science? There is no easy answer, no one correct response. Basic philosophical differences exist among scientists regarding the constructional processes composing science and theory. These differences stem from varying philosophical orientations — realism, idealism, pragmatism, and others — each with its own interpretation of reality.

To complicate the situation further, the many terms used to define theory can be bewildering. For example, words such as propositions, assertions, axioms, postulates and maxims, to name a few, are sometimes used interchangeably, at other times with different meanings. When one looks carefully, however, some common denominators of theory emerge. They are set, postulates, definitions, and hypotheses. Let us now briefly examine how each contributes to theory, and consequently, to science.

1. **Set.** Set is a well-defined collection of objects or elements. Facts, principles, and laws do not, in and of themselves, constitute theory. However, when a scientist selects particular facts, principles, and laws from the universal set (i.e., from the set of all elements under discussion) because of their interrelationships and relevance to the problem under investigation, he fulfills the requirements of set needed for theory development.
2. **Postulates.** The central core of a theory consists of its postulates. These are statements of general truth that serve as essential premises for whatever is being investigated. Postulates are usually stated as generalizations which are consistent with scientific evidence related to one's research problem. They form the essential presuppositions from which hypotheses are deduced and tested. Rogers (1970), for example, in developing her theoretical basis of nursing, identified four essential postulates about man. These postulates speak to man's wholeness, fluidity, sense of pattern and organization, and sentence.
3. **Definitions.** Definitions of terms are important for communication among scholars. Terms can be defined as primitive, theoretical, and key (ASCD Commission on Instructional Theory, 1968). Primitive terms are those which cannot be defined by specifying operations or by referring to other operationally defined terms. They represent entities which one can only intuitively experience. Purpose and need are examples of primitive terms. Theoretical terms are those which cannot be defined by pointing to particular operations, but which can be defined by their relationship to other terms which are operationally defined. Motivation is an example of a theoretical term. Key terms are those which can and must be operationally defined so that hypotheses under study can be tested. Learning is an example of a key term when it is essential to a hypothesis and can be operationally defined by use of valid and reliable instruments. Key terms are essential for replication research and theory verification.
4. **Hypotheses.** Hypotheses are predictions which have been deduced from a set of postulates and which state the relationship between two or more variables. They imply that the relationship between these variables can be observed and tested. This is no small matter, but one that is crucial in bridging theory and science. For if we cannot observe what we study, we cannot measure it. If we cannot measure it, we do not know whether or not it contributes to theory. If we do not know its impact on theory, we cannot know its potential contribution to science. Nurses are becoming more aware of these relationships. In a study of priorities in clinical nursing research, the highest priority in regard to "impact upon patient welfare" was given to items concerned with determining reliable and valid indicators of quality nursing care (Lindeman, 1975).

Because well stated hypotheses are based on observation of fact which permit them to be "proven" or "disproven," they are powerful instruments of science. Through systematic and rigorous testing of hypotheses, phenomena are explained and, depending on the amount of verifiable evidence, these phenomena have predictive ability, first as theory, then principles and laws (Weinland, 1975). Through the power of hypotheses, mankind's knowledge is increased, or at the very least in the case of disproven hypotheses, his ignorance is reduced.

If we now synthesize the above four common denominators of theory, we arrive at a workable definition: Theory refers to a **set** of related statements (most commonly, **postulates** and **definitions**) which have been derived from scientific data and from which plausible **hypotheses** can be deduced, tested, and verified. If verified, theory becomes part of the body of science from which other sets of postulates can be derived. The process of theory building, therefore, involves the formulation and testing of hypotheses which have been deduced from a set of statements derived from scientific knowledge and philosophical beliefs.

Implications for Nursing Research

When the research process is examined by studying the relationships among philosophy, science, and theory, one arrives at perspectives different from traditional viewpoints about the derivation and significance of nursing knowledge. These perspectives are discussed below:

1. **Ultimately, all nursing theory and research is derived from or leads to philosophy.** Traditionally, one is lead to believe that nursing research begins with theory. I believe it begins and ends with philosophy and this awareness enhances one's perspective about the research process.

   If one examines the four main branches of philosophy—logic, epistemology, metaphysics, and ethics—one begins to see the links between them and the process of nursing research. Through logic, researchers are able to establish the validity of various thoughts and the correctness of their reasoning. Germane to the research process is the ability to establish logical relationships between theory selection and problem identification, problem identification and hypothesis testing, hypothesis testing and derivation of valid conclusions.

   Epistemology, the study of the theory of knowledge, is also crucial to the process of nursing research. For is not the aim of research to discover, expand, or reaffirm knowledge? Yet, what constitutes knowledge is no simple matter. Inherent in the concept of knowledge are conditions of

truth, secure belief, and evidence (Scheffler, 1965). The truth condition claims that if one "knows" something to be true, he must be judged not to be in error. The belief condition stipulates if one "knows" something to be true, he also believes it to be true. The evidence condition states that one evaluates knowledge against all adequate standards of evidence at a particular time. Although nurse researchers have recognized the evidence condition of knowledge, they seemingly have paid less attention to the truth and belief conditions. By identifying and applying the contributions of epistemology to nursing, nurse researchers can gain further insights into the research process.

Metaphysics studies the most general concepts used in ordinary life and science by examining the internal structure of the language used in various disciplines (Harré, 1972). Of particular interest to the nurse researcher is an examination of the concept of causality. Questions the researcher might ask include: Is causality a necessary condition of objective experience? Can causality be demonstrated empirically? What are acceptable scientific criteria for the establishment of causality?

Finally, the study of ethics comes to grips with moral principles and values. Although all researchers are, I hope, familiar with the ethical requirements of informed consent and protection of the rights of human subjects, some, perhaps, have not considered other pertinent concepts. For example, what are ethical implications inherent in the nature of the research problem? What ethical considerations do advancements in science and technology present? What are the ethics involved in collaborative research and the reporting of research? To whom are researchers ultimately accountable? Although the "pure" scientist may argue that the use to which knowledge is put is not his business, I believe research cannot be conceived apart from its moral implications.

2. **Philosophical introspection and intuition are legitimate methods of scientific inquiry.** Historically and traditionally, nurses have been indoctrinated into a singular approach to the derivation of nursing knowledge—the scientific method. As early as the 1930s, scientific criteria were used to evaluate procedural demonstrations (Gortner & Nahm, 1977). In the 1960s, McCain (1965) stressed nursing by assessment, not intuition. This stress on the scientific method continues strongly today. For example, Riehl and Roy (1974), among others, express disapproval about nursing actions based on intuition. Gortner (1974) suggests that the logic of science is closed to intuition. In addition, many graduate nursing students have been indoctrinated into a methodology of nursing research which excludes anything but strict adherence to the scientific method.

The time has come to question this singular approach to the study of nursing knowledge. The time has come to value truths arrived at by intuition and introspection as much as those arrived at by scientific experimentation. For, in fact, the scientist has no greater claim to truth than does the theoretician or the philosopher. Yet, nurse scholars seem hesitant to acknowledge intuition and introspection as valid methods of acquiring knowledge.

However, what we scorn, others praise. Burner (1977), for example, tells us that the development of intuitive thinking is an objective of many highly regarded teachers and is considered to be a valuable asset in science. Intuition is not knowledge arrived at out of nothing; rather, it is knowledge arrived at by a deep grasp of a subject, although one may not be able to articulate the process by which a conclusion is reached. The derived knowledge may not always be correct, but neither is knowledge arrived at with all the advantages of the scientific method. The large numbers of unsubstantiated hypotheses support this assertion.

In addition, knowledge gained through introspection cannot be overlooked as it constitutes one of the major approaches to the derivation of knowledge—rationalism. The prime example, of course, is mathematics where truth is deduced from reasoning and not contingent on observation or experience. According to Scheffler, mathematicians conduct no experiments, surveys, or statistics, yet "they arrive at the firmest of all truths, incapable of being overthrown by experience" (Scheffler, 1965, p. 3).

The point to be made here is that we must keep our minds open to all potential avenues which lead to advancement of nursing knowledge. We must be careful not to impose our value judgments about the research process on others if, in the end, we narrow their thinking and undermine their creativity. For example, during the conduct of my dissertation, although never explicitly stated, it was inferred time and again that the experimental research design with its emphasis on causality is superior to all other types of research. Descriptive, historical, and other valuable types of research were quietly but steadfastly refuted.

3. **Nursing knowledge arrived at by the scientific method too often sacrifices meaningfulness for rigor.** Although rigorous research designs are praiseworthy, if not used judiciously, they can impede rather than enhance the research process. Too much rigor can (and often does) lead to trivial research problems with the logical outcome of trivial research results. The same is true of definition of terms and statistics. One can meticulously operationally define the independent and dependent variables in one's hypotheses, but if these definitions are so narrow that they have little or no meaning for nursing practice, what is the point? In terms of statistics, one can find statistically significant differences among groups (if they exist) if a large enough sample is used. However, for practical purposes, the differences may be so small as to be negligible. Such statistics can be impeccably and rigorously applied, yet offer little to the advancement of nursing knowledge and, at best, be misleading.

Although one expects sufficient rigorism of design so that there is confidence in the results, the pursuit and worship of rigorism and experimentation for their own sake—as at times seems the case—needs questioning. Cook and LaFleur (1975) maintain that experimentation (with its implications for rigorism) as an exclusive method of obtaining knowledge is becoming a dead end as too little meaningful behavior can be understood by this method alone.

How can this situation be improved? As previously noted, researchers can begin to examine other ways to derive nursing knowledge. This does not necessarily mean that we give up a method we believe in, only that we open our minds to other approaches. Most of us, for example, have traditionally considered probability theory as the basis for accepting or rejecting hypotheses. Yet, Frank (1957) discusses another option: logical probability. Instead of reducing probability statements to statements about relative frequencies, one uses inductive logic to arrive at the probable truth or falsity of the data. The statements of inductive logic are purely logical and say nothing about physical facts; that is, they are not statements that are derived from observations. The basic premise is as follows: The inductive probability of a hypothesis **h** on the basis of a certain evidence **e** is high; or stated in another way, the evidence **e** confirms to a high degree the hypothesis **h**. Although the precise logical formulations derived to arrive at the above premise are beyond the scope of this paper, the possibilities of validating hypotheses in non-traditional ways are interesting to ponder.

In summary, when nurse researchers examine the total philosophy-science-theory triad, they develop a more holistic and less traditional approach to the possibilities of deriving nursing knowledge. They are more open to contributions of other disciplines and less likely to see the research process as though through a glass darkly.

References

Andreoli, K.G., & Thompson, C.E. (1977). The nature of science in nursing. *Image, 9*, 32–37.

Association for Supervision and Curriculum Development Commission on Instructional Theory (ASCD). (1968). *Criteria for theories of instruction.* Washington, DC: National Education Association.

Bruner, J. (1977). *The process of education.* London: Harvard University Press (Originally published 1960).

Burns, E.M. (1955). *Western civilization: Their history and their culture* (4th ed.). New York: W.W. Norton.

Cook, D.R., & LaFleur, N.K. (1975). *A guide to educational research* (2nd ed.). Boston: Allyn and Bacon.

Frank, P. (1957). *Philosophy of science: The link between science and philosophy.* Englewood Cliffs, NJ: Prentice-Hall.

Gortner, S. R. (1974). Scientific accountability in nursing. *Nursing Outlook, 22*, 764–768.

Gortner, S.R., & Nahm, H. (1977). An overview of nursing research in the United States. *Nursing Research, 26*, 10–33.

Hardy, M.E. (1974). Theories: Components, development, evaluation. *Nursing Research, 23*, 100–107.

Harré, R. (1972). *The philosophies of science: An introductory survey.* London: Oxford University Press.

Jacox, A. (1974). Theory construction in nursing: An overview. *Nursing Research, 23*, 4–13.

Kerlinger, F.N. (1973). *Foundations of behavioral research* (2nd ed.). New York: Holt, Rinehart, and Winston.

Kneller, G.F. (1971). *Introduction to the philosophy of education* (2nd ed.). New York: John Wiley & Sons.

Labovitz, S., & Hagedorn, R. (1976). *Introduction to social research* (2nd ed.). New York: McGraw-Hill.

Leininger, M. (1968). Conference on the nature of science and nursing: Introductory comments. *Nursing Research, 17*, 484–486.

Lindeman, C.A. (1975). Delphi survey of priorities in clinical nursing research. *Nursing Research, 24*, 434–441.

McCain, R.F. (1965). Nursing by assessment—not intuition. *American Journal of Nursing, 65*, 82–84.

Riehl, J.P., & Roy, C. (1974). *Conceptual models for nursing practice.* New York: Appleton-Century-Crofts.

Rogers, M.E. (1970). *An introduction to the theoretical basis of nursing.* Philadelphia: F.A. Davis.

Scheffler, I. (1965). *Conditions of knowledge: An introduction to epistemology and education.* Glenview, IL: Scott, Foresman.

Van Laer, P.H. (1963). *Philosophy of science: An introduction to some general aspects of science* (2nd ed.). Pittsburgh: Duquesne University Press.

Walker, L.O. (1971). Toward a clearer understanding of the concept of nursing theory. *Nursing Research, 20*, 428–435.

Weinland, J.D. (1975). *How to think straight.* Totowa, NJ: Littlefield, Adams (Originally published 1963).

The Author Comments

This article in *Image* was adapted from a manuscript of mine written in the fall of 1972 as part of a doctoral course requirement in "Research Methods and Materials." The theme of the manuscript was influenced by three factors. First, since 1960 I have had an active interest in philosophy and in synthesizing seemingly disparate philosophical themes. Second, in the early 1970s I was aware of the growing emphasis in the nursing profession on formulation of theoretical models of nursing and on metatheory. Both trends interested me because of their conceptual approaches and yet, because my doctoral studies were not in nursing, I felt apart from them. And third, before the course on "Research Methods and Materials," I had already taken three research courses in quantitative methods that emphasized experimental design and inferential statistics. Yet, the type of nursing research problems that interested me most were descriptive in nature—clearly not well suited to an experimental design.

The *Image* article, therefore, represented my effort to integrate these three factors. I wanted to stress that nursing research does not begin in a philosophical vacuum but is linked to theory and philosophy of science even if implicit or unrecognized by the researcher. Furthermore, I wanted to stress that although the methods of the philosopher and the scientist may seem at odds at times, each shares a common goal of increasing human knowledge. Consequently, mutual respect and tolerance is needed.

And finally, I wanted to raise questions about the limitations of quantitative research methods and inferential statistics to study problems of significance in nursing. The article was a challenge to write because of the newness of much of the material to me and the considerable conflicting information about it. Nevertheless, through its writing, I reestablished my closeness to nursing and my commitment to it.

—MARY CIPRIANO SILVA

Chapter 59

The Relationship Between Theory and Research: A Double Helix

Jacqueline Fawcett

Both theory development and research, when isolated endeavors, are excursions into the trivial. What could be less important than a theory about sweet peas or research that involved mating the peas? Yet Mendel combined these seemingly trivial activities and formulated classic genetic theory (Gardner, 1968). And what could be less meaningful than trying to interpret x-rays of sugars and proteins, drawing pictures of protein pairs and tinkering with cardboard and tin replicas of the substances? Yet from these activities emerged an understanding of the double helix structure of DNA (Watson, 1968). Thus only when theory and research are integrated do both become non-trivial; and only then can they contribute to the advancement of science.

The relationship between theory and research may be thought of as a double helix, much like DNA. Theory is one helix, spiralling from the conception of an idea through modifications and extensions to eventual con-

firmation or refutation. Research is the second helix, spiralling from identification of research questions through data collection and analysis to interpretation of findings and recommendations for further study. The core of the double helix is the pairing of theory development with the research process. In the core, theory directs research and research findings shape the development of theory. It is this core that avoids the potential triviality of the separate helices.

The Theory Helix

The primary function of the theory helix is the development of theory. It is also concerned with such philosophic issues as "truth, the nature of reality, the processes of knowing, and the logic of meaning statements"(Dubin, 1978, p. 17).

A theory is defined as "a set of interrelated [concepts], definitions, and propositions that present a systematic view of phenomena by specifying relations among variables"(Kerlinger, 1973, p. 9). An empirically testable theory is composed of concepts that are narrowly bounded, specific and explicitly interrelated.

Content and Structure of Theory

As noted, a theory comprises concepts, definitions and propositions. A concept is an abstract idea expressed in words, a generalization from observed events which may range from a single word to several sentences to entire paragraphs. Concepts enable scientists to categorize, interpret and structure events and objects, helping them to make some sense of their world. Concepts refer to properties of things, not to the things themselves. Usually, they represent phenomena that vary in some manner and are thus referred to as variables (Burr, 1973; Dubin, 1978).

Concepts are the basic building blocks of theories and must therefore be precisely and explicitly defined to enable scientists to distinguish between the meanings of one concept and another. Concepts are defined constitutively and operationally. The constitutive definition, also referred to as the rational approach or the nominal definition, provides meaning for a concept by defining it in terms of the other concepts; it is a circular definition. The operational definition, in contrast, gives concepts empirical utility by linking them with the real world. These definitions, also called real definitions, rules of correspondence or rules of interpretation, define concepts in terms of observable data; i.e., the activities necessary to measure the concept or manipulate it.

Constitutive definitions facilitate communication about the meaning of concepts. Without them, as circular and imprecise as they are, it would not be possible to construct meaningful, logical theories. A theory composed of undefined concepts would be unintelligible, while one composed of only operationally defined concepts would probably be so complex that it too would be unintelligible. While all concepts in a theory should be defined constitutively, such a theory can be evaluated only on logical grounds and cannot be considered scientific. Therefore, for a theory to be empirically testable, operational definitions are required of at least some of its concepts. The operationally defined terms are called empirical indicators. Each is fully specified in terms of its measurement and is therefore clearly differentiated from others. It is important to point out that while constitutive definitions are a distinct part of a theory, operational definitions may be thought of as standing just outside the theory, serving as a link between it and research (Burr, 1973; Hempel, 1952; Torgerson, 1958).

Concepts are connected in a theory by verbal or mathematical statements called propositions. Propositions described the theoretical linkages between concepts. Two types of propositions are generally found in a theory. Axioms, or initial propositions, are the starting points for derivations; they are not to be tested, but rather are taken as givens in the theory. In contrast, postulate, also called deduced propositions or theorems, are statements of supposition regarding the type of relation between the concepts of the theory. A theory's explanatory power is found in its postulates (Burr, 1973; Skidmore, 1975).

The hypothesis is a postulate containing operationally defined terms. It is a descriptive, predictive or prescriptive statement about the presumed relations between the values of two or more empirical indicators. Like the operational definitions they contain, hypotheses are not part of a theory, but are derived from it. The theory is the explanation of relations between concepts; this explanation is tested through the tests of hypotheses (Dubin, 1978).

Theory-Building Strategies

Knowing what the elements of theory are does not, by itself, ensure adequate theory construction. For theory does not emerge out of a random selection and combination of concepts, definitions and propositions; it must be carefully constructed according to a defensible plan. Burr (1973) identified a taxonomy of theory building which includes strategies to assist the scientist to create, extend, integrate or modify theories.

Inductive strategies of theory building use relatively specific, concrete ideas to generate more general, abstract ideas. One such strategy is Glaser and Strauss's (1967) grounded theory, which requires scientists to immerse themselves, without preconceived ideas, in the data (preferably qualitative) of a research project in an attempt to generate new theoretical notions.

Merton (1957) describes another inductive strategy, codification; this is the process of systematizing apparently different empirical generalizations and using them as the basis for inducing new propositions. A third inductive approach is Zetterberg's (1965) definitional reduction in which several variables are redefined, or "collapsed," into a single variable. Thus a new theoretical formulation, more general than the original notions, is suggested.

A fourth theory-building strategy is Zetterberg's (1965) propositional reduction. This approach requires the scientist to select some of the original propositions as general axioms and then to derive other statements of relationships in a logical manner. This strategy qualifies as an inductive one because some propositions are taken to be more general than others.

Deductive strategies of theory building involve starting with relatively abstract, general propositions as the basis for logically deducing new theories that are more specific. One such strategy involves borrowing propositions from one discipline and applying them in another. However, this approach is appropriate only when the initial propositions are rather general and logically congruent with other knowledge in the discipline (Aldous, 1970; Jacox, 1969).

Another deductive strategy is the process of constructing a new theory by deductively extending an already established one. Zetterberg (1965) alludes to this approach, but it is not fully described in the literature.

Other theory-building strategies are not clearly classifiable as either inductive or deductive. The retroductive strategy, described by Hanson (1958), combines the two methods for the purpose of expanding theory. This approach requires the scientist to identify many specific propositions and then induce a more general proposition from which new, specific ones are deduced. Gibson's (1960) factor strategy is similar to induction and generates new theories by examining the interactions and contingencies of various independent variables and their influence on one or more dependent variables.

The final strategy in Burr's taxonomy is theory reworking, or the modification of a theory in light of new methodological tools, new conceptualization, new insights or new empirical data. Burr commented that while this strategy may not increase the amount of theory, "it can build theory in the sense of improving such things as the clarity, testability, communicability, parsimony, and heuristic value" (Burr, 1973, p. 281).

Burr (1973) also identified other activities that are indispensable to theory building. These include development of conceptual models; gathering of empirical data to generate, test of modify theory; improvement of data retrieval systems; and improvement of measurement instruments. However, the discussion of these techniques is beyond the scope of this article.

The ultimate purpose of theory is to order and systematize empirical observations. The scientist desires theory that is highly predictive and thus narrowly bounded; at the same time, he seeks theory that is highly explanatory and thus broad in scope. Since it is not possible to have both at once, decisions must be made as to which type of theory is most needed at any given time in the evolution of a science.

Merton's is perhaps the most popular solution for this paradox. He urged construction of "theories of the middle range"(Merton, 1957, p. 9)—that is, theories that focus on and are applicable to somewhat limited ranges of data. Such theories have some explanatory power and some predictive precision. Moreover, they are more readily testable than either grand theories that are initially too abstract for empirical testing, or partial theories that lack sufficient specification for empirical testing.

If scientists follow the procedures outlined above, they will produce theories that will probably have a degree of esthetic appeal. However, such theories could still be trivial. The theory helix becomes nontrivial only when theory is tested in the real world and modified accordingly.

The Research Helix

The primary function of the research helix is the development of prescriptions for empirical investigations. Its foci are measurement issues, translation of propositions into testable hypotheses and reliability of empirical indicators (Dubin, 1978).

Kerlinger defined scientific research as the "systematic, controlled, empirical, and critical investigation of hypothetical propositions about the presumed relations among natural phenomena" (Kerlinger, 1973, p. 11). Scientific research is systematic and controlled in that observations are sufficiently disciplined so that the investigator has confidence in the research outcomes. Systematization and control come from application of the "max-con-min principle" by which the investigator maximizes the variance of the variables of the research hypothesis, controls the variance of extraneous variables, and minimizes the error variance (Kerlinger, 1973, p. 306).

The empirical and critical nature of scientific research requires scientists to compare subjective belief against objective reality. They must continually subject their ideas to empirical inquiry and view their own and others' findings hypercritically.

Scientific research is a multiphase process which proceeds through several well-known stages: (a) formulation of a research issue, (b) identification of a specific research problem, (c) development of an appropriate research design, (d) selection of research instruments, (e) sampling of units of interest, (f) collection and analysis of data, (g) interpretation of findings and (8) dissemination of results.

Formulating Research Issues and Problems

The choice of research issues is typically based on scientists' current interests and their perceptions of what the crucial questions are in their discipline. Webb (1961) pointed out that scientists commonly base studies on: (a) their interest in the issues, (b) their belief that the answers to the problems inherent in the issues are available, (c) their compassion for society, (d) their belief that these issues will lead to expensive (and therefore important) studies, (e) their belief that the research will yield substantial personal rewards, (f) and their knowledge that everyone else is doing similar work. He noted that while each of these reasons may result in investigations of significant issues in the discipline, more often they result in delineation of pedestrian problems and trivial results.

Research Design and Instruments

The empirical expressions of research issues are the specific research problems, which state the relation between two or more variables. These statements should clearly indicate the scope of the research and should imply possibilities of empirical testing. Research design is the translation of research issues and derived problems into action. As noted above, scientific research attempts to deal with all sources of variance. The "max-con-min principle" is the basis of Campbell and Stanley's classic monograph comparing various research designs with regard to their likelihood of yielding valid inferences. Their work provides specific guidelines for research free from threats to internal and external validity (Campbell & Stanley, 1963).

The instruments selected for a particular study obviously should measure the variables identified in the problem statements. A major concern at this stage of the research process is the evaluation of instrument validity and reliability—their sensitivity in detecting significant differences or relations; their applicability to and appropriateness for the population of interest; and their objectivity. (Fox, 1976).

Sampling

Sampling techniques allow scientists to select for study groups of subjects that permit generalizations to the population of interest. While random samples are traditionally the most valued, they are not the ones that are most precise and they cannot be used under some circumstances. It is therefore not surprising to find an increased interest in sampling methods that are more generally applicable and which yield more precise estimates of the population (Kish, 1965). Sample size must also be considered. Various techniques exist for the determination of optimum sample size and are documented in the literature (Cohen, 1969).

Data Collection and Analysis

Data collection, of course, directly depends on the research problems and instruments. However, it is not unusual in the course of a study for the scientist to collect data that are only indirectly related to specific study problems. As will be seen later, often these additional data ultimately prove more valuable in terms of the overall research issue.

Data analysis is a focal point of contemporary research. As more sophisticated and complex analyses are facilitated by the use of computers, it becomes increasingly possible for scientists to examine more sources of variance among study variables. However, it is important that they not be so seduced by advanced analytical methods as to lose sight of the original study issues and problems.

Interpretation and Dissemination of Findings

Interpretation of research findings follows the rules of logic explicit in the statistical procedures used in the investigation. Objectivity is a key component of this stage of the research process. While statistical significance of findings is almost always reported, few scientists consider the strength of association between variables, despite repeated urging by experts to do so (Dunnette, 1966).

The scientist has not completed the research helix until findings are reported to peers. The purpose of the research report is to communicate as precisely, concisely and clearly as possible "what was done, why it was done, the outcome of the doing, and the investigator's conclusions" (Kerlinger, 1973, p. 694). The readers must then make their own judgments regarding the adequacy and validity of the study.

Relating Research to Theory

If scientists apply the research process carefully, it is likely they will conduct sophisticated investigations free from methodological flaws. However, it is quite possible the studies will be irrelevant, for, just as the theory helix is trivial in isolation, so is the research helix. Knowledge of research methodology, no matter how extensive, is meaningless unless it can be utilized in the design and conduct of investigations that are grounded in theory.

The ultimate purpose of a research study, according to Popper (1965), is to refute the theory on which the study is based. The Popperian stance focuses on improving rather than proving a theory. This approach allows all data collected during an investigation to be used, giving "particular attention to deviant cases and nonfitting data that feed back immediately into the theory-building process by resulting in theory modifications" (Dubin, 1978, p. 232). From this perspective, it is impossible to discuss research without discussing theory.

The Core of the Double Helix

The double helix has as its core the interrelation between theory and research. As in DNA, the core is essential for structure and function. Merton emphasized this point by noting, "It is commonplace that continuity, rather than dispersion, can be achieved only if empirical studies are theory-oriented and if theory is empirically confirmable" (Merton, 1957, p. 100). Thus the body of knowledge of a science must rely on the repeated investigation of theoretically based problems that are redefined as research results accumulate. Theory should guide all phases of the research process, from choice of research issue to dissemination of results. All research, in turn, should be directed to one of two goals—theory building or theory testing.

Types of Theory-Related Research

Theory-building research has as its primary purpose the discovery of relations between variables on the basis of empirical observations. Once observations are made, they are analyzed and examined for generalizations that might lead to formulation of concepts and propositions. Traditionally, these activities have been labeled theoretical, descriptive, inductive or hypothesis-generating research. This type of research stems mainly from and relies heavily on inductive strategies of theory building to create new theories or to modify existing ones.

Theory-testing research, on the other hand, seeks to confirm or refute previously postulated relations between variables. Its major function is to determine the degree of correspondence between predicted and observed relations. These activities are usually labeled empirical, deductive or hypothesis-testing research. Predominantly through deductive theory-building strategies, hypotheses are formulated and tested in the real world (Dubin, 1978).

It should be clear that the two types of research are inextricably bound to theory and are differentiated only by the direction of movement between observation and theory within the double helix. It should also be obvious that all phases of the research process should be based on theory. Of course, research can be conducted without an explicit theoretical base. However, according to Popper (1965), even the most creative induction is based on observations made within some theoretical frame of reference.

Designing and Implementing Theory-Related Research

Since there is some evidence that scientists are not highly successful in uniting theory and research in their work, and since few research or theory construction texts consider this in any detail, the content of the double helix core needs to be examined.

The formulation of a research issue may justifiably stem from either theoretical or pragmatic concerns of the scientist. If theoretical interest is the point of departure, the research may lead to theory building or theory testing, depending on the state of theory in the discipline. Pragmatic concern, on the other hand, often leads initially to theory-building research, since frequently there is no prior theory bearing on this issue available for testing.

Many failures to integrate theory and research occur when the research impetus is pragmatic and the scientist "does not bother" to develop a theory to explain results. Such research may be very important in practical terms, but it is likely to be sterile and not advance the discipline. However, a theoretical interest can also get in the way of integration when scientists put all their energies into constructing elegant theoretical edifices which they do not trouble to test, or which, even worse, may be untestable.

Once the research issue has been identified, specific research problems must be outlined. The relation between theory and research is perhaps more clearly illustrated at this point than at any other in the double helix core. The specific problems ultimately derive from theory and prior research. Scientists should take care at this stage to explicitly relate the present study to the larger body of knowledge in the discipline. Furthermore, they should take care to either state the propositions of the theory being tested and to clearly derive hypotheses from them, or to identify specific observations expected to lead to propositions of the theory being built. The expression of the research problem is the culmination of the theoretical process, "the final step in the unfolding of the logic that provides the foundation for the empirical phase of research" (Batey, 1977, p. 329).

The specific research problems will suggest the research design to be used in conducting the investigation. The level of knowledge from which the research problem is derived is even more influential in selecting the design. For instance, if a review of the literature reveals no previous study of the relations between variables of interest, an exploratory theory-building study might be undertaken. Such a study enables the investigator to collect preliminary data which can then be used to formulate specific concepts and propositions using inductive theory-building strategies. However, if the literature indicates a well-developed body of theory, the research might focus on derivation of hypotheses using deductive strategies and empirical testing of hypothesized relations.

The choice of research instruments should also be guided by the study's theoretical base. Extreme care must be taken to select tools that are valid and reliable empirical indicators of the relevant concepts. It is important to recognize that the tools of a research project are the links between "a theoretically formulated research problem and the data to be gathered from observations" (Lin, 1976, p. 10).

Sampling, too, is based on the theory underlying the investigation. The majority of theories should be limited to certain populations. The scientist who wishes to build or test a theory must therefore be explicit about its boundaries. Furthermore, if the research is designed to extend a theory, the scientist must be certain it has been confirmed in one population before testing it in another.

The data analysis stage links research problem and the raw data. The form of analysis is also dictated by the theoretical base of the study. The statistics used in the analysis should come as no surprise to the reader, since the hypotheses should reveal these, at least in the broad categories of analysis of relations or of difference. Once data analysis is completed, the task is to interpret the findings. Theory serves to order the findings and to place them in context. Research findings should be clearly and explicitly related to the theory being built or tested.

Interpreting Theory-Related Research

The results of research lead directly to confirmation or rejection of hypotheses. If they are confirmed, the scientist should plan even more stringent tests of the theory or studies which will continue to build it. If, on the other hand, the hypotheses are rejected and the scientist is convinced the study was a legitimate test of the theory, it is probable the theory requires modification and subsequent rigorous testing.

Regardless of the outcomes of the study and of the care taken to integrate theory and research, several additional should be considered at this point in the research process. Those relating mainly to the theory include reexamination of the causal structure and of variables identified as causes and effects. (Although the scientist may not have considered his theory as causal, these factors require examination because causal thinking and theory cannot be separated.) Factors relating primarily to reexamination of the data include scale of measurement assumed, coding procedures used and validity of the data as empirical indicators of the concepts (Smelser & Warner, 1976). The conclusions which may be reached from such a critical review include: (a) the data are faulty and cannot be relied on; (b) the theory is faulty and should be discarded; (c) the data are accurate and the theory requires modification; and (d) the data are accurate but have no relevance to the theory (Downs, 1973).

Ultimately, a theory can never be confirmed or refuted. Since hypotheses are tested in a probabilistic manner, and since the probability of error in inference is normally never zero or one, it is always possible that replications of a study will yield different results. Moreover, there is always the possibility of other logical explanations why the data of one study provided or failed to provide support for the hypotheses. Any theory can therefore be considered no more than an approximation of the real world or a plausible explanation of events. As Selltiz and her associates commented:

> . . . the most plausible theory is the one for which we have the strongest evidential support. And it is this theory that is to be provisionally "believed" or "accepted" until another theory gains superior evidential support. Scientific knowledge is knowledge under conditions of uncertainty (Selltiz, Wrightsman, & Cook, 1976, pp. 47–48).

Theory and Research in Nursing Science

Nursing Theory

Nursing theory is not trivial; it is practically nonexistent. The nursing literature yield little evidence of formulations that might be considered nursing theory, that is, "a set of interrelated propositions and definitions which present a systematic view of one or more of the essential [concepts] of nursing—person, environment, health, nursing—by specifying relations among relevant variables" (Fawcett, 1978, p. 26).

Currently, nursing science has not progressed much beyond a knowledge base composed of conceptual models. A conceptual model is a highly abstract umbrella of related multidimensional concepts that provide a broad perspective for scientists, telling them what to look at (Reilly, 1975). The conceptual models of nursing certainly are not trivial, since they have a demonstrated usefulness in guiding nursing practice, research and education (Riehl & Roy, 1974). However, they cannot be empirically tested because of the abstract nature of their concepts. Nursing science thus remains essentially devoid of any substantive nursing theories that could be related to nursing research.

Nursing's theory helix has received considerable attention over the past several years. Nurse scholars have offered definitions of nursing theories and urged their construction; they have described techniques of theory formalization and construction; and they have cited the advantages and disadvantages of theory-building strategies using borrowed theories (Cleland, 1967; Hardy, 1974; Jacox, 1974; Silva, 1977). More recently, it has been advocated that nursing theories be derived from the conceptual models of nursing and that theory construction follow the master plan offered by Dickoff and James' (1968) four levels of theory (Fawcett, 1978; Menke, 1978).

Nursing scholars are essentially in agreement on the need for nursing theory and the strategies for its construction. They even seem to agree that nursing knowledge may be a synthesis of theory borrowed from other disciplines. What, then, has been the payoff for the theory helix of nursing science? Apparently, it has been almost nil. As Menke stated:

> Thus far there has been a dearth of theory developed for nursing. Efforts have not been organized in any specific manner. The theory that has been developed has followed a laissez-faire route or has not necessarily been focused in any specific direction (Menke, 1978, p. 218).

It may be concluded than that while knowledge of the content of the theory helix exists in nursing science, the application of that knowledge is not evident.

Nursing Research

The content of the research helix of nursing science is better developed. Even a cursory review of nursing research publications and presentations reveals increasing attention to the cornerstones of scientific research, i.e., systematization, control, empiricism and critical review. Despite this, given the preceding discussion, it should be clear that most nursing research must be trivial, since it is not connected to theory in any discernible way. This assertion is supported by Batey's (1977) review of 25 years of research published in *Nursing Research*, which discovered few explicit theoretical bases for the research. Batey's findings suggest that while nurse researchers may know that theory and research should be interrelated, they apparently do not comprehend this, or do not accept it, or do not know how to apply this knowledge.

The Theory-Research Core

It should by now be apparent that the double helix core is essentially nonexistent in nursing science. While this situation is not unique to nursing, as pointed out earlier, it is important that some rapid progress be made if nursing is to retain and increase its respectability as a science.

The underdevelopment of the theory helix of nursing science is obviously the main factor impeding the development of the double helix core. For without nursing theory, it is rather difficult, if not impossible, to design theoretically based nursing research. A review of the literature has identified several other factors retarding the development of the double helix core of nursing science.

First, nursing has no scientific heritage. There is no comprehensive body of knowledge or research tradition on which to construct a core of unified theory and research (Johnson, 1974). Second, although the derivation of research problems from the conceptual frameworks of nursing has been advocated (Schlotfeldt,

1975), here is little evidence that nurse researchers have adopted this strategy, perhaps because of the effort required to deduce a theory and relevant empirically testable problems from these highly abstract models.

Third, the favoring of experimental research as the best way to test theories and of research with direct clinical practice implications has led away from basic descriptive studies that might provide the baseline data crucial for theory building. These research biases have, unfortunately, encouraged nurses to conduct "more sophisticated" studies that lack a firm theoretical foundation.

Fourth, the value placed on creativity, together with a "do your own thing" orientation in nursing, has inhibited study replication research that might provide empirical data needed for modification, extension or refutation of theories.

Fifth, since nurses are oriented to doing, it is evidently difficult for them to value "the time-consuming analysis and testing demanded by research before action is initiated" (Martinson, 1978, p. 159).

Sixth, as long as editorial reviews of research reports are less rigorous regarding theory helix content than for research helix content, it is doubtful that nurse researchers will be motivated to carefully delineate the type of research (theory building or theory testing) they are conducting or to explicitly integrate theory with research (Batey, 1977).

Finally, as long as published research is not related to theory, an implicit message of "why bother" is given to those who might otherwise attempt to relate theory to research and research to theory. Or, even worse, the effective message may be that this is not necessary.

Many other sciences have gone through a similar phase before the double helix core has come into being. For instance, only in the past decade has the literature of many of the behavioral sciences revealed integration of theory and research. It should not be surprising then that such integration has not yet occurred in the embryonic science of nursing. And it is probable that nursing's current preoccupation with this lack is the result of its quest for recognition as a distinct science, particularly in academe, but also in hallways of practice settings.

References

Aldous, J. (1970). Strategies for developing family theory. *Marriage and the Family, 32*(2), 250–257.

Batey, M.V. (1971). Conceptualization: Knowledge and logic guiding empirical research. *Nursing Research, 26*(5), 324–329.

Burr, W.R. (1973). *Theory construction and the sociology of the family.* New York: John Wiley & Sons.

Campbell, D.T., & Stanley, J.C. (1963). *Experimental and quasi-experimental designs for research.* Chicago: Rand McNally.

Cleland, V.S. (1967). The use of existing theories. *Nursing Research, 16*(2), 118–121.

Cohen, J. (1969). *Statistical power analysis for the behavioral sciences.* New York: Academic Press.

Dickoff, J., & James, P. (1968). A theory of theories: A position paper. *Nursing Research, 17,* 197–203.

Downs, F.S. (1973). Elements of a research critique. In F.S. Downs & M.A. Newman (Eds.), *A source book of nursing research.* Philadelphia: F.A. Davis.

Dubin, R. (1978). *Theory building* (rev. ed.). New York: Free Press.

Dunnette, M.D. (1966). Fads, fashions, and folderol in psychology. *American Psychologist, 21*(4), 343–352.

Fawcett, J. (1978). The 'what' of theory development. In *Theory development: What, why, how?* New York: National League for Nursing.

Fox, D.J. (1976). *Fundamentals of research in nursing* (3rd ed.). New York: Appleton-Century-Crofts.

Gardner, E.J. (1968). *Principles of genetics* (3rd ed.). New York: John Wiley & Sons.

Gibson, Q. (1970). *The logic of social enquiry.* New York: Humanities Press.

Glaser, B.G., & Strauss, A.L. (1967). *The discovery of grounded theory: Strategies for qualitative research.* Chicago: Aldine.

Hanson, N.R. (1958). *Patterns of discovery.* New York: Cambridge University Press.

Hardy, M. (1974). Theories: Components, development, evaluation. *Nursing Research, 23*(2), 100–107.

Hempel, C.G. (1952). *Fundamentals of concept formation in empirical science.* Chicago: University of Chicago Press.

Jacox, A. (1969). Issues in construction of nursing theory. In C. M. Norris (Ed.), *Proceedings, First Nursing Theory Conference.* Kansas City: University of Kansas Medical Center Department of Nursing Education.

Jacox, A. (1974). Theory construction in nursing. An overview. *Nursing Research, 23*(1), 4–13.

Johnson, D.E. (1974). Development of theory: A requisite for nursing as a primary health profession. *Nursing Research, 23*(5), 372–377.

Kerlinger, F.N. (1973). *Foundations of behavioral research* (2nd ed.). New York: Holt, Rinehart and Winston.

Kish, L. (1965). *Survey sampling.* New York: John Wiley & Sons.

Lin, N. (1976). *Foundations of social research.* New York: McGraw-Hill.

Martinson, I. (1978). Why research in nursing? In N.L. Chaska (Ed.), *The nursing profession: Views through the mist.* New York: McGraw-Hill.

Menke, E.M. (1978). Theory development: A challenge for nursing. In N.L. Chaska (Ed.), *The nursing profession: Views through the mist.* New York: McGraw-Hill.

Merton, R.F. (1957). *Social theory and social structure* (rev. ed.). New York: Free Press.

Popper, K.R. (1965). *Conjectures and refutations: The growth of scientific knowledge.* New York: Harper and Row.

Reilly, D.E. (1975). Why a conceptual framework? *Nursing Outlook, 23*(8), 566–569.

Riehl, J.P., & Roy, C. *Conceptual models for nursing practice.* New York: Appleton-Century-Crofts.

Schlotfeldt, R.M. (1975). The need for a conceptual framework. In P.J. Verhonick (Ed.), *Nursing Research, Vol 1.* (pp. 3–24). Boston: Little, Brown.

Selltiz, C., Wrightsman, L.S., & Cook, S.W. (1976). *Research methods in social relations* (3rd ed.). New York: Holt, Rinehart and Winston.

Silva, M.C. (1977). Philosophy, science, theory: Interrelationships and implications for nursing research. *Image, 9*(3), 59–63.

Skidmore, W. (1975). *Theoretical thinking in sociology.* New York: Cambridge University Press.

Smelser, N.J., & Warner, R.S. (1976). *Sociological theory: Historical and formal.* Morristown, NJ: General Learning Press.

Torgerson, W.S. (1958). *Theory and methods of scaling.* New York: John Wiley & Sons.

Watson, J.D. (1968). *The double helix.* New York: New American Library.

Webb, W.B. (1961). The choice of the problem. *American Psychologist, 16*, 223–227.

Zetterberg, H.L. (1965). *On theory and verification in sociology* (3rd ed.). Totowa, NJ: Bedminster Press.

Reactions

Advances in Nursing Science, April 1979, *1*(3), viii.

. . .[In]"Theory and Research: A Double Helix," Jacqueline Fawcett noted that Marge Batey's review of 25 years of research published in *Nursing Research* discovered few explicit theoretical bases for research. Hopefully, members of editorial review teams in nursing journals will heed Dr. Fawcett's admonishments, namely factors six and seven listed as retarding nursing. Journals reporting nursing research must act to allow the researcher to delineate relevant theory as explanation of relations between concepts in presenting empirical tests of these relationships.

BETTY D. PEARSON, R.N., Ph.D.
Associate Dean
Graduate Program in Nursing
School of Nursing
University of Wisconsin
Milwaukee, Wisconsin

On the "Relationship Between Theory and Research," *Advances in Nursing Science*, April 1979, *1*(3), x–xi.

To the Editor:

"The Relationship Between Theory and Research: A Double Helix" by Jacqueline Fawcett clearly identifies many important issues and concerns regarding relationships between theoretical and research components and the need for unification of these elements.

I would agree with the author that integration of theory development and research is paramount to a highly productive approach toward scientific advancement, this being particularly true for nursing in its embryonic theoretical state. However, while the integration of the two is highly desirable, lack of such integration need not deem such research to be trivial if by trivial one means of little importance or worth. While benefits of such research are greatly minimized, no valid scientific effort is without some significant value.

As was noted by the author, other sciences have experienced a process analogous to nursing's prior to integration of theory with research. Those sciences were also initially concerned with development of a knowledge base and survival as a profession much as nursing is. Perhaps this evolutionary process is indispensable to emerging sciences . . . is in fact a necessary part of that science's evolution. All previous nursing research, for example, with or without implications for practice, has significance in that it has increased skills of nurse investigators and has broadened the scope of nursing research. Both theory and research are valuable in and of themselves for the new avenues, ideas and implications for further research they may afford, and we should not be demoralized by the slow progress to date.

The various parts comprising the whole may lead to vistas unrecognized at earlier stages, as Dr. Fawcett noted when she described Mendel's combination of seemingly trivial activities which led to formulation of classical genetic theory. The pulling together of pieces of accumulated knowledge led ultimately to significant theory. Perhaps nursing has not yet recognized possible theoretical bases within its own accumulating body of knowledge; perhaps there are unidentified links or connections in research already done. While forging ahead we would do well to systematically evaluate connections in research which has already been documented. One wonders what contributions to theory building might be made out of existing empirical data, whether in fact we have not connected possible existing theoretical concepts.

The greater issue is not triviality so much as the need for nursing to decide whether it will take the position of firmly specifying directions for nursing research in the future. On the one hand we can continue the evolutionary course we have followed in the past, progressing at a snail's pace towards substantive theory, as it will take an inordinate amount of time to connect isolated research findings to theory development. On the other hand, we can purposely choose the fastest, most productive route towards theory building.

Nursing does not have the luxury of unlimited time; there is need to survive as a viable scientific discipline. Therefore the tremendous need for theory development behooves us to choose the most productive of the two approaches. Empirical research which tests theories and allows us to confirm, refute or modify those theories is of greatest value for steady, cumulative progress in nursing science. Isolated endeavors may indeed prevent us from "seeing the forest for the trees." Yet each tree is an integral, viable part of the forest, and in that sense nontrivial to its growth and development. Isolated theory and research indeed contribute to the advancement of science by providing new answers to questions. The larger issue is whether nursing, in developing its theoretical base, feels it is more valuable to speed this evolutionary process by consciously and consistently integrating the two.

CAROLYN ERICKSON D'AVANZO, M.S., R.N.
Bolton, Connecticut
Student, Doctor of Nursing Science Program
Boston, University
Boston, Massachusetts

The Author Comments

Doctoral coursework with Florence S. Downs at New York University sensitized me to the need for a strong and explicit theoretical base for empirical research and to the implications of research findings for theory development. However, no publications explained the close connection between theory and research in any detail. An invitation from Peggy L. Chinn to submit an article for the first issue of *Advances in Nursing Science* provided me the opportunity to share my ideas about the relationship between theory and research with my peers. Further development of those ideas has been motivated by students' questions and comments and appear in the book that I co-authored with Florence S. Downs, *The Relationship of Theory and Research* (Norwalk, CT: Appleton-Century-Crofts, 1985). The second edition of this book currently is being prepared and will be published by F.A. Davis Company.

—JACQUELINE FAWCETT

REFERENCE

Fawcett, J., & Downs, F.S. (1985). *The relationship of theory and research.* Norwalk, CT: Appleton-Century-Crofts.

Chapter 60

Nursing Philosophy and Nursing Research: In Apposition or Opposition?

Patricia L. Munhall

Expressions found in nursing philosophy should have logical congruency, coherence, and continuity with expressions found in nursing research.

Research paradigms guide and perpetuate nursing practice and the linguistic components of the paradigm should demonstrate contextual and syntactical parallelism with beliefs and values of the discipline. If the language of both represent conflictual ideologies, alternative paradigms should be explored and added to the research repertoire of nurses.

The scientific method is the most prevalent, encouraged and rewarded model used in nursing research for understanding man's place in the world.

Nurse researchers acquire the know-how of working out problems by doing variations on the dominant paradigm—the scientific method. Kuhn (1970) suggests that a paradigm is a discipline's specific method of solving a puzzle, of viewing a man's experience, and of structuring reality. Indeed, the paradigm structures the questions to be asked, while systematically eliminating those kinds of questions that cannot be stated within the concepts and tools the paradigm supplies. In these ways the paradigm preserves and perpetuates the disciplinary matrix of nursing.

The paradigm, because of its significance in perpetuating and preserving the nature of nursing, should have at its roots values and beliefs that are congruent with nursing philosophy. A problem occurs when analysis of the paradigm and the discipline's philosophy reveal basic incongruities, paradoxes, and conflicting ideologies. The question arises: Are nursing philosophy and nursing research in apposition or opposition? If a paradigm guides and perpetuates practice, it is essential to analyze where it takes the profession in relation to

About the Author

PATRICIA L. MUNHALL is interested in ambiguities, contradictions, and incongruities. She worries about implementing advance technology and then asking ethical questions after the fact. She has served as director of the graduate program and associate dean at Seton Hall University, and currently is a professor in the graduate program at Hunter College, Hunter-Bellevue School of Nursing.

Dr. Munhall has presented papers and published articles on research methods, ethics, and moral reasoning in *Image*, *Journal of Nursing Education*, *Topics in Clinical Nursing*, *Nursing Research*, and *Advances in Nursing Science*. With Dr. Carolyn Oiler, she co-authored a textbook titled *Nursing Research: A Qualitative Perspective*, published in 1986. The book received an AJN Book of the Year Award.

Her interests include nursing research and theory, ethics, feminist theory, role development in nursing, philosophy, psychoanalysis, children, and friends. She is appreciative of her friends in nursing and believes that the hope of the health care system in this country is clearly centered in the nursing profession.

the profession's stated beliefs and values. This article is an exploration of the contextual parallelism and logical congruency between the scientific method and nursing philosophy. Expressions found in nursing philosophy are examined for philosophical "fit" with expressions found in the scientific method.

Nursing Philosophy

Nursing is a profession that identifies itself as humanistic, and adheres to a basic philosophy that focuses on individuality and the belief that the actions of men are in some sense free. Free will is grounded in a world view of man where man acts upon his experience. He chooses, is self-determined, and is, in essence, an active organism. Inherent to humanism are philosophical beliefs and values, and these are sprinkled throughout contemporary nursing literature, and are found in such expressions as becoming, freedom, self-determination, autonomy, and human potential.

Nursing philosophy almost universally includes a belief about holistic man. The holistic view of man insists that man possesses an integration that does not allow analysis by breaking him down into reducible parts and piecing him back together. Man must be assessed simultaneously at a multitude of levels and perspectives: physical status, self-knowledge, goals, environmental surroundings, and so on. Man is an open

system possessing the capability of unlimited growth. He is evolving and emerging in mutual interaction with his environment. Nursing philosophies purport that man is unique. Individual uniqueness is valued and spoken about in terms of cultural, socio-economic, religious, and experimental relativism. According to this holistic, open-system, unique view of man, each person experiences his own "reality." The experience may be shared, but the individual is ultimately the one who interprets his own experience and gives meaning to it. In essence, he is autonomous.

In nursing philosophies the nurse is the advocate of the individual's autonomy and acts to safeguard the patient's rights. The nurse does not choose for the patient but educates and supports him in his choices, to insure that the patient's right of self-determination be upheld and to insure that he has the opportunity to participate or not in plans for his own health care.

The Scientific Method

The scientific method has been found to be the most effective way of determining relationships between variables, and thus enabling understanding, prediction, and to a degree control. The scientific method can be examined as a process, each step reflecting a belief that contributes to the philosophy of science and to a particular way of viewing the world. The scientist chooses what to study, then engages in a process of self-generated reductionism. By choosing an observable or measurable part of an individual's environment, the scientist sets limits on the problem. This is the first requisite of the scientific method.

The scientist usually becomes distant from the problem in order to be objective about the phenomena under study. The investigator is objective and what is studied becomes objectified, an object of study. The delimited problem must be defined and the definitions be made operational, therefore observable and/or measurable. Reality is reduced to the measurable and the empirical, with further definition according to the experience of the researcher, who has assigned meaning to the phenomenon, rarely having experienced it.

Controls and "controls for" are set for intervening or otherwise extraneous variables. In each group individuals are as much alike as possible to eliminate the influence of confounding variables. The experiment is performed, variables manipulated, and/or the instrument administered, measured and statistically analyzed. Measurements of central tendency often dictate upholding or rejecting of hypotheses. Results apply not to all cases tested, but to the mean of all cases tested. Theory is generated "on the average," for the "average person." Categorization, labeling, and further manipulation to enable prediction and control follow.

The basic premises of the scientific method are: individuals are alike according to categories, experience is quantifiable, and human and environmental constancy and passivity can be produced. The end result is a situation-producing theory that is deterministic, atomistic, and scientific. The basic world view is mechanistic: the individual reacts to predetermined stimuli to produce a desired outcome as set by the nurse.

Logical Congruency: "The Fit"

Are contemporary nursing philosophy and nursing research relevant to each other? Do they yield explanatory equivalence and possess the same syntactical relationship? Are they taking the profession in the same direction or do they represent opposing ideologies and are in conflict?

If the individual has free will and is self-determined, why should he be controlled behaviorally? For his own good? And who determines "good"?

If man's integration defies explanation by understanding of the parts, why reduce him to limited "discrete" variables in an attempt to study the whole. Why choose to study man, an open system, with the same method used to study "closed" systems? Man is unique, an individual. Why choose a method that ultimately categorizes him and encourages us to label him, as though labeling and categorizing brings with it understanding? In the search for categories and labels, man is depersonalized.

In nursing philosophy, the individual the nurse encounters is the focus of consideration, whereas, in nursing research, the researcher is the prime mover. The nurse researcher defines the problem, operates within the definitions of selected variables, chooses a framework from which to study the problem, decides what treatment might be helpful, chooses the answer (forced choice), and sets the categories.

The researcher interprets the data, makes recommendations, and speaks in a language distinct and apart from the subject. Scientific protocol is operative; the assumption is that human behavior is orderly, lawful, and predictable.

Data subjected to statistical analysis produces theory that is descriptive of or predictive of the average person. But doesn't nursing philosophy value the uniqueness of individuals? What gets lost in statistical analysis are alternative explanations for those individuals who reacted differently from the "mean." Perhaps as important, alternative interpretations of the findings are lost as well.

Implications

Are nursing philosophy and nursing research vis-à-vis the scientific method ideologically and philosophically opposed? Despite nurse researchers' humanistic intentions for their scientific endeavors, historically the intentions of scientists are considered incidental and not part of the scientific enterprise.

Qualitative research methods, particularly in theory development, may be more consistent with nursing's stated philosophical beliefs in which subjectivity, shared experience, shared language, interrelatedness, human interpretation, and reality as experienced rather than contrived are considered. (See Table 60–1.) Understanding and explanation come from a holistic

Table 60-1

Expressions of Contemporary Nursing in Philosophy

Humanism	Uniqueness
Individualism	Relativism
Self-determinism	Autonomy
Active Organism	Advocacy
Open System	Organismic
Holism	

Expressions of the Scientific Method

Reductionism	Theory for the Average
Objectivity—Positivism	Categorization
Delimited Problem	Prediction
Reality Reduced to the	Control
Empirical	Mechanistic
Human and Environmental	
Passivity	
Manipulation	

Contextual Parallelism

NURSING PHILOSOPHY	NURSING RESEARCH
Individualism —	Commonalities
Uniqueness —	Generalizations
Relativism —	Categorization
Open System —	Closed System
Holism —	Reductionism
Individual Interpretation —	Statistical Analysis
Active Organism —	Re-active Organism
Organismic —	Mechanistic
Self-Determination —	Control

analysis of that portion made up of: (a) a time frame and development (history), (b) diversity, shared interpretation of experiences (ethnography and phenomenology), (c) the sharing and interpreting of language (analytical), and (d) getting in the midst of the data without limitations of a predetermined problem and criteria that could make the study self-fulfilling.

The use of the scientific method as the only serious model for understanding man's place in the world is being questioned today by scientists as well as humanists. Bullock says that "the positivist view of science itself may be out of date and misleading" (Bullock, 1980, p. 184). Chargaff writes that "the over-fragmentation of the vision of nature—or actually its complete disappearance among the majority of scientists—has created a Humpty-Dumpty world that must become increasingly unmanageable as more and tinier pieces are broken off 'for classification,' from the continuum of nature. . . . The wonderful, inconceivably intricate tapestry is being pulled out, torn up, and analyzed; and at the end even the memory of the design is lost and can no longer be recalled" (Chargaff, 1978, pp. 55-56).

And Bullock asks, "Who is going to take the time or trouble to worry about individual human beings or even individual groups?" (Bullock, 1980, p. 184).

The nursing profession has made this commitment. To do so we must question aggregates, averages, fragmentation, standardization, classification, categorization, and generalization. Let us not compromise our values, instead let us look to other congruent methods for theory building.

References

Bullock, A. (1980). Future of humanistic studies. *Teacher's College Record, 82*, 173–190.

Chargaff, E. (1978). *Heraclitean fire: Sketches from a life before nature*. New York: Rockefeller University Press.

Kuhn, T.S. (1970). *The structure of scientific revolutions* (2nd ed.). Chicago: University of Chicago Press.

The Author Comments

First Edition

My interest in metaphorical language sometimes sparks a synapse connection when the page before me, as well as the mind, is blank. I am focusing on the word "table," as in "Table of Contents," and am pondering the possible ways this word began to be used descriptively to connote "a body of ideas."

As in an analogy to a richly served banquet at a "table" of committed and caring scholars of nursing theory, I feel at once a bit out of place (do I belong with such an erudite group?) and gladdened to be included. The origins and ideas for this article came from what is served at this table and exchanged by the participants. "Food" for thought includes stimulation, dedication, provocation, intellectualization, clarification, conceptualization, and demystification. As in any lively dialogue, some contradictions begin to emerge—hence the origin of ideas in this article flows from the dialogue illustrated in the table of contents.

Sometimes I wish for an original thought but it is most apparent, at least to me, how indebted I am to those who ventured on the initial maiden voyage of exploration. The participants within this volume have initiated the dialogue that provided a wealth of knowledge for me to ponder and, perhaps more important, the opportunity for me to offer their ideas and perspectives when graduate students and I sit at "tables" to continue the dialogue and dialecticism essential for intellectual life—"food" for the mind.

The Author Comments

Second Edition

This article was written 10 years ago and I hope it continues to serve a purpose of differentiating between worldviews. However, as I reread it today, the article seems to illustrate a piece of our research history and research evolution. I find it most interesting that graduate students today are hardly aware that qualitative methods of inquiry were not always part of nursing theory development.

—PATRICIA L. MUNHALL

Chapter 61

Toward a New View of Science: Implications for Nursing Research

Mindy B. Tinkle

Janet L. Beaton

It was her first dissertation committee meeting. The topic of discussion was her proposed research methodology. Two of the committee members (well-known for their "hard" research) began to dialogue about the "softness" of the approach in the proposal before them—the lack of control, the lack of quantitative measurement, and the lack of manipulation of variables. Before long, the committee was in accord about the relatively low scientific merit of this type of research methodology as opposed to an experimental approach. The student found herself agreeing to shift her methodology to one involving experimental manipulation.

The above scenario typifies the view held by many members of the scientific community that hard research is more rigorous, more objective, and hence more worthy of being done than so-called soft research. It highlights the value placed on the experimental method at the expense of devaluing other approaches involving naturalistic observation and qualitative patterning of phenomena. Bakan has cogently described this valuing of method as the "disease of methodolatry, the worship of method." He states that "when there is

worship of these methods themselves rather than that to which they are directed, then indeed does science become idolatrous" (Bakan, 1966, p. 8).

This value orientation is only a part of a much broader conception of what is proper or real science. It is a view that is influencing the development of nursing's body of knowledge. As nursing's sophistication in research and theory building grows, it is imperative that the dominant concept of what is proper science with its concomitant values not to be borrowed and

About the Authors

MINDY B. TINKLE currently is an Associate Professor at the University of Texas at El Paso, College of Nursing and Allied Health. A native Texan, she was born in Abilene, grew up in Houston, and currently lives in El Paso. Dr. Tinkle is a graduate of Texas Women's University (B.S., 1976), the University of Texas Health Science Center at San Antonio (M.S.N., 1980), and The University of Texas at Austin (Ph.D., 1985).

Dr. Tinkle's area of clinical interest is women's health care. She is an advanced women's health care nurse practitioner and has worked clinically in labor and delivery, postpartum, newborn nursery, and most recently in the primary care of women. She has held faculty appointments at the University of Texas at Austin and the University of Texas Health Science Center at Houston, teaching graduate and undergraduate students in the areas of obstetrics, pediatrics, and perinatal nursing. Before arriving in El Paso in July, 1990, Dr. Tinkle practiced as a women's health care nurse practitioner in the U.S. Army Nurse Corps in Nuremberg, West Germany.

JANET L. BEATON resides in Winnipeg, Manitoba, Canada, and is on the faculty of the School of Nursing of the University of Manitoba, where she has been teaching since 1974. Previously, she held a faculty appointment at the University of Washington. Clinically, Dr. Beaton is interested in maternal-child health and has worked in the newborn nursery, labor and delivery, and postpartum areas. She is a graduate of the University of Manitoba (B.N., 1969), the University of Washington (M.A., 1972), and the University of Texas at Austin (Ph.D., 1986).

When asked about personal interests, Dr. Beaton responded "I have always been interested in history and am an avid reader of historical biography. The interaction between personality and historical context fascinates me and I suppose in no small way has shaped my concern for the importance of contextual variables in nursing research and practice."

Dr. Beaton has coauthored (with Lesley Degner) a book, *Life-Death Decisions in Health Care* (Washington, D.C.: Hemisphere, 1987). She comments that "not only did this book mark the culmination of a 6-year field work investigation of the process of life-death decision making across a wide range of treatment settings and patient groups, it also represented a truly collaborative effort whereby the final product was indeed greater than the sum of the parts. Working together on virtually every word and sentence, bouncing ideas back and forth, we were able to achieve a level of integration that would not have been possible had we each worked independently on separate sections of the book. The intensity of that experience was immensely satisfying and profoundly gratifying."

adopted without introspection about the adequacy of this approach to meet nursing's most substantive problems.

Two Views of Science

Paradigm I

Sampson (1980) has eloquently described the long-standing controversy between two camps in regard to the definition of science. He has labeled these two positions paradigm I and paradigm II, a distinction that will be used throughout this article. Paradigm I, often termed hard science, (Baumrind, 1980), the positivist-empiricist approach, (Baumrind, 1980) or natural-law thought, (Wolf, 1971), is the dominant conception of science. This paradigm adopts the view that there is a body of facts and principles to be discovered and understood that are independent of any historical or social context. This search for truth seeks principles that are abstract, general, and universal. The critical assumption of this position is the belief in the existence of an independent, autonomous ordering of facts that area historical and acontextual.

Several authors have expounded on the constellation of characteristics that distinguish paradigm I science (Baumrind, 1980; Parlee, 1979; Sampson, 1980; Sheriff, 1979). The experimental methodology is typically employed with the purpose of inferring unambiguously the existence and direction of causal relations. The assumption of linearity is also synonymous with this view. Research is generally conducted in artificial contexts, and the influence of sociohistorical factors is considered a source of error. Context-free generalizations are then formulated to apply to all individuals with little regard to situation.

Paradigm II

In contrast, paradigm II views science as necessarily historical. Facts and principles are inextricably embedded in a particular historical and cultural setting. All forms of knowledge are historically generated and rooted. According to this paradigm, truth is dynamic and is to be found only in the interactions between persons and concrete sociohistorical settings (Sampson, 1980).

Guided by this view, research is often conducted in naturalistic settings, using observational methods. Investigations are often unguided by any hypotheses and uncontaminated by structured experimental designs imposed prior to data collection (Bronfenbrenner, 1977). The influence of sociohistorical factors is not considered a source of error, but rather an integral part of the phenomenon being studied.

Basis for Dominant Approach

Beyond a mere description of these two conceptions of science lies a subtle paradox. The dominant paradigm I view of science, while loudly proclaiming its objective and universal nature, is itself an evolutionary product of a particular sociohistorical context. Sampson, in a synthesis from the works of several writers, has proposed that contemporary paradigm I science has grown and developed as a result of the nourishment it has received from a "male-dominant, Protestant-ethic oriented, middle-class, liberal, and capitalistic society" (Sampson, 1980, p. 1332). The philosophy of rugged individualism and the Protestant work ethic have signif-

icantly influenced scientific thought by dictating a science that is divorced from the influences of social context and by advocating an instrumental, utilitarian approach to scientific inquiry.

Similarly, the point that paradigm I science is a male model of scientific pursuit has been made by several authors (Baumrind, 1980; Bernard, 1973; Parlee, 1979; Sampson, 1980; Sheriff, 1979). Carlson (1971) has used Bakan's (1966) original terminology of agency and communion to describe paradigm I and II science. Agentic or more masculine science (paradigm I) can be described as individualistic, achievement-mastery oriented, and detached from feelings or impulses. Communal or more feminine science (paradigm II) can be characterized as attached, organic, reflective, and relational.

Bernard (1973) makes the crucial point that the dominant male ideal of science has been catapulted to the position of standard science. It has become the touchstone against which scientific endeavors are measured. The sociohistorical, relational conception of science has meanwhile been relegated to an inferior and secondary, if not suspect, position. By maintaining this power balance, paradigm I science is able to reaffirm its value orientation and maintain the status quo. By ignoring the sociocultural context in which facts and scientific truths are embedded, paradigm I science perpetuates its own values and traditions. New information is fitted into pre-existing schemas. On the other hand, paradigm II science places environmental and cultural influences within the purview of proper science, thereby fostering social criticism, innovation, and change.

With growing numbers of nurses pursuing graduate education, the belief that paradigm I science is the best way of perceiving and doing proper science may become solidly entrenched. Values about the research process, including the appropriate framing of research questions and methodologies, are generally formed in graduate school. Many nurses gain their knowledge about research from other fields in which the dominant paradigm I view is exclusively held. Nurses may also be schooled in the research process by other nurses who were themselves taught the positivist-empiricist approach. The entrenchment of the belief that there is only one acceptable method for the acquisition of scientific truth can have profound implications for the development of nursing's body of knowledge and for its relationship as a practice discipline to the rest of society.

Implications for Nursing

Uncritical, unilateral acceptance of the paradigm I view of science has important implications for nursing research and practice. These implications extend from the type of variables deemed important concerns for nursing research to the impact that research findings ultimately have on health care delivery and social policy.

The paradigm I conception of science asserts that scientific truths, by virtue of their abstract, universalistic nature, are value free; that is, they exist independently of the particular sociohistorical context in which they are discovered. As has already been discussed, there is a relationship between models for the acquisition of scientific knowledge and the value orientation of a society. Not only do scientific paradigms reflect the dominant values of society, but they also serve to reinforce and reaffirm those values. It follows that scientific research will never and can never be entirely value free.

Relevance of Values

For those who embrace the paradigm I conception of scientific truth as ahistorical and acontextual, questions of the values and biases underlying research endeavors have no meaning. Indeed, they are largely irrelevant. Implicit value assumptions are not made explicit. They are either taken for granted as a priori truths or are ignored altogether. The danger in denying the influence that values can exert on scientific truth lies in the fact that it can produce a distorted view of social reality.

In psychology, for example, the pervasive yet subtle manner in which implicit methodological biases have worked against the accumulation of accurate knowledge about women has only recently been recognized (Frieze, Parsons, Johnson, et al., 1978). Frieze et al.

have stated that "one of the latent functions of most research on women and sex differences has always been to support the researcher's political position on the status of women in society" (Frieze, Parsons, Johnson, et al., 1978, p. 15). Conclusions thus reached could hardly be said to represent acontextual universal truths. Yet, frequently they have been presented and accepted as such by the scientific community and have all too frequently hindered rather than furthered an understanding of women and the social issues affecting them.

Recognition of Research Biases

As a social phenomenon, nursing is no less value laden than psychology, patients are no less vulnerable to distorted representation than are women, and the dangers of actually preventing or ignoring needed changes in the contextual variables affecting patient care are no less real. To accurately evaluate the results of research studies, nursing must make explicit the values on which its research methodologies are based. Otherwise, nursing will be blind to its own biases.

If, for example, patients are found not to participate in decision making regarding their care, the question could be raised as to whether this is a reflection of the natural order of things—i.e., that patients are by definition passive—or whether it is a function of other social, cultural, or economic factors that are amenable to change. When patient passivity is coupled with an underlying belief that decision making in health care is a professional prerogative for which patients should not really assume responsibility, such a finding can be used to reaffirm and justify the status quo. Patients are passive because that is their choice. Therefore, there is no reason to involve them in decision making or to question further the cause of their passivity beyond an investigation of intrapsychic variables.

This is not to say that an understanding of intrapsychic variables is not important nor that it is impossible to control for the influence of contextual variables to arrive at a valid conclusion that patients do indeed wish to remain passive with regard to decision making. Rather, situation-person interactions are less likely to be considered important within a scientific frame of reference that is focused exclusively on a paradigm I conception of proper science. Similarly, the influence of implicit professional biases is less likely to be acknowledged as a factor of the interpretation of research results. In this regard, paradigm I science has the potential to be less objective than that of paradigm II.

Frame of Reference

The acontextual nature of the paradigm I conception of science negates the involvement of the consumer in determining which questions are important areas for nursing research. Research interests will necessarily reflect the investigator's rather than the consumer's interests, values, and frame of reference. Considerations of social relevancy are unimportant to a science that emphasizes the pursuit of scientific truth as ahistorical and asocial.

No science is in reality value free. The only values that can be reflected by paradigm I research are those of the investigator. Consequently, not only is it likely that such research will suffer from a profound professional bias regarding what are the really important issues, it will also be severely limited in the scope of the issues that can be researched. When question generation is dependent solely on the values and experience of the investigator, a narrow science emerges (Wallston, 1981). It is also a science that tends to tacitly accept the status quo because those are the values on which it is based. Such an orientation is apt to favor retention of traditional modes of research and practice rather than experimentation with new ideas and methodologies.

Professional Relationships

At its most basic level, nursing is a relational profession. It exists by virtue of its commitment to provide care to others. If the concerns and perceptions of the recipients of nursing services are considered unimportant factors in nursing research, then nurses may indeed be providing nursing care that is more meaningful to themselves than to patients. Similarly, if research studies regarding patient behavior fail to ascertain the patients' perception of the rationale for their own ac-

tions, interpretation of research results will reflect only a one-sided bias in favor of what the nurse thinks the patient thinks.

Studies that fail to acknowledge the research subject's perception of the environment are said to lack ecological validity (Bronfenbrenner, 1977). According to Bronfenbrenner, the ecological validity of a study "refers to the extent to which the environment experienced by subjects in a scientific investigation has the properties it is supposed or assumed to have by the investigator" (Bronfenbrenner, 1977, p. 516). Research dominated by a paradigm I conception of science would have difficulty meeting Bronfenbrenner's criteria for ecological validity because it would not be concerned with the research subjects' definition of their situation. Nursing studies that fail to consider the patient's perspective could therefore be considered ecologically invalid.

Studies of the Real World

The goal of paradigm I science is to minimize the influence of contextual variables so that the results of a study may be generalized to all individuals without regard to age, sex, or situation (Baumrind, 1980). This goal is usually sought by means of experimental control and manipulation of situational variables. Unfortunately, this often results in research that is so tightly controlled that it bears little resemblance to what actually transpires in the real world (Baumrind, 1980; Bronfenbrenner, 1977). Rather than increasing the generalizability of research findings, the interpretation of the results of such studies must be limited to the artificial contexts in which they occur. In this regard, the methods employed by paradigm I science are self-defeating.

If a goal of nursing research is to provide findings that will have an impact on the delivery of health care services, then the exclusive use of methodologies typical of paradigm I science is obviously inappropriate. Similarly, research findings resulting from methodologies that ignore the importance of person-situation interactions are of limited utility in the formulation of social policy. The necessary data on which to base policy recommendations will not exist. If nursing is concerned about the strength of its voice in decision making regarding improvements in health care services, then it would do well to evaluate carefully the limitations placed on this ability by a paradigm I conception of the constituents of proper science.

Nursing's View of Science

Following the delineation of the implications an overvaluation of paradigm I science has for nursing, it is germane to examine the views of science most commonly held by nursing theorists and researchers. After a review of some of the classic metatheoretical pieces and papers on nursing research, a striking conflict emerges. This conflict involves a wide discrepancy between the conceptualization of nursing and the definition of science. Almost without exception the nurse authors, in talking about the goals and purposes of nursing, the content of nursing theory, and the criteria by which to evaluate nursing theory, emphasize the importance of sociohistorical contexts or person-environment interactions. There is strong evidence of a deep commitment to nursing conceptualized in a relational sense.

However, as the authors turn from conceptualization of nursing and nursing theory to definitions of science and the research process, the overvaluation of paradigm I science is blatant. Indeed, this view of science is presented as synonymous with true science, as little or no debate about an alternative view is evident. To illustrate this conflict, and overview of the major ideas posited in the nursing literature concerning theory, science, and the research process will be briefly sketched.

Human as Holistic Being

The overarching conceptualization of nursing that can be abstracted from many of nursing's theorists is centered around the view of human as a holistic being (Ellis, 1968; Fawcett, 1978; Johnson, 1974; Neuman, 1974; Rogers, 1970). Nursing involves treating those factors affecting the patient's health that emerge from each one's unique biopsychosocial context. There is concern for the whole person. Ellis (1968) suggests that nursing must examine and treat the variables that affect a patient's health in combination or in interaction with each other versus separately or in isolation. This combination of variables is often represented as greater than the sum of each part, a systems model approach (Ellis, 1968; Rogers, 1970).

The impact of the environment on patients and their health status is a recurrent theme in the nursing literature. Fawcett (1978) postulates that as skill in theory development matures, nursing theories will emerge that fully appreciate the continuous person-environment interaction and its relationship to health. The patient's environment is not restricted to one setting; it includes several levels of analysis—the individual level, the family level, and the community level. King (1964) extends the patient's environment within the domain of nursing beyond the community level to include those more distant social institutions that impinge on individual functioning.

Sociocultural Context

The import of the patient's sociocultural context is evident in the evaluative criteria for nursing theories. Johnson (1974) suggests that the criteria of "social congruence," "social significance," and "social utility" be used to assess the significance of a theory for nursing. These criteria address specifically the embeddedness of the individual as well as the nursing profession itself in a unique and specific social context. Hardy (1974) alludes to this dynamic and changing social context in discussing the tentative nature of theories. She posits that theory cannot be assessed without an examination of the cultural and societal values that are inextricably linked with theory development.

A synthesis of these perspectives on the goals of nursing and the context and evaluative criteria for nursing theory portrays a profession committed to the values embraced by the paradigm II view of science. These values include an appreciation of both the socio historical context in which an individual exists and the organismic or relational nature of the practice of nursing. However, these values are not congruent with the definitions of science and the descriptions of the research process most prevalent in the nursing literature. The paradigm I conceptualization is the model for proper science.

Empirical Reality

Jacox (1974) and Johnson (1974) describe the main purpose of science as the discovery of truths about the world. There is a knowable empirical reality to be discovered. Scientific knowledge is expressed in general, abstract, and universal laws. These universal statements are devoid of any sociohistorical context. Silva (1977) further asserts that the scientist is primarily concerned with establishing cause and effect relationships.

The experimental method is also held in the highest regard. Several authors describe a progression for research designs based on the amount of knowledge available in a discipline (Fawcett, 1978; Hardy, 1974). According to this progression, descriptive or qualitative research should be undertaken when there is little information available or when a science is young. Correlational research can then follow when the essential characteristics of a phenomenon under study are known. Finally, and most important, the experimental method can be utilized when these two lower levels have been explored. The experimental method is portrayed as the most appropriate design in testing theory (Brown, 1964).

Superiority of Paradigm I

There is some evidence within the nursing literature that this exclusive approach to science might be somewhat dissonant with dominant nursing values. However, following the explication of an alternative method of pursuing science, the superior or more rigorous nature of the experimental approach is usually reaffirmed. For example, Quint (1967) proposes that grounded theory or the field approach of Glaser and Strauss (1967) have much to offer in the development of nursing knowledge but views the outcome of these types of research only as the grounds for more rigorous or refined scientific endeavors. Walker identifies the

strength of this grounded theory approach as an opportunity for the researcher "to really see what's going on out there" (Walker, 1980, p. 5). However, she warns that the findings from an investigation of this sort should only be used in the context of discovery and not in the context of verification. As Sampson (1980) points out, this distinction grants final authority and superiority to paradigm I science.

Clearly what is needed is a more balanced and convergent perspective on what constitutes proper science. It is not that paradigm I values should be dismissed as useless and false, but rather that these values should no longer be dominant in nursing education and nursing research endeavors.

Toward a Convergent Definition of Science

The preceding discussion should not be interpreted as a total condemnation of paradigm I science. Nor should it be interpreted as the wholehearted endorsement of paradigm II. It is the position of the authors that neither paradigmatic stance by itself is sufficient. Indeed what is proposed is a blending of both methodologies to produce a science that retains a critical concern for the objectivity traditionally associated with paradigm I while ensuring that the research it produces has some validity in the real world and that the influence of contextual variables on research findings is acknowledged and made explicit. Such a synthesis requires the granting of equal status to each paradigmatic view, not the negation of one in favor of the other (Sampson, 1980).

If as a profession nursing does indeed possess its own body of knowledge, it would seem reasonable to expect that it may well have to develop its own unique research strategies to develop that body of knowledge. Nursing's research methodologies should reflect its theoretical propositions about the nature of its science. Borrowing methodologies from other disciplines with a different conceptual base may not only retard the development of nursing theory but will almost certainly dilute its uniqueness as well.

Nursing would do well to learn from other disciplines to avoid the pitfalls of "physics envy" and the concomitant devaluing of "soft" research to validate itself as a scientific discipline. In psychology, for example, Wallston (1981) has pointed out how an overvaluing of agentic approaches has retarded the understanding and integration of major concepts related to the study of women. She calls for the synthesis of agentic and communal science as a means of gaining additional information.

"Whole" Person in Context

Nursing theories and models for practice expound on the importance of considering the "whole" person in the sociocultural-biological context. Yet how often do nursing research questions, designs, and methodologies reflect this perspective? Too often nursing has taken a stance based on the prior belief that one methodological approach is by definition necessarily superior to another. All too often that beliefs has reflected nurses' desire to prove themselves as real scientists rather than a concern for the ability of the methodology to answer the research question. Insistence on the supremacy of one scientific paradigm over another commits the researcher to the view that there is only one right way to do research. Such a position is only slightly removed from a procedure manual approach to nursing research.

Dialectical Synthesis of Approaches

When paradigms I and II are granted equal status, the door is opened to a critical dialogue from which a dialectical synthesis of the two approaches can emerge. Sampson (1980) has argued that this new synthesis will not consist of the use of paradigm II methods in the context of discovery and the use of paradigm I methodologies in matters of verification. Rather, a convergence of paradigm I and paradigm II conceptions of science will involve the "higher organization of the opposites in both paradigms" (Sampson, 1980, p. 1312). Perhaps the true opportunity for nursing to develop a body of knowledge that is uniquely its own lies in this type of synthesis.

The development of a more convergent definition of science has the potential to enhance the impact that nursing research has on health care delivery and social policy. A new emphasis on contextual variables would force a closer examination not only of those theories that nursing currently utilizes to explain what happens in practice settings, but of the practices and their settings as well. A more functional integration of theory and practice can be achieved, and change and innovation in nursing practice can be facilitated. Similarly, when there is an increased awareness of the importance of contextual variables, policy implications are more likely to be considered and recommendations made.

The real value of a convergent definition of science for nursing, however, lies in the opportunity it provides to draw from a variety of sources to develop new methods and approaches specifically tailored to investigate questions of concern to nursing while remaining flexible and creative enough to avoid the "disease of methodolatry."

References

Bakan, D. (1966). *The duality of human existence: An essay on psychology and religion.* Chicago: Rand McNally.

Baumrind, D. (1980). New directions in socialization research. *American Psychologist, 35,* 639–652.

Bernard, J. (1973). My four revolutions: An autobiographical history of the ASA. *American Journal of Sociology, 78,* 773–791.

Bronfenbrenner, U. (1977). Toward an experimental ecology of human development. *American Psychologist, 32,* 513–531.

Brown, M. (1964). Research in the development of nursing theory. *Nursing Research, 13,* 109–112.

Carlson, R. (1971). Sex differences in ego functioning: Exploratory studies of agency and communion. *Journal of Consulting and Clinical Psychology, 37,* 267–277.

Ellis, R. (1968). Characteristics of significant theories. *Nursing Research, 69,* 1434–1438.

Fawcett, J. (1978). The relationship between theory and research: A double helix. *Advances in Nursing Science, 1,* 49–62.

Frieze, I.H., Parsons, J.E., Johson, P.B., et al. (1978). *Women and sex roles.* New York: Norton.

Glaser, B.G., & Strauss, A.L. (1967). *Discovery of grounded theory: Strategies for qualitative research.* Chicago: Aldine.

Hardy, M.E. (1974). Theories: Components, development, evaluation. *Nursing Research, 23,* 100–107.

Jacox, A. (1974). Theory construction in nursing: An overview. *Nursing Research, 23,* 4–13.

Johnson, D.E. (1974). Development of theory: A requisite for nursing as a primary health profession. *Nursing Research, 23,* 372–377.

King, I.M. (1964). Nursing theory—problems and prospect. *Nursing Science, 2,* 394–403.

Neuman, B. (1974). The Betty Neuman health care systems model: A total person approach to patient problems. In J. Riehl & C. Roy (Eds.), *Conceptual models for nursing practice.* New York: Appleton-Century-Crofts.

Parlee, M.B. (1979). Psychology and women. *Signs, 5,* 121–133.

Quint, J.C. (1967). The case for theories generated from empirical data. *Nursing Research, 16,* 109–114.

Rogers, M.E. (1970). *An introduction to the theoretical basis of nursing.* Philadelphia: F.A. Davis.

Sampson, E.E. (1980). Scientific paradigms and social values: Wanted—A scientific revolution. *Journal of Personality and Social Psychology, 35,* 639–652.

Sheriff, C.W. (1979). Bias in psychology. In J.A. Sherman & E.T. Beck (Eds.), *The prism of sex: Essays in the sociology of knowledge.* Madison, WI: University of Wisconsin Press.

Silva, M.C. (1977). Philosophy, science, theory: Interrelationships and implications for nursing research. *Image, 9,* 59–63.

Walker, L.O. (1980, June). Inductive approaches to theory development in nursing. Unpublished manuscript.

Wallston, B.S. (1981). What are the questions in psychology of women? A feminist approach to research. *Psychology of Women Quarterly, 5*(4), 597–615.

Wolf, K.H. (1971). Introduction. In K. Mannheim, *From Karl Mannheim.* New York: Oxford University Press.

The Authors Comment

First Edition

The stimulus for the article came from a course on the psychology of women in which both Mindy Tinkle and I were enrolled in our final year of doctoral study at the University of Texas at Austin. The articles we read for the course focused our attention for the first time on how the adoption of a "hard" science approach could produce a distorted and limited view of women and the issues affecting them. Mindy and I were both impressed by the parallels between the debate being waged in psychology over the validity of "soft" research strategies and the pressures we and many of our classmates felt to prove ourselves as researchers by using so-called "pure" science approaches in our dissertations. We were also struck by the similar potential for misrepresentation of the problems confronting women and those experienced by patients when contextual variables and the perspective of the research subject are ignored. Much of what we were reading in our psychology course seemed to apply equally well to nursing.

After several discussions, Mindy and I decided that the issues raised in our psychology course had sharpened and brought to the surface many of our concerns about the development and direction of nursing science. As we talked, it became apparent that we felt strongly enough about these concerns to commit them to paper before a wider audience. For a while, we struggled with a competing demand on our time—namely, the preparation of our dissertation proposals. In the end, the need to formalize our ideas won out and we wrote the article.

—JANET L. BEATON

Since this article was published, I have heard its theme sounded repeatedly in research conferences and in private conversations among peers. I think that nurses interested in research are coming to see the two paradigms in action more and more. They are also seeing the obvious bias that exists in the scientific community. It remains to be seen what shape our research questions and methodologies take in the future. There always will be the need to write proposals with funding restrictions, etc., in mind. But if the two views of science are at least conceptualized, it is a step in the right direction.

Second Edition

During the period when this article was written, a virtual flood of dialogue regarding a balanced view of science was just entering the nursing literature. Currently, there is much evidence of a synthesis of the two paradigms of science in the literature. Many studies demonstrate a blended qualitative and quantitative approach, giving rise to rich knowledge and theory building.

—MINDY TINKLE

Chapter 62

Scientific Inquiry in Nursing: A Model for a New Age

Holly A. DeGroot

Despite the acknowledged need for widespread and rapid scientific advancement in nursing, little system-atic attention has been paid to the progenitor of research, the individual investigator. The nature of scientific problem solving as the fundamental process of research practice is explored, and a model of scientific inquiry is proposed. Variables in the model are discussed in relation to their potential effect on the inquiry process, and strategies that facilitate the practice of research are identified.

Concern with the growth of nursing science has received full attention from nursing scholars over the past decade. The need for nursing theory as a foundation for nursing science and professional growth has been repeatedly acknowledged by contemporary nursing authors (Donaldson & Crowley, 1978; Hardy, 1983). Roy (1983) considers theory development as the number one priority for this decade. Current economic pressures have added unprecedented urgency to this scientific quest as health care policy makers and administrators demand research verification of nursing's disciplinary contribution.

Theory development literature in nursing has largely focused on theory construction (Dickoff, James, & Weidenbach, 1968; Jacox, 1984; Meleis, 1985), the nature of nursing's scientific advancement (Hardy, 1983; Newman, 1983), and the identification of conceptual and methodological deficiencies (Batey, 1977; Gortner, 1977; Jacobsen & Meininger, 1985). Despite agreement that creative strategies are required to resolve these theoretical inadequacies (Carper, 1978; Oiler, 1982), surprisingly little attention has been paid to the process and practice of scientific inquiry with the individual investigator as the unit of analysis. An understanding of the nature of scientific activity and the factors that influence individual inquiry and research practice is essential if nursing is to exercise its fullest intellectual power for theory development.

About the Author

HOLLY A. DEGROOT currently is the senior managing partner in Catalyst Systems, Mill Valley, California, a patient care services consulting firm. Her responsibilities include strategic planning, financial management, sales, marketing, product development, contracts, and resource allocation. Before taking this position, Dr. DeGroot was the special projects coordinator at Marin General Hospital, Greenbrae, California, a position she held from 1981–1987.

Dr. DeGroot's educational background includes an A.A. (1969) from Contra Costa College, San Pablo, California; a B.S.N. and a B.A. in Psychology from Sonoma State University in 1977; and a M.S. (1979) and a Ph.D. (1989) from the University of California, San Francisco. When asked about nursing as career, Dr. DeGroot commented "It has been a privilege to participate in such a growing, leading edge profession with such limitless opportunities. The work of nursing, and thus its science, is meaningful, worthwhile and highly gratifying." When asked about the future, she responded, "The greatest challenge facing nursing now is the unprecedented demand for rapid scientific advancement. Sound knowledge about our care delivery processes, practices, effectiveness, cost and quality are key to our professional survival and the health of the world community."

On a personal note, Dr. DeGroot notes that her long-standing interest in playing the guitar and writing music has fostered a personal understanding of creative processes and how they are likely to occur.

The Nature of Scientific Activity

Science has been characterized as a "creative and imaginative human activity" (Goldstein & Godstein, 1978, p. 4) and as a form of contemplative wisdom (Weiskopf, 1973). Bronowski observes that "all science is the search for unity and hidden likenesses" (Bronowski, 1965, p. 14). As the method of inquiry employed in this quest, the research process is virtually indistinguishable from what Bigge (1982) calls reflective thinking. This is "a reflective process within which persons either develop new or change existing tested generalized insights or understanding. So construed, reflective thinking combines both inductive—fact gathering— and deductive processes in such a way as to find, elaborate and test hypotheses" (Bigge, 1982, p. 105).

It is clear that the research process and the reflective thinking process constitute parallel attempts directed toward problem solving. Polanyi (1962) distinguishes between two phases of problem solving: an initial stage of perplexity and a subsequent stage of taking action directed toward dispelling the perplexity. Polanyi summarizes the four well-known stages of discovery in problem solving: (a) stage of preparation, during which a problem is initially recognized; (b) stage of incubation, which is an unconscious preoccupation with the problem; (c) stage of illumination, characterized by the tentative discovery of a possible solution; and (d) stage of verification, during which the solution withstands tests of practical reality. Implicit in this notion of scientific activity as a process of reflective thinking and of problem solving is the fundamental relationship of both to creativity. Bronowski (1965) asserts that while science is involved in a search for hidden likenesses, creativity is the discovery of hidden likeness.

Creativity can be viewed as a five-step process that is triggered by identifying or sensing a problem (Mackinnon, 1979). The first stage is called the period of preparation, during which experience, cognitive skills, and problem-solving techniques are acquired. The second stage, or period of concentrated effort, is often accompanied by frustration that results from unsuccessful attempts to solve the problem. Next comes a period of withdrawal, which is akin to the incubation stage of problem solving. In this stage the problem and its possible solutions are considered on a conscious as well as subconscious level. This stage is characterized by what Worthy (1975) has termed "fruitful obses sion." The fourth stage, or moment of insight, is accompanied by a feeling of exhilaration that comes from the sudden discovery of a solution to the problem. Worthy calls this "aha thinking," which results in intuitive leaps and sudden insights related to problem solution. The last step in the creative process, the period of verification, is characterized by the elaboration of the newly created insight or solution and its subsequent testing, refinement, extension, and evaluation. The attainment of this fifth and final step in the creative process forms the foundation and the starting point for further creative activities. That this creative process bears a striking resemblance to the problem-solving and reflective thinking processes of scientific activity, as outlined earlier, is central to the discussion of scientific inquiry.

Since scientific problem solving necessarily involves an individual's contribution to the creative process, characteristics of creative persons and their work are also important to consider. Creativity in individuals has been associated with divergent thinking, intelligence, commitment or involvement, and a preference for complexity from which simplicity and order may be derived (Nicholls, 1983). The willingness to take risks (Albert, 1983) and to use imagination and intuition (Yukawa, 1973) are other fundamental characteristics of creative individuals. Introversion, playfulness, and a well-developed sense of humor also figure heavily with these individuals (Worthy, 1975).

Characteristics of the outcomes or products of creative problem solving (e.g., research findings and theories) have also been identified Mackinnon, 1979). Originality and the ability of the solution to actually solve an existing problem are key characteristics. In addition, the solution must be "produced," which implies development, refinement, and communication of the problem solution. Additional criteria have relevance if nursing theory is considered to be the creative "product." These criteria are that the creative outcome or theory contains truth and beauty and that it contributes to the quality of human existence. It has also been observed that creativity can be generated as much by the nature of the problem as by the person attempting to solve it (Albert, 1983; Yukawa, 1973). Creative

problem solving has beneficial psychological effects on others who are exposed to the process by encouraging and engaging them in more imaginative and creative activity. Although creativity alone does not ensure successful problem solving, it is a vital ingredient for the theoretical complexity of knowledge generation in human sciences. It should be remembered that less than successful problem solving can be equally rich in stimulating creative scientific problem solving because it forces the consideration of alternative possibilities (Yukawa, 1973).

Phases of Inquiry

It is clear from this discussion that the quintessence of scientific inquiry is creative problem solving conducted through the research process. Scientific inquiry thus comprises at least four interrelated phases: (a) formulation of the research problem, (b) method selection, (c) method implementation, and (d) communication of findings. Each of these phases shares common characteristics that have implications for a model of scientific inquiry. Although these phases are typically presented as the orderly and normative approach to inquiry, it has been pointed out that the actual research process has little resemblance to such a rational model (Martin, 1982). The inquiry process has been aptly described as a series of dilemmas that can be neither solved nor avoided (McGrath, 1982).

Problem Formulation

The pivotal point for a system of scientific inquiry is the research problem, question, or hypothesis, for it reflects all that came before and directs all research activity that will follow. Kerlinger goes a step further, calling the research problem or hypothesis the "working instrument of theory"(Kerlinger, 1973, p. 20). The research problem (a term to be used alternatively with "research question" or "research hypothesis," denoting the same or similar entity) is a highly subjective construction. As such, it is an intensely personal and intimate creation because of its contextual and historical proximity to the very essence of its creator. Not surprisingly, Polanyi calls research problems "intellectual desires" (Polyani, 1962, p. 152), noting that in any scientific controversy personal attacks rather than scientific arguments are the norm because intellectual passions, not reason, are truly at odds.

Since the formulation of a research question is a creative effort based on imagination, ingenuity, and insight (Polit & Hungler, 1983), the research results stemming from it ultimately reflect the intellectual power of the question and, undeniably, the researcher. Research problem selection is closely related to personal values (Kaplan, 1964; Tucker, 1979) and actually discloses the direction of human will and intuition (Noddings & Shore, 1984). Runkel and McGrath observe that as a researcher attempts to formulate the research problem, "he begins with his own previous way of thinking about things; he seeks help in organizing his complexities from literature and colleagues; finally, he is inevitably affected by his own personal experience as he interacts with the world"(Runkel & McGrath, 1972, p. 13). Not surprisingly, this characteristic of subjectivity is inherent in the other phases of inquiry as well.

Selection of Methods

Although Kaplan (1964) acknowledges at least four distinct usages of the term "methodology," only the fourth is inclusive enough for a discussion of the process of scientific inquiry. This definition incorporates specific techniques and procedures as well as abstract philosophical imperatives. Kaplan asserts that the use of this expanded meaning allows for the inclusion of a wide range of activities, including concept delineation, hypothesis formation, observation and measurement, and model and theory construction, as well as explanation and prediction. The advantage of such a definition is that it treats all tools that a researcher has at his or her disposal (including the conceptual and the concrete) and the research implementation phases, such as data collection and analysis, as interrelated components of inquiry. Conceived in this way, factors influencing problem formulation directly or indirectly influence all phases of inquiry.

The implications of this expanded and integrated view of research methodology are not universally appreciated. At the very least, authors agree that the methods are dictated by the research question (Kerlinger, 1973; Kaplan, 1964; Runkel & McGrath, 1972; Wilson, 1985). However, there seems to be tacit endorsement of a greater rationality and objectively of method selection than actually exists. For example, some authors (Polit & Hungler, 1983) subscribe to a design selection hierarchy, usually with experimental designs at the top and nonexperimental approaches clearly at the bottom. This view implies that the selection of design methodology is based primarily on whether the research can meet the three requirements for a true experiment, namely, the ability for manipulation, control, and randomization. If these requirements can be met by the proposed study, the choice of methods is clear. If researchers are somehow unable to meet these requirements for experimentation, they are at once relegated to the realm of nonexperimental methodology. Kerlinger (1973) goes as far as to categorize nonexperimental methods as "compromise designs," consigning them rather casually to the bottom of the design hierarchy. Unfortunately this stance serves to create a methodological double bind: Methods are purportedly dictated by the question, but it is less desirable to ask questions that must be answered by "lower-order" designs and methods.

Brink and Wood (1983) propose a similarly straightforward and deductive approach to method selection based on the level of the research question. These levels are a function of existing amounts of knowledge related to the phenomena of interest. These authors also suggest that selection of methods may be based primarily on the existence of valid and reliable measures. Little attention is given to other factors that may influence the selection of research methods.

Method Implementation and Communication of Findings

How methods are implemented through the use of data collection techniques and analytical strategies is affected by the same subjective considerations inherent in problem formulation and method selection phases of inquiry. There is a wide range of methodological possibilities open to experimental and nonexperimental approaches, with choices to be made at each juncture. Whether one decides to use open-ended interview ν standardized questionnaire, grounded theory ν hermeneutic interpretation, analysis of covariance (ANCOVA) techniques ν multiple regression correlation (MRC), or a convenience ν a stratified random sample is influenced by a combination of interrelated factors. Even the communication of research findings is similarly influenced as choices are made about which journal to submit the results to, what information should be included in the report, how conservative or liberal the interpretations will be, and what the theoretical implications of the findings are.

Despite the rigorous assertions that method selection and implementation are primarily rational processes, some authors concede the influence of subjective factors on these phases of inquiry (Martin, 1982; Kuhn, 1970; Luria, 1973; Polkinghorne, 1983). These include factors such as disciplinary norms, personal research style, funding realities, and other value-laden considerations. Tucker (1979) points out that scientific activity is essentially a process involving a series of value decisions to be made by the researcher and that perhaps the largest number of these decisions is made in relation to methodological issues. Polkinghorne goes one step further, asserting that "particular methods do not operate independently of a system of inquiry" and in fact "the use of a method changes only as a researcher uses it in different systems of inquiry" (Polkinghorne, 1983, p. 6). This perhaps is the most important point of all, for it posits the inextricable relationship between each phase of inquiry and the subjective factors that necessarily influence each phase.

A Model of Scientific Inquiry

The model proposed here is fundamentally a systems/process model applied to a human system of inquiry (see Figure 62-1). As such, the system comprises six interrelated influencing variables, subdivided into four intrapersonal factors and two extrapersonal factors (see

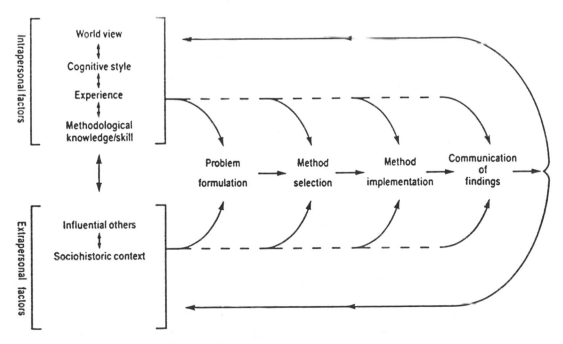

Figure 62-1 *A model of scientific inquiry.*

Major Factors Influencing Scientific Inquiry in Nursing

Intrapersonal factors

World view
  Nature of human beings
  Nature of knowledge and truth
  Nature of nursing science
Cognitive style
Experience
  Life experience
  Professional nursing experience
  Research experience
  Theoretical experience
Methodological knowledge and skill

Extrapersonal factors

Influential others
  Individual
  Institutional
Sociohistorical context

---

box). The six factors are assumed to be in constant and mutual interaction, and when there is a change in one variable the other variables are affected. There are four basic phases to the inquiry process, and each phase is influenced by the six variables. Accordingly, the cumulative effect of the variables on the system as a whole is greater than the sum of the influence of the individual variables.

The system is characterized by continual change and is directed toward growth and increasing sophistication. In addition, it operates according to the principal of equifinality (Von Bertalanffy, 1968), which asserts that the same final or end state can be achieved from different beginnings and by different paths or routes. Even though there is never a final state in the research process for the researcher, this proposed inquiry system accepts and encourages individual differences throughout the practice of research, since each path chosen can get equally close to the "truth." The six factors or influencing variables are not intended to represent all intrapersonal or extrapersonal possibilities. Rather they should be viewed as a major class of

variables that operate in addition to other factors such as personality, intelligence, or other values and beliefs. In addition, individual investigators vary in their awareness of the existence and nature of these variables as well as in the relative degree of influence any one factor may exert on the inquiry process.

Intrapersonal Factors
World View

The first personal variable that influences the process of inquiry is called world view, which consists of the researcher's general philosophical orientation, or world view, of the nature of human beings, the nature of knowledge and truth, and the nature of nursing science. Beliefs about human nature are fundamental to the development of the researcher's theoretical leanings, to the delineation of appropriate research questions, and, ultimately to the selection of research methodology. Relevant beliefs about human nature include such considerations as whether human beings are considered to be rational or irrational, whether human behavior is predetermined, and what the basis is for motivation of behavior. For example, are human motivations primarily conscious or unconscious? Is human behavior dictated by the need for growth or by the deprivation humans feel? Research questions generated will differ sharply, depending on whether human beings are viewed as highly self-directed individuals constantly striving for self-actualization v individuals who are at the mercy of their subconscious and who are constantly suppressing the primal urges the subconscious seeks to satisfy. Tucker points out that these latter beliefs as espoused by Freud and others, for example, have very specific implications for research methodology as well. He reminds us that the belief that one cannot ask a person directly about his or her thoughts and feelings provided the primary impetus for the development of popular psychological methods that employ unobtrusive and often deceptive testing techniques (Tucker, 1978).

Other beliefs related to a researcher's world view include how human beings are perceived in relation to their environment. For example, are people viewed as primarily passive reactors to events that impinge on them, or are they seen as proactive or mutually interactive with the environment? Does the human boundary end at the skin, or does the human field extend, as Rogers (1970) insists, beyond the skin to actually merge with the environmental field? Other perceptions that contribute to a researcher's world view relate to the multidimensionality of human beings. Are people seen as the popularized "biopsychosocial" beings, or are they seen as "biopsychosocial-spiritual-cultural" beings? The very nature of the research questions would be altered by these two alternative views in that they would contain a very different constellation of variables and possible methodological implications.

These beliefs form the basis for establishing theoretical congruence, or the degree to which prevailing theories comfortably conform to one's world view. For example, if one believed that human beings were passive reactors to their environment and that behavior is motivated by the desire to avoid discomfort, it is unlikely that a systems perspective or symbolic interaction-based method would be very appealing. In this way beliefs about human nature delimit the realm of theoretical possibility in the practice of research.

Beliefs about the *nature of knowledge and truth* also affect a researcher's world view and thus the process of inquiry. Two major competing schools of thought best illustrate the diversity of these beliefs. Logical positivism, later known as the received view, asserts that objective, axiomatic truth exists that is discoverable and able to be verified by hypotheticodeductive methods (Suppe, 1977). Only certain methods that are objective and produce sense data can appropriately demonstrate this truth with any certainty, and only that knowledge derived in this manner counts as true scientific knowledge. The received view, as the dominant contemporary conception of science, conflicts sharply with what Polkinghorne (1983) calls the postpositivist view. A postpositivist conception of scientific knowledge and truth has evolved in reaction to the rather obvious limitations of the received view, especially for the human sciences. This view holds that the pursuit of knowledge and truth is necessarily historical,

contextual, and theory laden. It claims no access to certain truth or knowledge but rather accepts certain knowledge to be "true" if it withstands practical tests of reason and utility. In this way, although knowledge may be useful, it is still fallible. Postpositivism does not cling to any one method of science and in fact encourages the use of the most appropriate method for the particular research question. Polkinghorne notes that "those methods are acceptable which produce results that convince the community that the new understanding is deeper, fuller, and more useful than the previous understanding" (Polkinghorne, 1983, p. 3).

The received view, or logical positivist approach to science, conforms closely to the correspondence norms of truth (Kaplan, 1964). What constitutes truth is the degree of correspondence between facts and their related theories and the degree to which propositions can be verified or shown to be false. Truth can be achieved only when it is shown that a proposition cannot be falsified. The received view also relies, in part, on the coherence theory of truth and its appreciation of theoretical aesthetics and logical simplicity in content and form. The postpositivist view, on the other hand, aligns itself with the pragmatic theory of truth, which emphasizes practical utility in problem solving and the degree of community consensus about that utility.

In the conduct of research positivism lends itself to reductionistic observables that must be quantified and verified, while postpositive concerns can be deductive or inductive in nature and can use either quantitative or qualitative strategies. It is clear that whether a researcher has positivist or postpositivist leanings and consciously or unconsciously subscribes to one theory of truth over another, these beliefs have a major effect on the formulation of the research question and the methodological strategy chosen. Thus it is unlikely that a researcher steeped in positivistic principles would ever ask a research question requiring the existential research methods of hermeneutic analysis.

A researcher's world view is also shaped by his or her beliefs about the *nature of nursing science*. Whether or not one believes that nursing is a "science of human health and behavior across the life span"

Gortner, 1983, p. 5) and is specifically concerned with "the diagnosis and treatment of human responses to actual or potential health problems" (American Nurses' Association, 1980, p. 9) has ultimate implications for the types of events, states, and situations perceived to be problematic. Although client, nursing, environment, and health have all been considered phenomena central to nursing (Fawcett, 1978), one might disagree as to the emphasis that one component has in relation to another or on whether some or all of these concepts must be included in a theoretical formulation for nursing. For example, Stevens (1979) deemphasizes the environmental aspects, while Fawcett (1978) states that at least one or more of the four concepts must be present if the theory is to be called a nursing theory. Flaskerud and Halloran (1980) insist that the concept of nursing must always be included in any theoretical formulation for it to be considered nursing theory, while Conway (1985) believes the inclusion of nursing is inappropriate.

Whether nursing science is believed to conform more to a human science model (postpositivist) or to a natural science model (positivist) also has implications for the formulation of research problems. As a human science nursing must take into account various characteristics of the human realm. For example, the systemic character of human phenomena and the unclear nature of their boundaries are important to consider (Polkinghorne, 1983). The former necessitates investigating the whole by looking at the whole rather than its individual parts, while the latter implies acceptance of indistinct conceptual boundaries. The process nature of the human realm must also be taken into consideration, as it signifies continual growth and repatterning over time. This implies the use of longitudinal or time series designs to fully explicate our phenomena of interest (Metzger & Schultz, 1982).

Fundamental to human sciences is the additional awareness that our perceptions about human phenomena are limited by our perceptions as human beings. Total objectivity is an unattainable ideal because "there is no absolute point outside phenomena from which to investigate. Moreover, the knowledge gained in the investigation changes the character of what has been in-

vestigated" (Polkinghorne, 1983, p. 263). It also is not possible to directly access the human realm by direct observation. Rather, it must be observed indirectly through our interpretation of human behavioral expressions. This is an important point, since one of the major forms of human expression is through language. This implies that access to human phenomena is rightly obtained from written or oral expressions, for example. Credibility is thus established for subjective data collection methods that include interviews and questionnaires. A natural science model, however, dictates a hypotheticodeductive approach to research with reliance on objective quantitative methods.

This notion of nursing as a human science—one modeled after a natural science—also has implications for expectations regarding nursing's scientific advancement. Some authors (Hardy, 1983; Newman, 1983) propose carte blanche acceptance of Kuhn's model for scientific growth, even though Kuhn clearly indicates that the model was developed for natural sciences (Kuhn, 1970). Expecting periods of normal science that will be periodically interrupted by scientific revolutions is perhaps unrealistic for nursing as a human science (Meleis, 1985). It may, in fact, lead to erroneous conclusions about scientific progress and, worse yet, hopelessly distort nursing's future direction. Kuhn points out that the rigid pattern of education for normal activity in the natural sciences "is not well designed to produce the man who will easily discover a fresh approach" (Kuhn, 1970, p. 166). It might well be that alleged patterns of revolution in natural science exist only because there is no other way for creative change to occur or for discoveries to be incorporated in such severely structured disciplines. It is clear that an investigator's fundamental beliefs about the nature of human beings, the nature of knowledge and truth, and the nature of nursing science contribute mightily to the definition of a research problem and ultimately to its solution.

Cognitive Style

It has long been observed that individuals have a preferred style of problem solving (Bloom & Broder,

1950) and that this style is a major factor in successful problem solving (Shouksmith, 1970). These cognitive styles "represent a person's typical modes of perceiving, remembering, thinking and problem solving" (Messick, 1970, p. 188). As such, cognitive styles exert a major influence on both the identification of a research problem and the ultimate approach to a solution.

In his theory of experiential learning, Kolb (1981) conceives of learning as a fourstage cycle that includes observations and reflections, formation of abstract concepts and generalizations, testing of implications of concepts and new situations, and concrete experience. Four kinds of abilities are required if this process is to be effective. Concrete experience (CE) is characterized by open, unbiased involvement, while the second ability, reflective observation (RO) involves considering experiences from many perspectives. Abstract conceptualization (AC) involves formulation and integration of concepts into logical and sound theories, and active experimentation (AE) reflects the ability to apply these theories in decision making and problem solving. These abilities can be considered polar opposites on two bisecting dimensions with CE and AC on either end of one continuum and AE and RO as opposites on the other. Kolb points out that the most sophisticated and highly evolved ability, that of creative insight, actually involves synthetic interaction between these abstract and concrete dimensions. In addition, individuals appear to develop cognitive styles that generally emphasize some abilities over others, and those abilities remain remarkably stable over time. It can be demonstrated, however, that styles tend to become somewhat more reflective and analytical as an individual gets older.

Through his research Kolb identifies four cognitive styles. *Convergers* operate predominantly between abstract conceptualization and active experimentation, with an aptitude toward practical application of ideas. These persons approach problems in a hypotheticodeductive way, focusing on a single solution to a problem, often preferring to deal with nonhuman entities. The opposite of convergers are *divergers*, whose abilities lie in concrete experience and reflective observation.

These people are "idea generators" who have strong and active imaginations and who are able to connect many unrelated but specific instances into a meaningful whole. Divergers are social and aesthetic in orientation and are often drawn to the humanities and the liberal arts. *Assimilators* operate predominantly in the abstract conceptualization and reflective observation modes and thus show great strength in inductive reasoning and theory formulation. These people are drawn to the logical and the abstract, with little attention to the need for practical application. *Accommodators*, operating on the opposite dimension from assimilators, are adept at concrete experience and active experimentation. These are action-oriented, risk-taking individuals who are often involved in implementation of an idea or a study. Accommodators are highly adaptive to changing situations and use the trial and error approach to problem solving.

These cognitive styles provide a useful way to conceive of general learning and problem-solving styles in individuals. Kolb (1981) warns against strict stereotyping, however, noting that research on cognitive style has consistently demonstrated how diverse and complex these processes actually are in real life. For example, cognitive function will vary in an individual according to the cognitive domain or situational demand.

The four cognitive styles described by Kolb (1981) can be related to inquiry norms in an academic discipline as well. Natural sciences and mathematics generally fall into the abstract-reflective quadrant; science-based professions are abstract-active; and social professions are more concrete-active. The concrete-reflective quadrant is characteristic of humanities and social sciences. Interestingly, in one study of a single university setting described by Kolb (1981), nursing fell into the abstract-active quadrant (converger), while in a much larger study nursing students and faculty fell into the concrete-reflective (diverger) category.

Kolb also proposes a typology of knowledge structures and inquiry processes in academic disciplines, suggesting that "forms of knowledge in different fields can be differentially attractive and meaningful to individuals with different learning styles" (Kolb, 1981, p. 245). That convergers would be drawn to or flourish in science-based empirical disciplines devoted to discrete analysis and conformance to correspondence norms is not surprising, nor is the attraction that the humanities and social science hold for divergers who profess to humanism, norms of coherence, and the conduct of research by historical analysis, field study, or clinical observation. That individuals with various cognitive styles would be attracted to nursing is also not surprising given the acknowledged complex and multifaceted nature of nursing's domain of interest. Certain cognitive styles are undoubtedly drawn to some scientific inquiry strategies more than others. For instance, the assimilator style might prefer theory generation using grounded theory methodology (Glaser & Strauss, 1967), while the accommodator style might choose involvement in clinical trials or intervention studies. A researcher whose predominant style is that of a converger might choose to be involved in theory-testing physiological research with animal subjects, while divergers might be drawn to phenomenological studies. Cognitive style appears to be a variable with major influence in a model of scientific inquiry.

Experience

The role of personal experience in scientific inquiry should not be underestimated. Both *life experience and professional nursing experience* provide fertile ground for problem awareness to grow. Problem identification and formulation of the research question become the fruit of that experience. Evidence of the verification or refutation of theories in the real world is also provided by this experience. Theories that work well are easily identified, while theories that fall short can be revised, extended, or discarded. Anomalous cases become readily apparent, as do continuing perplexities that remain unexplained by existing theories. One's sense of substantive significance stems from this experience, and intuition serves as a guided to the problems that have the most personal and professional meaning.

Prior *research experience* is also an important aspect of this variable, for it is through this experience that investigators learn which questions are able to be answered by current methods, which research approaches have worked in the past, and which ones have not. Experience also teaches what research needs to be conducted in the future and how it might best be accomplished. It also tells researchers whether prior research endeavors fit well enough with what Luria (1973) calls their research style. If prior research experience has been satisfactory and successful, an attempt will be made to replicate aspects contributing to that success, whether substantive or methodological in nature. While research success teaches investigators to utilize similar problem solving strategies in the future, less than successful research is often as instructive because of the demand for increasingly novel and creative approaches in subsequent studies.

Theoretical experience is another type of experience that affects the process of inquiry. One aspect of this experience relies upon the existing knowledge base in a substantive area and the researcher's individual perception of that knowledge base. Theoretical experience allows the researcher to identify the existing gaps in knowledge and the significant areas that remain unexplored or unexplained. Individual researcher perception is important in this type of experience, for it is that perception that drives interest in unexplored domains. Scientific advancement depends on theoretical experience over time because of the necessarily progressive nature of research questions based on prior studies. Insight gained from long-standing familiarity with theoretical issues is of inestimable value and contributes to the overall level of understanding about the phenomenon of interest. This level of understanding in turn affects the content and level of subsequent research questions.

A second aspect of theoretical experience relates to the degree to which the researcher has been open to various theoretical approaches and intellectual strategies related to the exploration of the research problem area. If the researcher remains intellectually open to diverging and opposing views, the quality of theoretical understanding will be affected even though initial theoretical orientation may be maintained. Obviously the greater the clarity of understanding of the problem area the greater the possibility of significant answers. This type of intellectual exploration also allows for greater problem tension to exist, which in turn results in greater efforts to resolve the problem (Polyani, 1962). Bruner (1966) points out that it is precisely this dialectical tension between the concrete and the abstract that allows for creativity in problem solving.

Methodological Knowledge and Skill

The level and type of methodological knowledge and skill possessed by a researcher have a major influence on the process and product of scientific inquiry. Since the seeds of the answer lie in every research question (Mackinnon, 1979) and it is asserted that researchers have a preferred style of problem solving (Kolb, 1981), it is natural that researchers pose research questions that they will be able to answer. Kaplan calls this the "law of the instrument" and observes that "it comes as no particular surprise to discover that a scientist formulates problems in a way which requires for their solution just those techniques in which he himself is especially skilled" (Kaplan, 1964, p. 28). He also points out that the cost of becoming an expert in any one research area results in what can be called a "trained incapacity." That is, the more expert one becomes in something the harder it is to solve a problem any other way. Maslow agrees, asserting that "it is tempting, if the only tool you have is a hammer, to treat everything as if it were a nail"(Maslow, 1966, pp. 15-16).

It would seem that the relationship of methodological skills to the formulation of the research question and the process of inquiry for a single investigator study is closer than is often admitted. This limitation may be easier to overcome in larger studies with more than one investigator or over many studies, each conducted by different investigators. Capitalizing on the methodological strengths of multiple investigators to study complex nursing phenomena allows for greater theoretical possibilities through the use of multiple research methods. Polkinghorne points out that multiple methods allow more to be learned about a research problem than could be discovered from any one procedure or method alone (Polkinghorne, 1983).

Extrapersonal Factors

Two classes of extrapersonal variables are proposed to relate to the process and practice of scientific inquiry: influential others and the sociohistoric context.

Influential Others

Two major types of influence on scientific inquiry are inherent in the variable of influential others: individual and institutional. Individual influences are initially conveyed primarily by mentors and other professors in graduate school, the primary wellspring of research values and training for the budding nursing scientist (Tinkle & Beaton, 1983). Here, individual faculty methodological preferences and research values are made known implicitly or explicitly, and disciplinary norms are passed on (Kuhn, 1970). Expectations regarding appropriate methods of scientific inquiry are embedded in each experience and are reinforced at every juncture. It is the prevailing "faculty view" that determines the ultimate breadth and depth of curricular exposure to various research strategies, and it is faculty expertise that delimits actual research opportunities for students. It is here in graduate research training that a nursing scientist's individual research style is born (Luria, 1973).

While the acquisition of disciplinary norms is unquestionably important, the notion implies existing disciplinary consensus on what those norms actually are. Nursing has not quite come to such a conscious consensus, although there is no evidence of the consistent use of diverse research methods to study nursing's complex phenomena (Jacobson & Meininger, 1985). When disciplinary research norms are not collectively shared, Toulmin points out that "theoretical debate in the field becomes largely—and unintentionally—methodological and philosophical; it is directed less at interpreting particular empirical findings than at debating the general acceptability (or unacceptability) of rival approaches, patterns of explanation and standards of judgment."(Toulmin, 1972, p. 380). The result is, of course, adamant assertions about one method over another, and the student scientist may be forced early on to align with one camp or another. Thus the norms that are acquired become not disciplinary but methodological and evaluative in nature. Kaplan calls this the "myth of methodology" and warns that "by pressing methodological norms too far, we may inhibit bold and imaginative adventure of ideas. The irony is that methodology itself may make for conformism—conforming to its own favored reconstructions" (Kaplan, 1964, p. 25). Polkinghorne (1983) points out that overall conceptual capacity, or what he calls "conceptual instruments," is also acquired by researchers in their graduate research training. However, he also notes that the unfortunate tendency is for these conceptual abilities to remain relatively unimproved throughout one's research career, even though the scientist may be exposed to diverse inquiry strategies throughout his or her research life. This notion lends support to the considerable influence of faculty norms on student scientists and to the relative strength of the other variables in the model of scientific inquiry as well.

Institutional influences, whether local, regional, or national in origin, also affect the process of scientific inquiry in a similar manner. Institutional norms function as operational imperatives for disciplinary activity in a given setting. Faculty researchers are thus expected, to some degree, to conform to these institutional norms, thus ensuring personal and professional prestige and survival. For example, on a large health science campus where the received view dominates the general conception of science, the faculty and student research in a school of nursing must reflect quasi conformance to these norms to exist at all. In the absence of such conformity university and extramural funding for the school and its research-related activities would be virtually impossible to secure. However, serious scientific repercussions can result when methodological conformity becomes the unquestioned status quo. Thompson (1985) warns that nurse researchers may not even be aware of the extent to which their research questions are prejudiced by the prevailing view. Martin (1982) notes the related influence of resource availabil-

ity on the selection of the research problem, choice of methodology, and, less commonly, the interpretation of research findings. It is essential to recognize these theoretical and methodological prejudices and the extent to which they enable or disable nursing's scientific progress.

Luria reminds us that "research in a university is free to the extent that the university itself is free"(Luria, 1973, p. 82). The same can be said for research in a school of nursing. Diverse faculty research expertise and activity are characteristic of research climates that are intellectually free. It has also been observed that "the progress of science, good science, depends on novel ideas and intellectual freedom" (Feyerabend, 1981, p. 165). Innovative inquiry and methodological diversity among faculty beget similar opportunity and ability in student scientists. It is upon this foundation of scientific inquiry that the most important advancements in nursing science will be made.

Sociohistorical Context

Sociohistorical influences also affect the process of scientific inquiry in two significant ways. First, significant research problems are often sociohistorically defined and prioritized, thus affecting health policy decisions and funding levels. One obvious example is the current and intense research interest in the causes, cure, and treatment for acquired immune deficiency syndrome (AIDS). This disease has existed in less virulent forms throughout the world for a long time. However, it was the sudden and virulent occurrence of AIDS in western urban population centers, predominantly in otherwise healthy young males, that prompted research interest and subsequent funding by virtue of its threat to public health. Other examples of sociohistorically defined research problem areas include the current focus on quality of life issues, such as stress and coping, as well as the management of chronic illness. These current research concerns are a natural focus in a society that has conquered communicable disease and has extended the human life span. As the aging population grows, so also grows involvement in gerontological health concerns and research problems ultimately related to controlling or decreasing health care expenditures for the elderly.

The second way that the sociohistorical context affects the conduct of inquiry is a function of the idiosyncratic relationship of research style to disciplinary fashion (Luria, 1973). Kaplan wryly observes that "the pressures of fad and fashion are as great in science, for all its logic, as in other areas of culture" (Kaplan, 1964, p. 28). Contemporary scientific fashion alone has the power to dictate substantive focus, theoretical perspective, and methodological approach. For individuals and disciplines in search of academic prestige or research funding, the pressures and priorities of fashion often prove too great to resist. These influences may have the intended effect of stimulating creativity and the solution of significant problems, or they may serve to stultify research activity and to make it less creative than usual.

It is clear from this discussion that the intrapersonal factors of world view, cognitive style, experience, and methodological knowledge and skill as well as the extrapersonal factors of influential others and sociohistorical context together exert a major influence on the progress of scientific inquiry. In the proposed model the process of scientific inquiry is thus depicted as evolutionary emergent, fueled by continual feedback and ultimately directed toward growth and self-actualization. In this way individual research programs develop and progress throughout a scientific career.

Implications for Nursing Science

Several assumptions are fundamental to a discussion of the implications of the model of scientific inquiry for nursing. It will be helpful to state them explicitly:

- The model of scientific inquiry is a reasonable representation of reality.
- As such, the model can be considered to be an existing disciplinary norm for research problem solving in nursing.
- The demand for methodological diversity is implicit in this model or norm because of the complex and multifaceted nature of nursing phenomena and the nature of the individual inquiry process.

- The progress or success of nursing science must be judged by the degree to which the most significant disciplinary problems are actually solved.

These assumptions carry certain implications for nursing science. For example, that this model can be viewed as a norm of nursing science implies ultimate respect for the individual researcher's personal process of problem formulation and resolution. Action that enhance this personal process ultimately will positively affect the development of nursing theory and science, while actions that interfere or interrupt this process will adversely affect the developing science.

Creativity

The assumption of methodological diversity implies certain mandates for student scientists, their graduate school professors and mentors, and for schools of nursing and other institutions. It has been established that science, at its best, demands the highest degree of creativity in problem solving. Nursing science, in its quest for rapid scientific advancement, is bound even closer than usual to this "constraint of creativity." Creativity coupled with sound methodological expertise is the rightful key to scientific progress. It is hypothesized that a creative scientist using a creative process and operating in a creative situation or climate is more likely to produce research results or theories that answer significant disciplinary questions. Fortunately there are several ways to enhance this creativity, beginning (for the purposes of this article) in doctoral study.

Creativity flourishes in a climate of intellectual freedom and open exploration. Creative problem solving must begin with self-exploration and self-knowledge. Student scientists should be provided with planned opportunities or activities designed for systematic, philosophical self-exploration so that one's world view can be explored and made known. This would contribute to more conscious decision making related to theoretical alignment, research methods, and the like. Opportunities to share and to discuss one's world view with peers and professors are also fundamental to scientific self-acceptance and acceptance of others. This obviously contributes to an academic atmosphere of openness and intellectual freedom.

Intuition

Intuition is ultimately associated with creativity and must be actively encouraged through the use of intuition-acknowledging and enhancing techniques. Students' exploration of their own pattern of receptivity and creativity should be part of every doctoral curriculum, as well as exposure to the processes of other creative thinkers. Faculty should share their own intuitive and creative processes freely, acknowledging the starts, stops, and detours inherent in the process. Other intuition-enhancing techniques can be employed throughout the educational experience as well. These include providing initial problem contexts or situations and encouraging students to explore the research problem, reformulating it in a manner appropriate to their experience and insight. Involvement in heuristic arguments, exercises in induction, and reasoning by analogy or metaphor all are activities directed toward increasing intuitive and receptive ability (Noddings & Shore, 1984). Ignoring the relationship of intuition to creativity or stifling its natural inclination exacts a terrible price from nursing theory development. To avoid the widespread underuse of such an obvious personal and professional resource implies ultimate acceptance of intuition as a legitimate partner to scholarly creativity and successful scientific enterprise. That intuition and creativity have "female" connotations should not worry those seeking scientific status, for it is relevant only to the observation that female scientists may be superior scientific problem solvers.

Cognitive Style

Assessment of personal cognitive style is also a highly useful strategy for beginning scientists so that existing abilities can be strengthened and weaker ones identified for possible intervention. Although there are obvious advantages and disadvantages to matching cognitive style of students and faculty, it has been proposed that the benefits of matching might be more related to

the purpose of the student-faculty relationship (Rogers, 1970). If the relationship is instrumental, or for the purpose of learning particular skills, as in a research residency or mentor relationship, matching cognitive styles may be productive. If the purpose of the relationship is developmental and aimed at developing critical thinking skills, for example, then a mismatch of cognitive styles might be more productive because of the exposure to diversity in thinking. Cognitive style assessment would provide useful baseline information upon which later decisions about course work, mentor relationships, research strategies, and the like might be made. The important point is that the assessment process should be a purposive activity within the doctoral curriculum.

Another important consideration related to cognitive style is the degree to which reflective thinking processes are enhanced or encouraged. Although creative and intuitive processes are important to scientific problem solving, critical thinking and analytical ability are equally important (Bigge, 1982). Inherent in reflective thinking is the ultimate balance between the cognitive and affective domains, the rational or analytical intuitive modes, the abstract and concrete levels of thinking, and, finally, the deductive and inductive approaches. Ideally these abilities would exist in exquisite balance in each researcher, but a more realistic focus would be to develop these abilities in each individual as much as possible. Fortunately many of the strategies directed toward enhancing intuition, creativity, and scientific problem solving also serve to improve reflective thinking abilities. Obviously if student scientists are to have adequate opportunity to refine these thinking skills in doctoral study, a faculty similarly skilled must be available to model and engage the students in appropriate exercise. If students are afforded the chance to increase skill in both analytical and intuitive modes, the gaps and flaws in existing theoretical conceptualizations will be easier to see and to overcome. Encouraging such creative yet critical thinking skills is the obvious antidote for nursing education's "long history of squelching curiosity and replacing it with conformity and a non-questioning attitude" Meleis, 1985, p. 37).

Methodological Diversity

Because the demand for methodological diversity is based as much on researcher characteristics as on the phenomenon of interest, opportunities for exposure to all types of research methods are essential. Thus a faculty must be carefully constructed so that quantitative and qualitative expertise exist side by side. This does not imply that a university cannot develop a research reputation for excellence in certain methodological strategies or theoretical orientation, merely that it should not gain it at the expense of other approaches. If faculty with varied philosophical orientation, cognitive styles, and methodological expertise are not available, then students are forced to match their process of inquiry to that of the available faculty. This can result in rather dire and sometimes dramatic consequences if a gross mismatch exists. At the outset the basic assumptions of the model of scientific inquiry are violated. Since the research problem that is formulated may not be a product of that intensely personal interactive process, there may be less investment in the research problem (Bigge, 1982). With decreased personal investment there may be diminished intellectual desire to solve the problem. When this natural obsession with one's problem is lost, so is what Polanyi calls "the mainspring of all inventive power" (Polyani, 1962, p. 127). Once this power is lost, the research problem is essentially relegated to the routine, and it becomes a chore instead of an exciting process of discovery. One wonders if the plethora of one-shot studies in nursing is in part a function of this lack of investment in the research problem.

When prevailing scientific attitudes and norms directly conflict with the intellectual-intuitive orientations of the researcher or student scientist and no safe haven for one's methodological leanings exists, interest is lost and so is another opportunity for scientific advancement. Jacox warns that "we have to be careful not to catch students and others who express these alternative views of science in our own somewhat narrower interpretations of science and theory. We must be cognizant that students may be in some jeopardy from faculty not knowledgeable or not accepting of emerging alternative views of science" (Jacox, 1981, p. 20). When it comes to the degree of faculty influence on a student scientist's process of inquiry, it is wise to take heed of Feyerabend's advice: "The hardest task needs the lightest hand or else its completion will not lead to freedom but to a tyranny much worse than the one it replaces"(Feyerabend, 1981, p. 167).

Nursing scientists are a scarce national resource and as such their scholarly productivity must be promoted whenever possible. The ultimate success of nursing science depends wholly on the ability to answer significant disciplinary questions. A creative research effort at all levels of theory building is required to accomplish this formidable task. This demands the existence of an intellectual climate most conducive to creative scientific problem solving and must allow a full array of cognitive and methodological possibilities for use by nursing's budding scientists. This climate should be responsive to individual differences in cognitive style, methodological preference, and the like but should simultaneously foster a fundamental appreciation for divergent approaches and styles.

Admittedly the costs of creating such a climate might appear to be high initially. In the extreme, widespread and epistemological anarchy and methodological revolution might result. At the very least it will require renouncement of scientific conformism, a return to individualism, and acceptance of methodological relativism. In either case the investment will yield a critical mass of highly committed and creative nursing scientists who are intrigued by nursing's scientific complexities and who are fully engaged in finding their solutions. In addition, an increasingly diverse pool of applicants will be attracted to doctoral study in nursing because of the increasing disciplinary consonance with a wide range of philosophical and intellectual possibilities. This can only further enhance the ability to address all levels of theory development.

Once the tremendous force of nursing's unclaimed creative potential is unleashed, a new age of inquiry in nursing science will be born. This new age of inquiry will be characterized by the generation of sophisticated methodological strategies suited to the complexities of a human science, the existence of sound theoretical formulations, and the general societal acknowledgement of nursing's sizable contribution to human welfare. A renewed sense of professional pride will prevail and nursing's scientific competence will be rightly judged by the ability to solve the discipline's most significant problems.

References

Albert, R.S. (Ed.). (1983). *Genius and eminence: The social psychology of creativity and exceptional achievement.* Oxford, England: Pergamon Press.

American Nurses' Association (1980). *Nursing: A social policy statement.* Kansas City: Author.

Batey, M.V. (1977). Conceptualization: Knowledge and logic guiding empirical research. *Nursing Research, 26*(5), 324–329.

Bigge, M. (1982). *Learning theories for teachers* (4th ed.). New York: Harper & Row.

Bloom, B., & Broder, C. (1950). *The problem solving process of college students.* Chicago: University of Chicago Press.

Brink, P., & Wood, M. (1983). *Basic steps in planning nursing research, from question to proposal* (2nd ed.). Monterey, CA: Wadsworth.

Bronowski, J. (1965). *Science and human values.* New York: Harper & Row.

Bruner, J. (1966). *The process of education.* New York: Atheneum.

Carper, B.A. (1978). Fundamental patterns of knowing in nursing. *Advances in Nursing Science, 1*(1), 13–23.

Claxton, C., & Ralston, Y. (1978). *Learning styles: Their impact on teaching and administration.* Washington, DC: The American Association for Higher Education.

Conway, M. (1985). Toward greater specificity in defining nursing's metaparadigm. *Advances in Nursing Science, 7*(4), 73–81.

Dickoff, J., James, P., & Weidenbach, E. (1968). Theory in a practice discipline: Part I—practice oriented theory. Nursing Research, 17(5), 415–435.

Donaldson, S.K., & Crowley, D.M. (1978). The discipline of nursing. *Nursing Outlook, 26*(2), 113–120.

Fawcett, J. (1978). The relationship between theory and research: A double helix. *Advances in Nursing Science, 1*(1), 49–62.

Feyerabend, P. (1981). How to defend society against science. In I. Hacking (Ed.), *Scientific revolutions.* London: Oxford University Press.

Flaskerud, J.H., & Halloran, E.J. (1980). Areas of agreement in nursing theory development. *Advances in Nursing Science, 3*(1), 1–7.

Glaser, B., & Strauss, A. (1967). *The discovery of grounded theory: Strategies of qualitative research.* New York: Aldine.

Goldstein, M., & Goldstein, I. (1978). *How we know: An exploration of the scientific process.* New York: Plenum Press.

Gortner, S., & Nahm, H. (1977). An overview of nursing research in the United States. *Nursing Research, 26,* 10–33.

Gortner, S. (1983). The history and philosophy of nursing science and research. *Advances in Nursing Science, 5*(2), 1–8.

Hardy, M. (1983). Metaparadigms and theory development. In N.L. Chaska (Ed.), *The nursing profession: A time to speak* (pp. 427–435). New York: McGraw-Hill.

Jacobsen, B., & Meininger, J. (1985). The design and methods of published nursing research: 1956–1983. *Nursing Research, 34,* 306–311.

Jacox, A. (1974). Theory construction in nursing: An overview. *Nursing Research, 23*(1), 4–13.

Jacox, A. (1981, June). *Competing theories of science.* Paper presented at the 1981 Forum on Doctoral Education in Nursing, Seattle, WA, June 1981.

Kaplan, A. (1964). *The conduct of inquiry.* New York: Harper & Row.

Kerlinger, F. (1973). *Foundations of behavioral research* (2nd ed.). New York: Holt, Rinehart & Winston.

Kolb, D. (1981). Learning styles and disciplinary differences. In A. Chickering (Ed.), *The modern American college* (pp. 232–255). San Francisco: Jossey–Bass.

Kuhn, T.S. (1970). *The structure of scientific revolutions* (2nd ed.). Chicago: University of Chicago Press.

Luria, S.E. (1973). On research styles and allied matters. *Daedalus, 102*(2), 75–84.

Mackinnon, D. (1979). Creativity: A multifaceted phenomenon. In J.D. Roslansky (Ed.), *Creativity* (pp. 19–32). Amsterdam: North-Holland.

Martin, J. (1982). A garbage can model of the research process. In J. McGrath, J. Martin, & R. Kulka (Eds.), *Judgment calls in research* (pp. 17–39). Beverly Hills, CA: Sage.

Maslow, A.H. (1966). *The psychology of science: A reconnaissance.* South Bend, IN: Gateway Editions.

McGrath, J.E. (1982). Dilemmatics: The study of research choices and dilemmas. In J. McGrath, J. Martin, & R. Kulka (Eds.), *Judgment calls in research* (pp. 69–102). Beverly Hills, CA: Sage.

Meleis, A.I. (1985). *Theoretical nursing: Development and progress.* Philadelphia: J.B. Lippincott.

Messick, S. (1970). The criterion problem in the evaluation of instruction: Assessing possible, not just intended extremes. In M. Wittrock & D. Riley (Eds.), *Evaluation of instruction: Issues and problems.* New York: Holt, Rinehart & Winston.

Metzger, B., & Schultz, S. (1982). Time series analysis: An

alternative for nursing. *Nursing Research, 31*(6), 375–378.

Newman, M.A. (1983). The continuing revolution: A history of nursing science. In N.L. Chaska (Ed.), *The nursing profession: A time to speak* (pp. 385–393). New York: McGraw-Hill.

Nicholls, J.G. (1983). Creativity in the person who will never produce anything original or useful. In R.S. Albert (Ed.), *Genius and eminence: The social psychology of creativity and exceptional achievement* (pp. 265–279). Oxford, England: Pergamon Press.

Noddings, N., & Shore, P. (1984). *Awakening the inner eye intuition in education.* New York: Teachers College Press.

Oiler, C. (1982). The phenomenological approach in nursing research. *Nursing Research, 31*(3), 178–181.

Polanyi, M. (1962). *Personal knowledge.* Chicago: University of Chicago Press.

Polit, D., & Hungler, B. (1983). *Nursing research: Principles and methods* (2nd ed.). Philadelphia, J.B. Lippincott.

Polkinghorne, D. (1983). *Methodology for the human science systems of inquiry.* Albany, NY: State University of New York Press.

Rogers, M.E. (1970). *A theoretical basis for nursing.* Philadelphia: F.A. Davis.

Roy S.C. (1983). Theory development in nursing: Proposal for direction. In N.L. Chaska (Ed.), *The nursing profession: A time to speak* (pp. 453–465). New York: McGraw-Hill.

Runkel, P., & McGrath, J. (1972). *Research on human behav-ior: A systematic guide to method.* New York: Holt, Rinehart & Winston.

Shouksmith, G. (1970). *Intelligence, creativity and cognitive style.* New York: Wiley Interscience.

Stevens, B. (1979). *Nursing theory: Analysis, application, evaluation.* Boston: Little, Brown.

Suppe, F. (1977). *The structure of scientific theories* (2nd ed.). Chicago: University of Illinois Press.

Thompson, J. (1985). Practical discourse in nursing: Going beyond empiricism and historicism. *Advances in Nursing Science, 7*(4), 59–71.

Tinkle, M.B., & Beaton, J.L. (1983). Toward a new view of science: Implications for nursing research. *Advances in Nursing Science, 5*(2), 27–36.

Tucker, R. (1979). The value decisions we know as science. *Advances in Nursing Science, 1*(2), 1–12.

Toulmin, S. (1972). *Human understanding* (Vol. 1). Oxford, England: Clarendon Press.

Von Bertalanffy, L. (1968). *General system theory.* New York: George Braziller.

Weiskopf, V. (1973). Introduction. In H. Yukawa (Ed.), *Creativity and intuition: A physicist looks east and west* (J. Bester, trans.). Tokyo: Kodansha International.

Wilson, H.S. (1985). *Research in nursing.* Menlo Park, CA: Addison-Wesley.

Worthy, M. (1975). *Aha! A puzzle approach to creative thinking.* Chicago: Nelson Hall.

Yukawa, H. (1973). *Creativity and intuition: A physicist looks at east and west* (J. Bester, trans.). Tokyo: Kodansha International.

The Author Comments

This work arose from an intensely passionate intellectual process that kept me in its grips for the first two years of doctoral study at the University of California, San Francisco. Coursework in theory development, the philosophy of science, and research methods had challenged my assumptions about the research process, forcing a reflective process unlike any I had ever experienced.

In order to understand my role as a budding nurse scientist and how I might best contribute to nursing's knowledge base, I struggled with the question "How does science really happen?" and more specifically, "What factors affect the conduct of research?" It seemed reasonable that insight into the many influences and pressures I was facing in defining my own research interests would be inherent in the resolution of these questions.

One of the primary dilemmas stemmed from two rather disparate notions with ultimately similar consequences. First, the customary portrayal of scientific activity as a rational, objective process was distressing because of its prescriptive, positivistic connotations. However, the view that nursing science should build its descriptive base first, using qualitative strategies, was equally linear, dogmatic, and disturbing. Both positions seemed to ignore the inclination and desire of those individuals who actually conduct the research and thus serve as the architects of the disciplinary knowledge base.

The process of resolving this dilemma was largely one of self discovery, problem-solving, and risk-taking, liberally leavened with lessons in humility. Besides reading everything I could get my hands on that was even remotely related, I challenged my own preconceptions as well as the ideas of others.

Initially considered to be time-consuming and somewhat uncomfortable, introspection became a close ally in my crusade.

As is often the case with processes, the final step signals the beginning of yet another related process. In this instance, it culminated in the desire to formally characterize my conclusions and insights related to the process of scientific inquiry in a way that could be communicated to others. The first step was to develop a visual or graphic representation of the model of scientific inquiry. This assisted me in refining my thinking and clarifying relationships among the variables in the model.

The drive to complete the accompanying narrative explanation was so strong that at times I felt that the paper chose me as the vehicle for expression rather than the other way around. I somehow came to an intuitive understanding that my personal process of inquiry and understanding would not be complete until the paper was finished. I sensed that, as with any labor of love, a certain peace and satisfaction would accompany the insight and direction gained from the process. I was not disappointed.

—HOLLY A. DEGROOT

Author Index

A

Aamodt, A. M., 310
Abdellah, F. G., 18, 38, 39, 231, 244, 251, 269, 271
Adams, M., 142
Adelman, L., 553
Albert, R. S., 676
Aldous, J., 643
Alexander, S., 346
Allen, D., 126, 183, 296
American Academy of Nursing, 183
American Association of Neuroscience Nurses, 310
American Association of Spinal Cord Injury Nurses, 310
American College of Nurse Midwives, 310
American Nurses' Association, 126, 145, 174, 183, 527, 676
American Nurses' Association Cabinet on Nursing Research, 310
American Nurses' Association Commission on Nursing Research, 619
American Organization of Nurse Executives, 310
Andreoli, K. G., 231, 244, 561, 634
Archbold, P. G., 174

Argyris, C., 215
Armiger, B., 215
Armstrong, D., 27
Ashley, C. C., 626
Association for Supervision and Curriculum Development Commission on Instructional Theory (ASCD), 634
Auger, J. R., 389
Avant, K. C., 167, 270
Ayer, A. J., 269

B

Baer, D. M., 341
Baer, E. D., 126
Baider, L., 142
Bailey, J. T., 415
Bakan, D., 659
Bakwin, H., 194
Baldwin, B., 167, 251, 287, 363, 371
Bales, R. F., 467
Baltes, M. M., 174
Baltes, P. B., 174
Barash, N., 132
Barber, B., 311
Barnard, K. E., 142, 231, 258, 627

Baron, R. J., 447
Batey, M. V., 83, 183, 237, 415, 604, 643, 676
Baumrind, D., 659
Beaton, J. L., 270, 652, 677
Becker, H. S., 203
Becker, M. H., 441
Beckstrand, J., 166, 237, 286, 529, 538, 542, 543, 561, 562, 571
Beckwith, J., 244
Beland, I. L., 231
Bellah, R. N., 174
Benner, P., 142, 166, 183, 271, 286, 296, 298, 311
Benoliel, J. Q., 161, 237, 244, 286, 299, 621, 627
Berardo, F. M., 431
Bergson, H., 346
Bergstrom, N., 311
Bernard, J., 659
Bernstein, A., 142
Bernstein, R. J., 166, 183
Berthold, J. S., 223
Bigge, M., 676
Bijou, J. W., 341
Bishop, B., 244

679

Subject Index